Handbook of
Experimental Pharmacology

Continuation of Handbuch der experimentellen Pharmakologie

Vol. 75

Toxicology of Inhaled Materials

General Principles
of Inhalation Toxicology

Contributors

I.Y. R. Adamson · B. D. Beck · M. R. Becklake · J. D. Brain
J. D. Crapo · R. T. Drew · D. L. Dungworth · A. B. Fisher
T. E. Gram · P. J. Hakkinen · J. A. Last · M. Lippmann
M. G. Mustafa · K. E. Pinkerton · C. E. Plopper · K. M. Reiser
S. A. Rooney · B. T. Smith · J. M. Sturgess · W. S. Tyler
P. A. Valberg · H. P. Witschi

Editors

H. P. Witschi and J. D. Brain

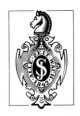

Springer-Verlag Berlin Heidelberg New York Tokyo

HANSPETER WITSCHI, M.D.
Section Head, Toxicology, Biology Division,
Oak Ridge National Laboratory, P.O. Box Y,
Oak Ridge, TN 37831, USA

JOSEPH D. BRAIN, S.D. in Hyg.
Professor of Physiology,
Director, Respiratory Biology Program,
Department of Environmental Science and Physiology,
Harvard University School of Public Health,
665 Huntington Ave., Boston, MA 02115, USA

With 80 Figures

ISBN 3-540-13109-4 Springer-Verlag Berlin Heidelberg New York Tokyo
ISBN 0-387-13109-4 Springer-Verlag New York Heidelberg Berlin Tokyo

Library of Congress Cataloging in Publication Data. Main entry under title: Toxicology of inhaled materials. (Handbook of experimental pharmacology; vol. 75) Bibliography: p. 1. Aerosols–Toxicology. 2. Gases, Asphyxiating and poisonous. 3. Toxicology, Experimental. I. Adamson, I.Y.R. II. Witschi, Hanspeter. III. Brain, Joseph D. IV. Series: Handbook of experimental pharmacology; v. 75. [DNLM: 1. Environmental Pollutants–toxicity. 2. Respiratory Tract Diseases–chemically induced. 3. Toxicology. W1 HA51L v. 75/WA 671 T755] QP905.H3 vol. 75 615′.1s [615.9′1] 84-20202 [RA1270.A34] ISBN 0-387-13109-4 (U.S.)

Typesetting, printing and bookbinding: Brühlsche Universitätsdruckerei, Giessen
2122/3130-543210

List of Contributors

I. Y. R. Adamson, Department of Pathology, Faculty of Medicine, University of Manitoba, 770 Bannatyne Avenue, Winnipeg, Manitoba, Canada, R3E OW3

B. D. Beck, Department of Environmental Science and Physiology, Harvard School of Public Health, 665 Huntington Avenue, Boston, MA 02115, USA

M. R. Becklake, Department of Epidemiology and Health, McGill University, 3775 University Street, Montreal, Quebec, Canada H3A 2B4

J. D. Brain, Director, Respiratory Biology Program, Department of Environmental Science and Physiology, Harvard University School of Public Health, 665 Huntington Avenue, Boston, MA 02115, USA

J.D. Crapo, Department of Medicine, Chief, Division of Allergy, Critical Care and Respiratory Medicine, Duke University Medical Center, P.O. Box 3177, Durham, NC 27710, USA

R. T. Drew, Medical Department, Brookhaven National Laboratory, Associated Universities, Inc., Upton, L. I., NY 11973, USA

D. L. Dungworth, School of Veterinary Medicine, Department of Pathology, University of California, Davis, CA 95616, USA

A. B. Fisher, University of Pennsylvania, Department of Physiology, School of Medicine, G-4, 37th & Hamilton Walk, D-404 Richards Bldg., Philadelphia, PA 19104, USA

T. E. Gram, Head, Biochemical Toxicology Section, Laboratory of Medicinal Chemistry and Pharmacology, National Cancer Institute, National Institutes of Health, Bldg. 37, Rm. 6D-28, Bethesda, MD 20205, USA

P. J. Hakkinen, University of Tennessee-Oak Ridge Graduate School of Biomedical Sciences and Biology Division, Oak Ridge National Laboratory, Oak Ridge, TN 37830, USA
Present address: The Procter & Gamble Company, Sharon Woods Technical Center, Cincinnati, OH 45241, USA

J. A. Last, Department of Internal Medicine, Division of Pulmonary Medicine and California Primate Research Center, University of California, Davis, CA 95616, USA

M. Lippmann, Department of Environmental Medicine, Institute of Environmental Medicine, New York University Medical Center, 550 First Avenue, New York, NY 10016, USA

M. G. Mustafa, Division of Environmental and Occupational Health Sciences, School of Public Health, and Division of Pulmonary Disease, Department of Medicine, University of California, Los Angeles, CA 90024, USA

K.E. Pinkerton, Department of Pathology, Duke University, Medical Center, P.O. Box 3177, Durham, NC 27710, USA

C.E. Plopper, Department of Anatomy and California Primate Research Center, University of California, Davis, CA 95616, USA

K. M. Reiser, Department of Internal Medicine, Division of Pulmonary Medicine and California Primate Research Center, University of California, Davis, CA 95616, USA

S. A. Rooney, Division of Perinatal Medicine, Department of Pediatrics, Yale University School of Medicine, P.O. Box 3333, New Haven, CT 06510, USA

B. T. Smith, Joint Program in Neonatology, Harvard Medical School, 75 Francis Street, Boston, MA 02115, USA

J. M. Sturgess, Warner-Lambert/Parke-Davis Research Institute, 2270 Speakman Drive, Sheridan Park, Mississauga, Ontario, Canada, L5K 1B4

W. S. Tyler, Department of Anatomy and California Primate Research Center, University of California, Davis, CA 95616, USA

P. A. Valberg, Department of Environmental Science and Physiology, Harvard University School of Public Health, 665 Huntington Avenue, Boston, MA 02115, USA

H. P. Witschi, Biology Division, Oak Ridge National Laboratory, P.O. Box Y, Oak Ridge, TN 37831, USA

Preface

This book deals with the methods and scientific basis of inhalation toxicology. It describes devices and facilities needed to expose animals to inhaled particles and gases as well as approaches to estimating or measuring the fraction of the inhaled material that is retained in the respiratory tract. The book then reviews the evergrowing repertoire of techniques that can be used to measure the responses elicited by the exposure. Quantitative and qualitative anatomical, physiological, and biochemical strategies are discussed in detail.

We believe that the toxicology of inhaled materials is an important and timely topic for several reasons. During the past decade, morbidity and mortality attributable to cardiovascular disease have significantly decreased. Progress in combatting cancer, the second most important cause of death, has been slower, and lung cancer actually became the leading cause of death in men and the second leading cause of cancer death in women. In addition, the incidence of non-neoplastic respiratory diseases such as emphysema, fibrosis, and chronic bronchitis has increased the past decade. In the United States, the National Institutes of Health (NIH) has recently reported that chronic obstructive pulmonary disease affects nearly 10 million persons and accounts for 59,000 deaths yearly; indeed, it ranks as the fifth leading cause of death. Because the incidence is increasing, the NIH estimates that it may become the nation's fourth or even third leading cause of death by the year 2000.

There is increasing awareness that this rising incidence in respiratory diseases is attributable to the inhalation of particles and gases in urban and work environments and especially to the use of tobacco products. Pulmonary diseases are of concern because they are difficult to treat and because they frequently manifest themselves only after decades of apparently innocuous exposure. For these reasons, the science of inhalation toxicology has emerged as an important specialty. The development of methods that permit the study of human respiratory disease experimentally in animals has gained importance, especially because of increasing concern about environmental lung disease.

A consideration of the biological issues also makes it apparent that the science of inhalation toxicology is an important one. The lungs have a unique proximity to the environment not shared by other organs of the body. The same thinness and delicacy that make the air-blood barrier ideal for the efficient exchange of oxygen and carbon dioxide reduce its effectiveness as a barrier to inhaled toxic particles and gases. Adults, depending on their size and physical activity, move from 10,000 to 20,000 liters of air daily in and out of their lungs. Inspired air frequently contains particles and gases which are hazardous. Among the purposes of this book are to describe various techniques that are used to expose animals to aerosols characteristic of the environment and to explore the diverse physiological and pathological mechanisms which take place as inhaled particles and gases interact with the respiratory tract and the body. Particular emphasis has been placed on quantitative methods that can be used to assess the eventual damage caused in pulmonary tissue by such agents. It is our hope that a better understanding of these mechanisms of lung injury will ultimately permit the design of more effective strategies to prevent and ameliorate respiratory diseases.

When we accepted the invitation to edit a handbook on *The Toxicology of Inhaled Materials,* we were aware of the magnitude of the task. To cover the whole field in detail would be difficult. However, we were convinced it would be extremely valuable to bring together the experience of many different experts. We hope that their collective wisdom will help crystallize the present state of knowledge and facilitate the entry of scientists who want to begin work in this area. The substantial increase in the number and variety of approaches in inhalation toxicology makes it all the more critical that work in this field be evaluated in a comprehensive way. It has been our aim, therefore, to assist scientists in assimilating and evaluating a rapidly growing body of knowledge; thus, the book is intended to be both scholarly and practical.

After careful consideration of each major area, we recruited authors who could summarize each topic and anticipate new directions of study. Each contributor has identified central issues against the context of a broad core of published papers. No obligation was felt to mention all the existing literature in the field; rather, the authors were encouraged to be selective. It is our hope that this book will be a chronicle of significant past work, a stimulus for their rapid and thoughtful application, and a guide for future work. We are indebted to all the authors for their outstanding contributions.

HANSPETER WITSCHI
JOSEPH D. BRAIN

Contents

Exposure Techniques

General Assessment of Toxic Effects

CHAPTER 6

The Isolated Perfused Lung. A. B. FISHER. With 5 Figures

CHAPTER 7

Pulmonary Cell and Tissue Cultures. B. T. SMITH

CHAPTER 8

Bronchoalveolar Lavage. J. D. BRAIN and BARBARA D. BECK. With 6 Figures

Morphologic Techniques

CHAPTER 9

Morphological Methods for Gross and Microscopic Pathology
D. L. DUNGWORTH, W. S. TYLER, and C. E. PLOPPER. With 6 Figures

CHAPTER 10

Morphometry of the Alveolar Region of the Lung
K. E. PINKERTON and J. D. CRAPO. With 9 Figures

Biological and Biochemical Analysis

CHAPTER 11

Cellular Kinetics of the Lung. I. Y. R. ADAMSON. With 8 Figures

CHAPTER 12

Mucociliary Clearance and Mucus Secretion in the Lung
JENNIFER M. STURGESS. With 11 Figures

CHAPTER 13

General Enzymology of the Lung. M. G. MUSTAFA. With 2 Figures

CHAPTER 14

The Pulmonary Mixed-Function Oxidase System
T. E. GRAM. With 10 Figures

CHAPTER 15

The Surfactant System of the Lung. S. A. ROONEY. With 1 Figure

CHAPTER 16

Effects of Pneumotoxins on Lung Connective Tissue
J. A. LAST and K. M. REISER

Exposure Techniques

CHAPTER 1

The Design and Operation of Systems for Inhalation Exposure of Animals

R. T. DREW

A. Introduction

The need to assess health effects of airborne chemicals has caused the evolution of a variety of inhalation exposure systems. The development has proceeded in two directions: constructing chambers for immersion of the whole animal in a cloud of the test agent (whole body exposure systems), and building systems that limit the exposure to the head or nose or, in some cases, to a smaller portion of the respiratory tract (hereinafter referred to as limited exposure systems). This chapter will describe the design of both simple and complex whole body exposure systems, outline some of the standard operational procedures, including calibration, review the development of head and nose exposure systems, and describe some of the advantages and potential problems of operating limited exposure systems. The subject is restricted to exposure systems since methods for generation and characterization of particles and vapors are covered elsewhere in this book. Three books have appeared on this subject in the last 5 years (DREW 1978; WILLEKE 1980; LEONG 1981), and for additional reviews the reader is referred to FRASER et al. (1959), DREW and LASKIN (1973), PHALEN (1976), and LIPPMANN (1980).

B. Design

I. Facilities

Inhalation studies are best undertaken in facilities specifically designed for that purpose. Ceilings should be high enough to allow for clearance above the chambers. Balconies with the tops of the chambers protruding into the balcony are very useful for location of the generation and monitoring equipment. When designing facilities, the researcher has the choice of putting a number of chambers in a large room or a few chambers, or even one, in a small room. While in the past the author has constructed large rooms with many chambers, he has come to believe that the best arrangement for chronic studies is to have one chamber in a room with enough space in the room to house the animals when they are not being exposed. With acute or subacute studies, this is not so important, primarily because the investment in subacute studies is far less than in chronic studies.

A constant supply of clean filtered air should be available with facilities for control of both temperature and humidity. The temperature inside inhalation chambers is controlled mainly by the temperature in the chamber rooms (BERN-

STEIN and DREW 1980). Two approaches for supplying chamber air are possible. A separate supply system can be used, or, alternatively, the chamber can get its air from the room. In either case, the air should be cleaned by both high efficiency particulate air filters and charcoal before entering the chamber. Accurate regulation of airflow is essential. In most facilities, chambers are connected to a common exhaust system. This system should be sized so as to be able to handle the maximum flow rate of all the chambers on that system. A high degree of negative exhaust duct pressure is necessary to minimize the effects of one chamber on another. In some facilities (COATE 1978, personal communication; REID et al. 1981), there are positive displacement exhaust pumps for each chamber. While this is initially expensive, it makes each chamber independent of all the others. If a pump or fan fails, it is easily replaced without affecting other chambers. When systems with large common air supply and exhaust systems fail, the entire facility is affected.

If at all possible, the floor above inhalation chamber rooms should be a mechanical room. This will allow installation of all the necessary heating, ventilation, and air conditioning equipment in an organized manner. This feature can be included by building a penthouse above the chamber room or by the recent technique of including an interstitial mechanical space between each floor. This arrangement allows for easy alterations and is very economical in the long run.

II. Simple Systems

The basic concept of a dynamic inhalation exposure is simple enough; one puts animals into a closed volume or chamber and passes air containing the test material through the chamber. The test agent is mixed with the incoming air, passed through the chamber and then through an air cleaning device to remove the test agent before discharging the air. The driving force for such systems is a pump or fan which pulls air through the chamber, allowing the chambers to be maintained at a pressure slightly less than that of the surrounding environment.

Systems for the controlled exposure of animals were described as early as 1865 (EULENBURG 1865). These early systems were usually cylindrical or cuboidal in shape and some type of mixing device was often included. In many cases, preexisting containers such as bell jars (VON OTTINGEN et al. 1936), battery jars (SPIEGL et al. 1953), cubes (FRASER et al. 1959), and even 50-gallon ($\sim$ 190-l) drums (STEAD et al. 1944) were used. One widely used system described in detail by LEACH (1963) consists of a cylindrical glass battery jar mounted horizontally in a frame with the open end sealed off with a panel. The panel has the necessary intake and exhaust ports and also ports for measuring pollutant concentration, pressure, etc. Figure 1 shows battery jars located inside a hood at Brookhaven National Laboratory. They are very convenient for short-term studies. Other investigators have used large cylinders (FERON and KRUYSSE 1977), small transparent plastic cylinders (DREW and LASKIN 1971), glass pipe (BLAIR and REES 1975), plastic hemispheres (STUART 1970), and even iron lungs (THIEDE et al. 1974).

BARROW and STEINHAGEN (1982) recently described the design, construction, and operation of an exposure system fabricated from a glass aquarium. They fabricated a top from acrylic plastic lined with a 3-mm sheet of Teflon (polyte-

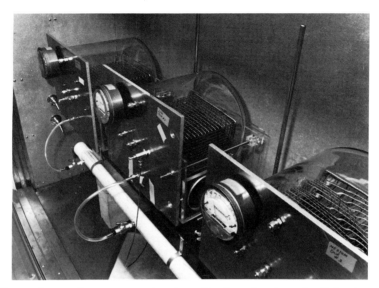

Fig. 1. Battery jars used as exposure chambers. The front face is made of aluminum which seals against the glass with a rubber gasket. Parts for intake and exhaust and sampling are provided in the aluminum plate

trafluoroethylene) and held in place with stainless steel screws. The entire inside surface was composed of glass, Teflon, and stainless steel, thereby being virtually inert. The chamber was made of a 100-gallon ($\sim$ 380-l) tank, but smaller tanks have also been used (SPIVAK and CONNOR 1977). A somewhat more complicated system described by MONTGOMERY et al. (1976) was made of plastic with a secondary plastic container allowing for individual housing of about six rats. The investigator has access to the animals to perform injections, etc. All of these small systems are relatively inexpensive and provide the ability to conduct acute or limited inhalation studies. Since mixing is probably less than ideal, the time required to reach equilibrium concentration will probably be greater than that calculated from theory. Provided the investigator understands the systems and their limitations, they can be very useful.

III. Current Chamber Design

The studies at the University of Rochester on the toxicity of materials relating to the Manhattan Project represent the beginning of modern chamber technology (STOKINGER et al. 1949). The original chambers were cubes ranging in size from 1.2 to 2.75 m and were constructed of a variety of materials, including wood, glass, and stainless steel, depending on the material being tested. They provided facilities for both whole body and head exposure to several species of animals. However, uniformity of aerosol distribution was a problem. Therefore, these early investigators began to experiment with vertical cylindrical systems with cones on the top and bottom. Since it was difficult to get good seals on curved surface, the shape was modified to provide a hexagonal cross section with pyramidal ends

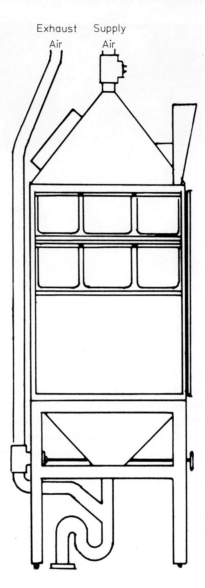

Exhaust   Supply
Air   Air

Fig. 2. The NYU chamber

(Wilson and Laskin 1950). This chamber design is generally known as the Rochester chamber (Leach et al. 1959). Further modification consisted of switching to a square cross section while retaining the pyramidal shape on the ends (Fig. 2). Modifications on the shape of the top, providing for a tangential entry, and the bottom, providing for a U-shaped exhaust, were described by Hinners et al. (1968) who published plans for several chambers of different sizes, ranging in width from 0.7 to 1.5 m.

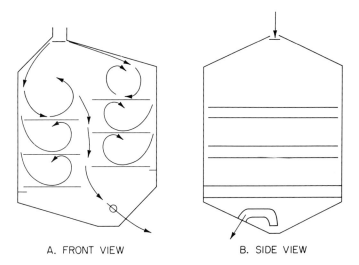

A. FRONT VIEW   B. SIDE VIEW

Fig. 3. The Battelle chamber

These chambers were used to expose a variety of animals to airborne agents. They often contained several layers or tiers of wire mesh cages, allowing exposure to many more animals than a single tier could accomodate. One major drawback to those systems was that in order to maintain uniform particle distribution in the chamber, the systems did not usually include pans between the tiers to catch urine and feces. This arrangement undoubtedly imposed an added stress on the animals. Recently, scientists at Battelle Northwest (Moss 1978, 1980) modified the standard chamber design to allow inclusion of catch pans while retaining a uniform particle distribution. The design (Fig. 3) provided for asymmetric pyramids on the top and bottom with the intake and exhaust offset from each other and also for the cages on one side offset in height from the chambers on the other side. This chamber has been thoroughly evaluated (Moss et al. 1982; GRIFFIS et al. 1981) and does provide reasonably uniform particle distributions. However, these evaluations do suggest that the cages should be rotated to even out any bias due to location. The airflow pattern in the chamber is controlled, in part, by the gap between the catch pan and the chamber side. Current developments in chamber design include maintaining two or three different concentrations in one chamber by controlling the gap between the side and the pan and also using simple rectangular systems (Moss 1982, personal communication). These systems need critical evaluation before they can be used with confidence. It seems ironic that we started with rectangular systems and are now going back to the original design.

IV. Rooms as Chambers

In some cases, laboratories have used actual rooms as exposure chambers. The inhalation toxicology facility at the Environmental Protection Agency, Research Triangle Park, North Carolina, uses environmental rooms as exposure rooms.

These rooms were built to provide close control of temperature and humidity and have been modified for chronic exposure of oxidant gases such as nitrogen dioxide and ozone. Inhalation exposure facilities at Washington University, St. Louis, Missouri (HARTROFT et al. 1977) also used whole rooms as exposure chambers and introduced the pollutants into the air duct supplying conditioned air to the room. Exposure rooms are also in use at Dow Chemical Company, Midland, Michigan (MACEWEN 1978) with another room above the exposure room for generating the pollutant being studied. Perhaps the most complex exposure room system is the one in operation at Wright-Patterson Air Force Base, Ohio. This exposure facility contains eight domes, 3.7 m in diameter, and 2.4 m tall, which can be entered through an airlock below each dome (THOMAS 1965). They were originally built to study effects of reduced pressures, but have been used for the last decade at ambient pressure. When necessary, the entire dome can be raised in order to facilitate cleaning and installation of equipment between studies. These systems can be operated 24 hours per day, 7 days per week, for as long as necessary.

V. Isolation Systems

The exposure of rodents to highly toxic particles presents special problems. The atmospheric concentration of such agents will return to zero after stopping the aerosol generator. However, after exposure, surfaces inside the chamber are coated with the material being studied. Subsequent handling of animals, cages, racks, etc., presents many opportunities to spread the test agent around the laboratory. For personnel protection, these agents must be contained. Possible solutions to this problem include the use of isolation systems and nose exposure systems (to be discussed in Sect. D.). Isolation systems consist of completely closed systems with access only through pass boxes and manipulations being performed with gloves which themselves constitute part of the barrier.

Several such systems have been described in the literature (LASKIN et al. 1970; KIMMERLE 1979; Leong et al. 1981). The isolation unit described by LASKIN et al. (1970) allows for exposure in a chamber within a chamber and provides several other glove boxes for aerosol generation, air cleaning, and rodent housing. Other systems mount living chambers adjacent to exposure chambers. Animals must be handled with gloves and when they are moved back and forth from exposure chamber to living chamber, a barrier must always be maintained between the contaminated animals and the operator. All these systems suffer from the same drawbacks. They are expensive to build, labor intensive, and can only expose a limited number of animals.

VI. General Design Features

The specific design of a chamber may often depend on the physical restraints imposed by the planned location of the chamber. The Battelle chamber was designed to fit into an existing rack washer. Chamber size varies with the intended use. Chambers for acute exposures tend to be small since the number of animals is usually small. At Brookhaven, chambers that are 0.68, 0.91, and 1.52 m wide with total volumes of 0.38, 1.4, and 4.5 m³ are being used. Two recent publications describe large chambers of 9.3 m³ (PULLINGER et al. 1979) and 12.6 m³ (SCHRECK et al. 1981). Researchers should think twice about installing such large systems. In the author's experience, the 4.5 m³ chambers are not often filled to their capacity.

CARPENTER and BEETHE (1978) discussed the effects of various cone shapes. The goal is to design a chamber which insures a uniform concentration of test material throughout. Modifications such as putting cones below the air intake and deflectors along the sides will increase turbulence and thereby decrease the time to reach equilibrium. It is important to mix the pollutant with the incoming air before it enters the chamber. One good way to do this is to provide opposing entry ports in the supply air duct and either split the test agent air to both ports or provide clean air on one side. This process provides good turbulence and therefore mixing before the air enters the cone in the chamber. The angle of the cone is also important; the higher the cone, the better the mixing. These subjects are covered in more detail in DREW (1978). Most chambers have their air intake at the top and exhaust at the bottom with the net movement of air in the downward direction. The flow is usually turbulent, although in at least one system, air straighteners were provided in the upper cone to provide laminar or plug flow through the main body of the chamber (HOLMBERG et al. 1981). Two horizontal flow systems have also been described (FERIN and LEACH 1980; HEMENWAY and MACASKILL 1979).

The chamber can be portable with wheels and quick-disconnect fittings so that the chamber can be disconnected and rolled into washing facilities. Fittings can also be permanently mounted and plumbed to the house drains for removal of wash water and wastes. In cases where highly hazardous materials are being used, it may be necessary to collect the wash water for decontamination or disposal elsewhere.

If the chambers are permanently installed, there must be facilities for cleaning them. In some cases, spray rings or rotators are included in the top of the chamber for cleaning. Rings have also been included at the bottom to flush urine and feces down the drain. In the author's experience, these rings have been inadequate and a high pressure hot water system equipped with a soap dispenser and a rigid wand is used to clean chambers. Portable steam generators are also useful.

C. Operation

I. Static Systems

Inhalation systems are considered to be static when the agent is introduced into the chamber as a batch and then mixed with the air in the closed system. The duration of static exposures is limited by: (a) the gradual depletion of oxygen; (b) the accumulation of carbon dioxide; (c) the accumulation of water vapor; (d) the gradual rise in temperature inside the chamber; and (e) the loss of the test agent via settling, wall loss, etc. In spite of these limitations, static systems can be useful in assessing acute toxicity, particularly when only a limited supply of the test material is available. Procedures similar to those described by Draize et al. (1959) have been very useful in screening compounds for toxicity. Many of the early test protocols were designed around the use of such systems. Static systems are also useful for exposure of animals to biologic aerosols because of the difficulty in continuously generating viable aerosols. In spite of the fact that most protocols call for use of dynamic chambers, there is at least one recent paper (DeWeese and Dews 1979) describing the use of a static system.

II. Dynamic Systems

Inhalation exposure systems are considered to be dynamic when the airflow and the introduction of the pollutant are continuous. The buildup and loss of the test agent in dynamic inhalation systems were originally described and verified by Silver (1946). The theoretical concentration of material in a chamber can be calculated as follows

$$\text{Concentration} = \frac{\text{flow of chemical}}{\text{flow of air}}.$$

Many factors including wall loss, animal uptake, variations in flow, etc., contribute to differences between the theoretical and the actual concentration in a chamber. Therefore, it is absolutely essential to measure the actual chamber concentration of a test agent with appropriate methods. It is not acceptable to report a nominal concentration derived from dividing the amount of pollutant expended by the volume of air passing through the system.

When material is introduced into a chamber, the concentration increases until it reaches a constant value. If perfect mixing occurs, the concentration can be calculated according to the following equation

$$C_t = (w/b)(1 - \exp(-bt/a)) \tag{1}$$

where C_t is the concentration of material at time t, w is the amount of material introduced per unit time, a is the volume of the chamber, and b is the airflow through the chamber.

The fraction of the equilibrium concentration (w/b) attained is

$$C_t/(w/b) = 1 - \exp(-bt/a) \tag{2}$$

and the time required to reach 99% (T_{99}) of the equilibrium (Fig. 1) can be determined:

$$0.99 = 1 - \exp(-bT_{99}/a)$$
$$\exp(-bT_{99}/a) = 1 - 0.99 = 0.01 \tag{3}$$
$$-bT_{99}/a = \ln 0.01 = -4.6052$$
$$T_{99} = 4.6052\, a/b.$$

This equation may be given the general form

$$tx = K(a/b), \tag{4}$$

where x is the percentage of the nominal equilibrium value attained and $K = \ln(100-x)/100$. Thus, T_{95}, for example, would be

$$T_{95} = \ln(100-95)/100(a/b)$$
$$= \ln 0.05(a/b)$$
$$= 2.9957 \, a/b.$$

The time to reach equilibrium is dependent only on the volume of the chamber and the flow rate. For example, if the flow rate through a 1-m^3 chamber is 250 l/min, $T_{95} = 3 \times 1\,000 \, l/(250 \, l/min) = 12$ min. MacFarland (1976) has demonstrated the impact of changing the flow rate on T_{99}. Notice that the term "air change" has not been used in this discussion. This is a misleading term and should not be used when describing chamber airflow (Drew 1981). When describing inhalation studies, both the chamber volume and the flow rate should be given.

These equations are derived on the assumption that perfect mixing occurs. If perfect mixing does not occur, T_{99} will be greater than shown in the equations. Recently, there has been much concern about the uniformity of aerosol or vapor distribution in inhalation chambers (Moss 1978; Carpenter and Beethe 1978; Griffis 1982). Hemenway et al. (1982) have defined the dead space in a chamber as representing areas in the chamber that come to equilibrium much more slowly than would be expected. MacFarland (1981 a) does not feel that the aerosol uniformity is a problem because of the degree of turbulence in the chamber, and correctly notes that it is impossible for local concentrations to exceed the equilibrium concentration. This is true if the pollutant is uniformly mixed in the incoming airstream. Clearly, there will be some areas in the chamber that are slower to come to equilibrium than others. Thus, it is wise to keep T_{99} short compared with the overall exposure duration.

III. Chamber Concentration

Figure 4 is a schematic representation of the concentration in a chamber with the generator being turned on at t_a and off at t_b. It can be seen that the exposure after t_b is equal to that missing during the buildup of the concentration. Notice also that T is long compared with T_{99}. MacFarland (1981 b) has suggested that the daily exposure duration should be greater than or equal to $13\, T_{99}$. If one adheres to this suggestion, the minimum flow rate through a chamber would be 10 chamber volumes per hour for a 6-h exposure. The duration of the exposure T is usually defined by $t_b - t_a$. However, the most recent National Toxicology Program protocol suggests that the duration of the exposure be defined as the time from t_a to t_c, the time when the concentration becomes low enough for the chamber to be opened safely. In the author's opinion, this is a mistake. The exposure duration should be considered as the time from when the generator is started to when it is turned off.

The question of what is an acceptable variation in chamber concentration is very difficult. Vapors are usually fairly easy to generate and to control. After a few weeks of experience with most vapor generators, the standard deviation on

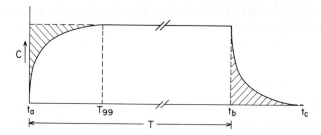

Fig. 4. A schematic representation of chamber concentration. C is concentration, t_a is the time the generator is turned on, T_{99} in the time required to reach 99% of the equilibrium value, t_b is the time the generator is turned off, T is the duration of the exposure, and t_c is the time when the chamber can be opened

a series of measurements through the day should be less than 10% of the mean value. Similarly, from day to day, the mean daily concentration should not vary by more than 10%.

Particle generators on the other hand are not easy to control. ALARIE (1981) has indicated that variations of as much as 20% are acceptable. Many factors other than concentration, including the animal's breathing rates and volumes, anatomic variations, etc., determine the actual dose delivered to the target tissue. Often, the variation in these factors is greater than the variation in the concentration. For these reasons, fine tuning the concentration variation may not be worthwhile. Standard deviations in the order of 10% of the mean should be sought. However, if during a subchronic study, the high dose chamber reached only 60%–70% of the target value one day, this is no reason to cancel the study. While the total accumulated exposures (concentration × time) should certainly come close to those called for in the protocol, an occasional value 40% or even 50% above or below the target value is no reason by itself to terminate a study.

IV. Airflow

Airflow can range from 8 to 60 chamber volumes per hour. At Brookhaven, the norm is 15 chamber volumes per hour. To some degree, the test agent will govern the flow. For example, in a study with chlorine, an airflow of 18 chamber volumes per hour was used to minimize ammonia buildup. In another study with only a few animals in a large chamber, an airflow of 8 chamber volumes per hour was used.

Measurement of airflow can be accomplished in many ways. HINNERS et al. (1968) described the design of a venturi flow meter. Orifice meters with a sensitive pressure gauge being used to measure the pressure drop across the orifice are commonly used. After installation they can be calibrated against an electronic flow computer (Autotronic Controls Corporation, El Paso, Texas) placed in the chamber at the entrance to the exhaust duct.

V. Static Pressure

Inhalation chambers are usually operated at a pressure 1–2 cm H$_2$O less than the pressure in the room. Measurement of chamber static pressure is fairly easy. Sensitive pressure gauges are readily available and have sufficient sensitivity to detect pressure differences as low as 1 mm H_2O. They can be calibrated easily using manometers or, for more sensitivity, incline manometers.

VI. Temperature and Humidity

Temperature and humidity should be measured and recorded frequently. Many devices can be used to measure temperature. Semiconductor analog temperature transducers (PC2626K, Analogue Devices, Norwood, Massachusetts) coupled to a computerized data management system are in use at Brookhaven. They can be calibrated by using ice water for one temperature point and a small constant temperature bath for the other point. Measurement of humidity is more difficult. At Brookhaven a wet-bulb, dry-bulb method, similar in concept to that described by HINNERS (1978), is being used. Air is drawn over a thermocouple covered by a wet wick. The humidity is calculated from the difference between the wet-bulb and dry-bulb temperatures. Automatic recording devices are available and should be considered. The method chosen will be a function of the investigator's experience with such devices.

VII. Exposure Duration

The duration of an exposure depends on the objectives of the study. Historically, acute studies have used either 1-hour exposures or 4-h exposures to assess acute inhalation toxicity. The 1-h exposures were used in static systems. More recently, the norm for single acute exposures in dynamic chambers has become 4 h. This is reasonable in light of the chamber dynamics already described. However, acute studies to assess the uptake distribution, retention, and excretion of an inhaled chemical may require shorter exposures. Such studies are usually done in systems capable of nose exposure or in units with drawers to allow rapid exposure and removal of the test animals.

Studies of subchronic and chronic toxicity fall into two categories: those where the exposure simulates that of a working day, usually for 6 or 7 hours per day, 5 days per week, and those which are performed continuously for 22–24 hours per day, 7 days per week, allowing a short time for servicing the animals. In both cases, the animals are exposed to a fixed concentration of the test agent. Neither situation approximates the actual human exposure where concentrations of pollutants continuously fluctuate over 1–2 orders of magnitude. One major difference between intermittent and continuous exposures is that with the former there is a 17- to 18-h recovery period between each exposure and a longer recovery period over the weekend. The choice depends on the objectives of the study and the human experiences that are being simulated.

VIII. Noise

Very little has been written about chamber noise. SCHRECK et al. (1981) measured noise levels in large (12.6-m^3) stainless steel and glass chambers and found that the chambers had to be modified to reduce noise levels from 75 to 65 dBA. The major source of the noise was the exhaust fan with its aerodynamic air noises in the chamber exhaust system. They adjusted the fan operation to avoid pulsations at low fan speeds. They also added acoustic baffles inside a plenum and replaced gate valves with damper valves. Most often the noise results from the movement of air through the controlling valves. This can sometimes be reduced by decreasing the chamber flow or changing the type of valve.

IX. Animal Loading

In his original article, SILVER (1946) suggested that the volume of animals in the chamber not exceed 5% of the volume of the chamber. Thus, for a 1-m^3 chamber, the animal volume should not exceed 50 l (equivalent to 50 kg or 100 rats each weighing 500 g, assuming unit density). This degree of animal loading does not cause thermal problems or untoward loss of aerosol on skin, and the rule of thumb is still useful today.

X. Cages and Racks

Inhalation exposure should be in six-sided wire cages to minimize particle deposition and maintain uniformity of concentration. To avoid two daily cage changes and thereby minimize labor costs, it is desirable to expose animals in the same cage in which they live. The cages must therefore have watering systems built in or be stored on a rack with water nipples which protrude into the cage. Cages are commercially available in which eight or more individual cages are arranged in a unit (cage pack) with common walls and individual watering nipples in each

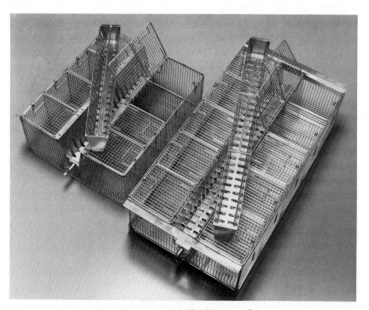

Fig. 5. Multicage units, showing the removable feeder troughs

cage. These cage packs have a trough down the center which accepts a matching feeder trough (Fig. 5). The troughs have slots which are aligned so that the animals can gnaw at the pellets contained in the trough. At Brookhaven, the area of an individual cage is sufficient to house one rat, two hamsters, or three mice and still conform to the guidelines promulgated by the American Association for Accreditation of Laboratory Animal Care (AAALAC).

It is convenient to have large chambers mounted in pits in such a fashion that racks containing tiers of wire cages can be wheeled directly into the exposure chamber. Alternatively, separate racks can be purchased which store cage packs at the same height as the chamber supports, thereby allowing cage packs to slide easily off the rack and into the chamber and vice versa. If water hookups are provided in the chambers, animals can be housed in chambers or in adjacent rooms during nonexposure periods.

At Brookhaven, the normal operating practice is to house animals in the 5-m³ chambers. The chambers are opened in the morning to change pans and remove the food troughs. In general, unless performing continuous exposures, it is not a good idea to allow food in the chambers during exposure. It will become contaminated with aerosols and may absorb vapors, rendering it unpalatable. After the exposure, the chambers are opened again to replace the food troughs. These operations are accomplished rapidly, allowing for efficient operation.

D. Limited Exposure Systems

Limited exposures are appropriate when: (a) the test agent is in short supply or very expensive; (b) the test agent is highly toxic and handling contaminated animals represents a significant hazard; (c) it is necessary to minimize skin absorption and/or ingestion due to preening; (d) such exposures most nearly represent human exposure such as with cigarette smoking; and (e) the protocol calls for exposures of a very short duration such as with studies on metabolism. Systems for head- or nose-only exposure were described as early as 1912 (SAITO 1912). STOKINGER et al. (1949) described chambers with openings for head exposures and HENDERSON (1952) described a cylindrical chamber with similar openings. Two divergent but practical needs spurred the development of nose exposure systems: the need to expose animals to cigarette smoke in a manner simulating the way humans smoke and the need to assess health effects of inhaled radionuclides.

Cigarette smoking machines have been described by many authors (HOFFMAN and WYNDER 1970; STUART et al. 1970; HOMBURGER et al. 1967; DONTENWILL et al. 1967; DONTENWILL 1970) with one more recent device described by BEVEN (1976). Most of these systems pull a fixed amount of air (usually 35 cm³) through a burning cigarette, dilute it (usually tenfold) and keep the diluted smoke in contact with the nose of the animal for a fixed interval (usually 30 s). In order to avoid CO asphyxia, these 30-s smoke exposures must be alternated by exposure to fresh air. Cigarettes are cycled through the system to allow the burning tip to cool between puffs. In most cases, the animals are restrained in tubes with their noses protruding slightly into the chamber which collects the smoke. In one system, mice were restrained in stocks which forced their noses into the smoke chamber

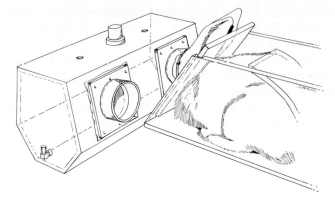

Fig. 6. A schematic representation of a nose exposure system for rabbits

(HENRY et al. 1981). This system allowed the body of the mouse to be open to room air, thus avoiding any temperature buildup in the restraint tubes.

A new series of tobacco smoking machines using peristaltic pumps has recently been developed by scientists at the Tobacco and Health Research Institute, University of Kentucky, Lexington, Kentucky. These machines can be used to expose in vitro systems or live animals to whole cigarette smoke, the gas phase, or sidestream smoke. Rather than using the sequence already described, one system uses a recycling dilution loop, exposing the test organism to 50% smoke for the first 2 s and then diluting the smoke with air such that the average age of the smoke is 3 s and the smoke is 99% diluted in 16 s. The machine is cycled once per minute. All of the necessary parameters such as puff volume, dilution time, etc., can be controlled.

One simple technique for limiting the exposure to the nose only was to enclose the animal in a tube and then place the entire tube in a chamber. This approach was followed by THOMAS and LIE (1963), who used plastic baby bottles as exposure tubes. Coca Cola bottles (180-ml) have also been used. Investigators have also used rubber face masks with small breathing holes cut around the nose (BOECKER et al. 1964; BAIR et al. 1969). A system of this sort for nose exposure of rabbits is shown schematically in Fig. 6. In most cases, the rubber mask fits into an opening fashioned from rubber dam which provides a good seal between the animal's nose and the chamber. Head-only systems have not been used in the recent past because of the difficulty in getting a good seal around the neck. Head exposure systems also result in skin contamination around the head of the animal.

Until fairly recently, exposure of rodents in tubes was limited to a few hours duration because of the stress imposed on the animals by restraint in the tubes. However, reports have begun to appear where animals are kept in nose tubes for 6–7 h/day without untoward effects (STAUFFER and RIEDWYL 1977; SMITH et al. 1980). SMITH et al. (1980) modified a 0.69-m chamber to accept a rack containing nose exposure tubes. One chamber could be used to expose 90 hamsters or 64 rats. Each animal was restrained in a polycarbonate exposure tube which was reported to minimize heat buildup inside the tube. These systems have been in operation for over 3 years with no untoward effects on animals. A similar system was described by HEWITT et al. (1978).

The actual shape of the tube is important. The polycarbonate tubes used by SMITH et al. (1980) have a symmetric conical end with an angle of 63 ° from the nasal end. BRIGHTWELL (1981, personal communication) and KUTZMAN et al. (1980) used tubes with asymmetric ends and both claim the animal is easier to restrain. Interestingly, in Brightwell's tube, the hole is closer to the bottom of the tube, while in Kutzman's, it is near the top. In any case, if designing a nose exposure tube, consideration should be given to asymmetric cones.

Another point to consider is the presence of ventilation slots in the exposure tubes. If there is a poor seal around the nose, air could easily pass through these slots up around the animal's nose and into the exposure chamber (assuming the chamber is at slightly negative pressure with respect to the outside of the tube). This would probably result in a decreased exposure to that animal. One would think that sealed tubes would minimize leaks and therefore potential contamination. However, it has been shown (OBERDORSTER et al. 1983) that the surface contamination on an animal is much greater in sealed tubes than in slotted tubes. When an animal exhales from a sealed system, it draws air around its nose and into the tube, resulting in substantial skin contamination. This does not happen when the tubes are ventilated.

Nose exposure systems which include plethysmographs have been described by RAABE et al. (1973), CUDDIHY and BOECKER (1973), and ALARIE (1973). MOKLER et al. (1979) suggest using such systems to improve measurement of the inhaled dose by using both the concentration and the minute volume to estimate the dose. The system described by Alarie has been used to assess sensory irritation in mice (BARROW et al. 1977; NIELSON and ALARIE 1982) and to evaluate toxicity of combustion products (ALARIE and ANDERSON 1979).

The current assessment of toxicity includes studies on uptake distribution, retention, and excretion of toxic agents. Such studies of inhaled materials often require very short exposures. Three systems have recently been described (KUTZMAN et al. 1980; KENNEDY and TROCHIMOWICZ 1982; LAWRENCE and DOROUGH 1981). These systems set up a dynamic exposure system and bypass the generator containing the test agent. Kutzman's system uses a Harvard pump to provide contaminant-laden air to the rat's nose while Kennedy's system uses the rat's own breathing rate to pull air through the contaminant generator. These systems expose only one animal at a time. A system using a large funnel and a plastic plate for the rapid exposure of a dozen rodents was described by HOBEN et al. (1976).

In spite of data reported by SMITH (1981) demonstrating no effects of restraint on the animals, a word of caution is necessary. LAPIN and BURGESS (1981) reported that restraint markedly alters the acute toxicity of carbon monoxide. The 1-h lethal concentration (LC_{50}) of CO was 1950 ppm in restrained rats and 3950 ppm in unrestrained rats. The possibility that the reason for the enhanced toxicity in restrained rats was due to the novel situation was investigated (DREW 1982). After acclimating rats in tubes for 2 months, a 1-h exposure to 3900 ppm killed all of five restrained rats, but none of five unrestrained rats. This difference is not demonstrable in naive rats if the LC_{50} is assessed after a 6-h exposure (SHIOTSUKA and DREW 1983, unpublished data). Head-only exposure was compared with whole body exposure by Sachsse et al. (1980) who measured the toxicity of five particulate agrochemicals. They saw little difference in the two modes of exposure and recommended head-only exposure for aerosols and whole body exposure for vapors and gases. The influence of stress on toxicity is a subject which has not received a great deal of attention. However, it has been shown (Riley 1981) that stressful situations can enhance the development of tumors. The interactions between stress and toxicity may be a very fruitful avenue of research.

E. Summary

This chapter summarizes the development, design, and operation of systems for exposure of animals to airborne pollutants. The most significant point is that there are no set ways to perform inhalation studies. Many methods and techniques are acceptable. The specific protocol developed depends on the objectives of the study or the questions being asked. Many chamber designs and operations are suitable to answer specific questions. The most important point for an investigator to understand is the limitations of the system chosen. A wide variety of chamber shapes and sizes are currently in use and are appropriate under certain circumstances. In conclusion, those beginning to design facilities or chambers are encouraged to consult with those who are currently operating such systems prior to beginning construction.

References

Alarie Y (1973) Sensory irritation of upper airways by airborne chemicals. Toxicol Appl Pharmacol 24:279–297

Alarie Y (1981) Inhalation and toxic responses. Presented at Mid-America toxicology course. Klassen CD Director, Kansas City, MO, p 286

Alarie YC, Anderson RC (1979) Toxicologic and acute lethal hazard evaluation of thermal decomposition products of synthetic and natural polymers. Toxicol Appl Pharmacol 51:341–362

Bair WJ, Porter NS, Brown DP, Wehner AP (1969) Apparatus for direct inhalation of cigarette smoke by dogs. J Appl Physiol 26:847–850

Barrow CS, Steinhagen WH (1982) Design, construction and operation of a simple inhalation exposure system. Fundam Appl Toxicol 2:33–37

Barrow CS, Alarie Y, Warrick JC, Stock MF (1977) Comparison of the sensory irritation response in mice to chlorine and hydrogen chloride. Arch Environ Health 32:68–76

Bernstein DM, Drew RT (1980) The major parameters affecting temperature inside inhalation chambers. Am Ind Hyg Assoc J 41:420–426

Beven JL (1976) Inhalation toxicity studies on cigarette smoke. I. A versatile exposure system for inhalation toxicity studies on cigarette smoke. Toxicology 6:189–96

Blair D, Rees HJ (1975) The generation and administration of atmospheres containing dichlorvos for inhalation studies. Am Ind Hyg Assoc J 36:385–397

Boecker BB, Aguilar FL, Mercer TT (1964) A canine inhalation exposure apparatus utilizing a whole body plethysmograph. Health Phys 10:1077–1089

Carpenter RL, Beethe RL (1978) Cones, cone angles, plenums, and manifolds. In: Drew RT (ed) Inhalation chamber technology. BNL Formal Report No 51318. Brookhaven National Laboratory, Upton, NY

Cuddihy RG, Boecker BB (1973) Controlled administration of respiratory tract burdens of inhaled radioactive aerosols in beagle dogs. Toxicol Appl Pharmcol 25:597–605

DeWeese J, Dews PB (1979) A simple apparatus for exposing a mouse to different atmospheric environments. J Physiol (Lond) 296:6–7

Dontenwill W (1970) Experimental investigations on the effect of cigarette smoke inhalation on small laboratory animals. In: Hanna MG Jr, Nettesheim P, Gilbert JR (eds) Inhalation carcinogenesis. Clearinghouse for federal scientific and technical information, NBS, US Deptartment of Commerce, Springfield, VA

Dontenwill W, Reckzeh G, Stadler L (1967) Smoking machine for laboratory animals. Beitr Tabakforsch 4:45–49

Draize JH, Nelson AA, Newburger SN, Kelley EA (1959) Inhalation toxicity studies of six types of aerosol hair sprays. Proc Sci Sect Toilet Goods Assoc 31:28–32

Drew RT (ed) (1978) Proceedings of a workshop on inhalation chamber technology. Brookhaven National Laboratory, Formal Report No 51318, Upton, NY

Drew RT (1981) Post symposium correspondence. In: Leong BKJ (ed) Inhalation. Toxicology and technology. Ann Arbor, Ann Arbor, MI pp 299–307

Drew RT (1982) Acute carbon monoxide toxicity in restrained vs unrestrained rats. Toxicologist 2:13

Drew RT, Laskin S (1971) A new dust-generating system for inhalation studies. Am Ind Hyg Assoc J 32:327–330

Drew RT, Laskin S (1973) Environmental inhalation chambers. In: Gay WI (ed) Methods of animal experimentation, vol 4. Academic, New York, pp 1–41

Eulenberg H (1865) Die Lehre von den schädlichen und giftigen Gasen. Vieweg, Braunschweig

Ferin J, Leach JF (1980) Horizontal airflow inhalation exposure chamber. In: Willeke K (ed) Generation of aerosols and facilities for exposure experiments. Ann Arbor, Ann Arbor, MI, pp 517–523

Feron VJ, Kruysse A (1977) Effects of exposure to acrolein vapor in hamsters simultaneously treated with benzo(a)pynene or diethylnitrosamine. J Toxicol Environ Health 3:379–394

Fraser DA, Bales RE, Lippmann M, Stokinger HE (1959) Exposure chambers for research in animal inhalation. U.S. Public Health Service Publication no 57, US Government Printing Office, Washington DC

Griffis LC, Wolff RK, Beethe RL, Hobbs CH, McClellan RO (1981) Evaluation of a multitiered inhalation exposure chamber. Fundam Appl Toxicol 1:8–12

Hartroft PM, Gregory RO, Gardner RA, Tansuwan C, Freeman S (1977) A system for the long-term continuous exposure of laboratory animals to mixtures of air pollutants. J Environ Sci Health [A] 12(6):225–257

Hemenway DR, MacAskill SM (1979) Design development and test results of a horizontal laminar flow inhalation toxicology facility. Presented at the annual meeting of American Industrial Hygiene Association, Chicago

Hemenway DR, Carpenter RL, Moss OR (1982) Inhalation toxicology chamber performance: a quantitative model. Am Ind Hyg Assoc J 43:120–127

Henderson DW (1952) Apparatus for study of airborne infection. J Hyg 50:53–68

Henry CA, Lopez A, Dansie DR, Avery MD, Whitmire CE, Caton JE, Stokely JR, Guerin MR, Currin RD, Kouri RE (1981) The distribution and clearance of three cigarette smoke constituents, dotriacontane (DCT), nicotine (NIC) and benzo (a) pyrene (BP), after exposure of mice to whole cigarette smoke. Toxicologist 1:139

Hewitt PJ, Hicks R, Lam HF (1978) The generation and characterization of welding fumes for toxicological investigations. Ann Occup Hyg 21:159–67

Hinners RG (1978) A system for automatically monitoring chamber temperature humidity and pollutant concentrations. In: Drew RT (ed) Proceedings of a workshop on inhalation chamber technology. Brookhaven National Laboratory Formal Report 51318, Upton, NY, pp 89–92

Hinners RG, Burkart JK, Punte CL (1968) Animal inhalation exposure chambers. Arch Environ Health 16:194–206

Hoben HJ, Ching S, Casarett LJ (1976) A study of the inhalation of pentachlonophenol by rats. II. A new inhalation exposure system for high doses in short exposure time. Bull Environ Contam Toxicol 15:86–92

Hoffman D, Wynder EL (1970) Chamber development and aerosol dispersion. In: Hanna MG Jr, Nettesheim P, Gilbert JR (eds) Inhalation carcinogenesis. Clearing house for federal scientific and technical information NBS, US Department of Commerce, Springfield, VA, pp 173–191

Holmberg RW, Moneyhun RW, Dalbey WE (1981) An exposure system for toxicological studies of concentrated oil aerosols. In: Leong BKJ (ed) Inhalation toxicology and technology. Ann Arbor, Ann Arbor, MI, pp 53–62

Homburger F, Bernfeld P, Bogdonoff P, Kelley T, Walton R (1967) Inhalation by small animals of fresh cigarette smoke generated by new smoking machine. Toxicol Appl Pharmacol 10:382

Kennedy GI Jr, Trochimowicz HJ (1982) Inhalation toxicology. In: Hayes AW (ed) Principles and methods of toxicology. Raven, New York, pp 185–208

Kimmerle G (1977) Inhalation chamber for the study of potentially carcinogenic polycyclic hydrocarbons in small laboratory animals. IARC Sci Publ 16:49–51

Kutzman RS, Meyer GJ, Wolf AP (1980) Biodistribution and excretion of (^{11}C)benzaldehyde by the rat after two-minute inhalation exposure. Xenobiotica 10:281–288

Lapin CA, Burgess BA (1981) The effects of restraint on the acute toxicity of carbon monoxide. Toxicologist 1:138–139

Laskin S, Kuschner M, Drew RT (1970) Studies in pulmonary carcinogenesis. In: Hanna MG Jr, Nettesheim P, Gilbert JR (eds) Inhalation carcinogenesis. Clearing house for federal scientific and technical information NBS, US Department of Commerce, Springfield, VA, pp 321–351

Lawrence LJ, Dorough HW (1981) Retention and fate of inhaled hexachloropentadiene in the rat. Bull Environ Contam Toxicol 26:663–668

Leach LJ (1965) A laboratory test chamber for studying airborne materials, AEC Progr Rep UR629. University of Rochester, Rochester, NY

Leach LJ, Spiegl CJ, Wilson RH, Sylvester GE, Lauterbach KE (1959) A multiple chamber exposure unit designed for chronic inhalation studies. Am Ind Hyg Assoc J 20:13–22

Leong BKJ (ed) (1981) Inhalation toxicology and technology. Ann Arbor, Ann Arbor, MI

Leong BKJ, Powell DJ, Pochyla GL, Lummis MG (1981) An active dispersion inhalation exposure chamber. In: Leong BKJ (ed) Inhalation toxicology and technology. Ann Arbor, Ann Arbor, MI, pp 65–76

Lippmann M (1980) Aerosol exposure methods. In: Willeke K (ed) Generation of aerosols and facilities for exposure experiments. Ann Arbor, Ann Arbor, MI, pp 443–458

MacEwen JD (1978) Nonconventional systems. In: Drew RT (ed) Proceedings of a workshop on inhalation chamber technology. BNL Formal Report 51318, Brookhaven National Laboratory, Upton, NY, pp 9–17

MacFarland HN (1976) Respiratory Toxicology. In: Hayes WJ Jr (ed) Essays in toxicology, vol 7. Academic, New York, pp 121–154

MacFarland HN (1981 a) A problem and a nonproblem in chamber inhalation studies. In: Leong BKJ (ed) Inhalation toxicology and technology. Ann Arbor, Ann Arbor, MI, pp 11–18

MacFarland HN (1981 b) Post-symposium correspondence. In: Leong BKJ (ed) Inhalation toxicology and technology. Ann Arbor, Ann Arbor, MI, pp 299–307

Mokler BU, Damon EG, Henderson TR, Carpenter RL, Benjamin SA, Rebar AH, Jones RK (1979) Inhalation toxicology studies of aerosolized products. LF 66 FDA No. PB-80-108509 National Technical Information Service, Springfield, VA

Montogomery MR, Anderson RE, Mortenson GA (1976) A compact, versatile inhalation exposure chamber for small animal studies. Lab Anim Sci 26(3):461–464

Moss OR (1978) A chamber providing uniform concentration of particulates for exposure of animals on tiers separated by catch pans. In: Drew RT (ed) Proceedings of a conference on inhalation chamber technology. BNL Formal Report 51318. Brookhaven National Laboratory, Upton, pp 31–38

Moss OR (1980) Exposure chamber. US Patent 4216741

Moss OR, Decker JR, Cannon WC (1982) Aerosol mixing in an animal exposure chamber having three levels of caging with excreta pans. Am Ind Hyg Assoc J 43:244–249

Nielsen GD, Alarie Y (1982) Sensory irritation, pulmonary irritation and respiratory stimulation by airborne benzene and alkylbenzenes: prediction of safe industrial exposure levels and correlation with their thermodynamic properties. Toxicol Appl Pharmacol 65:459–477

Oberdorster G, Meinhold SM, Marcello NL (1983) Reducing external body contamination from radioactive aerosols in nose only inhalation experiments in rats. Toxicologist 3:119

Phalen RF (1976) Inhalation exposure of animals. Environ Health Perspect 16:17–24

Pullinger DH, Crouch CN, Dare PR (1979) Inhalation toxicity studies with 2,3-butadiene – I Atmosphere generation and control. Am Ind Hyg Assoc J 40:789–795

Raabe OG, Bennick JE, Light ME, Hobbs CH, Thomas RL, Tillery MI (1973) An improved apparatus for acute inhalation exposure of rodents to radioactive aerosols. Toxicol Appl Pharmacol 26:264–273

Reid WB, Klok JR, Leong BKJ (1981) Hazard containment in an inhalation toxicology laboratory. In: Leong BKJ (ed) Inhalation toxicology and technology. Ann Arbor, Ann Arbor, MI, pp 1–10

Riley V (1981) Psychoneuroendocrine influences on immunocompetence and neoplasia. Science 212:1100–1109

Sachsse K, Zbinden K, Ullmann L (1980) Significance of mode of exposure in aerosol inhalation toxicity studies – Head only versus whole body exposure. Arch Toxicol (Suppl) 4:305–311

Saito Y (1912) Experimental investigations on the quantitative absorption of dust by animals at accurately known concentrations of dust in air (in German). Arch Hyg 75:134–151

Schreck RM, Chan TL, Soderholm SC (1981) Design operation and characterization of large volume exposure chambers. In: Leong BKJ (ed) Inhalation toxicology and technology. Ann Arbor, Ann Arbor, MI, pp 29–52

Silver SD (1946) Constant flow gassing chambers: principles influencing design and operation. J Lab Clin Med 31:1153–1161

Smith DM, Ortiz LW, Archuleta RF, Spalding JF, Tillery MI, Ettinger HJ, Thomas RG (1980) A method for chronic "nose-only" exposures of laboratory animals to inhaled fibrous in aerosols. In: Leong BKJ (ed) Inhalation toxicology and technology. Ann Arbor, Ann Arbor, MI, pp 89–105

Spiegl CJ, Leach LJ, Lauterbach KE, Wilson R, Laskin S (1953) Small chamber for studying test atmospheres. AMA Arch Ind Hyg Occup Med 8:286–288

Spivak JL, Connor E (1977) A simple hypoxic chamber. J Lab Clin Med 89:1375–1378

Stauffer HP, Riedwyl H (1977) Interaction and pH dependence of effects of nicotine and carbon monoxide in cigarette smoke inhalation experiments with rats. Agents Actions 7(5–6):579–588

Stead FM, Dernehl CU, Nau CA (1944) A dust feed apparatus useful for exposure of small animals to small and fixed concentrations of dust. J Ind Hyg Toxicol 26:90–93

Stokinger H, Baxter RC, Dygert HP, Labelle CW, Laskin S, Pozzani UC, Roberts E, Rothermel JJ, Rothstein A, Spiegl CJ, Sprague GF III, Wilson HB, Yaeger RC (1949) Toxicity following inhalation. In: Voegtlin C, Hodge HC (eds) Pharmacology and toxicology of uranium compounds, vol 3, 1st edn. McGraw-Hill, New York, NY, p 423

Stuart BO, Willard DH, Howard EB (1970) Uranium mine air contaminants in dogs and hamsters. In: Hanna MG, Nettesheim P, Gilbert JR (eds) Inhalation carcinogenes, Conf-691001. Clearing house for federal scientific information, US Department of Commerce, Springfield, VA, pp 413–428

Thiede FC, Hackney JD, Linn WS, Spier C, House W (1974) Animal atmosphere exposure chamber system using a modified tank respirator. Am Ind Hyg Assoc J 35-6:370–373

Thomas AA (1965) Low ambient pressure environments and toxicology. AMA Arch Environ Health 2:316–322

Thomas RG, Lie R (1963) Procedures and equipment used in inhalation studies on small rodents. US Atomic Energy Commission Research and Development Report, Lovelace Foundation Report LF-11, Albuquerque, NM

Von Oettingen WF, Hueper WC, Deichmann-Gruebler W, Wiley FH (1936) R-chlorobuta-
    diene (chloroprene) its toxicity and pathology and the mechanism of its action. J Ind
    Hyg Toxicol 18:240–270
Willeke K (ed) (1980) Generation of aerosols and facilities of exposure experiments. Ann
    Arbor Science Publishers, Ann Arbor, MI
Wilson RH, Laskin S (1950) AEC Proj Rep UR-116. University of Rochester, Rochester,
    NY, p 80

CHAPTER 2

Gases and Vapors: Generation and Analysis

M. LIPPMANN

A. Introduction

The generation and measurement of exposure atmospheres for inhalation studies is, in principle, quite simple, especially for gases and vapors where all of the molecules of a given material have independent motion and the same properties. When the molecules are clustered in particles of varying sizes and aerodynamic properties, their generation, measurement, and toxic properties are more difficult to describe and control.

Since inhalation exposures require relatively dilute solutions of gas and vapor molecules in air at temperatures and pressures close to those normally encountered indoors at sea level, some convenient simplifications can be made. All such mixtures have essentially the same gas density and properties as pure air, and therefore the small changes in temperature, pressure, and density which we produce in handling them are governed by the ideal gas laws.

Vapors are the gas phase of materials which can exist in the liquid phase at or near normal temperatures and pressures. Thus, inorganic compounds such as ammonia (NH_3) and sulfur dioxide (SO_2), which can be used as refrigerant fluids, are vapors, as are organic solvents such as alcohol, acetone, and benzene. Gases such as oxygen (O_2), nitrogen (N_2), and carbon monoxide (CO) can also be liquefied, but only at very low temperatures. The distinction between gases and vapors is usually not very important in the monitoring of exposure concentrations. However, it may be important in exposure atmosphere generation, where it may be convenient to use a liquid feed or reservoir in generating a vapor, or where losses of material can occur by condensation of the vapors on cool surfaces.

The concentrations of gases and vapors in air can be expressed in terms of volume fractions or mass concentration per unit volume. Volumetric ratios are generally more convenient operationally and more understandable in the conceptual sense of toxic effects relating to molecular interactions at deposition, absorption, or interaction sites. Among the commonly used volumetric concentrations are molar ratio, percentage, parts per million by volume (ppm_v), and parts per billion (ppb_v). These are related to one another, differing respectively by dilution ratios. Thus, percentage is $10^{-2} \times$ of molar ratio, ppm_v is 10^{-6}, and ppb_v is 10^{-9}.

In inhalation toxicology, the highest concentration that one is likely to use is 5 g/m^3, an arbitrary and probably excessive upper concentration range for product safety evaluations specified by regulatory agencies. More typically, mass concentrations used in inhalation studies will be expressed in mg/m^3 or $\mu g/m^3$, which are related to g/m^3 by factors of 10^3 and 10^6, respectively. To convert a mass concentration, such as $5\,g/m^3$ to volumetric concentration, we must know the molecular weight M and molar volume at the exposure conditions. The molar volume of a gas or vapor at the standard conditions used in chemistry (0 °C, 1 atm) is 22.4 l. Since the typical inhalation exposure condition is 25 °C and 1 atm; the molar volume of interest can be easily determined:

$$22.4 \times \frac{(273+25)}{273} = 24.5\,\text{mol/l}.$$

To illustrate the volumetric concentrations equivalent to $5\,g/m^3$, let us consider a variety of vapors of different molecular weights (Table 1). The volume occupied by 5 g at chamber conditions is

$$\left(\frac{5}{M}\,\text{mol} \times 24.5\,\text{l/mol} \right)$$

Table 1. Volume occupied by various gases (5 g) at 25 °C and 1 atm

Vapor	Molecular weight	Volume (1)	Percentage	ppm
Ammonia	17	7.21	0.72	7,200
Formaldehyde	30	4.08	0.41	4,100
Nitrogen dioxide	46	2.66	0.27	2,700
Benzene	78	1.57	0.16	1,600
Perchlorethylene	166	0.74	0.074	740

Almost all inhalation toxicology is done with dynamic flow systems in which the inlet airstream is maintained at a constant concentration and flow rate. The continuous flow permits maintenance of steady state conditions with respect to temperature, humidity, CO_2, and other animal-generated contaminants. Since the volumetric rate of flow of the air feed into an inhalation chamber is generally relatively low in relation to the volume of the chamber, there will usually be a finite time required to achieve a steady state concentration within the chamber. Furthermore, since the inlet air does not flow uniformly across the chamber cross section, the time required to reach a steady state concentration is always longer than that calculated on the basis of perfect mixing.

In those studies where it is necessary to have well-defined brief exposures, there are several options. One is to use an airlock system in order to insert a group of animals rapidly into a chamber, and later withdraw them from an established concentration. Another is to have a higher flow rate to chamber volume ratio and a well-mixed chamber concentration. In some cases, especially when the feed material is in very limited supply and/or expensive, and the exposure period is brief, it may be necessary to resort to static chamber exposures.

Static mixtures can also be used for nonchamber inhalation exposures. When exposing individual animals or humans via masks, mouthpieces, or catheters, a premixed exposure atmosphere can be drawn from a reservoir. If the reservoir is a flexible plastic bag, then the concentration can remain constant until the volume of the bag is exhausted. Static or fixed volume atmospheres may also be useful as calibration atmospheres for gas and vapor samplers and monitors, especially those sampling at low flow rates.

B. Generation and Atmospheres

Methods of producing known concentrations are usually divided into two general classifications: (a) static or batch systems; and (b) dynamic or continuous flow systems. With static systems, a known amount of gas is mixed with a known amount of air to produce a known concentration. Static systems are limited by two factors, loss of vapor by surface adsorption, and by the finite volume of the mixture. In dynamic systems, air and gas or vapor are continuously metered in the appropriate proportion to produce the final desired concentration. They provide an unlimited supply of the test atmosphere and wall losses are negligible after equilibration has taken place.

I. Static Systems

Rigid containers such as 5-gallon ($\sim$ 19-l) bottles can be used for static systems. The bottles are usually equipped with an inlet tube, valve, and outlet tube. A third port may also be provided for introduction of the contaminant. In practice, after the mixture has come to equilibrium, samples are drawn from the outlet side while replacement air is allowed to enter through the inlet tube. Thus, the mixture is being diluted while it is being sampled.

Under ideal conditions, the concentration remaining is a known function of the number of air changes in the bottle. If one assumes instantaneous and perfect mixing of the incoming air with the entire sample volume, the concentration change, as a small volume is withdrawn, is equal to the concentration multiplied by the percentage of the volume withdrawn:

$$dC = C \, dV/V_o.$$

This integrates to

$$C = C_o \exp(-V/V_o)$$

or

$$2.3 \log_{10} C_o/C = V/V_o,$$

where: C is the total concentration at any time; V is the total volume of sample withdrawn; C_o is the original concentration; and V_o is the volume of the chamber. Thus, if one extracts a gas volume equal to one-tenth the container volume

$$2.3 \log_{10} C_o/C = 0.1$$
$$\log_{10} C_o/C = 0.1/2.3 = 0.0435$$
$$C_o/C = 1.1053$$

or

$$C/C_o = 0.9047.$$

The average concentration of the sample withdrawn is $(1 + 0.9047)/2 = 0.9524$. If instantaneous mixing does not occur, and the inlet and outlet port are separated, the average concentration may be even higher.

If one were interested in a maximum of 5% variation from the average concentration, only about 10% of the sample could be used. Setterlind (1953) has shown that this limitation can be overcome by using two or more bottles of equal volume V_o in series, with the initial concentration in each bottle being the same. When the mixture is withdrawn from the last bottle, it is not displaced by air, but by the mixture from the preceding bottle. If, as stated, a maximum of 5% variation in concentration can be tolerated, two bottles in series provide a usable sample of 0.6 V_o. With five bottles, the usable sample will increase to about 3 V_o. A table in Setterlind (1953) gives both residual concentration and average concentration of the withdrawn sample as a function of the number of volumes withdrawn for each of five bottles in series.

A rigid system can also be modified to give greater usable volumes by attaching a balloon to the inlet tube inside the bottle. Air from the bottle can then be displaced without any dilution by merely inflating the balloon. Many of the difficulties associated with the dilution of rigid systems can be overcome with nonrigid plastic bag systems. These systems allow withdrawal of the entire sample without need of replacement air and dilution. One, however, has to have assurance that the chemical does not permeate through the bag, or is not sorbed by the bag. A variety of available plastic films, including Mylar (polyethylene terephthalate polyester), aluminized Mylar, polyethylene, and Teflon (polytetrafluoroethylene) are useful for such systems. The bags generally have a wall thickness of 0.03–0.13 mm, thus allowing flexibility for inflation. For additional strength and impermeability to moisture, the polymer is often laminated to aluminium. Polyethylene is simple to use, but many gases and vapors either diffuse through it or are absorbed onto the walls. Mylar and aluminized Mylar are less permeable. The polyfluorocarbons are generally the most resistant chemically and most resistant to absorption and diffusion over a wide range of compounds.

Prior to the introduction of any component into a nonrigid system, the bag should be evacuated as thoroughly as possible and then the component and any dilution gas metered very carefully. Calibrated syringes provide a simple method for introduction of materials, either gaseous or liquid, into static systems. The syringe should be flushed several times with the component of interest and then injected through a soft septum material through which the syringe needle can be inserted and then removed without leakage.

Another approach is to use a rigid-walled pressure vessel which can be evacuated, filled with a measured volume of gas or liquid, and then repressurized with compressed air or other carrier gas to produce the concentrations required. This mixture can then be used to fill a static chamber either directly, or after further dilution. A number of gases and vapors are available in different concentrations from a variety of suppliers. Analysis, usually gravimetric, is provided on request.

These should always be checked since the trace gas may not be adequately mixed, or may be partially lost owing to wall adsorption.

II. Dynamic Systems

In dynamic systems, the rate of airflow and the rate of addition of contaminant to the airstream are both carefully controlled to produce a known dilution ratio. Dynamic systems offer a continuous supply of material, allow for rapid and predictable concentration changes, and minimize the effect of wall losses as the contaminant comes to equilibrium with the interior surfaces of the system. Both gas and liquid feeds can be used with dynamic systems. With liquids, however, provisions must be available for conversion to the vapor state.

1. Gas Dilution Systems

A simple schematic view of a gas dilution system is shown in Fig. 1. Air and the contaminant gas are metered through restrictions and then mixed. The output can be used as is, or further diluted in a similar system. In theory, this process can be repeated until the necessary dilution ratio is obtained. In practice, series dilution systems are subject to a variety of instabilities which make them difficult to control. Figure 2 describes a system for compensation of back pressure. Both the air and contaminant gas flows are regulated by the height of a water column which, in turn, is controlled by the back pressure of the calibration system. Thus, an increase in back pressure causes an increase in the delivery pressure of both air and contaminant gas.

The ppm Maker (Calibrated Instruments, Incorporated, Ardsley, New York) consists of a four-output positive displacement pump and two mechanized four-way stopcocks with single bore plugs. The bore is normally aligned with the carrier gas flow. When activated, the stopcock is rotated 180°, momentarily aligning

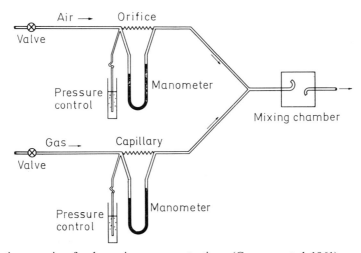

Fig. 1. Continuous mixer for dynamic gas concentrations. (COTABISH et al. 1961)

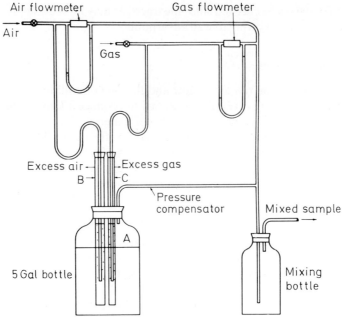

Fig. 2. Modified Mase gas mixer for compensation of back pressure. (COTABISH et al. 1961)

the bore with the contaminant gas airflow and delivering a precise volume to the carrier gas. A mixing chamber downstream mixes the carrier gas and the contaminant. The mixture is then pumped through a second identical system. By varying the flow rates of the carrier gas, dilution ratios of the order of $1:10^9$ can be achieved. The stepwise increments of the pumps and the stopcocks provide more than 10,000 different concentration ratios.

Another device for constant delivery of a pollutant gas was described by GOETZ and KALLAI (1962). It consists of a large gas-tight syringe with a centrifugal rotor attached to the piston so that the piston rotates around its axis. The rotation, caused by a jet of air directed tangentially toward the rotor, is nearly friction-free and induces a constant pressure in the gas. The outlet of the syringe is connected on one side of a glass T-tube. Dilution air is piped into the base of the T and the mixture exits the T-tube from the other side arm.

2. Vaporization of Liquid Feed Stream

When the contaminant is a liquid at normal temperature, a vaporization step must be included. One procedure is to use a motor-driven syringe, and meter the liquid onto a wick or a heated place in a calibrated airstream. NELSON and GRIGGS (1968) described a calibration apparatus which makes use of this principle (Figs. 3 and 4). The system consists of an air cleaner, a solvent injection system, and a combination mixing and cooling chamber. A large range of solvent concentrations can be produced (2–2,000 ppm). The device permits rapid changes in the concentrations and is accurate up to about 1.0%. It also can be used to produce gas dilutions with an even wider range of available concentrations (0.05–2,000 ppm).

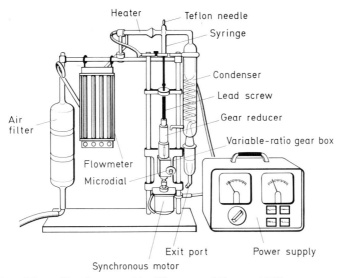

Fig. 3. Syringe drive calibration assembly. (Nelson and Griggs 1968)

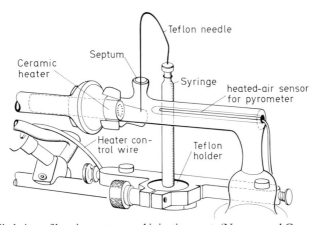

Fig. 4. Detailed view of heating system and injection port. (Nelson and Griggs 1968)

A second vapor generation method is to saturate an airstream with vapor and then dilute with makeup air to the desired concentration. The amount of vapor in the saturated airstream is dependent on both the temperature and vapor pressure of the contaminant and can be precisely calculated. A simple vapor saturator is shown in Fig. 5. The inert carrier gas passes through two gas washing bottles in series which contain the liquid to be volatilized. The first bottle is kept at a higher temperature than the second one which is immersed in a constant temperature bath. By using the two bottles in this fashion, saturation of the exit gas is assured. A filter is sometimes included to remove any droplets entrained in the airstreams as well as any condensation particles. A mercury vapor generator using this principle was described by Nelson (1970).

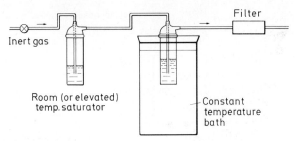

Fig. 5. Vapor saturator. (COTABISH et al. 1961)

Diffusion cells have also been used to produce known concentrations of gaseous vapors. In this case, the liquid diffuses up a center tube and into a mixing chamber through which air is passed. Devices of this type can be used with dynamic systems. They are, however, limited to low flow rates. O'KEEFE and ORTMAN (1966) developed a technique for dispersing vapors of any material whose critical temperature was above 20–25 °C. The material is sealed in Teflon tubing and permeates the walls of the tube, diffusing out at a rate dependent upon wall thickness and area (fixed parameters) and temperature. At constant temperature, the rate of weight loss is constant as long as there is liquid in the tube. In use, precautions are necessary to assure constant temperatures since, for example, the sulfur dioxide permeation rate more than doubles for every 10 °C increase in temperature. Sulfur dioxide permeation tubes have been most commonly used. Nitrogen dioxide tubes are also available, however, the NO_2 may affect the permeability of the Teflon walls. In addition, permeation tubes of hydrogen sulfide, chlorine, propane, butane, and methyl mercaptan are available (AIR SAMPLING INSTRUMENTS COMMITTEE 1983).

C. Monitoring and Control of Concentrations

There have been great advances in gas and vapor monitoring technology in recent years. The availability of instantaneous and rapid response concentration sensors makes it possible to achieve close control of concentrations as well as accurate measurement and recording of exposure variables. Rapid response sensors, in conjunction with modern feedback control circuitry, make it possible to have continuous automatic adjustment of feed rates, as well as an ability to shut off feed systems and actuate automatic vent systems and alarms.

For some gases and vapors, rapid response monitors are not available, and the characterization of chamber concentration is dependent on the periodic collection of air samples and analysis of the collected samples. In such cases, adjustment of feed rates is a manual operation and substantially greater concentration excursions can be expected. It may be desirable to use some secondary indicator to maintain a constant concentration, such as the rate that the feed chemical is dispensed, and to use periodic samples collected from the chamber to determine the average concentration actually inhaled by the animals.

I. Basic Considerations in Monitoring

In some respects, gas and vapor monitoring in exposure chambers is simpler than monitoring community air and occupational exposures, but in others, it is more difficult. Among the favorable factors are: chamber concentrations are likely to be higher, and there will be less chemical interference. Also, there will usually be fewer limitations on instrument size and weight, since portability is generally not a requirement, and less likelihood of limitations imposed by extremes in temperature and other environmental variables. On the other hand, it may be more difficult to locate the sensor at the position where the concentration of interest is located, and the use of sampling probes or lines may produce sampling artifacts and/or lags in instrument response times.

1. Sensitivity

Most direct reading gas and vapor monitors developed for industrial hygiene and air pollution measurements are adaptable to inhalation toxicology. In some cases, instruments designed for measuring higher concentrations in stack gas and process gas streams can also be adapted to exposure monitoring. The sensitivities of a wide variety of such instruments are summarized in *Air Sampling Instruments* (AIR SAMPLING INSTRUMENTS COMMITTEE 1983).

2. Specificity

Since most inhalation studies involve only one agent at a time, many nonspecific sensors can be used without concern for interference. For example, heat of combustion instruments can be used for a wide variety of organic vapors, and electrical conductivity analyzers can be used for various ionizable species collected by gas washing. For aerosol exposures, it may be possible to monitor and control concentrations using nephelometers or accumulated mass sensors such as the quartz crystal microbalance or the β-attenuation meter. Whenever nonspecific sensors are used to monitor exposures, they should be supplemented with specific chemical analyses of periodically collected samples of the exposure atmospheres to document that the nonspecific factor being monitored is a suitable surrogate for the agent of interest.

3. Temporal Response

The temporal responses of the various direct reading gas and vapor detectors vary considerably. For those detectors which measure a spectral absorption within a defined sensing zone, such as infrared (IR) and ultraviolet (UV) detectors, the temporal response is limited by the size and configuration of the sensing zone and the flow rate of the stream passing through it. It is also affected by the delay introduced by the time needed for the sampled stream to pass through the inlet probe, sampling lines between the probe and the instrument inlet, and pipes or tubes between the instrument inlet and the sensing zone. For instruments with sequential sample collection and analysis, such as colorimetric and conductivity analyzers, the temporal responses are considerably slower.

4. Calibration and Maintenance

All monitoring instruments will need periodic calibration and maintenance to ensure reliable performance, and to serve as parts of a quality assurance program for the study as a whole. There should be provision for delivery of clean air to the sensor for verification and/or adjustment of the zero reading. There should also be provision for delivering one or more known concentrations of the agent of interest to the sensor to check and/or adjust the instrument response characteristics. Some instruments have built-in span checks, which generally involve either the output indicator response to an electronic signal simulating the sensor output, or to the insertion of a filter into the sensor which mimics the absorption of a sample in the sensor. Such span checks are useful and convenient, and provide good checks on many elements in the overall system. They can supplement, but not completely replace, periodic calibration tests with known concentrations of the gas or vapor of interest. The techniques for generating gas and vapor atmospheres for instrument calibration are the same as those previously described for generating exposure atmospheres, especially those that produce relatively low flow rates.

II. Control of Concentration

The adjustment of exposure concentration within a chamber or mask can be made manually or automatically. Manual adjustments consist of throttling the flow or feed rate of either the gas stream or the dilution air on the basis of either direct reading monitors or the results of the analysis of spot samplers. The proper calibration and use of automated air sampling instruments depends upon an understanding of the types of output signals through which the data are handled. WILLARD et al. (1981) have reviewed the basic considerations of digital electronics, signal modifying circuits, and computer aided analysis as they apply to instrumental methods of analysis.

In most systems used with air monitoring instruments, the detector in the instrument produces an analog voltage which is proportional to the pollutant concentration. The analog voltage can be read on a meter, or a digital output can be obtained by the use of an analog-digital converter. This interprets the analog voltage in terms of binary numbers which are powers of 2. The most commonly used code for representing binary numbers is the ASCII (American Standard Code for Information Interchange), which uses seven bits to represent each character, and an eighth bit (parity bit) for error checking.

The signals from the monitoring instrument can be transmitted by either parallel or serial transmission. Parallel transmission uses a number of wires (one for each bit plus one additional wire for a clock signal) to transmit an entire character at one time. Therefore, transmission of an ASCII coded character requires eight wires, one for each of the seven bits plut the parity bit. Parallel transmission can be used at very high rates of transmission. With serial transmission of data, only two wires are used, one to transmit the data, and one wire to serve as a common signal ground. The eight bits of an ASCII character are transmitted serially, one at a time. In general, parallel transmission is used internally in a computer or over very short distances where extremely high rates of transmission are necessary. Serial transmission is more often used for communication over long distances. This is the most common and most practical method of communication between computerized instrumentation.

Binary information, such as contained in the eight bits of an ASCII character, is in the form of zeros (0) or ones (1) only. Serial transmissions, such as over a telephone line, are a continuum of analog voltage. Therefore, to accomplish serial transmission of binary data, a device has been developed which first converts the binary data from the sender into an analog signal. This can be transmitted over the phone line (modulated) and then converted at the receiving end, back into binary data (demodulation). Such a device is known as a Modem. There are two standard methods which are used to convert data in this manner. One method varies the current, while the other method varies the voltage, to transmit the binary zeros and ones.

In a 20-mA current loop, binary information is transferred by turning a 20-mA current on and off. When the current is on, a binary 1 bit is sent, and when the current is off, a binary 0 is sent. While this method of transmission is less susceptible to voltage-induced noise, it was not designed for use with modems, and has limited applications for long distance transmission.

The Electronics Industry Association (EIA) has established a standard system known as RS-232C which incorporates modem control information needed for transmission. The standard specifies that both the sender and receiver have male connectors, and that modems have female connectors. Therefore, to connect two EIA devices a null modem must be used which allows the connection of the two male plugs. Data is transmitted with this system by reversing the polarity of the voltage on a DC serial line. A positive voltage denotes a 0 bit while a negative voltage denotes a 1 bit.

III. Types of Monitors

1. Electromagnetic Gas Phase Sensors

In these monitors, the sampled stream is passed continuously through a sensing zone which is traversed by a stream of photons, part of which is absorbed or scattered by the pollutant of interest. Most applications involve absorption of IR, visible, or UV radiation. Recent advances in spectroscopy have introduced a number of techniques that are being adapted to gas analyses (HANST 1970). These include microwave radiation, correlation spectroscopy, Raman radiation, laser sources, solid state detectors, derivative spectroscopy, and Fourier transform spectroscopy. Some of these techniques are being applied to emission and scattering of electromagnetic waves by pollutant gases in addition to the absorption phenomena.

These electro-optic techniques offer a broad range of applications, some of which cannot be achieved by any other method. For example, long path in situ gas analyses, as well as remote sensing, can be conducted by electro-optic methods only. This discussion considers three basic molecular phenomena under which these methods fall, namely, absorption, emission, and scattering. A discussion on the various spectroscopic schemes by which these phenomena are detected and analyzed will follow.

Molecules characteristically absorb, scatter, and emit electromagnetic radiation. The unique relationship of the radiation involved in any of these processes with the molecular structure permits qualitative identification and quantitative concentration measurements to be made. Gas molecules *absorb* incident electromagnetic energy at wavelengths corresponding to the change in energy states of a given molecule. Gas molecules *emit* at wavelengths corresponding to the change in energy states of a given molecule. Absorbing wavelengths are identical to emitting wavelengths for a specific change in the energy state of a molecule. Absorption constitutes an increase in energy; and emission, a decrease in energy. In emission, the source of energy can be internal, such as thermal emission, or external, such as chemiluminescense by chemical interaction. Energy absorbed and reemitted at new wavelengths is referred to as fluorescence. The shift in wavelength, indicating some loss of energy, is toward longer wavelengths.

Incident radiation can be *scattered* as well as absorbed, or it may be absorbed and reemitted at a different wavelength. Energy scattered by molecules at the same wavelength as the incident wavelength is referred to as Rayleigh scattering. In Raman scattering, the incident radiation causes a virtual transition in the molecular energy states, with reemission of radiation at both longer and shorter wavelengths than that of the incident radiation. Raman scattering does not require the incident radiation to be at or near the absorbing wavelength of the gas, and can thus take place at any wavelength. The intensity of Raman scattering, however, increases inversely as the fourth power of the wavelength of the incident radiation. Consequently, the UV region is a more attractive region for Raman scattering than the IR portion of the spectrum. Raman scattering is further enhanced by a factor of 100 or more when the incident radiation is near the absorbing wavelength of the gas. This is referred to specifically as resonance Raman scattering.

a) Infrared Photometry

α) *Nondispersive Methods.* Many pollutant gases have characteristics absorption lines in the IR region of the electromagnetic spectrum. The nondispersive method avoids the use of dispersive optics, e. g., prisms or gratings. Selectivity in sensing the pollutant at its absorbing wavelength is achieved in one of several ways: by selective light sources (lasers), by selective detectors, by selective filtering of light sources, or by combinations of selective elements.

IR gas analyzers are available for measurement of CO, CO_2, and some hydrocarbons by selective detection using gas filters (BURCH and GRYVNAK 1974). In a typical analyzer, IR radiation from two hot filament sources passes through parallel tubes, one a reference cell (containing clean air) and the other the analysis or sample cell (containing the pollutant gas, e. g., CO in air). Some of the radiation is removed by the CO in the sample cell at its absorbing wavelengths, and the remainder passes on to the detector. The detector is made selective only to the absorbing wavelengths of CO by filling it with pure CO. The detector generates an electrical signal output based on the difference in absorption between the reference and sample cells. This output becomes a quantitative measure of the concentration of CO in the sample cell based on calibration of the output readout.

The availability of laser sources, offering monochromatic wavelengths and high beam intensities has stimulated new monitoring instrument developments. Although lasers are highly selective light sources, and the state of the art in developing lasers for operation at various wavelengths is advancing rapidly, there are still limitations on available wavelengths. The technique of selecting a laser line that coincides with an absorption line of a gas as a means of specific and sensitive gas analysis has been demonstrated (HANST 1971, 1968). Current developments in tunable dye lasers (BRADLEY et al. 1968) in the UV and visible, and tunable solid state diode lasers in the IR (HINKLEY and KELLEY 1971), offer great potential for a range of specific and sensitive gas analyzers with direct readout.

Selective filtering of light in nondispersive techniques can be achieved anywhere between the light source and the detector in the sensing of a pollutant at its absorbing wavelength. It is done most effectively with filters at the detector. Optical filters are available with various specifications on transmission, bandwidth, and location of central wavelength of transmission. Interference filters provide very narrow transmission bandwidths, but do not approach the wavelength resolution capability of dispersive techniques.

Resolution of filtering techniques in the IR is of the order of 10 cm^{-1} as compared with absorption linewidths that may be of the order of 0.1 cm^{-1}. Consequently, interference is possible because of overlapping absorption lines from other pollutant gases within the transmission band of the filter. This necessitates correcting for interference by additional measurements in adjacent spectral regions, and introduces more complexity in the analytical scheme and instrumentation. In comparison, the use of lasers as selective light sources offers the advantage of a very narrow line (of the order of 0.001 cm^{-1}) to give high discrimination against interference). On the other hand, selective light filtering and detection by gas filters offers the resolution of the absorbing gas itself and deletion of all the lines of the absorbing gas. This method is also referred to as gas correlation spectroscopy.

β) Dispersive Methods. Dispersive methods are used in spectrophotometers having optical elements such as prisms or gratings. These elements spatially disperse the light from a broadband source so that wavelength selection may be achieved by means of proper physical placement of mechanical slit openings. Resolution is related primarily to the slit width, the dispersive power of the optical element, and the optical configuration of the instrument. The limiting factor on resolution is the dispersive optical element. Gratings are available that permit resolution in the IR of the order of 0.1 cm^{-1} and less.

The dispersive technique permits continuous scanning of the spectrum within the wavelength region of the dispersive element. This is an advantage over fixed optical filter techniques. In the IR for example, a grating can cover the region 7–14 μm. Lasers fall in between, since they can have a single wavelength, or, as in the case of an isotopic CO_2 gas laser, have as many as 150 discrete lines. These lines fall within a narrow range of the spectrum, however, and being discrete, do not permit a continuous scan.

b) Ultraviolet Photometry

UV photometers operate on the characteristic of certain gases to absorb UV radiation. An appropriate wavelength is selected for the detector based on the absorption characteristics of the pollutant of interest. Mercury, for instance, has a strong absorption at 254 nm. The reduction of energy at this wavelength, transmitted to the photometer as a result of absorption by vapors in the gas samples, is a measure of mercury vapor concentration. Other spectroscopic techniques such as correlation and derivative techniques, as discussed in Sects. C.III.1.c.β and γ, are also applied to UV detectors.

c) Other Photometric Techniques

α) *Fourier Interferometry*. The interferometer-spectrometer is a dispersive instrument that permits an examination of a large portion of the spectrum, which eventually can be displayed as a function of wavelength. Unlike the grating dispersive technique, interferometry first generates a frequency spectrum by light interference in an optical system. The frequency spectrum is converted mathematically into the conventional wavelength spectrum by Fourier transforms. A conventional scanning dispersive spectrometer generates a spectrum by serially scanning the spatially dispersed wavelengths as a function of time. The interferometer has multiplexing capability, whereby all the wavelengths are scanned concurrently in time and are measured directly as a frequency spectrum.

The Michelson interferometer–spectrometer (Fig. 6) consists of two plane mirrors, M_1 and M_2, one of which is fixed, and two plane-parallel plates, G_1 and G_2. Light from an extended source is incident at 45° on plate G_1, partially silvered on the rear surface, and is divided into a reflected (path A) and a transmitted (path B) beam of equal intensity. The light reflected from M_1 passes through plate G_1 a third time before it reaches the detector. The light reflected from mirror M_2 passes back through G_2 a second time, is reflected from the surface of plate G_2, and into the detector. The two beams have a phase difference governed by the differences in the two paths. As incoming radiation is received by the interferometer, a fringe pattern is produced by interference in the two beams. When one of the mirrors is moved back and forth at a slow constant velocity, the motion is manifested as an alternate brightening and darkening of the central fringe. The detector records these signal changes. Incident radiation containing many wavelengths would generate a composite signal of all the sine waves that correspond to all the wavelengths in the source. A Fourier wave analysis of the signal produces a wavelength spectrum.

The maximum resolution of this interferometer depends upon the maximum travel of the movable mirror and is equal to the maximum travel distance divided by one-half the wavelength. Commercial interferometers are available with resolution approaching 0.5 cm^{-1} in the IR. Throughput and multiplexing capability of the interferometer offer an advantage over the conventional dispersive spectrometer in the speed with which a spectrum can be obtained. The Fourier transformation, however, is an involved procedure and adds to the complexity and cost of the instrumentation.

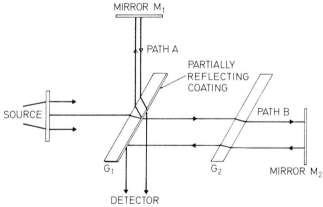

Fig. 6. Michelson interferometer

β) Correlation. Correlation techniques consist of matching a reference spectrum of the gas to be measured against the spectrum of the sampled gas to be analyzed (the sample spectrum). The reference spectrum may be generated by a photographic mask or by a gas cell whereby the techniques are referred to as optical correlation spectroscopy or gas correlation spectroscopy, respectively. The latter is also referred to as a matched filter technique or a gas filter technique and was discussed in Sect.C.III.1.a.α. The sample spectrum may be generated by dispersive optics or by nondispersive gas filters.

γ) Derivative Technique. The derivative technique consists simply in the processing of the transmission–wavelength function of an ordinary spectrometer into a signal proportional to the first, second, or *n*th derivative of this function. The derivative signal improves the detectability of overlapping spectral lines and bands, and suppresses the effects of a fluctuating light source. Thus, it enhances the signal:noise ratio, the resolution of the data, and the sensitivity. Instrument designs have involved different approaches in executing the derivative output. These include sinusoidal modulation and a difference measurement of flux at two adjacent wavelengths. Theoretical work has been conducted to evaluate the accuracy with which various approaches represent the derivatives (HAGER and ANDERSON 1970). A detrimental effect found in using higher derivatives is the decrease in signal.

δ) Hadamard Transform Technique. The Hadamard transform technique (DECKER and HARWIT 1969) is an analytic technique developed to overcome the energy limitations of frequency scanned spectrophotometers. Thus, it offers the advantages of the Michelson interferometer with its high energy input and multiplexing capability, but does not involve the usual Fourier transforms. This method consists of optically encoding the spectral output of a multislit spectrometer. The encoding involves sequential measurements of the total light intensity in combinations of selected spectral bands. The resulting encoded optical information is obtained as a set of simultaneous linear algebraic equations, and the spectral reconstruction is accomplished through the use of matrix inversion techniques.

2. Flow Reactions with Gas Phase Sensors

These monitors utilize emissive radiation that is detected by photometric techniques. The emission of radiation is stimulated either chemically by a gas-solid or gas-gas chemiluminescent interaction or thermochemically by a gas/hydrogen flame chemiluminescent interaction. An ozone analyzer, based on the chemiluminescent reaction of O_3 with rhodamine B absorbed on silica gel and on photometric detection of the resultant emission, gives a measure directly related to the mass of ozone flowing over the dye per unit time (Fig. 7). Emission is at 585 nm, and sensitivity of the method is 1.0–10 ppb. A gas-gas chemiluminscent reaction utilizes a similar approach in the photometric detection of the resultant emission. Ethylene-ozone and ozone-NO are reactions that have been developed for ozone and nitric oxide analysers, respectively. Sensitivities are in the 1.0–10 ppb range, and interference is generally negligible.

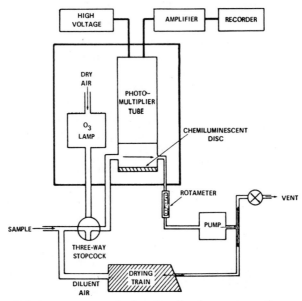

Fig. 7. Ozone analysis by ozone-organic dye chemiluminescent reaction and photometric detection

Flame photometric detection (FPD) based on strong luminescent emissions between 300 and 423 nm has been applied to sulfur compounds introduced into hydrogen-rich flames (Fig. 8). Use of a narrow-band optical filter with transmission at 394 ± 5 nm gives a specificity ratio of sulfur to nonsulfur compounds of 10^4. The method has a sensitivity for sulfur compounds (SO_2, H_2S, CS_2, CH_2SH) of the order of 1.0–10 ppb. Although the FPD method gives a measure of total sulfur primarily, this method combined with gas chromatography provides the capability to separate and measure each sulfur compound in a mixture of sulfur compounds. Since the response to the various sulfur compounds is not the same for equal concentrations, calibration of the system for each compound of interest is necessary.

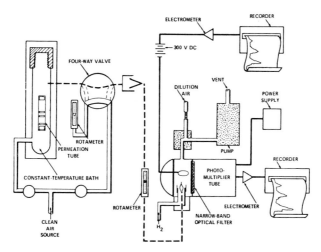

Fig. 8. Flame photometric detector for sulfur compounds

3. Electrical and Electrochemical Sensors

This category includes the various methods by which chemical and/or physical properties of the gaseous pollutant introduce changes in the electrical parameters of the input sensor, so that sensor output is related to the concentration being measured.

a) Conductivity

Gases that form electrolytes in an aqueous solution cause a change in the conductivity of the solution. Since the electric conductance of the solution is a summation of the effects of all ions present, the method is not specific. Assuming that concentrations of all other electrolyte gases are either constant or relatively insiginificant, then the observed conductance can be related to the concentrations of the gas being measured. Temperature control is important because, in electrolytic conduction, the temperature coefficient can be of the order of 2%/°C. Cabinets equipped with thermostats are sometimes used to maintain temperature equilibrium. To obviate the need for temperature control, electrical compensation is sometimes used. Variations in test solution temperature are accounted for automatically by a thermistor immersed in the test solution. The thermistor is part of the electrical circuit and is selected to have a temperature coefficient of resistance that will permit satisfactory compensation over a range of temperature variations.

b) Potentiometry

Gases that react with reagents in solution to change the pH of the solution produce a potentiometric change that reflects the concentration of the reacting gas. The potentiometric change is sensed by a galvanic cell commonly referred to as a pH electrode. The galvanic cell is basically a system in which energy associated with chemical reactions is converted into electrical energy in the form of an electromotive force (EMF). In analytic applications it depends primarily on concentrations of the substances involved in the electrode reactions.

To obtain a correct measure of the EMF sensed by a pH electrode, a potentiometric measurement is required. This is defined as a measurement in which there is no flow of current into or out of the cell being measured. Null balance potentiometers meet this requirement. Other techniques in use, such as vacuum tube voltmeters and pH meters, result in observations with relatively negligible current flow ranging from 10^{-6} to 10^{-14} A.

In principle, pH change, or potentiometry, is nonspecific. In practice, a certain amount of specificity may be introduced by the choice of reagents that are most conducive to the desired reaction for the gas to be sampled. The carbon dioxide analyzer developed by LODGE et al. (1962) is an example of potentiometric measurement of equilibrium pH in the reaction of CO_2 with a suspension of insoluble carbonate in the form of marble chips. The hydrogen ion activity gives a measure of the CO_2 concentration.

c) Coulometry

Coulometry is the measurement of the number of electrons in terms of coulombs transferred across an electrode–solution interface to carry to completion the reaction of a particular substance in a sample. In instrumental applications, the measurements involve an indirect determination of the number of coulombs required for the production of bromine that reacts with the sulfur dioxide being determined. The method is inherently sensitive, since a microcoulomb equivalent corresponds to nanogram amounts (or less) of most simple substances.

In principle, there is no restriction in coulometry relating to the volume of the sample or to the concentration of the substance in the sample. Furthermore, since the method basically involves a measurement of the number of coulombs required for a particular reaction, it does not include provision for determining the end point of the reaction. As a result, any of the known methods of end point detection may be utilized. The sensitivity of the end point detection technique, however, may become the limiting factor in the ability of the coulometric system to detect very low concentrations.

d) Ionization

Detection by ionization is based fundamentally upon making a gas conductive by the creation of electrically charged atoms, molecules, or free electrons, and the collection of these charged particles under the influence of an applied electric field. Various ionizing reactions used for the measurement of gas concentrations have been discussed in considerable detail by LOVELOCK (1961). Ionization is actually a special case of electrical conductivity as a physical method of detection. Since prime consideration is given to the ionizing reactions rather than the resulting conductivity, ionization is identified separately. As a conductivity measurement, the method is, in general, nonspecific. The nature of the ionizing reaction, however, may make the method more or less specific.

e) Flame Ionization

Flame ionization is a method that has been applied in commercial instruments (Fig. 9). The great increase in production of ions by introducing a volatile carbon compound into a hydrogen flame burning in air provides a sensitive method of ionization detection. No satisfactory explanation of the process leading to production of ions in this manner is available, although some explanations have been offered. This detector has a wide linear dynamic range and a response extending to a concentration of approximately 1.0%. It is insensitive to the presence of such contaminants as air or water vapor, but responds to most organic compounds. Response is depressed with compounds having electronegative atoms such as oxygen, sulfur, and chlorine. Changes in geometry, flow rate, and composition of the gases supplied to the flame alter the relative response of the detector to different compounds.

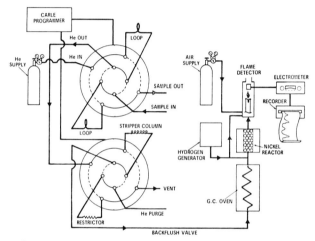

Fig. 9. Automated gas chromatographic flame ionization detection system for CO and CH_4 analysis

f) Special Case

An electrochemical technique may be combined with a selective sampling scheme to give better discrimination. For example, some commercial instruments sample through a gas-permeable membrane that is selected for its capability to be more highly specific in the gas or gases that can pass through it.

4. Other Rapid Response Sensors

a) Radioactive Tracers

Very small quantitites of radioactive substances can be detected by well-developed physical methods such as scintillation and Geiger counters. In a device reported by BERSIN et al. (1962), SO_2 breaks down $NaClO_2$ to release ClO_2, which breaks down a clathrate in which [85]Kr is contained. The released [85]Kr is detected by a Geiger counter, and the resulting count rate is related to the SO_2 concentration initiating the reaction. The method is sensitive to concentrations of the order of 1.0 ppm and is specific to the extent that the initial reaction is limited to the gas of interest.

b) Thermal Conductivity

The specific heat of conductance for a gas provides a physical method of quantitative measurement. The method is nonspecific, however, for a mixture of gases. Where mixtures are resolved into components, as in a chromatographic column, thermal conductivity is used extensively. When a combustible hydrocarbon is burned in air, the change in carbon dioxide is measured before and after combustion, and related to the hydrocarbon content. In applying this technique, one must consider the increased water vapor as a product of combustion. It can be accounted for either by drying or saturating the sampled airstream before and after combustion. Although carbon dioxide has low solubility in water, at very low concentrations such a procedure may present additional problems.

c) Heat of Combustion

The heat of combustion, a particular physical characteristic of combustible gases, also used for quantitative detection, suffers the same limitations as thermal conductivity. One type of thermal combustion cell involves a resistance bridge in which the arms of the bridge are heated filaments. The principle of operation consists of introducing the sample into the gas cell in which the combustible gas ignites upon contact with a heated filament. The resulting heat of combustion changes the resistance of the filament. The change in resistance is detected by conventional bridge measurement techniques and is related to the gas concentration on the basis of calibration standards.

Another combustion method uses catalytic heated filaments or oxidation catalysts, and detection is by change in resistance in a balanced bridge or by thermocouples, respectively. Combustion can be made more or less specific by operating specified filament temperatures so as to ignite the gas of interest and/or by selection of an oxidation catalyst favoring a desired reaction.

d) Paramagnetic Analyzers

The paramagnetism of oxygen, a conspicuously distinctive physical property of oxygen compared with other gases, provides a method by which it may be detected under the influence of a magnetic field. In practice, an air sample is introduced into an electrically heated cross tube of an annular chamber, half of which is exposed to the field of a strong magnet. As the oxygen molecules are attracted to the region of higher field strength, the resultant airflow partially cools the heating coil. The difference in the electrical resistances of both parts of the heating coil constitutes a measure of the oxygen concentration.

e) Mass Spectroscopy

In principle, mass spectroscopy consists of the deflection of ionized molecules subjected to a magnetic field and in their classification in accordance with their mass and charge. The current intensity detected is proportional to the number of particles in each class. The sample size required is very small, of the order of 1.0 μl. Specificity is high because individual particle classes are detected with instruments of high resolution capability. The detection limit for SO_2, for example, has been reported of the order of 0.001 μl. Mass spectrometry has been combined with gas chromatography for the identification of chromatographic fractions and peaks.

5. Analysis of Collected Samples

In these instruments, there is both a sample collecting component and an analytic component to measure the material which is collected. In such instruments, the response time is inevitably longer than in the gas phase sensors, and they are generally not suitable for feedback control of exposure concentration.

a) Colorimetry

Colorimetry is a method wherein the pollutant gas is sampled and reacted with a reagent. With selection of the proper reagent, the reaction is specific to the pollutant gas of interest and a unique color is formed. The absorption of electromagnetic radiation in the visible wavelengths by the reacted reagent is utilized to give a quantitative analysis. In addition, the intensity distribution of a range of transmitted wavelengths (referred to as the spectral characteristic of the absorbing medium) is unique to the absorbing medium and provides a qualitative analysis.

The measurement system consists of a source of radiant energy, the sample solution to be measured, and a detector for the unabsorbed or transmitted radiation. The usual radiant energy source in the visible range is the electric bulb with an incandescent tungsten filament. Special sources are used for UV and IR to provide sufficient energy at these wavelengths. Photocells are used as detectors and include three types: (a) photoconductive, (b) photovoltaic, and (c) photoemissive. The important point to consider with respect to the detector and source combination is that each has its own spectral characteristic; therefore, the optimum combination is one in which both have maximum response in the wavelength range of interest to obtain maximum sensitivity.

An important aspect of the instrumental design is the provision for operation in a given spectral region. This may be done in a number of ways, extending from the simple fixed-band filter to the relatively complex monochromator with an adjustable bandwidth and a wavelength drive to scan the entire spectrum. Calibration curves should be determined by the instrument operator for each specific instrument under its normal working conditions.

These chemicophysical systems do not have the relatively instantaneous response of the purely physical devices because of the time delay involved in the gas scrubbing process, the chemical reaction time, and the reagent flow system. Consequently, the 90% response times are of the order of 5–30 min compared with 5–30 s for the physical systems.

b) Gas Absorption Chromatography

In these instruments, the components of a mixture migrate differentially in a porous sorptive medium. The method does not serve directly for the detection of substances; nor does it provide an estimate in the absolute sense. Chromatography is primarily a method of resolving complex mixture, and this depends upon the differential migration of the components through the absorption column. Detection of the separated components takes place as the carrier gas emerges from the column.

As an analytic system, gas chromatography utilizes various sensitive detection techniques. The detection methods need not be specific because the chromatographic method itself is highly specific. Early detection was based on thermal conductivity cells. Since then, great strides have been taken to improve the sensitivity of detection so that extremely sensitive methods are now used to measure trace components of the order of $1.0–10^3$ ppb. These include the flame ionization method (Fig. 9), and the flame photometric method (Fig. 8) described earlier.

A chromatographic system, basically consisting of an absorption column and a detection unit, is selected on the basis of the following considerations: (a) the nature and concentration of the associated components in the mixture from which the separation is to be made; (b) the nature and concentration of the component to be measured; (c) the resolving ability of the absorbing column, its stability, contaminants, and temperature characteristics; and (e) the sensitivity of the detection cell, its reproducibility, stability, and response time.

Analysis for a specific component requires a method, either specific or nonspecific, for the detection and identification of the isolated components of a mixture. The use of a particular reference substance and the sorption time sequence technique are suitable methods. In addition, under standardized conditions, the relative migration of carrier gas and components can be used.

D. Sampling and Analysis

I. Sampling Procedures

There are two basic methods for collecting gaseous samples. In one, an actual sample of air is taken in a flask, bottle, bag, or other suitable container; in the other, gases or vapors are removed from the air and concentrated by passage through an absorbing, or adsorbing medium. The first method involved the collection of grab or instantaneous samples, usually within a few seconds, or a minute or two. This type of sampling is acceptable when the concentration of a pollutant is relatively constant, and is limited only by the detection limit of the analytic methods available. An important feature of grab samples is that their collection efficiency is normally 100%. However, sample decay does occur for various reasons, and this type of sampling must be used with this clearly in mind.

When the contaminant concentration varies with time, is very low, or when a time-weighted average exposure is desired, grab sampling is of questionable value, and continuous or integrated sampling is employed. The gas or vapor in these cases is extracted from air and concentrated by: (a) solution in an absorbing liquid; (b) reaction with an absorbing solution (or reagent therein); or (c) collection on a solid adsorbent. Collection efficiency of devices utilized for these sampling procedures is frequently less than 100% and therefore must be determined for each case.

Important criteria for selecting sampling devices are solubility, volatility, and reactivity of the contaminant and the sensitivity of the analytic method. Generally speaking, nonreactive gaseous substances may be collected as grab samples in a container of some type. Water-soluble gases and vapors, and those that react rapidly with absorbing solutions can be collected in simple gas washing bottles. Volatile and less soluble gaseous substances and those that react slowly with absorbing solutions require more liquid contact. For these substances, more elaborate sampling devices such as gas washing bottles of the spiral type or fritted bubblers may be required. Insoluble and nonreactive gases and vapors are collected by adsorption on activated charcoal, silica gel, or other suitable adsorbents. Frequently, for a given contaminant, there is a choice of sampling equipment; more than one of the devices mentioned may be suitable.

1. Grab Samplers

a) Evacuated Flasks

These are usually thick-walled containers of 200, 500, or 1.000 ml capacity. By means of a heavy-duty vacuum pump, the internal pressure is reduced practically to zero. The pressure need not be reduced to zero, but the degree of evacuation must be known. This information, along with the barometric pressure and temperature at the sampling site, is used to calculate the actual volume of air or gas collected.

b) Gas or Liquid Displacement Containers

Any ordinary sealable container can be used as a displacement sampler. Original air is replaced by test air. The volume of air swept out should be 10–15 times the container volume to achieve an equilibration of more than 99%. An alternative method for sampling with these containers is to fill them with water and allow the water to drain out slowly in the test area. Liquid is replaced by test air. Obviously, this procedure is not suitable for collecting soluble gases.

For soluble and reactive gases, an absorbent or reagent solution may be introduced into the gas displacement sampler. The usual procedure is to fill the sampler with test air and then add the absorbent. When dealing with partially or totally evacuated flasks, the reagent solution or absorbent is added before they are put under vacuum. In both cases, after the sample has been taken, the container is rotated to insure an even distribution of the reagent on the inside surface of the sampler.

c) Flexible Plastic Containers

Plastic bags are used to collect air samples and prepare known concentrations in the range from ppb to more than 10% by volume in air. They are commercially available in a wide variety of sizes, with 5- to 15-l bags being the most useful. These bags are constructed from a number of plastic materials including polyester, polyvinylidene chloride, Teflon, or other fluorocarbons. Aluminized Scotch Pak, and Mylar are trade names for the first type; Saran is an example of the second; Chemton, Kel F, FEP, Aclor, Kynar, and Tedlar are trade names for fluorocarbon plastics. Plastic bags have the advantages of being light, nonbreakable, inexpensive to ship, and simple to use. But they should be used with caution since storage stabilities for gases, memory effects from previous samples, permeability, precision, and accuracy of sampling systems vary considerably.

Before using them, plastic bags should be tested. Storage properties, decay curves, and other factors, however, will vary considerably from those reported for a given gas or vapor since sampling conditions are rarely identical. Each bag, therefore, should be evaluated for the specific gas for which it will be used. In addition, all bags should be leak tested, cleaned with compressed air, and conditioned before use or reuse.

d) Syringes

Syringes of 10–15 ml volume have been found satisfactory for air sampling. They are available in glass and disposable plastic. Gas and vapor storage and decay curves for these devices must be determined. Advantages are their low cost, convenience, and ease of use.

2. Continuous Samplers

a) Absorbers

The absorption theory of gases and vapors from air by solution, as developed by ELKINS et al. (1937) assumes that gases and vapors behave like ideal gases and dissolve to give ideal solutions. The concentration of the vapor in solution is increased during air sampling until an equilibrium is established with the concentration of vapor in the air. Absorption is never complete, however, since the vapor pressure is not reduced to zero, but only lowered by the solvent effect of the absorbing liquid. Some vapor will escape with continued sampling, but is replaced. Continued sampling, however, will not increase the concentration of vapor in solution once equilibrium is established.

The effeciency of vapor collection depends on: (a) the volume of air sampled; (b) the volume of the absorbing liquid; and (c) the volatility of the contaminant being collected. Efficiency of collection, therefore, can be increased by cooling the sampling solution (reducing the volatility of the contaminant), increasing the solution volume by adding two or more bubblers in series, or altering the design of the sampling device.

Absorption of gases and vapors by chemical reaction depends on the volume of air bubbles produced by the bubbler, the interaction of contaminant with reagent molecules, rapidity of the reaction, and a sufficient excess of reagent solution. If the reaction is rapid and a sufficient excess of reagent is maintained in the liquid, complete retention of the contaminant is achieved regardless of the volume of air samples. If the reaction is slow, and the sampling rate is not low enough, collection efficiency will suffer.

Four basic absorbers used for the collection of gases and vapors are: simple gas washing bottles, spiral and helical absorbers, fritted bubblers, and glass bead columns. The midget impinger is the most widely used in this group and is illustrated in Fig. 10. Friedrichs and Milligan gas washing bottles are examples of spiral and helical absorbers. They may be used for collecting gaseous substances that are only moderately soluble or slow reacting with reagents in the collection media. The spiral or helical structures provide for higher collection efficiency by allowing longer residence time of the contaminant within the tube. Slower acting and less soluble substances are permitted more time to react with the absorbing solution. Gases and vapors that are sparingly soluble in the collecting medium may be sampled in fritted bubblers. They contain sintered or fritted glass or multiperforated plates at the inlet tube. Air drawn into these devices is broken up into very small bubbles and the heavy froth that develops increases the contact of gas and liquid.

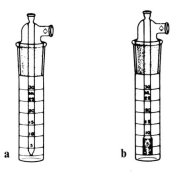

Fig. 10. a Midget impinger (Ace Glass Company, Vineland, New Jersey). **b** Midget gas bubbler: coarse frit (Ace Glass Company, Vineland, New Jersey)

Frits come in various sizes and grades, usually designated as fine, medium, and coarse. A coarse frit is usually best for gases and vapors that are appreciably soluble or reactive. A medium porosity frit may be used for gases and vapors that are difficult to collect, but the sampling must be adjusted to maintain a flow of discrete bubbles. For highly volatile gaseous substances that are extremely difficult to collect, a frit of fine porosity may be required to break the air into extremely small bubbles and insure adequate collection efficiency. Airflow, however, must be controlled to avoid the formation of large bubbles from the coalescence of small bubbles. There is little value, for example, in using a fine porosity frit if airflow is increased and a large bubble population is produced. The finer the frit, however, the higher the pressure drop. Selection of proper frit should be made with all these factors in mind. The collection efficiency of the sampling equipment must be determined for specific contaminants involved.

b) Cold Traps

Cold traps (see Fig. 11) are used for collecting materials in liquid or solid form primarily for identification purposes. Vapor is separated from air by passing it through a coil immersed in a cooling system, dry ice and acetone, liquid air, or liquid nitrogen. These devices are employed when it is difficult to collect samples efficiently by other techniques. They have the advantage that water is extracted along with organic materials and two-phase systems result.

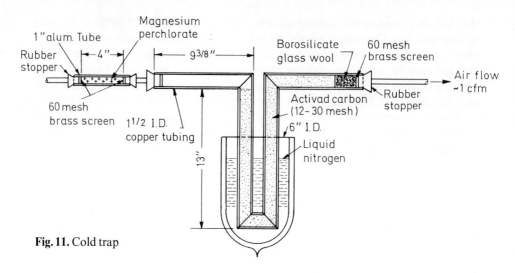

Fig. 11. Cold trap

c) Plastic Sampling Bags

Plastic bags can also be used for collecting integrated air samples.

d) Solid Adsorbents

Ordinary charcoal becomes activated charcoal by heating it to 800–900 °C with steam. During this treatment, a porous, submicroscopic internal structure is formed which gives it an extensive internal surface area, as large as 1,000 m^2/g, thus greatly enhancing its adsorption capacity. Activated charcoal is an excellent adsorbent for most organic vapors. It has the advantage over silica gel that humidity does not usually interfere in air sampling. Because of its nonpolar character, charcoal adsorbs organic vapors and gases in preference to atmospheric moisture. Organic vapors will not be trapped, however, if the amount of water in air is so great that it condenses in the charcoal sampling tube. Inorganic compounds such as ozone, nitrogen dioxide, chlorine, hydrogen sulfide, and sulfur dioxide react chemically with activated charcoal, and cannot be collected for analysis by this method.

Several types of charcoal are commercially available. The products most frequently employed for air sampling are derived from coconut shells and lignite. The final choice for a specific application should be made only after performance and recovery tests have been made. Sampling tubes for activated charcoal vary in shape and size. NIOSH (1975) recommended tubes measure 7 cm long with 6 mm internal diameter and contain two sections of 20–40 mesh activated charcoal separated by a 2-mm portion of urethane foam. The front end contains 100 mg charcoal, the backup section 50 mg. These tubes are commercially available from many chemical suppliers.

The volume of air that can be collected without loss of contaminant depends on the sampling rate, sampling time, volatility of the contaminant, and concentration of contaminant in the air. For many organic vapors, a sample volume of 10 l (1 l/min) can be collected without significant loss in NIOSH tubes. A breakthrough of more than 20% into the backup section indicates that some of the sample was lost. The sample volume for gases and highly volatile solvents must necessarily be smaller. A 3% breakthrough was found to occur on NIOSH tubes at 0.2 l/min for 15 min in an environment containing 5 ppm vinyl chloride. Losses occurred before 5 l sample was collected in a 200 ppm vinyl chloride environment at a sampling rate of 0.05 l/min (RECKNER and SACHDER 1975).

It is always best to refer to an established procedure for proper sampling rates and air sample volumes. In the absence of such information, breakthrough experiments must be performed before sampling is attempted. After the procedure has been checked out, chamber sampling may be performed. Immediately before sampling, the ends of the charcoal tube are broken, rubber or Tygon tubing (NORTON COMPANY, AKRON, OHIO) is connected to the backup end of the charcoal tube, and air is drawn through the sampling train with a calibrated suction pump. The duration of the sampling may be several minutes or hours depending on the information desired. In any case, airflow should be periodically checked with a flow meter when sampling is completed; plastic caps or masking tape, but not rubber caps, are placed on the end of the tube.

For each new batch of charcoal tubes, the aging, collection efficiency, and recovery characteristics for a given contaminant must be determined. This may be achieved by introducing a known amount of the contaminant into a freshly opened charcoal tube, passing clean air through it to simulate sampling conditions, and carrying through its analysis with the samples. Another charcoal tube, not used to sample, is oppened and used as a blank.

The next step in the analysis procedure is to remove the contaminant from the charcoal. The most frequently employed desorption technique uses carbon disulfide. Unfortunately, carbon disulfide does not always completely remove the sample from charcoal. Recovery varies for each contaminant and batch of charcoal used, its extent must be determined experimentally.

In some cases where the recovery is low, a combination of solvents will increase the yield. The following mixtures have been employed in NIOSH procedures: carbon disulfide + 5% 2-propanol; carbon disulfide + 1% methanol; carbon disulfide + 1% 2-butanol; 5% methanol in methylene chloride; ethyl acetate; tetrahydrofuran. Some organic substances are not removed from charcoal by any combination of solvents. For these, other sampling methods must be used.

The desorption step in charcoal analysis is critical since the initial heat of reaction upon the addition of carbon disulfide to charcoal may drive off the more volatile components of the sample. This can be minimized by adding charcoal slowly to carbon disulfide cooled with a dry ice–acetone slurry. Another technique is to transfer the charcoal sample to vials lined with Teflon septum caps and introduce the carbon disulfide with an injection needle. The sealed vial will prevent the loss of any volatilized sample. It should be emphasized that carbon disulfide is a highly toxic solvent. Care should be exercised in its handling, and the analytic procedure should be performed in a well-ventilated area.

Silica gel is an amorphous form of silica derived from the interaction of sodium silicate and sulfuric acid. It has several advantages over activated charcoal for sampling gases and vapors: (a) the contaminant is more easily removed from the adsorbent by a variety of common solvents; (b) the extractant does not usually interfere with wet chemical or instrumental analyses; (c) amines and some inorganic substances for which charcoal is unsuitable can be collected; and (d) the use of highly toxic carbon disulfide is avoided.

One disadvantage of silica gel is that it is selective to water adsorption. Silica gel is electrically polar and polar substances are preferentially attracted to active sites on its surface. Water is highly polar and is tenaciously held. If enough moisture is present in the air or if sampling is continued long enough, water will displace organic solvents, which are relatively nonpolar in comparison, from the silica gel surface. With water vapor at the head of the list, the descending order of polarizability is alcohols, aldehydes, ketones, esters, aromatic hydrocarbons, olefins, and paraffins. Thus, the volume of moist air that can be effectively passed over silica gel is limited.

In spite of this limitation, silica gel has proven to be an effective adsorbent for collecting many gases and vapors. Even under conditions of 90% humidity, relatively high concentrations of benzene, toluene, and trichlorethylene are quantitatively adsorbed on 10 g silica gel from air samples collected at the rate of 2.5 l/min for periods of at least 20 min or longer. Under normal conditions, hydrocarbon mixtures of C_2–C_5 paraffins, low molecular weight sulfur compounds (H_2S, SO_2, mercaptans), and olefins concentrate on silica gel at dry ice–acetone temperature if the sample volume does not exceed 10 l. Significant losses of ethylene, methane, ethane, and other light hydrocarbons occur if sampling volume is extended to 30 l.

Silica gel is available in a wide range of mesh sizes. Individual preference to some extent determines the final selection. It should be remembered that resistance to airflow increases with mesh number. New silica gel is conditioned by heating at 350 °–400 °C overnight in a dry atmosphere. After being allowed to cool to room temperature, it is stored in a sealed container. An economic advantage of silica gel is that it can be regenerated and reused. Used silica is washed, fines discarded, and treated as described.

Sampling devices for silica gel range from glass tubing to galvanized pipes. U-shaped calcium chloride tubes containing two columns of silica gel, 10 g each, which are separated by a wad of glass wool make good collectors. NIOSH (1975) recommends a 8-mm internal diameter 12.5-cm long Pyrex sampling tube packed with three sections of 45–60 mesh silica gel, 700, 150 and 150 mg, respectively, for sampling aromatic amines (WOOD and ANDERSON 1975).

After sampling, the silica from the front and back sections of the tube is poured into separate test tubes and stoppered, plastic-capped culture tubes serve well for this purpose. Analysis of the sample can be delayed several weeks since there is little tendency for loss of adsorbed vapor, even if the silica gel is kept in a capped container at room temperature. Factors affecting sampling time and breakthrough are humidity, concentration of contaminant, sampling rate, weight and depth of gel bed, and volatility of sample.

A moderate amount of humidity will not affect collection of most contaminants commonly encountered in exposure chambers, and 50–60 l of air sampled on 10 g silica gel is adequate for most solvent vapors. For others, the collectable volume may be much higher. Sometimes, introducing a drying agent before the silica gel will increase the collection efficiency. Magnesium perchlorate, calcium sulfate, and molecular sieves are efficient drying agents, but must be used with caution if it is not known they affect the collection of the contaminant of interest. Heat of adsorption and volatility of the sample are two other factors that may cause loss in collection efficiency, but it may be minimized by sampling on silica gel cooled in an ice or acetone–ice bath. High air flow also reduces collection efficiency, but the loss in sample can be reduced by increasing the silica gel mass and depth. A long column of silica gel, however, is more important than total mass.

After collection, the sample is recovered from the silica gel. This is achieved by thermal or solvent desorption. For thermal desorption, the silica gel is transferred to a tube furnace and flushed with carrier gas directly into a gas chromatograph or into a plastic bag and subsequently analyzed by gas chromatography or IR spectrophotometry. Most frequently, samples are recovered from silica gel by solvent desorption. Nonpolar solvents like hexane, pentane, and heptane are unsuitable for displacing aromatic hydrocarbons. However, the lower molecular weight ketones are removed completely in 1 h with water. Benzene is eluted with isopropyl alcohol or ethanol in about the same period of time, whereas toluene and xylene are desorbed more slowly, usually taking several hours or overnight (ELKINS et al. 1962; VAN MOURIK 1965). Trichlorethylene and 1,1,1-trichloroethane are desorbed in 10 min when silica gel is added to methanol (SIMMONS and MOSS 1973). Other desorbing agents mentioned in the literature for silica gel are acetone and dimethylsulfoxide. The latter is particularly useful if the analysis is performed by gas chromatography (WHITMAN and JOHNSON 1964). The usual procedure is to add the silica gel slowly to the solvent, almost grain by grain, to prevent a buildup of heat in the solution and avoid driving off some of the sample.

II. Sampling Train

Samplers (except grab sample devices) are always used in assembly with an air moving device and an air metering instrument. The order followed is: sampler, air metering device, and air mover.

III. Analysis of Gases and Vapors

Pertinent analytic information for the collection and analysis of a number of organic vapors which can be analyzed by gas chromatography can be found in the NIOSH (1975) analytic manual. Guidance for gases and vapors that are commonly analyzed by wet chemical methods or by UV spectrophotometry is available (AIR SAMPLING INSTRUMENTS COMMITTEE 1983).

E. Calibration and Record Keeping

I. Calibration Techniques

Calibrations are performed to establish the relationship between an instrument's response or analytic results and reference values of the parameter being measured. The parameter may be the pollutant concentration, particle size, or flow rate. The reference standards used must be accurate and precise to produce well-characterized and reproducible calibrations. Reference materials and instruments available from, or calibrated by, a recognized authority such as the National Bureau of Standards (NBS), Washington, D. C., should be used whenever possible.

Test atmospheres generated for the purpose of calibrating collection efficiency or instrument response should be checked for concentration using reference instruments or sampling and analytic procedures whose reliability and accuracy are well documented. The best procedures to use are those which have been referee or panel tested, i. e., methods which have been shown to yield comparable results on blind samples analyzed by different laboratories. Such procedures are published by several organizations (Table 2). Those published by the individual organizations are supplemented by those approved by the Intersociety Committee on Methods for Air Sampling and Analysis, a cooperative group formed in March 1963. This group is composed if representatives of the Air Pollution Control Association (APCA), the American Conference of Governmental Industrial Hygienists (ACGIH), the American Industrial Hygiene Association (AIHA), the American Public Health Association (APHA), the American Society for Testing and Materials (ASTM), the American Society of Mechanical Engineers (ASME), and the Association of Official Analytical Chemists (AOAC). "Tentative" methods endorsed by the Intersociety Committee have been published at random intervals since April 1969 in *Health Laboratory Science,* a publication of APHA. These "tentative" methods become "standard" methods only after satisfactory completion of a cooperative test program. Lists of published "tentative" and "standard" methods for air sampling and analysis are summarized in Table 3.

Two types of calibration can be used: static and dynamic. With dynamic calibration, a material which is the same as that being monitored is used. For example, when monitoring a gas in an exposure chamber, reference samples of the same gas within the same concentration range encountered in the chamber should be used. With the reference samples the relationship of the instrument's response to the actual concentration would be established with a calibration curve, or the instrument itself could be adjusted to produce a one-to-one linear relationship with the actual concentration.

Static calibrations are performed directly on the instrument, bypassing the air sampling system. Standard solutions may be used to simulate the same number of molecules of a gas that would be encountered by the airstream. This method is often used to calibrate gas chromatographs designed to sample airstreams whereby a known quantity of liquid sample is injected into the instrument to simulate a vapor concentration that would be encountered in the airstream. Other static methods include simulating equivalent optical density for spectrophotometric instruments or electrical signals to test the calibration and response of various electrical components in an instrument. While static calibrations are often easier to perform than dynamic calibrations, they have the drawback of not testing the instrument's response against the actual concentration in the airstream. Because one or more components of the sampling and monitoring systems are bypassed with static calibrations, there is more room for error.

Table 2. Organizations publishing recommended or standard methods and/or test procedures applicable to air sampling instrument calibration

Abbreviation	Full name and address
APCA	Air Pollution Control Association, 4400 Fifth Avenue, Pittsburgh, PA 15213
ACGIH	American Conference of Governmental Industrial Hygienists, 6500 Glenway Avenue, Bldg. D-5, Cincinnati, OH 45211
AIHA	American Industrial Hygiene Association, 475 Wolf Ledges Parkway, Akron, OH 44311
ANSI	American National Standards Institute, Inc., 1430 Broadway, New York, NY 10018
ASTM	American Society for Testing and Materials, D-22 Committee on Sampling and Analysis of Atmospheres, 1016 Race Street, Philadelphia, PA 19103
EPA	U.S. Environmental Protection Agency, Environmental Monitoring and Support Laboratory, Dept. E (MD-76), Research Triangle Park, NC 27711
ISC	Intersociety Committee on Methods for Air Sampling and Analysis, 250 W. 57th Street, New York, NY 10019
NIOSH	National Institute for Occupational Safety and Health, Center for Disease Control, Robert A. Taft Laboratories, 4676 Columbia Parkway, Cincinnati, OH 45226

Table 3. Summary of recommended and standard methods relating to air sampling and instrument calibration

Organization	No. of methods	Type of methods	Panel tested
ACGIH	19	Analytic methods for air contaminants [a]	Yes
AIHA	93	Analytic guides	No
ANSI	1	Sampling airborne radioactive materials	N.A.
APCA	3	Recommended standard methods for continuous air monitoring for fine particulate matter	N.A.
ASTM	37	Sampling and analysis of atmospheres	No [b]
ASTM	7	Recommended practices for sampling procedures, nomenclatures, etc.	N.A.
EPA	9	Reference and equivalent methods for air contaminants	No
ISC	4	Recommended methods of air sampling and analysis	Yes
ISC	121	Tentative methods of air sampling and analysis	No [c]
NIOSH	454	Analytic methods	No

[a] Methods developed prior to 1970 and no longer published by ACGIH
[b] Methods undergoing panel validation under ASTM Project Threshold
[c] All tentative methods will be panel tested before advancing to reference methods
N.A. Not applicable

Analysis of pollutant concentration, whether it be through direct reading instrumentation, wet chemical techniques, or indirect methods, is only as good as the calibration of the system. While a multipoint calibration may be performed periodically, it is necessary to ensure on a daily basis with a one- or two-point calibration check, that the system is functioning properly. A comprehensive review of calibration techniques, statistical considerations, and instrumentation follows.

II. Data Handling

In the past, the handling of data from air sampling systems was rather straightforward and usually involved the reading of an analog meter and the subsequent recording of that value in a notebook. This procedure, however, is extremely time consuming and subject to reading and transcription errors. Much of the interpretation and recording of air sampling and analytic instrument has been automated through the use of electronic systems such as analog–digital converters, microprocessors, mini computers, and their associated data storage devices, as discussed in Sect. C.

Because the accuracy of all sampling instruments is dependent on the precision of measurement of the sample volume, sample mass, or sample concentration involved, extreme care should be exercised in performing all calibration procedures. The following comments summarize the essentials of air sampler calibration:

1. Use standard devices with care and attention to detail.
2. Check all standard materials, instruments, and procedures periodically to determine their stability and/or operating condition.
3. Perform calibrations whenever a device has been changed, repaired, received from a manufacturer, subjected to use, mishandled, or damaged, and at any time when there is a question as to its accuracy.
4. Understand the operation of an instrument before attempting to calibrate it, and use a procedure or setup which will not change the characteristics of the instrument or standard within the operating range required.
5. When in doubt about procedures or data, assure their validity before proceeding to the next operation.
6. Make all sampling and calibration train connections as short and free of constrictions and resistance as possible.
7. Exercise extreme care in reading scales, timing, adjusting, and leveling, and in all other operations involved.
8. Allow sufficient time for equilibrium to be established, inertia to be overcome, and conditions to stabilize.
9. Obtain enough data to give confidence in the calibration curve for a given parameter; at least three readings per calibration point to ensure statistical confidence in the measurement.
10. Keep a complete permanent record of all procedures, data, and results. This should include trial runs, known faulty data with appropriate comments, instrument identification, connection sizes, barometric pressure, temperature, etc.

11. When a calibration differs from previous records, determine the cause of this change before accepting the new data or repeating the procedure.
12. Identify calibration curves and factors as to conditions of calibration, device calibrated and what it was calibrated against, units involved, range and precision of calibration data, and who performed the actual procedure. It is often convenient to indicate where the original data is filed, and to attach a tag to the instrument indicating this information.

F. Summary

The generation and measurement of the concentration of trace level contaminants in air is subject to numerous variables, many of which are difficult to control. Thus, it is prudent to perform frequent calibration checks on air sampling and monitoring instruments. Such calibrations should be based on sampling controlled test atmospheres generated at concentration levels comparable to those encountered in the exposure chambers. This chapter provides a review of available techniques for the production and monitoring of test atmospheres of gases and vapors, with diagrammatic sketches of some of the more useful techniques, and provides references and descriptions of other commonly used techniques.

References

Air Sampling Instruments Committee (1983) Air sampling instruments, 6th edn. American conference of governmental industrial hygienists, Cincinnati

Bersin RL, Brousaides FS, Hommel CO (1962) Monitoring atmospheric SO_2 employing inverse radioactive tracers. J Air Pollut Control Assoc 12:129–137

Bradley DJ et al. (1968) Characteristics of organic dye lasers as tunable frequency sources for nanosecond absorption spectroscopy. IEEEJ Quantum Electron QE-4

Burch DE, Gryvnak DA (1974) Cross-stack measurement of pollutant concentrations using gas-cell correlation spectroscopy. In: Stevens RK, Herget WF (eds), Analytical methods applied to air pollution measurements, sect 3. Ann Arbor, Ann Arbor, MI, pp 193–233

Cotabish HN, McConnaughey PW, Messer HC (1961) Making known concentrations for instrument calibration. Am Ind Hyg Assoc J 22:392–402

Decker JA, Harwit M (1969) Experiment operation of a Hadamard spectrometer. Appl Opt 8:2552–2555

Elkins HB, Hobby A, Fuller JE (1937) The determination of atmospheric contamination. I. Organic halogen compounds. J Ind Hyg 19:474–485

Elkins HB, Pagnotto LD, Comproni EM (1962) The ultraviolet spectrophotometric determination of benzene in air samples adsorbed on silica gel. Anal Chem 34:1797–1801

Goetz A, Kallai T (1962) Design and performance of an aerosol channel for the synthesis and study of atmospheric reaction product. J Air Pollut Control Assoc 12:427–433

Hager RN Jr, Anderson RC (1970) Theory of the derivative spectrometer. J Opt Soc Am 60:1444–1449

Hanst PL (1968) Detection and measurement of air pollutants by absorption of infrared radiation. J Air Pollut Control Assoc 18:754–759

Hanst PL (1970) Infrared spectroscopy and infrared lasers in air Infrared spectroscopy and infrared lasers in air pollution research and monitoring. Appl Spectroscopy 24:161–174

Hanst PL (1971) Spectroscopic methods for air pollution measurement. In: Pitts JN Jr, Metcalf RL (eds) Advances in environmental sciences and technology, vol 2. Wiley-Interscience, New York, pp 91–213

Hinkley ED, Kelley PL (1971) Detection of air pollutants with tunable diode lasers. Science 171:635–639

Lodge JP, Frank ER, Ferguson J (1962) A simple atmospheric carbon dioxide analyzer. Anal Chem 34:702–704

Lovelock JE (1961) Ionization methods for the analysis of gases and vapors. Anal Chem 33:162–178

Nelson GO (1970) Simplified method for generating known concentrations of mercury vapor in air. Rev Sci Inst 41:776–777

Nelson GO, Griggs KS (1968) Precision dynamic method for producing known concentrations of gas and solvent vapors in air. Rev Sci Instrum 39:927–928

NIOSH (1975) Manual of analytical methods. US DHEW publication 75–121

O'Keefe AE, Ortman GO (1966) Primary standards for trace gas analysis. Anal Chem 38:760–763

Reckner LR, Sachder J (1975) Charcoal sampling tubes for several organic solvents. US DHEW publication Niosh 75–184

Setterlind AN (1953) Preparation of known concentrations of gases and vapors in air. Am Ind Hyg Quart 14:113–120

Simmons JH, Moss IM (1973) Measurement of personal exposure to 1,1,1-trichloroethane and trichlorethylene using an inspective sampling device and battery operated pump. Ann Occup Hyg 16:47–49

Van Mourik JHC (1965) Experience with silica gel as absorbent. Am Ind Hyg Assoc J 26:498–509

Whitman ME, Johnson AE (1964) Sampling and analysis of aromatic hydrocarbon vapors in air: A gas-liquid chromatographic method. Am Ind Hyg Assoc J 25:464–469

Willard HH, Merritt LL, Dean JA, Settle FA (1981) Instrument methods of analysis. Van Nostrand, New York

Wood GO, Anderson RG (1975) Personal air sampling for vapors of aniline compounds. Am Ind Hyg Assoc J 36:538–548

CHAPTER 3

Determination of Retained Lung Dose

P. A. VALBERG

A. General Principles

The emphasis in this chapter is going to be primarily on measurement of particle retention in the respiratory tract, although many of the same considerations apply to gas uptake. Inhaled air, unless it has been previously filtered, contains airborne dust. Figure 1 shows the size range of some aerosols typically encountered in natural and occupational settings. In the process of respiration, air flows into the lungs where it is brought in close proximity to lung surfaces for the purpose of oxygen and carbon dioxide exchange. This same process also makes the lungs an excellent filter of the particles present in inhaled air, and a significant fraction do not exit upon exhalation. The total mass of air breathed daily can range from 10 to 25 kg. Even rural "clean" air has a particulate concentration of about 0.05 ppm (by weight). Hence, even if only half of these particles are deposited in the lung, this amounts to a *daily* accumulation of 0.5–1.25 mg potentially toxic material on delicate lung surfaces. During smog episodes, particulate concentrations have been measured to be as high as 3–4 ppm (GOLDSMITH and FRIBERG 1977), resulting in a *daily* accumulation of about 60 mg. The correlation between air pollution indices and chronic pulmonary disease has been examined (LAVE and SESKIN 1970; FERRIS 1978), and considerable attention is currently focused on the health effects of indoor air pollution (SPENGLER and SEXTON 1983). Types of inhaled particles for which measurement of retained dose is of major interest are briefly described in the following sections.

I. Types of Aerosols

1. Infectious Particles

Infectious aerosols can be produced during coughing, sneezing, or talking. Viable bacteria and viruses can also become airborne through both the action of air currents and production of mist by waves, waterfalls, and raindrops. Many artificial sources such as air conditioners also contribute to airborne infection as evidenced by Legionnaires' disease. The importance of airborne pathogens in infectious disease has been reviewed (LEEDOM and LOOSLI 1979). The risk of infection is related not only to retention of microorganisms in the lung, but also to the efficacy of mechanisms inactivating and killing bacteria and viruses (BRAIN et al. 1977).

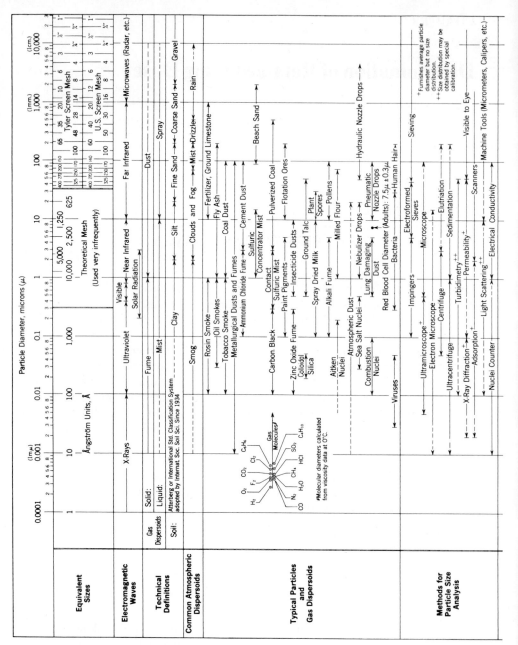

Fig. 1. Types and sizes of some commonly encountered aerosols. Reprinted courtesy of SRI International, Menlo Park, California

2. Allergens

Allergic diseases can result from the inhalation of pollen, spores, and fragments of plant and animal materials. A comprehensive description of types of pollen, their modes of distribution, and their pathogenic effects has been published by EDMONDS (1979). Most pollen particles are large, 20–60 µm diameter, and they would not be expected to penetrate deep into the lung (PATTERSON 1972). However, fragments of pollen particles may be carried much deeper into the respiratory tract before deposition. It has been reported that a significant fraction of the antigenicity of pollen can be found in small fragments (<5 µm), rather than whole pollen particles (BUSSE et al. 1972).

3. Occupational Dusts

In addition to the combustion products characteristic of any energy-consuming, industrialized society, there are aerosols that are unique to specific industrial processes. These particles present special hazards to plant employees and to the populations living nearby. Mines, cement mills, iron and steel mills, oil-processing plants, and factories of every kind often produce particles as an unwanted accompaniment to their primary product. Dusts containing silica, asbestos, metal fumes, organic matter, and synthetic chemicals are inhaled every day by millions of workers.

The respiratory tract is the most important route for the entry of toxic substances from occupational exposures. The long-term respiratory effects of these substances persist and may even grow worse after the exposure has stopped. The relationship between lung disease and inhaled asbestos, coal dust, beryllium, cotton dust, and silica has been the subject of considerable investigation (LANZA 1963; MORGAN and SEATON 1975; PARKES 1982).

4. Radioactive Particles

Weapons testing, electric power generation, and naturally occuring radon all contribute to radioactivity in the air. Mining, milling, and fuel fabrication can give rise to radioactive metallic oxides (EISENBUD 1977). The size distribution of radioactive aerosols ranges from 0.03 µm for radon daughter products up to about 1.0 µm for fission products recovered from the stratosphere (LOCKHART et al. 1965). Airborne radioisotopes can be inhaled and retained in the lung where they initiate disease processes (WALSH and HAMRICK 1977). The majority of the health risk from insoluble particles, which are cleared slowly from the lung, appears to be increased risk of lung cancer (LUNDIN et al. 1969; WALSH and HAMRICK 1977; JABLON and BAILAR 1980; SINCLAIR 1981).

5. Cigarette Smoke

An aerosol of particular importance to human health is tobacco smoke, which may contain particle concentrations as high as 40,000–70,000 ppm (50–90 g/m^3). Most smoke particles are 0.2–0.6 µm in diameter, with essentially none larger than 1 µm in diameter. Such small particles penetrate deep into the lung during inhalation. The size of smoke particles depends on the concentration of the smoke, because agglomeration is likely. HINDS (1978) reported that the mass median aerodynamic diameter of smoke decreased from 0.52 to 0.38 μm as the dilution of the mainstream smoke was increased from 10:1 to 700:1. Approximately 50%–80% of inhaled smoke is deposited in the lungs, resulting in the deposition of approximately 25 mg particulate matter per unfiltered cigarette (HOEGG 1972). The toxic effects of cigarette smoke are legion, including chronic bronchitis, pulmonary emphysema, cardiovascular disease, and lung cancer (DOLL 1971; USPHS 1979).

6. Therapeutic Aerosols

The respiratory tract provides a convenient route of access both for topical administration of drugs to lung surfaces and for systemic administration of drugs which are easily absorbed into the bloodstream. Inhalation of aerosols has become an established component of respiratory therapy and is discussed in most major texts (EGAN 1977). A major concern is whether the aerosol reaches the desired location. The primary considerations here are aerosol size (SWIFT 1980) and patient use (SELF et al. 1983). For example, there is evidence that in mist tent therapy only 5% of the nebulized activity actually entered the body, and that only 0.5% of the nebulized activity could be associated with intrapulmonary airways and lung alveoli (BAU et al. 1971). Thus, estimation of retained dose in the case of therapeutic aerorols is an important yet often neglected problem.

II. Description of the Aerosol

The goal of retention measurements is to be able to predict amount and location of lung retention from parameters that describe the exposure: particle size, breathing pattern, and respiratory system anatomy. For a given volume of inhaled air, the most complete aerosol description would be a tabulation of the number, size, shape, density, chemical composition, physical state, charge, and radioactivity of each particle. Fortunately, such a cumbersome compilation is not necessary for most purposes. In addition to measurement of mass, number, or activity concentration, the two most important parameters determining deposition are mean diameter and distribution of particle diameters. Aerosols with only particles of similar diameter are unusual and are called monodisperse. More typical aerosols are polydisperse, i.e., composed of particles having a range of diameters. For spherical particles, the definition of diameter is unambiguous; but for irregular particles, a variety of definitions exist. The most useful definition is the aerodynamic diameter, even though this measure may bear little relation to the physical appearance of the particle. The aerodynamic diameter is the diameter of a unit density sphere that has the same settling velocity as the particle in question.

Complete texts have been written on the characterization of aerosols (MERCER 1973; LUNDGREN et al. 1979; HINDS 1982), and only a few major principles will be presented here. Measuring the size distribution can rely on the mass of the particles (elutriators, cascade impactors, centrifuges, particle relaxation time analyzers), the optical appearance of the particles (microscopes, light scattering devices), or mobility of the particles (electrical mobility analyzers, diffusion batteries). After distribution of aerodynamic diameters in an aerosol is experimentally determined, a frequency distribution function can often be empirically derived. Many polydisperse aerosols fit a log-normal distribution in which a plot of particle number density (number of particles per given size interval) versus the logarithm of size produces a bell-shaped, normal distribution curve. Such aerosols can be effectively described by two numbers, the count median aerodynamic diameter (CMAD) and the geometric standard deviation (GSD or σ_g). CMAD represents the diameter of that particle in the middle of the number distribution, i. e., with half the total number of particles being larger in diameter and half smaller. The GSD is the ratio of the diameter of the particle that is larger than 84.2% of all others to the CMAD. If GSD $= 1$ or $1 < $ GSD < 1.2, then the aerosol is monodisperse, consisting of particles of a single diameter, or nearly so if GSD is in the range 1.0–1.2. For GSD > 1.2 the aerosol particles cover a distribution of sizes sufficiently large to be considered polydisperse. Aerosols with GSD > 3 are encountered only rarely. An advantage of the log-normal distribution is the fact that if particle size is log-normally distributed, so also are particle mass, particle surface area, and any other properties that are power functions of particle size. Therefore, all have the same GSD. These log-normal distributions are interrelated by the Hatch–Choate equations (see HINDS 1982, pp 91–100). For example, mass median aerodynamic diameter (MMAD) is related to CMAD by

$$\ln(\text{MMAD}) = \ln(\text{CMAD}) + 3 \, (\ln \text{GSD})^2, \qquad (1)$$

where ln is the natural logarithm. An important consideration is that MMAD is more heavily weighted toward the larger diameters than CMAD since it represents the diameter of that particle in the middle of the mass distribution of the total aerosol. The choice of diameter depends on how the physical properties of the aerosol particles determine their effect on the lung. If the activity of the particle is distributed throughout its volume, the mass median diameter is relevant. If activity is distributed only on the surface of the particle, then area median diameter is important. If the effect of deposited particles is determined not by their size, but only by the presence or absence of a particle, i. e., by the number of particles, then count median diameter is the size parameter of choice.

If an instrument other than the lung is used to sample an aerosol, attention must be paid to collecting a representative sample. Flows higher than those found in the lung may break up aggregates or collect particles before they are measured. Flows that are too low may cause large particles to settle out and small ones to diffuse to the walls. Factors influencing evaporation, condensation, polymerization, agglomeration, and disaggregation must be closely controlled. Also, the collection process should separate size fractions sharply, should not alter the particles physically or chemically, and should collect them in sufficient numbers to allow for physical or chemical analysis. A number of devices do mimic, to some degree, the collection characteristics of the lung or provide information about the aerodynamic size distribution of the particles. A discussion of respirable dust sampling has been published (LIPPMANN 1978), and the texts previously mentioned are excellent sources for a more general discussion of measurement of aerosol size distribution.

One example of an instrument that measures aerodynamic size directly is the aerosol centrifuge. It is particularly useful for submicrometer particles that settle slowly, and for delicate agglomerates that break up easily (and for which the aerodynamic behavior is impossible to predict from electron micrographs because of their complex shape and unknown density). It was designed by TILLERY (1974) and modified by HINDS (1978).

This aerosol spectrometer determines aerodynamic size distributions from observations of particle settling velocity in a centrifugal field. This instrument draws a sample of aerosol directly from the exposure area and, as shown in Fig. 2, enhances particle sedimentation velocity by flowing the sample into a rotating chamber and around a rectangular deposition channel concentric with the axis of rotation. Centrifugal forces arising from high speed rotation cause an acceleration of ~ 700 g at right angles to the aerosol flow down the channel. The particles are deposited on a removable strip that lines the outer wall of the channel. This collecting strip is metal, or paper impregnated with a solution of graphite, so that static charges are drained away and will not repel or attract particles as they approach. Aerodynamic size is correlated with the position of deposition along the strip relative to the point where the aerosol entered. Large particles are deposited soon after entry into the channel; small ones, further along the strip. Because aerodynamic size is defined in terms of settling velocity, the point of deposition can be derived mathematically, and calculations are found to agree with deposition of polystyrene and polyvinyltoluene spheres of known density and diameter.

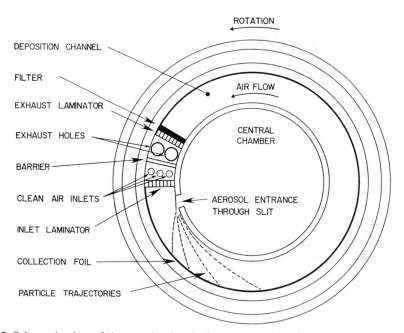

Fig. 2. Schematic view of the rotating head of the aerosol centrifuge. Aerosol is injected parallel to the inner surface of the channel and settles toward the outer channel while being carried along the channel by a clean airflow. Large particles settle early in the channel, and smaller particles at successively later points

III. Characterization of Retained Dose

The qualification of particle retention can rely on any measurable property such as optical appearance, radioactivity, chemical reactivity, radiation absorption spectrum, or magnetization. In tissue sections, particles may have a characteristic appearance identifiable in light or electron microscopy; they may be fluorescent or detectable by a variety of optical methods (SLAYTER 1976). Radioactive particles can be detected and localized by a wide variety of techniques (KNOLL 1979), some of which will be discussed in subsequent sections. The presence of particles can be revealed by analysis for the elements contained in them, which includes techniques such as colorimetry, atomic absorption spectroscopy. X-ray fluorescence (and absorption) spectroscopy, neutron activation, and nuclear magnetic resonance spectra. Analysis for the molecular and crystalline nature of particles utilizes such procedures as infrared spectroscopy, X-ray diffraction, and chromatography. In some cases, the particles are ferro- or ferrimagnetic, and magnetometry can be used to determine retention (VALBERG and BRAIN 1979).

1. Initial Deposition

The distinction between retention (the amount of an aerosol present at any time) and deposition (the initial collection of airborne particles by lung surfaces) should be kept in mind. Retention, but not deposition, is influenced by clearance and translocation. The exposure to the aerosol must be brief and the interval between death and analysis must be short if the results are to reflect deposition per se. Because of clearance and translocation, there may be loss and redistribution of deposited particles with time. If the animals are killed, it is important to avoid artifacts caused by agonal and postmortem changes, or those caused by fixation and other processes required for the preparation and examination of the specimens.

2. Clearance

Particles on lung surfaces generally do not remain at the site of initial deposition, but are redistributed or expelled from the lung by a variety of processes. Even the diseased and blackened lungs of miners who die of pneumoconiosis contain less than 2% of the dust originally deposited there (see HATCH and GROSS 1964, pp 69–73). The fundamental relationship that must be kept in mind is

Retention = deposition – net clearance

For continuous exposure, the relative rate constants of deposition and clearance will determine an equilibrium level of retention (BRAIN and VALBERG 1974). Pathways of clearance differ in various regions of the respiratory tract, and thus the pattern of removal will depend on the site of initial deposition (MORGAN et al. 1983). The pattern of removal will also depend on the physical and chemical properties of the particle such as solubility, size, surface character, and reactivity (MORROW et al. 1964).

Airways down to the level of terminal bronchioles are cleared primarily by mucociliary transport, and particles are removed by this system over time periods ranging from minutes to hours (see Chap. 12). Sneezing and coughing may also remove particles from airways capable of high velocity airflow (LEITH 1977). In those regions of the lung having no cilia (alveoli, alveolar ducts, respiratory bronchioles), phagocytosis by alveolar macrophages is the first step in removal of insoluble particles (SOROKIN and BRAIN 1975). These cells may find their way to the mucus blanket on ciliated airways and thus be carried to the pharynx (see Chap. 12). A small number of particles may enter lung epithelial cells (WATSON and BRAIN 1979) or penetrate epithelial barriers and become translocated to the lung lymph nodes (THOMAS 1976). For insoluble particles, alveolar clearance takes days rather than the hours characteristic of ciliated airways. For soluble particles, uptake of material into the blood can be a major clearance route.

3. Distribution of Retention

The toxic influence of inhaled materials will be determined not only by the amount of retention, but also by the site of retention. Much attention is devoted to describing response at the organ, tissue, cell, and subcellular level, and local deposited particle concentration is a key variable. Distribution of retention can be measured noninvasively, but not with as great a precision as by invasive methods. There are clear advantages to using nondestructive, noninvasive methods for detecting particle retention. Repeated measurements on the same animal are possible. For human experiments, such detection methods are essential except when autopsy material is available. Although gamma cameras, magnetometry, and other noninvasive approaches can give some information about the distribution of dose to structures of interest, the greatest precision is obtained by killing and dissecting animals. It is then possible to divide the respiratory tract into individual pieces and analyze the particle content of each piece. The precision here is limited only by one's patience and the sensitivity of the method of detection.

B. Predicting Dose from Exposure: Determining Factors

The respiratory system acts like a filter in that a significant fraction of the aerosol present in inspired air is removed during its movement into and out of the lungs. Several factors are important in determining the amount and site of lung aerosol retention. The characteristics of the airborne particles, the aerodynamics of ventilation, and the anatomy of the lung are all primary factors influencing aerosol collection on lung surfaces. Comprehensive treatises on aerosol behavior are available, and only major points will be noted here (MORROW 1960, 1974; FUCHS 1964; DAVIES 1966, MERCER 1964, HINDS 1982). The goal is to identify the role of particle character, airflow patterns, and airspace dimensions in producing patterns of lung deposition.

I. Deposition as Related to Particle Properties

1. Sedimentation

All particles with density (p_{part}) greater than that of air (p_{air}) experience a net downward force due to gravity. The magnitude of this force (F_{grav}) is calculated as follows

$$F_{grav} = V_{part}(\varrho_{part} - \varrho_{air})g, \tag{2}$$

where V_{part} is the volume of the particle and g is gravitational acceleration. A particle accelerates downward until its velocity increases to the point where the retarding force due to its motion through air just balances its weight. For spherical particles small enough so that viscous forces are the primary resistive forces, Stokes' Law can be used to predict the retarding forces

$$F_{resist} = \frac{3\pi\eta vd}{C_c}, \tag{3}$$

where d is the diameter of the particle, η the viscosity of air, and v is the velocity of the particle. C_c is the Cunningham correction factor necessary in Stokes' Law for particles whose diameter approaches the mean free path of gas molecules, λ. For particles down to 0.1 μm diameter this factor is given by

$$C_c = 1 + 2.52\frac{\lambda}{d}. \tag{4}$$

The velocity at which this resistive force equals the gravitational force is their terminal settling velocity, v_t

$$v_t = (\varrho_{part} - \varrho_{air})\frac{C_c gd^2}{18\eta}. \tag{5}$$

For example, for a unit density, 1-μm diameter sphere falling through air at atmospheric pressure and body temperature, the terminal velocity is 33 μm/s. This terminal velocity would be established in about 10 μs if the particle were started from rest.

For unit density particles settling in air, this form of Stokes' Law is valid for particles 0.1–40 μm in diameter. Correction factors can be included to extend the range of the equations from 0.001 to 200 μm (DAVIES 1966). With large particles, the retarding force is increased by the inertial effects of accelerating a mass of gas to push it aside. With a small particle, the retarding force is less than that predicted by Stokes' Law because the particle is comparable in size to the mean free path of air molecules, and the assumption of zero fluid velocity at the particle surface needs to be amended. The equation for the Cunningham correction factor becomes more complex than in Eq. (4). Although the terminal velocity of most irregularly shaped particles cannot be calculated directly from physical dimensions, such particles are often characterized by aerodynamic diameter. This is the diameter of a unit density sphere having the same v_t as the particle in question. Once distribution of particle aerodynamic diameters is experimentally determined, prediction of deposition behavior in the lungs becomes possible. An additional complication is that fiber particles and some particle aggregates assume a preferred orientation in flowing gas (DAVIES 1979).

2. Impaction

If a particle moving at velocity v is placed into still air in the absence of gravity, the drag forces will bring it to a stop. If the resistance to particle motion is given by Stokes' Law, this stop distance χ can be caluclated to be

$$\chi = v \left(\frac{v_t}{g} \right), \tag{6}$$

where v_t is the settling velocity given in Eq. (5). This is analogous to what occurs when an airstream moving at velocity u with aerosol particles moving along with it, makes a sudden change in direction by an angle θ. The particles suddenly obtain a velocity of magnitude $(u \sin\theta)$ at right angles to the airstream. Hence, from Eq. (6), the particle moves a total distance of

$$\chi = \frac{(u \sin\theta)v_t}{g} \tag{7}$$

across the direction of flow before it again comes to rest relative to the airstream. If traveling this distance bring it into contact with a wall, the particle is assumed to be deposited.

If a unit density 1-μm diameter sphere travels in an airstream moving at 1.0 m/s (typical air velocity in major bronchi), then a 30° change in the direction of airflow will move the particle 1.7 μm away from its previous streamline. This displacement increases with airstream velocity, angle of airstream deflection, and the square of the particle diameter (which affects v_t).

If we compare χ, the stop distance, to R, the radius of the tube, and replace the peak velocity u by twice the average velocity $\bar{v}$ this ratio is the Stokes number St, which is related to the probability of deposition by impaction

$$St = \frac{\chi}{R}. \tag{8}$$

3. Diffusion

The constant random collision of gas molecules with small aerosol particles pushes them about in an irregular fashion called Brownian motion. Thus, even in the absence of gravity, a particle in still air moves in a "random walk". This is a probabilistic process of random motion in three dimensions. The root-mean-square displacement from the origin Δ after a time t is given by

$$\Delta = \sqrt{6Dt}, \tag{9}$$

Table 1. Root-mean-square Brownian displacement in 1 s compared with distance fallen in air in 1 s unit density particles of different diameter[a]

	Diameter (µm)	Brownian displacement in 1 s (µm)	Distance fallen in 1 s (µm)
Settling greater in 1 s	50	1.7	70,000
	20	2.7	11,500
	10	3.8	2,900
	5	5.5	740
	2	8.8	125
	1	13.0	33
Diffusion greater in 1 s	0.5	20	9.5
	0.2	37	2.1
	0.1	64	0.81
	0.05	120	0.35
	0.02	290	0.013
	0.01	570	0.0063

[a] Temperature 37 °C; gas viscosity 1.9×10^{-5} Pa s. Appropriate correction factors were applied for motion outside the range of validity of Stokes' Law

where D is the diffusion coefficient of the particle. D can be expressed in terms of T, the absolute temperature; k the Boltzmann constant; η gas viscosity; and d particle diameter

$$D = \frac{kTC_c}{3\pi\eta d}. \tag{10}$$

At 37 °C in air 1 atm pressure, $D = 28$ µm/s² for a 1-µm sphere; it will move 13 µm in 1 s as a result of diffusion. It is important to remember that this displacement varies with the square root of time and increases as particle size decreases, independent of density. A comparison of settling and diffusion for a range of particle sizes is shown in Table 1.

4. Interception

Even if a particle does not deviate from its gas streamline, it may contact lung surfaces because of its physical size. This can result in particle collection in the lung because inspired air is brought in close proximity to a large surface area. As particles move into smaller and smaller air spaces, they may reach a point where the distance to a surface is less than particle dimensions; this contact is called interception. The importance of this mechanism can be estimated by calculating the volume from which deposition by interception can occur. If the surface area of the lung is assumed to be 70 m², then for particles with a diameter of 1 µm, collection will occur from the portion of the volume that is 1 µm away from this surface. This is equal to 70 ml, about 1.5% of total lung volume. Moreover, this calculation should be corrected for the fact that the fresh aerosol is not presented to lung surfaces; it is diluted by residual gas which also forms a barrier between fresh aerosol and the major surface area of the lung. In addition, convective flow cannot bring freshly inspired air to within micrometers of respiratory surfaces. However, for particles such as fibers, whose extreme dimensions are large, but whose aerodynamic diameter is small, interception can become important. Since fibers tend to align with gas streamlines, they will be carried into small airways where the probability of touching a surface is high (DAVIES 1979). In fact, experiments have shown that alveolar duct bifurcations are sites of asbestos fiber deposition (BRODY et al. 1981).

5. Hygroscopicity

The addition or removal of water can significantly affect the size of an aerosol particle. Aerosols composed of sodium chloride (NaCl) crystals avidly take up water, so that an aerosol that began as crystals becomes water droplets containing dissolved salt. CINKOTAI (1971) has discussed the growth of NaCl particles in moist air and has shown that the increase in diameter becomes particularly marked as the relative humidity increases above 95% and approaches 100%. At 95% humidity, a tripling in diameter of NaCl particles can be expected; at 100% humidity, the size of the NaCl particle can grow without bound. The exact relative humidity within airways is not known, and our understanding of the dynamic growth of inhaled hygroscopic particles in the respiratory tract is still inadequate. Dry atmospheric aerosols have been found to double in diameter when the relative humidity is increased to 98% (SINCLAIR et al. 1974). A theoretical study of the growth of dry salt particles of various kinds was undertaken by FERRON (1977). He found that the time allowed for hygroscopic growth is important, and that the assumption of hygroscopic particles reaching an equilibrium size is overly simplistic. SCHERER et al. (1979) have collected data on the growth and evaporation of hygroscopic aerosols in an airway model. Their experimental results were in good agreement with theoretical predictions.

On the one hand, it is clear that the hygroscopic character of some aerosols must be taken into account when attempting to predict how a particle will be deposited. On the other hand, droplets of pure water can evaporate rapidly, even under conditions of 100% humidity, because of increased pressure inside a small droplet caused by surface tension. For example, a 1-μm droplet of water will evaporate within 0.5 s at room temperature, even under saturated conditions. A 10-μm droplet will evaporate within approximately 1 min.

6. Electrostatic Attraction

The surfaces of the respiratory tract are uncharged, but electrically conducting. When an electrically charged particle approaches such a surface, it induces an "image charge" of the opposite polarity in the surface and is attracted toward it. This force becomes stronger as the particle approaches the surface, and hence deposition of charged particles is greater than that of neutral ones. If all of the aerosol particles have charges of the same polarity (unipolar), they will repel each other and accelerate deposition. These forces depend on the amount of charge on the particle; moreover, the enhancement of deposition increases with lower flow rates and smaller particle sizes.

Airborne particles can carry an excess of positive or negative charge acquired either in the process of formation or accumulated from the atmosphere. Charged particles discharge with a time constant of approximately 400 s, until they reach equilibrium. At equilibrium, the average number of excess positive or negative charges q is given by

$$q = 2.37 \sqrt{d}, \qquad (11)$$

where d is the particle diameter in μm (FUCHS 1964).

An electric charge on a particle affects its behavior in three ways: (a) the particle moves along electric field lines; (b) evaporation from and condensation (coagulation) onto the particle are altered; and (c) the particle is attracted to a neutral surface by the image charge induced. Because negligible electric fields exist within the air spaces of the respiratory system, the first consideration does not apply. Except for the collection of water, the second process is primarily important in altering the characteristics of the aerosol while it is still outside the respiratory tract. The image force effect is potentially an important process in enhancing deposition, and its operation in the respiratory tract has been analyzed theoretically and experimentally (MELANDRI et al. 1977; CHAN et al. 1978; CHAN and YU 1982). It appears that when the number of charges on the aerosol particle is ten or more, deposition is enhanced. Electric charge is primarily an important factor when dealing with highly charged, freshly generated particles.

Even when a neutral particle approaches a neutral surface at distances of the order or 1 of 2 μm, electric forces called van der Waals' forces cause an attraction between them. These forces are due to fluctuations in the positions of electric charges in the two bodies, and any electric dipole moment formed in one body will induce an attractive dipole moment in the other. These forces, in addition to the fact that most collisions are inelastic, insure that aerosol particles coming very close to or actually contacting a surface will adhere to it.

7. Magnetic and Other Effects

Deposition enhancement by magnetic forces has been reported experimentally (VALBERG and BRAIN 1979). Spontaneously breathing conscious rabbits were exposed to 300 mg/m^3 γ-iron oxide (γ-Fe$_2$O$_3$) aerosol for 1 h while a small 900-G (90-mT) permanent magnet was applied to the chest. A control rabbit was exposed while a piece of bronze was applied in a similar position to the chest. The magnetic content of the excised lungs was assayed with a magnetometer. Retention per unit weight of lung was fivefold greater in regions of lung near the magnet compared with those farther away. This enhancement is due to the force that the gradient of the magnetic field exerts on the magnetic particles. The force F is given by

$$F = (m \cdot V)B \qquad (12)$$

where m is the magnetic dipole of the aerosol particles, and B is the function that describes the spatial variation of the magnetic field. For monodomain particles

1 µm in diameter, the magnetic force in the vicinity of the permanent magnet can far exceed gravitational or diffusive effects.

Other forces acting to effect deposition, such as acoustic, thermal, and radiational, are normally not significant in the lung. The lifetime of an aerosol in the ambient atmosphere should also be considered, apart from the behavior of the particles once they are in the lung. The size range typical of aged aerosols is 0.2–0.5 µm. Although particles outside this size range may be copiously generated, larger particles precipitate out and smaller ones coagulate. The consequence of coagulation is an increase in the size of the smaller particles at the expense of particle number. Very small particles also serve as condensation nuclei for the absorption of water. Although size may determine the percentage of particles deposited in a given area, the mass of material delivered depends on the cube of particle diameter. Thus, deposition of 99% of 0.1 µm particles still delivers only 1/100th of the dose from the deposition of only 10% of the same number of 1-µm particles.

II. Pattern of Ventilation

In addition to the properties of the aerosol, the aerodynamics of breathing is another important factor in estimating retained dose from exposure. Inertial impaction depends on the velocity of the airstream. The effects of diffusion and settling increase with time. Hence, the breathing pattern influences the effectiveness of deposition mechanisms. Inertial impaction is important in upper airways, where velocities are high; diffusion and settling are important in lower airways, where residence time is longer. Minute volume determines the total particle burden that enters the respiratory tract. Hence, even if the deposition fraction is fixed, increasing minute volume results in an increased particle burden for the lung. But larger pulmonary volumes in the distal lung mean that distances to surfaces are increased, so that the fraction of aerosol deposited may decrease. An important consideration in aerosol deposition is the airflow profile. As minute volume and consequently, flow velocity increase, turbulent airflow may penetrate more deeply into the lung. To determine the nature of flow, it is useful to calculate the Reynolds number Re which is given by

$$Re = \frac{\varrho v d}{\eta}, \tag{13}$$

where d is the diameter of the tube; ϱ the density of the gas; v the flow velocity; η the viscosity of the gas. For the types of bifurcating tubes found in the respiratory tract, turbulent flow will develop if the Reynolds number exceeds 1,000. During normal viscous (laminar) flow, airflow is most rapid at the center of a tube, so that aerosol-laden air entering the airways is surrounded by a sheath of residual gas that contains a lower concentration of aerosol. Compared with the same volumetric laminar flow, turbulent flow causes more mixing within the airstream, and radial transport of aerosol into residual gas and onto the airway walls is accelerated. SWIFT et al. (1982) observed that total aerosol collection for human subjects depended on gas composition of the inhaled air, an effect that they attributed to the influence of gas composition on airflow profile.

DENNIS (1971) has reported that during exercise, the deposition fraction increases with minute volume, particularly for larger particles (1.0–3.0 μm). HARBISON and BRAIN (1983) have also reported that retention of particles increases more rapidly than minute ventilation, as gauged by oxygen consumption. Thus, with increased ventilation, the amount of aerosol deposited in the lung per unit time is increased both by the amount presented and by the percentage deposited.

Experimenting with 0.5-μm monodisperse particles, MUIR and DAVIES (1967) found that the percentage of particles deposited increased with tidal volume and decreased with the square root of breathing frequency. The effect of changes in tidal volume was very small. Later experiments (DAVIES et al. 1972; DAVIES 1982) incorporated the effect of expiratory reserve volume; the results showed that deposition decreased when the resting expiratory level was increased. PALMES et al. (1973) showed that loss of aerosol from inspired air was an exponential function of breath-holding time. Loss of aerosol also increased markedly with depth of inhalation.

Experiments measuring the effect of breathing pattern on the distribution of aerosol deposition are few. FOORD et al. (1978) administered monodisperse particles in the size range 2.5–7.5 μm to mouth-breathing subjects to study regional deposition, measured by comparing initial retention with 24-h retention. Regional deposition, compared with the sum of pulmonary and tracheobronchial deposition, was a monotonically decreasing function of the impaction parameter, d^2F where d was the aerodynamic diameter of the particle, and F was average inspiratory flow. VALBERG et al. (1982) reported experiments on excised dog lungs ventilated with radioactive aerosol according to various breathing patterns. After exposure, lungs were inflated, dried, and sliced transversely at 1-cm intervals. Distribution of deposited aerosol in each slice was measured by gamma camera, autoradiography, and dissection of each slice into pieces whose activity, weight, and airway content were recorded. Deposition efficiency was 32% for slow, deep breathing and 6% for rapid, shallow breathing. The results indicated that (a) total deposition decreases as breathing frequency increases; (b) slow, deep breathing produces uniform deposition throughout the lung, but with little aerosol collection in large airways; (c) rapid, shallow ventilation results in enhanced large airway deposition and marked heterogeneity in deposition distribution; and (d) slow, shallow breathing enhances small airway deposition.

Distribution of ventilation within the lung would clearly have an effect on distribution of aerosol deposition. SWEENLY et al. (1983) have used radioactive aerosols to show the existence of nonventilated areas in the lungs of anesthetized hamsters. However, measurements of ventilation distribution (HUBMAYR et al. 1983) seem not to correlate well with the distribution of deposition. The topographic localization of particle retention in the lungs is poorly understood and there may be a role for a number of factors: distribution of ventilation, local deposition efficiency, redistribution within the lung, and regional clearance differences (MORGAN et al. 1983).

III. Respiratory Tract Anatomy

Anatomic factors such as nasal versus oral breathing, numbers and angles of airway branching, and dimensions of airspaces contribute to determining aerosol retention. Inhalation of aerosols via the nasal route removes more particles than the oral route. Narrow cross sections and the resulting high linear velocities, sharp bends, and nasal hairs all promote impaction of large aerosol particles (PROCTOR 1974). Different species can be expected to have different patterns of deposition. STAUFFER (1975) has used dimensional analysis to predict that the probability of deposition of inhaled aerosols should be the same for different animals in the case of sedimentation-dominated deposition, but should scale as (body weight)$^{-0.1}$ for diffusion-dominated deposition. The predictions of MCMAHON et al. (1977) differ from those of STAUFFER (1975), and suggest that diffusion-dominated deposition is independent of body weight. MCMAHON et al. (1977) suggest specifying each of the physical mechanisms of particle deposition by identifying controlling dimensionless groups, e. g., Stokes number, Reynolds number, Froude number, etc. The predictions were tested in an experiment involving simultaneous exposure of six different species. The conclusion was that the collection efficiency of the lung alone and the collection efficiency of the entire respiratory tract are substantially independent of body size for aerosols of less than 1 μm diameter.

Animals differ not only in lung size and respiratory rate, but also in airway branching pattern. The human bronchial tree is more symmetric in its branching pattern than that of horses, dogs, cats, or rodents. The tracheobronchial geometries of different animal species have been measured, and the results have been incorporated into predictions of lung deposition (YEH 1980; SCHUM and YEH 1980). Different species have also been shown to have different clearance patterns (SNIPES et al. 1983). Even within species, anatomic considerations are important. An anatomic factor influencing deposition of aerosol in distal lung units is alveolar diameter. GLAZIER et al. (1967) measured the vertical gradient of alveolar size both in lungs of dogs frozen intact and in isolated lungs. For excised lungs they found no systematic differences in alveolar size, but for erect dogs apical alveoli had a diameter 1.5 times that of basal alveoli. The possibility that animal orientation relative to gravity might change retention patterns has been examined by SNEDDON and BRAIN (1981). They found that when rats spontaneously breathe small radioactive aerosols, more deposition goes to apical (cranial) lobes than to basal (caudal) lobes independent of the animal body position during inhalation: upright, inverted, or prone.

IV. Effect of Disease and Age

Deposition of aerosols is altered by pathologic changes in airways and parenchyma. LIPPMANN et al. (1971) have reported dramatically increased bronchial deposition in subjects with chronic bronchitis and asthma. Most abnormal states appear to enhance airway deposition at the expense of pulmonary deposition. For example, LOURENÇO et al. (1972) have shown that the deposition of 2-μm particles in patients with bronchiectasis is frequently more central than that in normal subjects. JAKAB and GREEN (1973) studied the retention of radiolabeled bacteria in normal mice and mice with pneumonia due to a previous infection with Sendai virus. The retention of bacteria was compared in consolidated and nonconsolidated areas of the lungs; 90% of the retained bacteria were deposited in the nonconsolidated areas, whereas only 10% were found in consolidated areas of similar volume.

The mechanisms responsible for these alterations in the pattern of deposition are numerous and complex. Airway obstruction diverts inspired flow to unobstructed airways. Decreased cross section of the airways increases linear velocity and turbulence, thereby enhancing inertial impaction and central deposition. Many diseases are also associated with alterations in alveolar dimensions that may alter the rate of deposition of particles. It is important to recognize that disease may affect not only deposition, but also clearance.

Most animals and human studies have been performed in adults. The mechanical properties of the lung are known to change with age both for humans (PERMUTT and MENKES 1979) and animals (MAUDERLY 1979). However, only fragmentary data exist on lung aerosol retention as a function of age. MUIR (1972) estimated that the filtration efficiency of airways in the newborn is similar to that of the adult. However, when SIKOV and MAHLUM (1976) studied the deposition of 1- to 3-μm aerosols in newborn (1-day-old) and adult rats, they found lower deposition fractions in the lungs of the immature animals.

V. Models of Lung Deposition

The first theoretical approach to predicting lung deposition was by FINDEISEN (1935). He used a nine-section model of the lung with dichotomous bronchial branching and 5×10^7 alveolar spaces. First, he calculated air velocities and times of transport in each airway, and then he developed mathematical expressions for particle deposition. Progress has generally been in one of these two areas, either a refined lung model or a revised analysis of deposition probability by impaction, sedimentation, and diffusion. LANDAHL (1950) used a different lung model and derived new expressions for deposition probabilities, and BEECKMANS (1965) extended the analysis to include the role of air mixing. The expressions for aerosol collection worked out by LANDAHL (1950) included a probability of deposition due to settling P_s

$$P_s = 1 - \exp\left(-0.8 v_t t \cos\varphi / R\right) \tag{14}$$

where the controlling variables are the particles settling velocities v_t, the time duration t, the angle of the airway to the horizontal φ, and the radius of the airspace R.

Inertial impaction is governed by the Stokes' number St defined in Eq. (8), and the probability of impaction is given by

$$P_I = \frac{St}{St + 1}. \tag{15}$$

Diffusion is governed by the expression for Brownian displacement Δ and the probability of deposition due to diffusion is

$$P_D = 1 - \exp\left(-0.58 \, \Delta / R\right). \tag{16}$$

The combined deposition probability is generally taken to be

$$P = 1 - (1 - P_s)(1 - P_I)(1 - P_D)$$ (17)

although this simple combination of the efficiencies has been questioned (Yu et al. 1977).

Models of the lung have become more sophisticated as morphometric techniques have become more advanced. The most widely used model is that of Weibel (1963) which is a dichotomous branching system with 23 generations. A more complete model recognizes the asymmetry of the branching system and the fact that alveoli can appear in early generations (Horsfield et al. 1971). A lobar model is that of Yeh and Schum (1980), which predicts more deposition in human lower lung lobes than upper lung lobes over a particle size range 0.01–10.0 μm. A theoretical evaluation of aerosol deposition in the rat predicts that apical lobes get more deposition than basal lobes (Schum and Yeh 1980).

The most important compendium of the influence of aerosol size distribution on lung deposition has been that of the International Commission on Radiation Protection (ICRP), which surveyed a large number of experimental and theoretical studies of lung deposition (Morrow 1966). A graphic summary of their findings is shown in Fig. 3. The range of these curves has been extended by Morrow (1974) to include particles of aerodynamic diameter 0.001–1,000 μm. Recent deposition calculations and experimental analysis have focused on the influence of aerosol polydispersity (Diu and Yu 1983), and on the effect of intrasubject variability (Davies 1982; Stahlhofen et al. 1981; Heyder et al. 1982). Although the main particle parameter governing aerosol deposition is MMAD, some influence

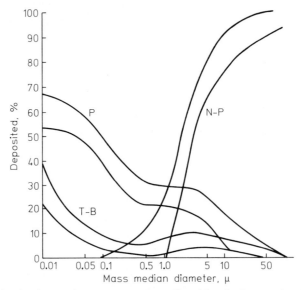

Fig. 3. Deposition in the respiratory tract, as predicted by the International Commission on Radiation Protection for three lung compartments show as a function of MMAD. The amount by which widely different GSDs affect the curves at a given MMAD is depicted by the width of the curves (Morrow 1966)

of geometric standard deviation, particularly for $\sigma_g > 2$, is predicted. Deposition data for spontaneously breathing humans continue to show large intrasubject variations, and the identification of the physiologic or anatomic parameters responsible for this has been difficult.

C. Dose by Measurement of Inspired and Expired Aerosol

I. Mass Balance Measurement

A simple approach is to measure the difference in the aerosol content between inspired and expired gas, i.e., its disappearance. If ventilation is known, one can determine the total amount of material deposited in the respiratory tract. However, no information is obtained regarding the site of deposition . Typically, an aerosol photometer is placed in line with the mouthpiece to monitor particle concentration constantly during breathing. The particles in the inspired and expired air pass through an optical chamber illuminated by a laser beam. The light scattered by the particles is detected by a photomultiplier tube, and the voltage is amplified and measured. Either the number of individual pulses or the total intensity of scattered light can be used to measure the number of particles present. If information about the angle of scattered light is included, a size distribution for both inhaled and exhaled aerosol can be derived so that lung retention of different particle sizes can be assessed.

II. Within-Breath Analysis

If assumptions about dead space and the extent of mixing are made, concentration of particles as a function of expired volume can be used to estimate regional deposition and study aerosol transport (TAULBEE et al. 1978). Conversely, the particle concentration profiles in exhaled air have been used to examine gas transport within the respiratory tract (HEYDER and DAVIES 1971). Particles below 1 µm in aerodynamic diameter serve as a tracer for gas flow patterns in the lung and can be used to test ideas concerning mixing processes in the lung. Yet another line of investigation has used measurement of exhaled aerosol to probe lung anatomy. PALMES et al. (1973) and GEBHART et al. (1981) used persistence of aerosol during breath-holding to estimate alveolar dimensions.

D. Infectious Particles

The fact that exhaled air is almost entirely free of airborne bacteria has been known for over a century (see HATCH and GROSS 1964, p 45). This fact has been used to assess lung deposition of infectious organisms (GREEN and KASS 1964; LAURENZI et al. 1964). The assay system here involves homogenizing the animal lungs at a series of times after exposure and determining the number of viable bacteria growing up cultured lung homogenate. This system is used primarily to study antimicrobial defenses, but it is also indicative of the retention of airborne infectious organisms in the lung (JAKAB and GREEN 1973; HUBER et al. 1977).

E. Techniques Utilizing Radioactivity

Radioactivity has frequently been used for studies of aerosol deposition because of its potential for noninvasive measurement as well as its sensitivity and resolution. Hundreds of radioisotopes are produced, and labeled compounds of every sort can be synthesized with a wide spectrum of energy, type of radiation (α-, β-, and γ-radiation, positrons, neutrons), half-lives, and doses. Several recent books summarize the medical applications of radiation detection (ROLLO 1975; KNOLL 1979).

I. Radiopacity

The chest radiograph is one of the mainstays for detecting pulmonary retention of inhaled dusts and for epidemiologic investigation of pneumoconioses (MORGAN and SEATON 1975). A chest film can provide not only a measure of the dust retained, but also a reasonable idea of distribution. The main shortcomings involve interpretation and quantification. Radiographic opacities can be produced not only by the retained dust, but also by the fibrogenic response to the dust. Efforts have been made to standardize interpretation of films by radiologists, but a wide latitude of subjectivity remains.

Some materials, such as tantalum, are highly opaque to X-rays and can be visualized sharply in radiologic studies (NADEL et al. 1968). Pulmonary retention and translocation have been studied for aerosolized tantalum dust using both radioactive tantalum and bronchography (MORROW et al. 1976). Other radiopaque particles such as those of antimony oxide, bismuth trioxide, and iron oxide are also suitable for such experiments (McCALLUM et al. 1971; FRIEDMAN et al. 1977; VALBERG and BRAIN 1979).

II. Whole Body Counting

Frequently it is of interest to know the total amount of material retained by an animal after exposure to a radioactive aerosol. In that case, the most useful approach for γ-ray emitters is to place the animal in a sodium iodide crystal that surrounds the entire body. A whole body count can then be obtained which reflects total retention (BOECKER et al. 1977). A variety of shielded whole body counters use large NaI crystals and appropriate lead shielding. It is not necessary to surround the subject completely (MORROW et al. 1964). Smaller detectors provide some information regarding the distribution of radioactivity in the body. One can distinguish material deposited in the upper airways, lung, and gastrointestinal tract (CUDDIHY and BOECKER 1973). Many devices use multiple detectors. MORSY et al. (1977) have described a system of four NaI crystals that provide excellent sensitivity.

III. Collimated Detectors and Gamma Cameras

Frequently, it is useful to restrict the field of view of the detector so that only the region of interest is seen. This is achieved by using a collimator that blocks most radiation, but allows radiation from one region of the body to reach the detector.

Collimators range from a simple cylindrical hole in a lead block to elaborate multihole shields. Resolution becomes increasingly better as the holes become smaller. However, for a fixed crystal size and shield thickness, smaller holes reduce detector sensitivity. A collimator is similar to the lens of a camera; it plays an important role in determining sensitivity, spatial resolution, and depth of field. STAHLHOFEN et al. (1980) have described a collimated detector suitable for determination of regional deposition in the human respiratory tract. The counter can separate activity present in the head, chest, and stomach and achieves a lower detection limit of about 4 nc.

A scintillation detector that actually produces an image of the radioactivity incident over a large area is the gamma camera, initially developed by H. O. Anger in 1956 (see ROLLO 1977, pp 231 ff). The gamma camera uses a single, large (approximately 25-cm diameter) scintillation crystal masked with a honeycomb, parallel hole lead collimator containing as many as 15,000 holes. Each part of the crystal looks at a small area of the patient or animal. An array of approximately three dozen phototubes 5 cm in diameter senses the distribution of light pulses produced in the crystal by incoming γ-rays. The relative pulse sizes from different photomultiplier tubes give the position of the scintillation. From this information, the distribution of radioactivity is extracted and displayed on a video screen or stored in a computer. The location of activity in lungs or lung slices can be determined from gamma camera images (VALBERG et al. 1982). An image consists of an array of 128×128 elements; each element represents an area approximately 3×3 mm. The counts sensed in each of these elements are converted to color on an intensity scale ranging from blue (low counts) to white (high counts), and the appropriate color is displayed in the radioactivity "picture". Associated computer systems allow identification of "regions of interest" on each picture by means of a joystick-controlled cursor. The activity in such regions can be correlated with activity in various anatomic compartments.

Most systems can detect and separate the simultaneous presence of two isotopes by differentiating their γ-ray energy spectra. Once an activity picture is taken with each isotope, the computer system permits addition, subtraction, multiplication, and division of these images so that differences in deposition pattern between the two isotopes can be detected. The resolution of the camera depends on the γ-ray energy, the collimator design, and the distance from the collimator to the source. The price paid for spatial resolution is lower counting efficiency, typically 5,000-fold less than for a well-type gamma counter.

IV. Tissue Samples and Dissection

When used with whole lungs or intact animals, collimated NaI crystals and gamma cameras can provide some information regarding the amount and distribution of deposited particles. In a gamma camera picture of a dog or human exposed to a radioactive aerosol, one can easily identify the lung contours and detect large shifts in the distribution of the aerosol. However, many important questions cannot be answered by examination of the whole lung. For example, it is nearly impossible to subdivide deposition into airway and parenchymal compartments or to describe gradients from apex to base. Interlobar differences cannot be detected, and it is impossible to identify nonventilated areas when they are small. Greater precision and resolution are available when lungs are made rigid by fixation, drying, or freezing and then sliced or dissected. More important, this permits correlation of the site of retention with the anatomic location.

1. Counting Retained Activity

Necropsy, organ separation, and radioactivity assay is a standard technique in determining distribution of inhaled aerosol retention (SNIPES et al. 1983). Separation of the lung into lobes further refines resolution of tissue retention (RAABE et al. 1977). Another procedure has been to inflate lungs, dry them in a microwave oven, and then dissect the rigid lung (VALBERG et al. 1982). Drying time for dog lungs is approximately 1 h, and this technique is valuable when short-lived isotopes such as ^{99m}Tc are used. An important advantage of this procedure is that retained activity is not moved about, as might be the case with fixation by fluid instillation into the airways. Inflated lungs can be embedded in polyurethane foam to permit precise orientation during slicing. Dried lungs can also be decorticated. Bits of parenchyma are picked away from the airway tree to expose it. The airways can then be dissected, and the precise of individual samples can be recorded. This strategy is appropriate for describing patterns of particle deposition along airways.

When analyzing aerosol content of lung pieces, it is frequently useful to normalize for the size of the piece. This helps evaluate how deposited activity is distributed throughout a lung or a lobe (BRAIN et al. 1976; VALBERG et al. 1982; SWEENEY et al. 1983). Such an evenness index (EI) is calculated by expressing the activity of each piece as cpm per milligram dried or frozen lung, and comparing this number with the activity per milligram whole lung

$$EI = \frac{(\text{cpm/mg lung piece})}{(\text{cpm/mg whole lung})}. \tag{18}$$

EI less than 1.0 indicates that the lung piece received less than an average share of radioactivity; similarly, a piece with EI greater than 1.0 received more than an average share of radioactivity. The degree of departure from 1.0 reflects heterogeneity in particle retention distribution. Figure 4 shows an example of this analysis for a lung slice. EI can also be calculated for the slices and lobes of each lung. EI can be correlated to anatomic information such as the fraction of each piece that is composed of airways.

As in the case of the gamma camera, the simultaneous distribution of two or more isotopes can be determined (SNIPES and CLEM 1981). For example, one can tag an aerosol first with ^{99m}Tc and in a later experiment with ^{67}Ga. Animals can then be exposed to the two aerosols sequentially under different experimental conditions. In this way, each animal can act as its own control when comparing the effect of the different experimental conditions. The deposition in the whole animal or in pieces of lung can be determined for each aerosol individually by separating the two isotopes on the basis of γ-ray energy spectrum, half-life, or both.

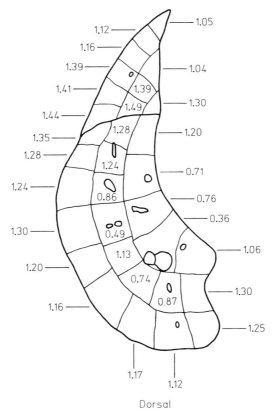

Dorsal

Fig. 4. An example of lung pieces dissected from a slice of dried dog lung. EI values show the relative local retention in this lung which was exposed to aerosol while being ventilated in a slow, deep breathing pattern. Retention is fairly uniform with slightly more retention in ventral as compared with dorsal pieces. Pieces containing airway have a very low EI because their weight is considerably larger than pieces without airways

2. Autoradiography

If the radioisotope involved has an α- or β-particle emission, distribution of activity in tissue samples can be obtained by autoradiography. Ionizing radiation exposes photographic film, and charged particles are more efficient than γ-rays (HERZ 1969; ROGERS 1978). α-Particle emitters or low energy β-particle emitters have a short range in tissue and film and provide the best resolution. In addition, the thinner the specimen and the thinner the photographic layer, the better the resolution. β-Particle autoradiographs on X-ray film have been used in studying ^{99m}Tc-labeled aerosol deposition in lung slices (VALBERG et al. 1982; SWEENEY et al. 1983). Although it is a low energy γ-ray emitter (140 keV), ^{99m}Tc also emits low energy electrons (1.6, 1.9 and 119 keV). Because these electrons are strongly ionizing, they are the predominant source of film exposure. Typically, 10^9 γ-ray photons/cm² are required to achieve unit optical density, whereas only 10^7 electrons/cm² are required to produce the same density. The short range of the elec-

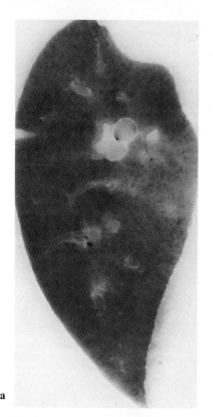
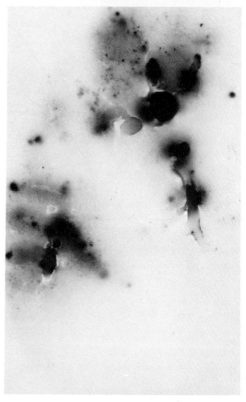

a   b

Fig. 5 a–c. Autoradiographs of lung slices following an inhalation exposure to aerosol (particles < 1 μm activity median aerodynamic diameter). Darkening on these images corresponds to photographic exposure caused by retained activity. Even though anatomic features are recognizable, it must be remembered that these are "radioactivity" pictures and not photographs. An autoradiograph of a lung slice with no activity would produce only a blank sheet.
a from a spontaneously breathing dog, within hours after inhalation exposure, note the fairly uniform distribution with some activity in airways which may represent the early stages of mucociliary clearance; **b** an excised dog lung which was exposed to aerosol while ventilated in a rapid, shallow fashion, note the highly heterogeneous pattern of retention with considerable collection of aerosol in airways as compared with parenchyma;

trons (90 μm in film) results in a crisp image of the distribution of radioactivity over the face of the slice. Figure 5 gives examples of autoradiographs of dried lung slices for a variety of exposure conditions. Film exposure is related to retention in lung tissue immediately adjacent to the film. The portions of the lung slice beyond the range of the electrons contribute negligibly to the exposure. The developed film is a compact record of the site (or sites) of deposition, with anatomic features readily visible. With an overlay tracing of the lung slice, the distribution of the retained dose can be mapped precisely. To convert this record into meaningful quantitative information, a computer assisted correlation of anatomic features with film density can be achieved using a scanning microdensitometer.

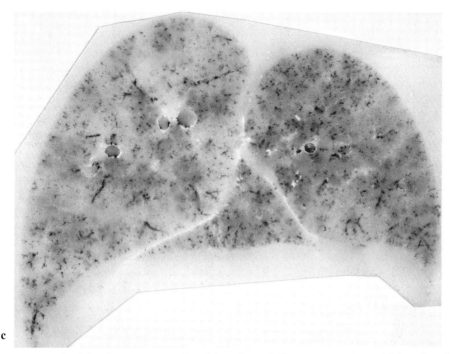

c

c these excised dog lungs were ventilated in a slow, shallow pattern at very high end expiratory volume ~90% of total lung capacity. Even though overall deposition is quite uniform, there appears to be enhanced aerosol collection in small (1–2 mm) airways

Autoradiography has been used to examine the effect of lavage treatment on lung retention (SNIPES et al. 1979) and changes of lung retention distribution with time (RHOADS et al. 1982; VALBERG et al. 1983). α-Particle emitters are useful for examining retention on a finer scale owing to the shorter range of the particle. Liquid emulsion autoradiographs have been used on lung sections to examine distribution of inhaled PuO_2 (DIEL et al. 1981) and to localize long-term particle retention in airway tissues (STIRLING and PATRICK 1980).

3. Neutron Activation

A variety of elements can be made radioactive by exposure to a neutron flux in a reactor core. Not only does this make nonradioactive substances detectable by γ-ray counting, but also the γ-ray spectrum can be used to identity the elements present (PARSONS 1976). This method has been used primarily to activate aerosols prior to inhalation (e. g., coal dust) (MORROW et al. 1982), but could in principle be used for activation of tissue samples.

4. Lung Lavage

Particles deposited on lung surfaces may either be free or ingested by pulmonary macrophages. Both pulmonary macrophages and free particles can be recovered from the lung by lavage (BRAIN and CORKERY 1977). If the particles are radioactive, their degree of association with pulmonary macrophages can be assayed, and retention in the macrophage compartment can be determined (VALBERG et al. 1983). Chapter 8 has more details on information available from lung lavage samples.

F. Morphological Methods

I. Measurement at Autopsy

For occupational, nonradioactive particle exposure, measurement of the mineral content of lungs obtained at autopsy has long been used as a measure of permanent retention within lungs or lung lymph nodes. Lungs are generally digested in acid to liberate retained dust, which can then be weighed and put through any number of analysis procedures to establish its identify. Often such results are used to correlate lung pathology with components of the dust. To mention but a few studies, work has been done on coal miners (DAVIS et al. 1977), ore miners (VERMA et al. 1982), and asbestos workers (MCDONALD et al. 1982).

II. Light and Electron Microscopy

Even with analytic approaches that depend on separating the lung into pieces, some questions still cannot be answered. It may be important to know with a precision of a few millimeters where the particles are in the lungs. For example, are particles still free or have they been ingested by pulmonary macrophages? Then, morphological studies using light and electron microscopy can be very useful. The localization of particles on alveolar duct surfaces can be identified in scanning electron microscopy (HOLMA 1969) and X-ray energy spectroscopy can be used to identify elements (BRODY et al. 1982). It may be important to identify cell types containing deposited particles. This kind of information is not easily obtained by other than morphological methods. There is increasing evidence that inhaled aerosols may penetrate airway and alveolar barriers (SOROKIN and BRAIN 1975; WATSON and BRAIN 1979; STIRLING and PATRICK 1980). Precise location of particles within the bronchial epithelium or beneath it, in lymph nodes, and the relationship between these particles and components of the immune system can only be demonstrated with morphological techniques. Thus, it is important to select the method used according to the type of information required.

III. Morphometry

As investigators become more demanding about the precision of deposited particle location, more sophisticated and quantitative techniques will be necessary. In order to express the association of particles with various lung structures accurately, the morphometric techniques described by WEIBEL (1979, 1980) will have to be employed. This involves careful and systematic tissue sampling procedures along with numerical scoring of particle location. Such rigorous analysis has been used in morphometric measurements of the lung (WEIBEL 1963), but has only found limited application in particle retention studies (DAVIES 1977).

G. Magnetopneumography

I. Retention from Occupational Exposure

Some mineral dusts are magnetizable, and sensitive magnetometry can be used to measure their concentration and distribution in the lungs (COHEN 1973, 1975). The technique consists of applying a magnetic field to the whole thorax or to localized areas and detecting the consequent alignment of ferromagnetic domains in retained lung particles. Accumulation of such particles has been measured in foundry workers, arc welders, coal miners, and asbestos miners (COHEN et al. 1981; KALLIOMÄKI et al. 1976, 1978, 1979, 1980, 1982; FREEDMAN et al. 1980, 1982). The greatest advantage of this technique is that measurements are not limited by a radioactive half-life and can be made as long as sufficient dust remains in the lung. Thus, one can noninvasively describe clearance kinetics over years. Two magnetic dusts suitable for studying retention of dust in the lung are Fe_3O_4 (magnetite) and γ-Fe_2O_3 (a magnetic form of hematite). Both are inert, relatively insoluble at physiologic pH, and can be produced in aerosol form (VALBERG and BRAIN 1979). These materials can be magnetized by application of an external field, so that magnetic domains of the particles are lined up to produce a remanent field that is measurable by sensitive magnetometers. The magnitude of the remanent field can be used to quantify the amount of dust remaining in the lungs.

II. Measurement of Lung Clearance

The deposition of 1–3 mg Fe_3O_4 is sufficient to describe clearance curvers in animals and humans by either fluxgate or superconducting magnetometers (COHEN et al. 1979; HALPERN et al. 1981; SCHLESINGER et al. 1982; BRAIN et al. 1983). The main drawback of this technique is the difficulty of correlating remanent magnetic field reading with distribution of retention in the lungs, a difficulty due to the vectorial nature of the field generated by the particles and its falloff with distance by an inverse cube law. Thus, redistribution of a constant amount of magnetic material in the lungs may cause the reading at a given point on the chest to go up or down in the absence of any net clearance. Also, the decrease in remanent magnetic field readings may be due not only to physical clearance, but also to conversion of the iron oxide to nonmagnetic forms, such as by solubilization. Contributions to the remanent field from ferromagnetic contaminants in the gut or on the fur and skin can also cause artifacts.

III. Particle Environment Measurements: "Relaxation"

As COHEN (1973) initially pointed out, lung retention of inhaled ferromagnetic dusts can be measured with a sensitive magnetometer. He also noted that the magnitude of the remanent field dropped by as much as a factor of six during the first hour after magnetization, a phenomenon he called "relaxation" and attributed to some viable process randomly rotating magnetic particles retained in the lungs. If particles, whose magnetic fields were initially aligned, rotate, the vector sum of magnetic field contributions from each particle decreases in proportion to the randomization caused by rotations. Initial remanent magnetic field strength can be restored by remagnetization. Kalliomäki et al. (1976) and others (Valberg and Brain 1979; Cohen et al. 1979; Brain et al. 1983) have published lung relaxation curves in both humans and animals. Possible mechanisms driving this relaxation are tissue movements, body fluid motions, particle diffusive motion, and cell motions. The character of the relaxation curve may provide information about the intrapulmonary location of particles, and it has been confirmed that the remanent field relaxation seen in intact animals exposed to magnetic reflects cytoplasmic movements within particle-containing macrophages (Valberg 1984). This technique may provide a useful in vivo probe of phagocytosis, but further investigation of the phenomenon remains to be done.

H. Tomography: the Imaging Problem

I. Computed X-Ray Transmission Tomography

Computed axial transmission tomography, also known as computerized axial tomography (CAT) has become a standard technique for imaging body tissues, and several texts discuss the capabilities of the technique (Sutton 1982; Lee et al. 1983). Recent reports have described application of the technique to mapping pulmonary ventilation (Pinsky et al. 1983), but application to particle retention measurements has not been forthcoming. Since the technique is sensitive enough to pick up differences in gas density, it would appear logical that radiopaque dusts (cf. Sect. E. I.) could be easily mapped.

II. Emission Tomography: γ-Ray and Positron

Radioactive emissions from particles deposited in lungs can be tomographically localized by rotating the subject relative to a gamma camera (Larsson 1980). This would give another dimension to the two-dimensional gamma camera pictures of retention that were discussed earlier. However, it is difficult both to rotate and to maintain strict body position during the time required to accumulate sufficient counts. This is another localization technique that remains to be exploited in lung retained dose measurements.

Some radionuclides emit positrons upon decay. The emitted positrons have a very high probability of being captured by an electron in the immediate vicinity of their origin. The ensuing annihilation process produces two γ-ray photons at $180°$ relative to each other. If the subject is surrounded by detectors capable of recording the site of interaction of these photons with a scintillation crystal, then the line along which decay events originate can be reconstructed. A mapping of the three-dimensional distribution of radionuclides is possible (Ter-Pogossian et al. 1981). This technique is being used to examine metabolic pathways in living tissue, but could also be used to reveal lung retention distributions.

III. Nuclear Magnetic Resonance

An even more novel imaging technique involves producing images from nuclear magnetic resonance (NMR) signals within the body. The frequency and decay rate of an NMR signal depend on the identity of the nucleus being probed and on the local magnetic environment. The subject is placed in a strong homogeneous magnetic field (0.1–1.0 T) in which nuclei with magnetic moments have a predictable precession frequency, or resonant frequency. When a short excitation pulse of radiofrequency radiation is applied at the nuclear resonance frequency, these nuclei are put in a radiative mode and the resulting "ringing" can be detected as an induced signal in the same coil that generated the pulse. If a known gradient is added to the homogeneous magnetic field, the signal frequency from a nucleus will depend on its location because of the spatial variation in the applied static field. By applying a series of gradient patterns, enough information can be collected for computer algorithms to generate an image of the density distribution of the probed nucleus. In addition to displaying the NMR observable density, additional information can be extracted by examining the decay time of the induced NMR signal. The immediate magnetic environment of a nucleus is influenced by the type of chemical compound in which it is located. NMR imaging was initiated over 10 years ago (LAUTERBUR 1973) and current images are comparable in resolution to other tomographic techniques (MORAN et al. 1983; KAUFMAN et al. 1981). This sophisticated technique is yet another imaging process that could be used to describe patterns of lung retention.

It is important to remember that exposure to an aerosol does not adequately define the dose produced, nor does it specify the anatomic distribution of that dose. Regardless of the aerosol exposure problem being studied, it is essential to quantify the dose. Investment in a thorough description of the location of aerosols in the respiratory tract will be rewarded, because improved understanding of the effects of aerosols stems from the recognition of factors important to their uptake and fate.

References

Bau SK, Aspin N, Wood DE, Levison H (1971) The measurement of fluid deposition in humans following mist tent therapy. Pediatrics 48:605–612

Beeckmans JM (1965) The deposition of aerosols in the respiratory tract. I. Mathematical analysis and comparison with experimental data. Can J Physiol Pharmacol 43:157–172

Boecker BB, Thomas RG, McClellan RO (1977) Accumulation and retention of 137-Cs fused aluminosilicate particles by beagle dogs after repeated inhalation exposures. In: Walton WH (ed) Inhaled particles IV. Pergamon, Oxford, pp 221–236

Brain JD, Corkery GC (1977) The effect of increased particles on the endocytosis of radiocolloids by pulmonary macrophages in vivo: competitive and toxic effects. In: Walton WH (ed) Inhaled particles IV. Pergamon Press, Oxford, pp 551–564

Brain JD, Valberg PA (1974) Models of lung retention based on the report of the ICRP task group. Arch Environ Health 28:1–11

Brain JD, Knudson DE, Sorokin SP, Davis MA (1976) Pulmonary distribution of particles given by intratracheal instillation or by aerosol inhalation. Environ Res 11:13–33

Brain JD, Proctor DF, Reid L (eds) (1977) Respiratory defense mechanisms, vol 5. In: Lenfant C (ed) Lung biology in health and disease. Marcel Dekker, New York

Brain JD, Bloom SB, Valberg PA, Gehr P (1984) Behavior of magnetic iron oxide particles deposited in the lungs of rabbits correlates with phagocytosis. Exp Lung Res 6:115–131

Brody AR, Hill LH, Adkins B, O'Connor RW (1981) Chrysotile asbestos inhalation in rats: deposition pattern and reaction of alveolar epithelium and pulmonary macrophages. Am Rev Respir Dis 123:670–679

Brody AR, Roe MW, Evans JN, Davis GS (1982) Deposition and translocation of inhaled silica in rats. Lab Invest 47:533–542

Busse WW, Reed CE, Hoehne JH (1972) Where is the allergic reaction in ragweed asthma? II. Demonstration of ragweed antigen in airborne particles smaller than pollen. J Allergy Clin Immunol 50:289–293

Chan TL, Yu CP (1982) Charge effects on particle deposition in the human tracheobronchial tree. Ann Occup Hyg 26:65–75

Chan TL, Lippmann M, Cohen VR, Schlesinger RB (1978) Effect of electrostatic charges on particle deposition in a hollow cast of the human larynx and tracheobronchial tree. J Aerosol Sci 9:463–468

Cinkotai FF (1971) The behaviour of sodium chloride particles in moist air. J Aerosol Sci 2:325–329

Cohen D (1973) Ferromagnetic contamination in the lungs and other organs of the human body. Science 180:745–748

Cohen D (1975) Measurement of the magnetic field produced by the human heart, brain, and lungs. IEEE Trans Magn 11:694–700

Cohen D, Arai SF, Brain JD (1979) Smoking impairs long-term dust clearance from the lungs. Science 204:514–517

Cohen D, Crowther TS, Gibbs GW, Becklake MR (1981) Magnetic lung measurements in relation to occupational exposure in asbestos miners and millers in Quebec. Environ Res 26:535–550

Cuddihy RG, Boecker BB (1973) Controlled administration of respiratory tract burdens of inhaled radioactive aerosols in beagle dogs. Toxicol Appl Pharmacol 25:597–605

Davies CN (ed) (1966) Aerosol science. Academic, New York

Davies CN (1979) Particle-fluid interactions. J Aerosol Sci 10:477–513

Davies CN (1982) Deposition of particles in human lungs as a function of particle size and breathing pattern, an empirical model. In: Walton WH (ed) Inhaled particles V. Pergamon, Oxford, pp 119–135

Davies CN, Heyder J, Ramu MCS (1972) Breathing of half-micron aerosols. I. Experimental J Appl Physiol 32:591–600

Davies P, Sornberger GC, Huber GL (1977) The stereology of pulmonary macrophages after prolonged experimental exposure to tobacco smoke. Lab Invest 37:297–306

Davis JMG, Ottery J, LeRoux A (1977) Effect of quartz and other non-coal dusts in coal worker's pneumoconiosis. In: Walton WH (ed) Inhaled particles IV. Pergamon, Oxford, pp 691–702

Dennis WL (1971) The effect of breathing rate on the deposition of particles in the human respiratory system. In: Walton WH (ed) Inhaled particles III. Unwin, Surrey, pp 91–102

Diel JH, Mewhinney JA, Snipes MB (1981) Distribution of inhaled 238-PuO$_2$ particles in Syrian hamster lungs. Radiat Res 88:299–312

Diu CK, Yu CP (1983) Respiratory tract deposition of polydisperse aerosols in humans. Am Ind Hyg Assoc 44:62–65

Doll R (1971) Cancers related to smoking. In: Richards RG (ed) Proceedings of the 2nd world conference on smoking and health. Pittman Medical, London, pp 10–23

Edmonds RL (ed) (1979) Aerobiology: the ecological systems approach. Dowden, Hutchison and Ross, Stroudsburg, PA

Egan DF (1977) Aerosol and humidity therapy. In: Fundamentals of respiratory therapy, 3rd edn. Mosby, St. Louis, pp 213–268

Eisenbud M (1977) The primary air pollutants – radioactive. In: Stern AC (ed) Air pollutants, their transformation and transport, vol 1, chap 5. Academic, New York, pp 197–231

Ferris BG (1978) Health effects of exposure to low levels of regulated air pollutants: a critical review. Air Pollut Control Assoc J 28:482–497

Ferron GA (1977) The size of soluble aerosol particles as a function of the humidity of the air: application to the human respiratory tract. J Aerosol Sci 8:251–267

Findeisen W (1935) Über das Absetzen kleiner, in der Luft suspendierten Teilchen in der menschlichen Lunge bei der Atmung. Pflügers Arch Physiol 236:367–384

Foord N, Black A, Walsh M (1978) Regional deposition of 2.5–7.5 μm diameter inhaled particles in healthy male non-smokers. J Aerosol Sci 9:343–357

Freedman AP, Robinson SE, Johnston RJ (1980) Non-invasive magnetopneumograph estimation of lung dust loads and distribution in bituminous coal workers. J Occup Med 22:613–618

Freedman AP, Robinson SE, Green FHY (1982) Magnetopneumography as a tool for the study of dust retention in the lungs. Ann Occup Hyg 26:319–335

Friedman M, Stott FD, Poole DO, Dougherty R, Chapman GA, Watson H, Sackner MA (1977) A new roentgenographic method for estimating mucous velocity in airways. Am Rev Respir Dis 115:67–72

Fuchs NA (1964) The mechanics of aerosols. Pergamon, Oxford

Gebhart J, Heyder J, Stahlhofen W (1981) Use of aerosols to estimate pulmonary airspace dimensions. J Appl Physiol 51:465–476

Gehr P, Brain JD, Bloom SB, Valberg PA (1983) Magnetic particles in the liver: a probe for intracellular movement. Nature 302:336–338

Glazier JB, Hughes JMB, Maloney JE, West JB (1967) Vertical gradient of alveolar size in lungs of dogs frozen intact. J Appl Physiol 23:694–703

Goldsmith JR, Friberg LT (1977) The effects of air pollution on human health. In: Stern AC (ed) Air pollution, the effects of air pollution, vol 2, chap 7, 3rd edn. Academic, New York, pp 457–610

Green GM, Kass EH (1964) Factors influencing clearance of bacteria by the lung. J Clin Invest 43:769–776

Halpern M, Williamson SJ, Spektor DM, Schlesinger RB, Lippmann M (1981). Remanent magnetic fields for measuring particle retention and distribution in the lungs. Exp Lung Res 2:27–35

Harbison M, Brain JD (1983) Effects of exercise on particle deposition in Syrian golden hamsters. Am Rev Respir Dis 128:904–908

Hatch TR, Gross P (1964) Pulmonary deposition and retention of inhaled aerosols. Academic, New York

Herz RH (1969) The photographic action of ionizing radiations. Wiley-Interscience, New York

Heyder J, Davies CN (1971) The breathing of half micron aerosols. III. Dispersion of particles in the respiratory tract. J Aerosol Sci 2:437–452

Heyder J, Gebhart J, Stahlhofen W, Stuck B (1982) Biological variability of particle deposition in the human respiratory tract during controlled and spontaneous mouthbreathing. In: Walton WH (ed) Inhaled particle V. Pergamon, Oxford, pp 137–147

Hinds WC (1978) Size characteristics of cigarette smoke. Am Ind Hyg Assoc 39:48–54

Hinds WC (1982) Aerosol technology. Wiley, New York

Hoegg UR (1972) Cigarette smoke in closed places. Environ Health Perspect 2:117–128

Holma B (1969) Scanning electron microscopic observations of particles deposited in the lung. Arch Environ Health 18:330–339

Horsfield K, Dart G, Olson DE, Filley GF, Cumming G (1971) Models of the human bronchial tree. J Appl Physiol 31:207–217

Huber GL, Johanson WG, LaForce FM (1977) Experimental models and pulmonary antimicrobial defenses. In: Brain JD, Proctor DF, Reid LM (eds) Respiratory defense mechanisms. Marcel Dekker, New York, pp 983–1009

Hubmayr RD, Walters BJ, Chevalier PA, Rodarte JR, Olson LE (1983) Topographical distribution of regional lung volume in anesthetized dogs. J Appl Physiol 54:1048–1056

Jablon S, Bailar JC (1980) The contribution of ionizing radiation to cancer mortality in the U.S. Prev Med 9:219–226

Jakab GJ, Green GM (1973) Effects of pneumonia on intrapulmonary distribution of inhaled particles. Am Rev Respir Dis 107:675–678

Kalliomäki PL, Karp PK, Katila T, Makipaw P, Jaar P, Tossavainen A (1976) Magnetic measurements of pulmonary contamination. Scand J Work Environ Health 4:232–239

Kalliomäki PL, Korhonen O, Vaaranen V, Kalliomäki K, Koponen M (1978) Lung retention and clearance of shipyard arc welders. Int Arch Occup Environ Health 42:83–90

Kalliomäki PL, Kalliomäki K, Korhonen O, Koponen M, Sortti V, Vaaranen V (1979) Lung contamination among foundry workers. Int Arch Occup Environ Health 43:85–91

Kalliomäki K, Kalliomäki PL, Kelha V, Vaaranen V (1980) Instrumentation for measuring the magnetic lung contamination of steel welders. Ann Occup Hyg 23:174–184

Kalliomäki PL, Aittoniemi K, Gustafsson T, Kalliomäki K, Koponen M, Vaaranen V (1982) Research on industrial ferrous metal aerosols. Ann Occup Hyg 26:337–345

Kaufman L, Crooks LE, Margulis AR (1981) Nuclear magnetic resonance imaging in medicine. Igaku-Shoin, New York

Knoll GF (1979) Radiation detection and measurement. Wiley, New York

Landahl HD (1950) On the removal of airborne droplets by the human respiratory tract. I. The lung. Bull Math Biophys 12:43–56

Lanza AJ (ed) (1963) The pneumoconioses. Grune and Stratton, New York

Larsson SA (1980) Gamma camera emission tomography. Acta Radiol [Suppl] (Stockh) 363:5–75

Laurenzi GA, Berman L, First M, Kass EH (1964) A quantitative study of the deposition and clearance of bacteria in the murine lung. J Clin Invest 43:759–768

Lauterbur PC (1973) Image formation by induced local interactions: examples employing nuclear magnetic resonance. Nature 242:190–191

Lave EB, Seskin EP (1970) Air pollution and human health. Science 169:723–733

Lee JKT, Sagel SS, Stanley RJ (1983) Computed body tomography. Raven, New York

Leedom JM, Loosli CG (1979) Airborne pathogens in the indoor environment with special reference to nosocomial (hospital) infection. In: Edmonds RL (ed) Aerobiology: the ecological systems approach. Dowden, Hutchison and Ross, Stroudsburg, PA, pp 208–210

Leith DE (1977) Cough. In: Brain JD, Proctor DF, Reid L (eds) Lung biology in health and disease, vol 5. Marcel Dekker, New York, pp 545–592

Lippmann M (1978) Respirable dust sampling. In: Air Sampling Instruments Committee. Air sampling instruments for evaluation of atmospheric contaminants, 5th edn. American Conference of Governmental Industrial Hygienists. Cincinnati, pp G1–G23

Lippmann M, Albert RE, Peterson HT (1971) The regional deposition of inhaled aerosols in man. In: Walton WH (ed) Inhaled particles III. Unwin, Surrey, England, pp 105–120

Lockhart LB Jr, Patterson RL Jr, Saunders AW Jr (1965) The size distribution of radioactive atmospheric aerosols. J Geophys Res 70:6033–6035

Lourenço RV, Loddenkemper R, Cargon RW (1972) Pattern of distribution and clearance of aerosols in patients with bronchiectasis. Am Rev Respir Dis 106:857–866

Lundgren DA, Harris FS, Marlow WH, Lippmann M, Clark WE, Durham MD (eds) (1979) Aerosol measurement. University Press of Florida, Gainesville

Lundin FE, Lloyd JW, Smith EN, Archer VE, Haladay DA (1969) Mortality of uranium miners in relation to radiation exposure, hard-rock mining, and cigarette smoking, 1950 through 1967. Health Phys 16:571–578

McCallum RI, Day MH, Underhill J, Aird EGA (1971) Measurement of antimony oxide dust in human lungs in vivo by X-ray spectrophotometry. In: Walton WH (ed) Inhaled particles III. Unwin, Surrey, pp 611–620

McDonald AD, McDonald JC, Pooley FD (1982) Mineral fiber content of lung in mesothelial tumors in North America. Ann Occup Hyg 26:417–422

McMahon TA, Brain JD, LeMott SR (1977) Species differences in aerosol deposition. In: Walton WH (ed) Inhaled particles IV. Pergamon, Oxford, pp 23–33

Mauderly JL (1979) Ventilation, lung volumes and lung mechanics of young and old Syrian hamsters. Exp Aging Res 5:497–508

Melandri C, Prodi V, Tarroni G, Formignani M, DeZaiacomo T, Bompane GR, Maestri G, Giacomelli Maltoni GR (1977) On the deposition of unipolarly charged particles in the human respiratory tract. In: Walton WH (ed) Inhaled particles IV. Pergamon, New York, pp 193–201

Mercer TT (1973) Aerosol technology in hazard evaluation. Academic, New York

Moran PR, Nickles RJ, Zagzebski JA (1983) The physics of medical imaging. Phys Today 36(7):36–42

Morgan WKC, Seaton A (1975) Occupational lung diseases. Saunders, New York

Morgan WKC, Clague HW, Vinitski S (1983) On paradigms, paradoxes, and particles. Lung 161:195–206

Morrow PE (1960) Some physical and physiological factors controlling the fate of inhaled substances. Health Phys 2:366–376

Morrow PE (1974) Aerosol characterization and deposition. Am Rev Respir Dis 110:88–99

Morrow PE, Chairman, Task group on lung dynamics (1966) Deposition and retention models for internal dosimetry of the human respiratory tract. Health Phys 12:173–207

Morrow PE, Gibb FR, Johnson L (1964) Clearance of insoluble dust from the lower respiratory tract. Health Phys 10:543–555

Morrow PE, Klipper RW, Beiter EH, Gibb FR (1976) Pulmonary retention and translocation of insufflated tantalum. Radioloy 121:415–421

Morrow PE, Gibb FR, Beiter H, Amato F, Yulie C, Klipper RW (1982) Pulmonary retention of coal dusts. Ann Occup Hyg 26:291–307

Morsy SM, Werner F, Stahlhofen W, Pohlit W (1977) A detector of adjustable response for the study of lung clearance. Health Phys 32:243–251

Muir DCF (1972) Deposition and clearance of inhaled particles. In: Muir DCF (ed) Clinical aspects of inhaled particles. Davis, Philadelphia, pp 1–20

Muir DCF, Davies CN (1967) The deposition of 0.5 µm diameter aerosols in the lungs of man. Ann Occup Hyg 10:161–174

Nadel HA, Wolfe WG, Graf PD (1968) Powdered tantalum as a medium for bronchography in canine and human lungs. Invest Radiol 3:229–238

Palmes ED, Chiu-Sen W, Goldring RM, Altshuler B (1973) Effect of depth of inhalation on aerosol persistence during breath holding. J Appl Physiol 34:356–360

Parkes WR (1982) Occupational lung disorders. Butterworths, Boston

Parsons ML (1976) Neutron activation. In: Winefordner JD (ed) Trace analysis: spectroscopic methods for elements. Wiley, New York, pp 151–208

Patterson R (1972) Aeroallergens. In: Patterson R (ed) Allergic diseases: diagnosis and management. Lippincott, New York, pp 87–123

Permutt S, Menkes HA (1979) Spirometry. In: Macklem PT, Permutt S (eds) The lung in the transition between health and disease. Marcel Dekker, New York, pp 113–152

Pinsky M, Gur D, Best K, Pennock RM, Herbert D (1983) Regional pulmonary ventilation mapping by non-radioactive xenon enhanced dynamic computed tomography. Am Rev Respir Dis 127:241(Abstract)

Proctor DF (1974) The upper respiratory tract and the ambient air. Clin Notes Respir Dis 12:2–10

Raabe OG, Yeh HC, Newton GJ, Phalen RF, Velasquez DJ (1977) Deposition of inhaled monodisperse aerosols in small rodents. In: Walton WH (ed) Inhaled particles IV. Pergamon, Oxford, pp 3–21

Rhoads K, Mahaffey JA, Sanders CL (1982) Distribution of inhaled 239-PuO/d2/u in rat and hamster lung. Health Phys 42:645–656

Rogers AW (1978) Techniques of autoradiography, 3rd edn Elsevier/North Holland, New York

Rollo RD (ed) (1977) Nuclear medicine physics, instrumentation and agents. CV Mosby, St. Louis

Scherer PW, Haselton Fr, Hanna LM, Stone DR (1979) Growth of hygroscopic aerosols in a model of bronchial airways. J Appl Physiol 47:544–550

Schlesinger RB, Halpern M, Lippmann M (1982) Long-term clearance of inhaled magnetite and polystyrene latex from the lung, a comparison. Health Physics 42:68–73

Schum M, Yeh HC (1980) Theoretical evaluation of aerosol deposition in anatomical models of mammalian airways. Bull Math Biol 42:1–15

Self TH, Brooks JB, Lieberman P, Ryan MR (1983) The value of demonstration and the role of the pharmacist in teaching the correct use of pressurized bronchodilators. Can Med Assoc J 128:129–131

Sikov MR, Mahlum DD (1976) Influence of age and physicochemical form on the effects of ^{239}Pu on the skeleton of the rat. In: Jee WSS (ed) The health effects of plutonium and radium. JW Press, Salt Lake City, pp 33–47

Sinclair DR, Countess J, Hoopes GS (1974) The effect of relative humidity on the size of atmospheric aerosol particles. Atmos Environ 8:111–117

Sinclair WK (1981) Effects of low-level radiation and compactive risk. Radiology 138:1–9

Slayter EM (1976) Optical methods in biology. Krieger, Huntington, New York

Sneddon SL, Brain JD (1981) Persistent apex to base gradients in aerosol deposition in rats. Respir Physiol 48:113–124

Snipes MB, Clem MF (1981) Retention of microspheres in the rat lung after intratracheal instillation. Environ Res 24:33–41

Snipes MB, Runkle GE, Muggenburg BA (1979) Influence of lavage treatment on the distribution patterns of inhaled, relatively insoluble particles in the lung. Health Phys 37:201–206

Snipes MB, Boecker BB, McClellan RO (1983) Retention of monodisperse or polydisperse aluminosilicate particles inhaled by dogs, rats, and mice. Toxicol Appl Pharmacol 69:345–362

Sorokin SP, Brain JD (1975) Pathways of clearance in mouse lungs exposed to iron oxide aerosols. Anat Rec 181:581–625

Spengler JD, Sexton K (1983) Indoor air pollution: a public health perspective. Science 221:9–17

Stahlhofen W, Gebhart J, Heyder J (1980) Experimental determination of the regional deposition of aerosol particles in the human respiratory tract. Am Ind Hyg Assoc J 41:385–398

Stahlhofen W, Gebhart J, Heyder J (1981). Biological variability of regional deposition of aerosol particles in the human respiratory tract. Am Ind Hyg Assoc 42:348–352

Stauffer D (1975) Scaling theory for aerosol deposition in the lungs of different mammals. J Aerosol Sci 6:223–225

Stirling C, Patrick G (1980) The localisation of particles retained in the trachea of the rat. J Pathol 131:309–320

Sutton D (1982) Radiology and imaging for medical students, 4th edn. Churchill Livingston, New York

Sweeney TD, Brain JD, LeMott S (1983) Anesthesia alters the pattern of aerosol retention in hamsters. J Appl Physiol 54:37–44

Swift DL (1980) Generation and respiratory deposition of therapeutic aerosols. Am Rev Respir Dis 122:71–77

Swift DL, Carpin JC, Mitzner W (1982) Pulmonary penetration and deposition of aerosols in different gases: fluid flow effects. Ann Occup Hyg 26:109–117

Taulbee DB, Yu CP, Heyder J (1978) Aerosol transport in the human lung from analysis of single breaths. J Appl Physiol 44:803–812

Ter-Pogossian MM, Mullani NA, Ficke DC, Markham J, Snyder DL (1981) Photon time-of-flight assisted positron emission tomography. J Comput Assist Tomogr 5:227–239

Thomas RG (1976) Uptake kinetics of relatively insoluble particles by tracheobronchial lymph nodes. In: ERDA (proceedings) Radiation and the lymphatic system. National Technical Information Service, Springfield, Va, pp 67–72

Tillery M (1974) A concentric aerosol spectrometer. Am Ind Hyg Assoc J 35:62–74

US Public Health Service (1979) Surgeon General's report on smoking and health. US DHEW publication PHS79–50066

Valberg PA (1984) Magnetometry of ingested particles in pulmonary macrophages. Science 224:513–516

Valberg PA, Brain JD (1979) Generation and use of three types of iron oxide aerosol. Am Rev Respir Dis 120:1013–1024

Valberg PA, Brain JD, Sneddon SL, LeMott SR (1982) Breathing patterns influence aerosol deposition sites in excised dog lungs. J Appl Physiol 53:824–837

Valberg PA, Wolff RK, Mauderly JL (1983) Redistribution of retained particles: effect of hyperpnea. Am Rev Respir Dis (in press)

Verma DK, Muir DFC, Stewart ML, Julian Ja, JA, Ritchie AC (1982) The dust content of the lungs of hard-rock miners and its relationship to occupational exposure, pathological and radiological findings. Ann Occup Hyg 26:401–409

Walsh PJ, Hamrick PE (1977) Radioactive materials: determinants of dose to the respiratory tract. In: Falk HL, Murphy SD (eds) Reactions of environmental agents. American Physiological Society, Bethesda, pp 233–242 (Handbook of Physiology, sect 9)

Watson AY, Brain JD (1979) Uptake of iron oxide aerosols by mouse airway epithelium. Lab Invest 40:450–459

Weibel ER (1963) Morphometry of the human lung. Academic, New York

Weibel ER (1979) Stereological methods, vol 1. Practical methods for biological morphometry. Academic, New York

Weibel E (1980) Stereological methods, vol 2. Theoretical foundations. Academic, New York

Yeh HC (1980) Respiratory tract deposition models. National Technical Information Service, Springfield, Va, LF-72; UC-48

Yeh HC, Schum GM (1980) Model of human lung airways and their application to inhaled particle deposition. Bull Math Biol 42:461–480

Yu CP, Liu CS, Taulbee DB (1977) Simultaneous diffusion and sedimentation of aerosols in a horizontal cylinder. J Aerosol Sci 8:309–316

General Assessment of Toxic Effects

CHAPTER 4

Animal Models *

P. J. HAKKINEN and H. P. WITSCHI

A. Introduction

Animal models are of great importance in the search for information relevant to the understanding, prevention, treatment, and eradication of human diseases. Both experimentally produced and spontaneous (naturally occurring) models are available which allow us to improve our understanding of the pathophysiology of lung diseases. An additional feature of the spontaneous models is that they allow the study of both the pathogenetic mechanisms and the pathologic features of a particular disease. Along this line, SLAUSON and HAHN (1980) have reviewed selected naturally occurring animal lung diseases that may serve as useful models of human chronic bronchitis, bronchiectasis, emphysema, interstitial lung disease, hypersensitivity pneumonitis, hyaline membrane disease, and bronchial asthma.

Criteria applied to the definition of an ideal animal model for the study of lung cancer etiology, as suggested by ROE (1966), may also be used more broadly. Such specifications, with appropriate modification pertinent to a generalized inhalation exposure animal model include use of small animal species so that large numbers of animals may be studied. Exposure of the animals should occur in as realistic a way as possible, assuming adequate anatomic and physiologic similarity between the respiratory tract of the animal model and humans. Other important considerations include similarities in the site of lesion development and the cell types affected. The end point chosen to determine toxicity should not occur, or occur only with low spontaneous incidence, in the controls. Finally, the potential animal model should biologically handle (absorption, metabolism, storage, and excretion) the material as similarly as possible to humans.

What types of information do animal models provide for the evaluation of inhalation hazards? Carefully executed experiments can identify specific cause-and-effect relationships along with possible effects on overall toxicity and mortality, define pathology and physiopathology of the respiratory tract, detect changes in pulmonary resistance due to infection, and detect extrapulmonary changes. Information is also provided on the maximum tolerated doses in various species, potential human target organs, and on the mechanisms of pulmonary or systemic toxicity.

---

* By acceptance of this article, the publisher or recipient acknowledges the U. S. Government's right to retain a nonexclusive, royalty-free license in and to any copyright covering the article

This chapter is a review of some advantages and disadvantages of different species used as models for inhalation toxicity testing. Where appropriate, specific selected animal models of human pulmonary disease will be discussed. General information on care, diseases, physiologic data, special procedures, spontaneous neoplasms, and genetics of various species of laboratory animals are available (MELBY and ALTMANN 1974a, b, 1976; ALTMANN and KATZ 1979a, b, c; HARKNESS and WAGNER 1977).

B. Advantages and Disadvantages of Different Species

I. Mice

The advantages of using mice in inhalation toxicity studies are their small size, the low purchase and maintenance costs, ready availability, and the ease by which they can be handled and exposed. Other major advantages are the vast amount of genetic, biochemical, physiologic, and pathologic information available on the numerous strains being used in biomedical research. General information on the more widely used or more unusual of the more than 300 inbred or clearly defined substrains is available (ALTMAN and KATZ 1976a, b, c; HEINIGER and DOREY 1980; CRISPENS 1975; FOSTER et al. 1981; MELBY and Altman 1976).

The small body size of mice is of some advantage in studies on cell renewal and cell turnover in lung with autoradiogrpahic techniques. Injection of $1–2$ µCi ^{3}H-labeled thymidine per gram body weight, $1–2$ h prior to killing usually provides sufficient labeled thymidine to keep exposure time of autoradiograms prepared from lung tissue within practical limits ($2–4$ weeks). Although data on cell turnover in larger species such as rat are available, most of the knowledge on cell turnover in lung has been obtained in mice (KAUFMANN 1980).

Small osmotic pumps (minipumps, Alza Corporation, Palo Alto, California) have become available which can be implanted subcutaneously or intraperitoneally. These pumps will deliver a continuous rate of solution for up to 2 weeks from models designed for small rats and mice and up to 1 month from models designed for larger animals. One use of minipumps in mice involves the continuous administration of thymidine ^{3}H to study the cumulative labeling index of mouse lung alveolar cells. This technique has been used to study the cell kinetics in lung injury produced by the antioxidant butylated hydroxytoluene (HASCHEK et al. 1983). Another use of osmotic pumps in lung research in mice involved bleomycin-induced pulmonary toxicity following continuous infusion compared with intermittent injection (SIKIC et al. 1978).

Because of their small size, short reproduction time, and the vast amount of genetic information available for the species, mice have been used for mutagenesis testing. The mouse spot test reflects the induction of mutations in several genes as manifested in the appearance of coat spots which are observable 2 weeks after birth following in utero treatment. While initially developed for radiation mutagenesis, it has now been used as a method for detection of chemically induced somatic mutations, including those following exposure to volatile mutagenic agents. The test provides an alternative or adjunct to microbial and cell culture assay systems with the advantage that in vivo assessment is made of the ability of a compound or active metabolite to cross the placental barrier and induce somatic mutations (reviewed by NEUHAUSER-KLAUS 1981; BUTTERWORTH 1981).

Certain genetically well-defined mouse strains may provide interesting models of pulmonary disease. The blotchy mouse is such an example of a genetically defined defect altering a biochemical response to a toxicant. Blotchy mice have a genetic defect that prevents formation of the lysine-derived aldehyde necessary for cross-linking of collagen and elastin. The lungs of this mouse strain show many morphological characteristics typical of emphysema and may serve as a useful spontaneous animal model for certain studies of emphysema (reviewed by SLAUSON and HAHN 1980). This strain has been used to produce accelerated development of emphysema and persistent bronchiolitis as a result of nitrogen dioxide inhalation (RANGA and KLEINERMAN 1981). Recently, a gene mutation of interest as a potential spontaneous model of interstitial lung disease has been described in mice. The "motheaten" mouse is homozygous for a single-gene recessive mutation and dies at 8 weeks of age from a noninfectious, chronic interstitial lung disease characterized by alveolar hemorrhage, macrophage neutrophil alveolitis, and fibrosis, along with localized immunologic alterations in the levels of T-cells, neutrophils, and immunoglobulin-secreting cells (ROSSI et al. 1982).

The mouse has also been the species most extensively investigated in the elucidation of the role of genetic factors in strain differences in toxicant metabolism and toxicity. Marked differences have been found in strain capacities to induce microsomal mixed-function oxidase (MFO) enzyme system activities following inducing agents. For instance, lung microsomal MFO (aryl hydrocarbon hydroxylase) activity in various mouse strains is induced to different degrees by cigarette smoke (ABRAMSON and HUTTON 1975). Furthermore, the mouse, along with the rat, have been the species most used in the study of the role of MFO-mediated formation of active metabolites from agents including 3-methylfuran, 4-ipomeanol, and carbon tetrachloride in lung injury (reviewed by BOYD 1980). Finally, in a five-species comparison (mouse, rat, hamster, rabbit, and guinea pig), all were found to have substantially less pulmonary enzyme activity than hepatic activity. Noteworthy was the observation that mouse lung was found to contain considerably more glutathione S-arylsulfatase activity than the other species (LITTERST et al. 1975).

Aside from MFO induction studies, mouse lung biochemistry has not been studied in great depth. However, it has been shown that when exposed to 95% oxygen, neonatal mice show rapid increases in lung antioxidant enzyme activities whereas adult mice show no enzyme response to hyperoxia (FRANK et al. 1978).

A disadvantage of using mice as a species for lung studies is the susceptibility of pulmonary infection, particularly by Sendai virus. Mouse strains vary widely in their susceptibility to Sendai virus infection. Compared with rats, hamsters, and guinea pigs, mice are susceptible to the greatest number of rodent viruses although it should be noted that such common rodent viruses such as Sendai virus, reovirus, and pneumonia virus of mice can infect all of these species (reviewed by JACOBY and BARTHOLD 1981).

Chronic Sendai virus-induced lesions may confuse the interpretation of respiratory toxicology experiments with the marked squamous metaplasia of the respiratory epithelium observed possibly appearing similar to lesions induced by inhalation of toxicants. Sendai virus infection may also alter the immune response of mice and rats (reviewed by Jacoby and Barthold 1981; Boorman 1981).

Mycoplasma pulmonis is the most common chronic microbial agent of mice and rats and induces a contagious, chronic inflammatory disease of the respiratory tract. Once a mouse or rat colony is infected, it remains infected. Like Sendai virus infection, M. pulmonis infection may confuse interpretation of experimentally induced lesions or enhance their severity. Mycoplasmosis can also increase the susceptibility of rodents to other microorganisms, resulting in the development of bacterial pneumonia together with mycoplasmal pneumonia (reviewed by Jacoby and Barthold 1981; Boorman 1981).

In contrast to other species of laboratory animals, such as the rat and rabbit, little work on isolated cells from mouse lungs has been done. BALB/c mice given injections of urethane develop lung adenomas with the morphological appearance of alveolar type II cells. These adenomas have been dissected and used for studies of surfactant production (Wykle et al. 1977, 1980; Voelker and Snyder 1979). Primary mixed monolayer cultures and explants of mouse lungs have also been studied (see Chap. 7).

Along with the development of animal models of human pulmonary disease, attempts have been made to develop and apply techniques of sampling and measurement of pulmonary disease that can be applied to humans (see for example Wilson et al. 1976; Hollinger et al. 1980; Roth 1981; DeNicola et al. 1981; Newman et al. 1981). In the case of mice, advantages such as low cost and ease of exposure are offset by difficulties of detecting damage by measuring pulmonary function changes owing to higher rates of respiration and smaller lung volumes. However, the use of whole body plethysmographs has shown that increases in respiratory rate correlated well with lung morphological changes (pneumonitis and fibrosis) following exposure to the antineoplastic agent cyclophosphamide or thoracic X-irradiation (Travis et al. 1979, 1980; Collis et al. 1980). Tidal volume and functional residual capacity can also be measured in conscious mice (Vinegar et al. 1979). Parameters of pulmonary function have also been studied in anesthetized mice (lung volumes, compliance) (Vinegar et al. 1979) and using excised mice lungs (compliance) (Weiss and Weiss 1976; Morstatter et al. 1976).

II. Rats

A comparatively larger body of information is available on rat lung physiology, biochemistry, and morphology compared with mice or other species. Basic physiologic, biochemical, immunologic, and other data can be found in Altman and Katz (1979 b) and in Melby and Altman (1976). Additional sources of information include Baker et al. (1979, 1980) and a recent review by Oser (1981). Finally, a recent review by Mondino (1980) partially focused on the history of the rat as the animal of choice in biomedical research and on strain and species differences in toxicity.

As with mice, the comparatively small size of the rat permits large numbers to be used in a study. Other advantages include low price due to widespread use, the short lifetime compared with larger experimental species (of use in lifetime studies), and their good disposition. Disadvantages such as lack of gallbladder and no emetic reflex may play more of a role in nonpulmonary toxicity studies (reviewed by BRIGGS and OEHME 1980; OSER 1981).

The larger size of the rat, compared with the mouse allows for more types of, and more extensive, laboratory procedures and perhaps surgery to be performed. Blood pressure and blood sampling are easily done and are well tolerated. Furthermore, rats are much easier to use than mice in studies in which lung function changes (respiratory rates, lung volumes, diffusing capacity, compliance, flow resistance) are used to detect damage (see for example O'NEIL 1981; DIAMOND and O'DONNELL 1977; HOLUB and FRANK 1979; TAKEZAWA et al. 1980; BEVEN 1980; SILVER 1981; KIDA and THURLBECK 1980).

Another advantage of using rats for an animal model of human lung disease is that the morphology is well known and that morphometric data, for normal and toxicant-exposed (O_2, NO_2) rat lungs are available (see for example KISTLER et al. 1967; HAIES et al. 1981; CRAPO et al. 1978, 1980).

Although the rat has been shown to have low pulmonary MFO activity in comparison with other common laboratory species, rats have been the subject of numerous investigations of lung oxidant metabolism (see Chap. 14). Furthermore, techniques are available which allow isolation of several purified lung cell populations from rat lung. Cell types isolated and, on occasion, maintained in culture include alveolar macrophages, alveolar type II epithelial cells, and endothelial cells. Such cells have helped in the study of lung metabolism, including MFO activity, and fatty acid and surfactant phospholipid synthesis. Cultured mesothelial cells and tracheal explants from rats have also been studied (see Chap. 7). Finally, although the advantages of isolated perfused lung preparations over intact animal experiments in the study of the nonrespiratory functions of the lung are not detailed here, it should be noted that rats and rabbits are the species most often used as a source of these preparations (reviewed by MEHENDALE et al. 1981).

Rats appear to behave somewhat differently toward oxygen toxicity than do most other small laboratory species. When various species are exposed to 95% or more of oxygen, differences arise as to the response of the lung antioxidant enzymes (superoxide dismutase, catalase, and glutathione peroxidase). Neonatal rats, mice, and rabbits show rapid and significant increases in the activities of these antioxidant enzymes during hyperoxia along with minimal evidence of lung pathology. Neonatal guinea pigs and hamsters show no lung antioxidant enzyme response to hyperoxia and die. In contrast, adult animals from all five species exposed to hyperoxia die within 3–5 days of $\geq 95\%$ oxygen exposure (FRANK et al. 1978). However, adult rats can tolerate 100% oxygen for long periods if they are preexposed to 85% oxygen for 5–7 days (ROSENBAUM et al. 1969) with at least partial explanation being increased activities of the lung superoxide dismutase (CRAPO et al. 1980). The other species cannot be made tolerant to oxygen.

Rats develop a wide variety of spontaneous lesions with the incidence of benign mammary gland tumors varying from 10% to 40%, depending on the age and strain of the rats (reviewed by BOORMAN 1981). This can be a serious obstacle if rats are to be exposed over a lifetime in a head-only inhalation chamber because to fit tumor-bearing animals into a holder, tumors must be removed.

It must be kept in mind that with a small number of human subjects in a toxicity study of inhaled materials, one may fail to include individuals such as asthmatics or members of the significant proportion of healthy humans who breath predominately orally at rest. These people are or may be unusually sensitive to air pollutants. Any results obtained in a limited study may underestimate the risk to sensitive individuals. For example, asthmatics develop bronchoconstriction at considerably lower concentrations of inhaled SO_2 than healthy people without asthma (SHEPPARD et al. 1980). This makes it somewhat difficult to extrapolate from laboratory studies to humans and to estimate fully and precisely the risk of chemical exposure to all segments of the population. To make such extrapolations easier, efforts to develop homogeneous populations of laboratory animals as models for human asthma have resulted in development of a rat strain which develops asthma-like symptoms upon antigen challenge (HOLME and PIECHUTA 1981).

It has been said that the susceptibility of the rat to chronic respiratory disease may make it necessary to keep the animals in inhalation studies under germ-free or specific pathogen-free conditions (ROE 1966). *M. pulmonis* appears to be the main, and in many cases, the sole agent causing chronic respiratory disease in rats (reviewed by SLAUSON and HAHN 1980; BOORMAN 1981). The advantage of using a species resistant to respiratory infections has been shown in a study which found that chronic respiratory disease in rats increased the susceptibility to lung cancer caused by a systemically administered carcinogen (SCHREIBER et al. 1972). However, it is of interest to note that the high susceptibility of rats to develop chronic respiratory disease may one day make this species useful in the study of the pathogenesis of chronic airway damage and bronchiectasis (reviewed by SLAUSON and HAHN 1980). Finally, in addition to being a mouse respiratory pathogen, Sendai virus has also been implicated in rat respiratory disease, although, in contrast to mice, increased mortality and clinical signs may not be observed (reviewed by BOORMAN 1981).

III. Hamsters

The Syrian golden hamster has been used in biomedical research for approximately 50 years. More than 25 inbred lines of hamsters are now available. They have been found to be well suited for a wide range of studies and have been used in cheek pouch tumor growth, transplantation and carcinogenesis studies, genetics and aging studies, cardiovascular research, and studies in virology, bacteriology, psychology, and other fields. Their larger size makes them far more suitable for biochemical and hematologic studies than the mouse. Hamsters are easily handled although their rudimentary tail makes it difficult to grab them or to perform intravenous injections (reviewed by STREILEIN 1979; HOMBURGER 1976). Hamsters have been said to be very susceptible to several bacterial and viral diseases. However, although they are susceptible to many experimental infections, they are said to be free of disease if adequate protection measures are provided (reviewed by HOMBURGER 1976).

A large amount of information is available on spontaneous tumor development, induced tumors, behavior patterns, biochemistry, and physiology of hamsters (ALTMAN and KATZ 1979 a, b, c). Additional information on spontaneous diseases of hamsters is available (POUR and BIRT 1979; ARNOLD and GRICE 1979).

The respiratory system of hamsters has recently been compared with that of other species (KENNEDY and LITTLE 1979).

The hamster has been shown to be the animal of choice for the development of an animal model for human bronchogenic carcinoma. This species was selected because of the low incidence of spontaneous lung tumors and also because, among the small laboratory animal species, it is the one most free of spontaneous respiratory disease. Intratracheal instillation of carcinogens gave up to 100% incidences of respiratory tract tumors (mostly bronchogenic carcinomas) which are histologically very close to those found in human lung cancers (SAFFIOTTI et al. 1968). However, the hamster does lack both tracheal and bronchial mucus glands and thus cannot develop a condition similar to human chronic bronchitis (ROE 1966).

The use of hamsters in the production of laryngeal cancer following exposure to cigarette smoke has been reviewed (HOMBURGER 1976; BERNFELD et al. 1979; HOFFMANN et al. 1979). Other data on the use of the Syrian hamster in inhalation toxicology research are available (WEHNER et al. 1979). Tests are available for the assessment of changes in hamster pulmonary function (diffusing capacity, lung volumes) (see for example TAKEZAWA et al. 1980; SNIDER et al. 1978; KOO et al. 1976; SNIDER et al. 1977).

Although rats and rabbits have been the species most often used for isolation of alveolar type II and other lung cells, PFLEGER (1977) reported success in the isolation of type II cells capable of phospholipid synthesis from Syrian hamsters. Epithelial cells from hamster trachea have been isolated and cultured, and the secretion of mucous glycoproteins has been studied. Hamster tracheal explants have also been studied (see Chap. 7).

Hamsters have been shown to be remarkably resistant to toxic inhalants such as bacterial aerosols, cigarette smoke or, 3-methylfuran and to systemically (intraperitoneally) administered toxicants such as nicotine tartrate, 4-ipomeanol, and methylcyclopentadienyl manganese tricarbonyl when compared with mice and/or rats (EHRLICH 1966; HOMBURGER 1976; DUTCHER and BOYD 1979; HAKKINEN and HASCHEK 1982).

IV. Rabbits

Two key sources of information on the rabbit as a laboratory animal are ALTMAN and KATZ (1979c) and WEISBROTH et al. (1974). Rabbits have an advantage of interest to pulmonary toxicologists: compared with rats, mice, hamsters, and guinea pigs, they have a much higher activity of the lung MFO system. This has been taken advantage of in numerous metabolic studies (see Chap. 14). The rabbit has also seen use as the animal of choice in numerous studies using isolated perfused lung preparations (reviewed by MEHENDALE et al. 1981).

The isolation of heterogeneous cell populations, alveolar macrophages, alveolar type I epithelial, type II epithelial, and nonciliated bronchiolar epithelial (Clara) cells from rabbit lungs have enabled the study of lung metabolism, MFO activity, surfactant phospholipid synthesis, and cellular membrane components associated with individual cell types (see Chap. 7). Tests are available for the assessment of changes in rabbit pulmonary function (diffusing capacity, lung volumes) (TAKEZAWA et al. 1980). Spontaneous neoplasms in laboratory and commercial rabbits are apparently low in incidence although bronchial carcinoma and epithelioma and lung carcinoma have been reported (reviewed by STEDHAM 1976).

V. Guinea Pigs

General information on biology of the guinea pig can be found in ALTMAN and KATZ (1979c) and in WAGNER and MANNING (1976). Guinea pigs are expensive, but easy to obtain, easy to handle, and have a body weight between that of the rat and rabbit. However, relatively few inbred strains and mutants are available and blood collection and intravenous injections are difficult owing to the absence of large superficial blood vessels. Guinea pigs are also said to be relatively susceptible to many infections. Among the small laboratory animals, the guinea pig is said to resemble humans most closely in hormonal balance, reproductive physiology, and immune response (reviewed by DE WECK and FESTING 1979).

Guinea pigs have been used in research on physiology, immunology, genetics, otology, infectious diseases, parasitology, nutrition (like humans and other primates they require vitamin C in the diet), and oncology. The use of the guinea pig in toxicity and teratology studies has been reviewed (HOAR 1976). With regard to inhalation toxicology, AMDUR and MEAD (1958) demonstrated that pulmonary function testing in guinea pigs was practical. They reported baseline values in unanesthetized animals for tidal volume, respiratory rate, minute volume, resistance, and compliance. Additional work by AMDUR et al. (1978a, b) described the effects of irritant gases in combination with aerosols, the effects of histamine aerosols and other inhaled gases and aerosols on lung physiology and pathology. Recent references for guinea pig pulmonary function assessment include TAKEZAWA et al. (1980), SKORNIK et al. (1981), and AGRAWAL (1981).

The guinea pig has been considered by some to be unsuitable for the study of the effects of inhaled materials because of a potential to respond to respiratory irritation by developing an asthmatic type of bronchial spasm (ROE 1966). However, strains of guinea pigs are now available which have bronchial walls that are either sensitive or insensitive to chemical mediators or have high and low responsiveness to ovalbumin-induced respiratory anaphylaxis (TAKINO et al. 1970; LUNDBERG 1979). A method has been described which allows testing of pulmonary function in guinea pigs without the need for restraint, anesthesia, and surgery (WONG and ALARIE 1982). A whole body plethysmograph was used to measure the tidal volume and respiratory rate during exposure to air or a mixture of 10% CO_2, 20% O_2, and 70% nitrogen. Inhalation of CO_2 produces an increase in tidal volume and respiratory rate in normal animals with increased lung flow resistance resulting in a diminished ventilatory response to CO_2. The applicability of this method to assess lung injury and recovery following exposure to an inhaled toxicant was shown by the production of concentration-related reductions in CO_2-induced increases in tidal volume and respiratory frequency following inhalation of a sulfuric acid mist.

In the guinea pig, spontaneous tumors are rare and spontaneous pulmonary tumors are of bronchial origin with adenomas far more common that adenocarcinomas. It is difficult to induce tumors with carcinogens in the guinea pig (reviewed by ROBINSON 1976; DE WECK and FESTING 1979). In the area of guinea pig lung biochemistry, an odd response has been noted of the MFO system to enzyme inducers such as cigarette smoke, benzo[a]pyrene, 3-methylcholanthrene, and Arochlor 1254 (see Chap. 14).

VI. Dogs

The dog has been said to be an unsatisfactory species for pulmonary carcinogenesis experiments because acute and chronic pneumonitis along with bronchial metaplasia often occur (RIDGON and CORSSEN 1963). However, it has also been said by S. W. Nielsen (quoted in STUART 1976) that "... the dog is of sufficient size and longevity to serve as an useful experimental model for various pulmonary physiological and pathologic studies, which may require training, surgical intervention, and other experimental techniques that cannot be done in the common small laboratory rodent. The dog, more than any other species, approximates man in its environment and living habits." Studies on aerosol deposition related to particle size, lung morphology, respiratory physiology parameters, and blood gas characterization also compare very favorably to that observed in humans (reviewed by STUART 1976).

Spontaneous pulmonary neoplasms found in dogs include malignant tumors of the nasal cavity, pharynx, larynx, trachea, lung, and bronchi. Of significance is the observation that the only two species of animals which have pulmonary anaplastic and squamous cell carcinomas are the animals most commonly associated with humans, the dog and cat (reviewed by NIELSEN 1976).

The dog was used as the donor in the first major demonstration of the utility of isolated perfused lungs in the study of the nonrespiratory function of the lung when it was shown that the lung was the major site of conversion of circulating angiotensin I to angiotensin II. This observation was followed by numerous other studies in several species of the possible uptake, metabolism, and release of compounds, including vasoactive amines, drugs, steroids, and prostaglandins (reviewed by ROTH 1979; MEHENDALE et al. 1981).

In research on chronic obstructive pulmonary disease, a canine model of functional α_1-antitrypsin deficiency has been produced by systemic administration of the oxidizing agent chloramine-T. The results suggest that loss of the elastase inhibitory site on α_1-antitrypsin can lead to spontaneous development of morphological changes associated with emphysema (ELIRAZ et al. 1980; DAMIANO et al. 1980).

Chronic bronchitis has been found to affect mainly smaller dogs of middle age or older and has been presented as a possible spontaneous pulmonary disease in dogs which closely resembles, both clinically and pathologically, human chronic bronchitis (reviewed by SLAUSON and HAHN 1980). Dogs also seem to be the only animals which develop a defined hypersensitivity disease related to airborne allergens, including ragweed pollen, grass, and house dust. In the laboratory setting, dogs with pollen allergy will almost always develop a respiratory response to aerosolized antigen (reviewed by SLAUSON and HAHN 1980). In particular, the Basenji-Greyhound dog, unlike the typical mongrel dog, displays nonspecific airway hyperreactivity which has led to its use in asthma research (see for example, Hirshman et al. 1981). The Basenji-Greyhound dog model of asthma is also said to provide an approach to the immunologic mechanisms involved in antigen-induced airway constriction independent of the effects of nonspecific airway hyperreactivity (Peters et al. 1982). Tests are available for the assessment of changes in dog pulmonary function (Robinson et al. 1972; Park et al. (1977). As with other large animals, exposure of dogs to aerosol can create some technical problems. Dogs have been exposed in large inhalation chambers as well as by face mask or even through tracheotomies.

VII. Cats

The cat has been deemed to be an inappropriate species for inhalation exposure studies because it may respond to respiratory irritation by producing an abundance of thin serous secretion in which it may "drown" (Roe 1966). However, in an effort to validate and extend to another species the vast body of work on exposure of guinea pigs to air pollutants, Corn et al. (1972) chose the cat owing to the availability of data on the mechanisms of bronchoconstriction and peripheral airway constriction in the cat and also because the techniques to be used were well developed.

The effects of ozone and sulfur dioxide inhalation on pulmonary function in cats have been studied (Corn et al. 1972; Watanabe et al. 1973) and the tests available for the assessment of changes in cat pulmonary function (volumes, diffusing capacity) have been detailed further by Watanabe and Frank (1975). Cats have also been studied for the effects of inhaled irritants including cigarette smoke, ammonia, and NO_2 on tracheal mucus transport rates (Carson et al. 1966).

VIII. Sheep

Sheep are rather docile, although on occasion stubborn creatures, and have been used mainly in studies on the physiology and pathophysiology of the pulmonary circulation (see for example Küng et al. 1978; Lock et al. 1980; Goetzman and Milstein 1980). Both drug- and antigen-induced bronchoconstriction have been recently studied in sheep (Wanner et al. 1979; Abraham et al. 1981). Sheep have also seen use in the development of a venous air emboli model in the study of lung microvascular permeability injury (Ohkuda et al. 1981). Fetal and newborn lambs have seen extensive use in studies of lung physiology, including prostaglandin action and surfactant and tracheal fluid production (see for example Jobe et al. 1980; Kitterman 1981). A study has validated the use of the respiratory inductive plethysmograph as a noninvasive monitor of pulmonary function (tidal volume, respiratory rate) in sheep (Abraham et al. 1981).

Calabrese et al. (1977) have identified people with a genetically inherited condition of glucose-6-phosphate dehydrogenase (G6PD) deficiency as a potential high-risk population for hemolytic anemia in response to elevated ambient levels of ozone. In efforts to develop animal models that simulate exposure of a human high-risk group to ozone, they have studied both mice and sheep with low levels of G6PD in their erythrocytes (CALABRESE 1978; MOORE et al. 1981). Both deficient species models have been shown to have G6PD levels comparable to that found in deficient humans. However, while G6PD-deficient humans also have significantly lower amounts of reduced glutathione (GSH) which protects erythrocytes from oxidative damage, G6PD-deficient mice actually have higher levels of GSH than their high G6PD counterparts. The validity of the mouse model in simulating exposure of a human high-risk group to ozone remains to be shown (CALABRESE 1978). Studies with the G6PD-deficient sheep found that the sheep were not as sensitive to ozone as predicted, with no statistically significant biochemical changes observed except for a significant GSH decrease with a high level ozone exposure (0.5 ppm for 2.75 h) (MOORE et al. 1981). It is also of interest to note that glutathione-deficient sheep do not show an increased sensitivity to oxidant drugs (SMITH 1976).

IX. Horses and Donkeys

Aerosol deposition and clearance studies have been done with the horse (reviewed by STUART 1976). Primary tumors of the lower respiratory tract of horses are rare with granular cell tumors being the most common (NICKELS et al. 1980). Among the best studied chronic lung diseases in horses is emphysema, a condition that is not well documented in other species (reviewed by SLAUSON and HAHN 1980).

The donkey has seen extensive use as a model for study of the effects of inhaled toxicants, including cigarette smoke and SO_2, on bronchial clearance (see for example ALBERT et al. 1974). Recently, long-term clearance of ferrimagnetic magnetite particles was studied using magnetic field detection on unsedated donkeys (HALPERN et al. 1981).

X. Goats

Goats, cattle, and sheep have been used extensively to study 3-methylindole-induced pulmonary toxicity (edema and emphysema) following intravenous and intraruminal administration (see for example HUANG et al. 1977; BRADLEY et al. 1978; DICKINSON et al. 1976; CARLSON et al. 1972, 1975). The morphology of the goat lung has also led to this species being suggested as a model for studies on high-altitude pulmonary adjustment and response to polluted environments (ATWAL and SWEENY 1971). The goat has also seen use as a model for pulmonary and systemic circulatory system studies (see for example CASSIN et al. 1979; CHAND 1981; LARSEN et al. 1981).

XI. Pigs

The pig has become a commonly used animal for hematologic, cardiac, and cardiovascular models. Miniature swine have been used in inhalation studies of potential toxicants for several decades. Advantages of the pig as a model for humans include its easy availability, body size, and long life span and the close similarities of the gastrointestinal, circulatory, skeletal, endocrine, reticuloendothelial systems, skin, and nutritional requirements to that of humans (reviewed by STUART 1976; DODDS 1982). The size and growth rate of the pig have also been cited as advantages for physiologic and surgical studies.

Because of its "vigorous response to hypoxia," the pig has been used for iso-lated perfused lung experiments in which the pulmonary vasodilator and constric-tor responses to hypoxia were studied (Sylvester et al. 1980). Both piglets and foals have been shown to develop naturally occurring hyaline membrane disease (reviewed by Slauson and Hahn 1980).

XII. Cattle

Cattle seem prone to develop interstitial lung disease with proliferative interstitial pneumonia which has morphological similarities to human interstitial pneumoni-tis. Hypersensitivity pneumonitis (extrinsic allergic alveolitis) has been best de-scribed in cattle and horses and is clinically, etiologically, immunologically, and morphologically similar to the human disease counterpart. Eosinophilic bron-chiolitis of cattle may represent a potential animal model for human bronchial asthma (reviewed by Slauson and Hahn 1980).

XIII. Nonhuman Primates

Nonhuman primates have seen extensive use as neurologic and physiologic mod-els for humans. The morphology of the nonhuman primate lung is very similar to that of humans and numerous studies with inhaled pollutants have been per-formed (reviewed by Stuart 1976). Spontaneous neoplasms in nonhuman pri-mates are not rare. Pulmonary neoplasms which have been described include sar-coma, carcinoma, and carcinoid and alveolar tumors (reviewed by Griesemer 1976).

The use of nonhuman primates (baboons, rhesus monkeys, and cynomolgus monkeys) as an animal model for human oxygen toxicity has been reviewed by Robinson et al. (1974). The baboon is the species of choice because both rhesus monkeys and cynomolgus monkeys have a greater frequency of naturally occur-ring pulmonary lesions from mite infestations. The similarity of the pathologic response of these nonhuman primates to human oxygen toxicity makes them the choice over other animal species (dog, rat, and mouse) (Robinson et al. 1974).

The difficulty and cost of obtaining and maintaining nonhuman primates are disadvantages of using these kinds of animals for experiments. In a study of ozone-induced alterations in pulmonary collagen metabolism in monkeys, lung biopsy specimens were taken for biochemical analysis before and after exposure to ozone (Last et al. 1981). Thus, each animal served as its own control, allowing fewer animals to be used in the study. In research on the development of an ani-mal model for chronic obstructive pulmonary disease, the feasibility of using chloramine-T to develop a monkey model of α_1-antitrypsin deficiency has been demonstrated (Cohen 1979).

C. Conclusions

Many factors are involved in the selection of an appropriate animal species for human lung disease. Differences in anatomy, physiology, and biochemical re-sponse to inhaled materials all play a role in deciding how appropriate a species is for study. It must also be kept in mind that strain differences in response may exist and that the age of the animal may also play a role in the potential development of disease.

In addition, the successful completion of an inhalation toxicity study is not just the product of using an appropriate animal species, but rather of careful generation and characterization of the inhaled material and close attention to the health of the animals before and after exposure, including minimization of uncontrolled variables such as concomitant respiratory infection. Numerous other factors can also significantly modify the biologic response of an animal to a toxicant, including the methods and amounts of handling, population density, cleanliness of the cage, cage type, bedding material, noise, light cycles, temperature, humidity, mixing of sexes within the same room, and the amount of adaptation time allowed after transfer from one location to another. Large day-to-day variations in microsomal enzyme activity can also occur (reviewed by LANG and VESELL 1976; VESELL et al. 1976). Thus, even if a suitable animal model for human lung disease is found, problems in producing a realistic exposure to an inhaled material may arise along with other problems.

Finally, as noted by REID (1980), it must be remembered that the usefulness of animal models is only limited by the questions that are asked of them. It should also be kept in mind that a model for a human pulmonary disease can result from as simple a treatment as starvation. Of interest as an animal model for human emphysema is the recent observation that starvation of rats until they lose 40% of their initial body weight leads to mechanical, morphological, and ultrastructural changes that are indistinguishable from naturally occurring or enzyme-induced emphysema. In fact, the starvation model holds the advantage over enzyme-induced emphysema in that, rather than involving severe initial injury, starvation-induced changes, like human emphysema development, occur gradually (SAHEB-JAMI and WIRMAN 1981).

Acknowledgements. This research was jointly sponsored by the Office of Health and Environmental Research, U.S. Department of Energy, under contract W-1405-eng-26, with the Union Carbide Corporation. P.J. HAKKINEN is a postdoctoral investigator, supported by subcontract 3322 from the Biology Division of Oak Ridge National Laboratory to the University of Tennessee.

References

Abraham WM, Watson H, Schneider A, King M, Yerger L, Sackner MA (1981) Noninvasive ventilatory monitoring by respiratory inductive plethysmography in conscious sheep. J Appl Physiol 51:1657–1661

Abramson RK, Hutton JJ (1975) Effects of cigarette smoking on aryl hydrocarbon hydroxylase activity in lungs and tissues of inbred mice. Cancer Res 35:23–29

Agrawal KP (1981) Specific airways conductance in guinea pigs: normal values and histamine induced fall. Respir Physiol 43:23–30

Albert RE, Berger J, Sanborn K, Lippmann M (1974) Effects of cigarette smoke components on bronchial clearance in the donkey. Arch Environ Health 29:96–101

Altman RL, Katz DD (eds) (1979a) I. Mouse. Inbred and genetically defined strains of laboratory animals, part 1. Mouse and rat. Federation of American Societies for Experimental Biology, Bethesda, Maryland, pp 9–232 (Biological handbooks, vol 3)

Altman RL, Katz DD (eds) (1979 b) II. Rat. Inbred and genetically defined strains of laboratory animals, part 1. Mouse and rat. Federation of American Societies for Experimental Biology, Bethesda, Maryland, pp 233–362 (Biological handbooks, vol 3)

Altman RL, Katz DD (eds) (1979 c) III. Hamster. Inbred and genetically defined strains of laboratory animals, part 2. Hamster, guinea pig, rabbit, and chicken. Federation of American Societies for Experimental Biology, Bethesda, Maryland, pp 425–504 (Biological handbooks, vol 3)

Altman RL, Katz DD (eds) (1979 d) IV. Guinea pig. Inbred and genetically defined strains of laboratory animals, part 2. Hamster, guinea pig, rabbit, and chicken. Federation of American Societies for Experimental Biology, Bethesda, Maryland, pp 505–563 (Biological handbook, vol 3)

Altman RL, Katz DD (eds) (1979 e) V. Rabbit. Inbred and genetically defined strains of laboratory animals, part 2. Hamster, guinea pig, rabbit, and chicken. Federation of American Societies for Experimental Biology, Bethesda, Maryland, pp 565–606 (Biological handbooks, vol 3)

Amdur MO, Mead J (1958) Mechanics of respiration in unanesthetized guinea pigs. Am J Physiol 192:364–368

Amdur MO, Dubriel M, Creasia DA (1978 a) Respiratory response of guinea pigs to low levels of sulfuric acid. Environ Res 15:418–423

Amdur MO, Bayles J, Ugro V, Underhill DW (1978 b) Comparative irritant potency of sulfate salts. Environ Res 16:1–8

Arnold DL, Grice HC (1979) The use of the Syrian hamster in toxicology studies, with emphasis on carcinogenesis bioassay. In: Homburger F (ed) The Syrian hamster in toxicology and carcinogenesis research. Prog Exp Tumor Res 24:222–234

Atwal OS, Sweeny PR (1971) Ultrastructure of the interalveolar septum of the lung of the goat. Am J Vet Res 32:1999–2010

Baker HJ, Lindsey JR, Weisbroth SH (eds) (1979) The laboratory rat, vol 1. Biology and diseases. Academic, New York, pp 1–435

Baker JH, Lindsey JR, Weisbroth SH (eds) (1980) The laboratory rat, vol 2. Research applications. Academic, New York, pp 1–276

Bernfeld P, Homburger F, Russfield AB (1979) Cigarette smoke-induced cancer of the larynx in hamster (cinch): a method to assay the carcinogenicity of cigarette smoke. In: Homburger F (ed) The Syrian hamster in toxicology and carcinogenesis research. Prog Exp Tumor Res 24:315–319

Beven JL (1980) A new system for monitoring respiratory patterns of small laboratory animals. Lab Anim 14:133–135

Boorman GA (1981) Spontaneous lesions of importance for long-term toxicity testing in rats and mice. In: Gralla EJ (ed) Scientific considerations in monitoring and evaluating toxicological research. Hemisphere, Washington, pp 89–121

Boyd MR (1980) Biochemical mechanisms in chemical-induced lung injury: roles of metabolic activation. CRC Crit Rev Toxicol 7:103–176

Bradley BJ, Carlson JR, Dickinson EO (1978) 3-methylindole-induced pulmonary edema and emphysema in sheep. Am J Vet Res 39:1355–1359

Briggs GR, Oehme FW (1980) Toxicology. In: Baker HJ, Lindsey JR, Weisbroth SH (eds) The laboratory rat, vol 2. Research applications. Academic, New York, pp 104–118

Butterworth BE (1981) Predictive assays for mutagens and carcinogens. In: Gralla EJ (ed) Scientific considerations in monitoring and evaluating toxicological research. Hemisphere, Washington, pp 157–177

Calabrese EJ (1978) Animal model of human disease. Increased sensitivity to ozone. Animal model: mice with low levels of G-6-PD. Am J Pathol 91:409–411

Calabrese EJ, Kojola WH, Carnow BW (1977) Ozone: a possible cause of hemolytic anemia in glucose-6-phosphate dehydrogenase deficient individuals. J Toxicol Environ Health 2:709–712

Carlson JR, Yokoyama MT, Dickinson EO (1972) Induction of pulmonary edema and emphysema in cattle and goats with 3-methylindole. Science 176:298–299

Carlson JR, Dickinson EO, Yokoyama MT, Bradley B (1975) Pulmonary edema and emphysema in cattle after intraruminal and intravenous administration of 3-methylindole. Am J Vet Res 36:1341–1347

Carson S, Goldhamer R, Carpenter R (1966) Responses of ciliated epithelium to irritants. Mucus transport in the respiratory tract. Am Rev Respir Dis 93 (Suppl):86–92

Cassin S, Tyler T, Leffler C, Wallis R (1979) Pulmonary and systemic vascular responses of perinatal goats to prostaglandins E_1 and E_2. Am J Physiol 236:H828–H832

Chand N (1981) 5-hydroxytryptamine induces relaxation of goat pulmonary veins: evidence for the noninvolvement of M and D-tryptamine receptors. Br J Pharmacol 72:233–237

Cohen AB (1979) The effects in vivo and in vitro of oxidative damage to purified α_1-antitrypsin and to the enzyme-inhibiting activity of plasma. Am Rev Respir Dis 119:953–957

Collis CH, Wilson CM, Jones JM (1980) Cyclophosphamide-induced lung damage in mice: protection by a small preliminary dose. Br J Cancer 41:901–907

Corn M, Kotso N, Stanton D, Bell W, Thomas AP (1972) Response of cats to inhaled mixtures of SO_2-NaCl aerosol in air. Arch Environ Health 24:248–256

Crapo JD, Marsh-Salin J, Ingram D, Pratt PC (1978) Tolerance and cross-tolerance using NO_2 and O_2. II. Pulmonary morphology and morphometry. J Appl Physiol 44:370–379

Crapo JD, Barry BE, Foscue HA, Shelburne J (1980) Structural and biochemical changes in rat lungs occurring during exposures to lethal and adaptive doses of oxygen. Am Rev Respir Dis 122:123–143

Crispens CG Jr (1975) Handbook on the laboratory mouse. Thomas, Springfield, Illinois, pp 1–267

Damiano VV, Sandler A, Abrams WR, Meranze DR, Cohen AB, Kimbel P, Weinbaum G (1980) Electron and light microscopic studies of the lungs of chloramine-T treated dogs. Bull Eur Physio-Pathol Respir 16 (Suppl):141–154

DeNicola DB, Rebar AH, Henderson RF (1981) Early damage indicators in the lung. V. Biochemical and cytological response to NO_2 inhalation. Toxicol Appl Pharmacol 60:301–312

De Weck AL, Festing MFW (1979) Guinea pig. In: Altman PL, Katz DD (eds) Inbred and genetically defined strains of laboratory animals, part 2. Hamster, guinea pig, rabbit, and chicken. Federation of American Societies for Experimental Biology, Bethesda, Maryland, pp 507–510 (Biological handbooks, vol 3)

Diamond L, O'Donnell M (1977) Pulmonary mechanics in normal rats. J Appl Physiol 43:942–948

Dickinson EO, Yokoyama MT, Carlson JR, Bradley BJ (1976) Induction of pulmonary edema and emphysema in goats by intraruminal administration of 3-methylindole. Am J Vet Res 37:667–672

Dodds WJ (1982) Symposium report. The pig model for biomedical research. Fed Proc 41:247–256

Dutcher JS, Boyd MR (1979) Species and strain differences in target organ alkylation and toxicity by 4-ipomeanol. Predictive value of covalent binding in studies of target organ toxicities by reactive metabolites. Biochem Pharmacol 28:3367–3372

Ehrlich R (1966) Effect of nitrogen dioxide on resistance to pulmonary infection. Bacteriol Rev 30:604–614

Eliraz A, Abrams WR, Meranze DR, Kimbel P, Weinbaum G (1980) Development of an animal model of functional alpha$_1$-antiprotease deficiency. Chest 77 (Suppl 2):278

Foster HL, Small JD, Fox JG (eds) (1981) The mouse in biomedical research, vol 1. History, genetics and wild mice. Academic, New York, pp 1–306

Frank L, Bucher JR, Roberts RJ (1978) Oxygen toxicity to neonatal and adult animals of various species. J Appl Physiol 45:699–704

Goetzman BW, Milstein JM (1980) Pulmonary vascular histamine receptors in newborn and young lambs. J Appl Physiol 49:380–385

Griesemer RA (1976) Naturally occurring neoplastic diseases. IX. Nonhuman primates. In: Melby EC, Altman NH (eds) CRC Handbook of laboratory animal science, vol 3. CRC Press, Cleveland, Ohio, pp 309–323

Haies DM, Gil J, Weibel ER (1981) Morphometric study of rat lung cells. I. Numerical and dimensional characteristics of parenchymal cell population. Am Rev Respir Dis 123:533–541

Hakkinen PJ, Haschek WM (1982) Pulmonary toxicity of methylcyclopentadienyl manganese tricarbonyl: nonciliated bronchiolar epithelial (Clara) cell necrosis and alveolar damage in the mouse, rat, and hamster. Toxicol Appl Pharmacol 65:11–22

Halpern M, Williamson SJ, Spektor DM, Schlesinger RB, Lippmann M (1981) Remanent magnetic fields for measuring particle retention and distribution in the lungs. Exp Lung Res 2:27–35

Harkness JE, Wagner JE (1977) The biology and medicine of rabbits and rodents. Lea and Febiger, Philadelphia, pp 1–152

Haschek WM, Reiser KM, Klein-Szanto AJP, Kehrer JP, Smith LH, Last JA, Witschi HP (1983) Potentiation of butylated hydroxytoluene-induced acute lung damage by oxygen. Cell kinetics and collagen metabolism. Am Rev Respir Dis 127:28–34

Heiniger HJ, Dorey JJ (eds) (1980) Handbook on genetically standardized jax mice, 3rd edn. Jackson Laboratory, Bar Harbor, Maine

Hirshman CA, Downes H, Leon DA, Peters JE (1981) Basenji-greyhound dog model of asthma: pulmonary responses after β-adrenergic blockade. J Appl Physiol 51:1423–1427

Hoar RM (1976) Toxicology and teratology. In: Wagner JE, Manning PJ (eds) The biology of the Guinea pig. Academic, New York, pp 269–280

Hoffmann D, Rivenson A, Hecht SS, Hilfrich J, Kobayashi N, Wynder EL (1979) Model studies in tobacco carcinogenesis with the Syrian golden hamster. Prog Exp Tumor Res 24:370–390

Hollinger MA, Giri SN, Patwell S, Zuckerman JE, Gorin A, Parsons G (1980) Effect of acute lung injury on angiotensin converting enzyme in serum, lung lavage and effusate. Am Rev Respir Dis 121:373–376

Holme G, Piechuta H (1981) The derivation of an inbred line of rats which develop asthma-like symptoms following challenge with aerosolized antigen. Immunology 42:19–24

Holub D, Frank R (1979) A system for rapid measurement of lung function in small animals. J Appl Physiol 46:394–398

Homburger F (1976) Potential contributions of inbred Syrian hamsters to future toxicology. In: Mehlman MA, Shapiro RE, Blumenthal H (eds) Advances in modern toxicology, vol 1, part 1. New concepts in safety evaluation. Hemisphere, New York, pp 35–60

Huang TW, Carlson JR, Bray TM, Bradley BJ (1977) 3-Methylindole-induced pulmonary injury in goats. Am J Pathol 87:647–666

Jacoby RO, Barthold SW (1981) Quality assurance for rodents used in toxicological research and testing. In: Gralla EJ (ed) Scientific considerations in monitoring and evaluating toxicological research. Hemisphere, Washington, pp 27–55

Jobe A, Ikegami M, Sarton-Miller I, Barajas L (1980) Surfactant metabolism of newborn lamb lungs studied in vivo. J Appl Physiol 49:1091–1098

Kaufman SL (1980) Cell proliferation in the mamalian lung. Int Rev Exp Pathol 22:131–191

Kennedy AR, Little JB (1979) Respiratory system differences relevant to lung carcinogenesis between Syrian hamsters and other species. Prog Exp Tumor Res 24:302–314

Kida K, Thurlbeck WM (1980) Lack of recovery of lung structure and function after the administration of β-amino-propionitrile in the postnatal period. Am Rev Respir Dis 122:467–475

Kistler GS, Caldwell PRB, Weibel ER (1967) Development of fine structural damage to alveolar and capillary lining cells in oxygen-poisoned rat lungs. J Cell Biol 33:605–628

Kitterman JA, Liggins GC, Clements JA, Campos G, Lee CH, Ballard PL (1981) Inhibitors of prostaglandin synthesis, tracheal fluid, and surfactant in fetal lambs. J Appl Physiol 51:1562–1567

Koo KW, Leith DE, Sherter CB, Snider GL (1976) Respiratory mechanics in normal hamsters. J Appl Physiol 40:936–942

Küng M, Reinhart ME, Wanner A (1978) Pulmonary hemodynamic effects of lung inflation and graded hypoxia in conscious sheep. J Appl Physiol 45:949–956

Lang CM, Vesell ES (1976) Environmental and genetic factors affecting laboratory animals: impact on biomedical research. Introduction. Fed Proc 34:1123–1124

Larsen JJ, Boeck V, Ottesen B (1981) Effect of vasoactive intestinal polypeptide on cerebral blood flow in the goat. Acta Physiol Scand 111:471–474

Last JA, Hesterberg TW, Reiser KM, Cross CE, Amis TC, Gunn C, Sterfey EP, Grandy J, Hendrickson R (1981) Ozone-induced alterations in collagen metabolism of monkey lungs: use of biopsy-obtained lung tissue. Toxicol Appl Pharmacol 60:579–585

Litterst CL, Mimnaugh EG, Regan RL, Gram TG (1975) Comparison of in vitro drug metabolism by lung, liver and kidney of several common laboratory species. Drug Metab Dispos 3:259–265

Lock JE, Hamilton F, Luide H, Coceani F, Olley PM (1980) Direct pulmonary vascular responses in the conscious newborn lamb. J Appl Physiol 48:188–196

Lundberg L (1979) Guinea pigs inbred for studies of respiratory anaphylaxis. Acta Pathol Microbiol Scand Sect C 87:55–66

Mehendale HM, Angevine LS, Ohmiya Y (1981) The isolated perfused lung – A critical evaluation. Toxicology 21:1–36

Melby EC Jr, Altman NH (eds) (1974a) CRC handbook of laboratory animal science, vol 1. CRC Press, Cleveland, Ohio, pp 1–451

Melby EC Jr, Altman NH (eds) (1974b) CRC handbook of laboratory animal science, vol 2. CRC Press, Cleveland, Ohio, pp 1–523

Melby EC Jr, Altman NH (eds) (1976) CRC handbook of laboratory animal science, vol 3. CRC Press, Cleveland, Ohio, pp 1–943

Mondino A (1980) The choice of animal species in experimental toxicology. In: Galli CL, Murphy SD, Paoletti R (eds) The principles and methods in modern toxicology. Elsevier/North Holland, Amsterdam, pp 259–275

Moore GS, Calabrese EJ, Schulz E (1981) Effect of in vivo ozone exposure to dorset sheep, an animal model with low levels of erythrocyte glucose-6-phosphate dehydrogenase activity. Bull Environ Contam Toxicol 26:273–280

Morstatter CE, Glaser RM, Jurrus ER, Weiss HS (1976) Compliance and stability of excised mouse lungs. Comp Biochem Physiol 54A:197–202

Neuhauser-Klaus A (1981) An approach towards the standardization of the mammalian spot test. Arch Toxicol 48:229–243

Newman RA, Hacker MP, Kimberly PJ, Braddock JM (1981) Assessment of bleomycin-, tallysomycin-, and polyamine-mediated acute lung toxicity by pulmonary lavage angiotensin-converting enzyme activity. Toxicol Appl Pharmacol 61:469–474

Nickels FA, Brown CM, Breeze RG (1980) Myoblastoma. Equine granular cell tumor. Mod Vet Pract 61:593–596

Nielsen SW (1976) Canine and feline neoplasia. In: Melby EC, Altman NH (eds) CRC Handbook of laboratory animal science, vol 3. CRC Press, Cleveland, Ohio, pp 887–943

Ohkuda K, Nakahara K, Binder A, Staub NC (1981) Venous air emboli in sheep: reversible increase in lung microvascular permeability. J Appl Physiol 31:887–894

O'Neil JJ, Raub JA, Mercer R, Miller FJ, Graham JA (1981) Pulmonary function changes in small animals following exposure to oxidant gases and in the presence of experimental emphysema. Proceedings of the 11th conference on environmental toxicology. Air Force Aerospace Medical Research Laboratory Report TR-80-125, Wright Patterson Air Force Base, Ohio, pp 105–113

Oser BL (1981) The rat as a model for human toxicological evaluation. J Toxicol Environ Health 8:521–542

Park SS, Kikkawa Y, Goldring IP, Daly MM, Zelefsky M, Shim C, Spierer M, Morita T (1977) An animal model of cigarette smoking in beagle dogs: correlative evaluation of effects on pulmonary function, defense, and morphology. Am Rev Respir Dis 115:971–979

Peters JE, Hirshman CA, Malley A (1982) The Basenji-greyhound dog model of asthma: leukocyte histamine release, serum I_gE and airway response to inhaled antigen. Am Rev Respir Dis 125 (no 4, part 2):64 (Abstract)

Pfleger RC (1977) Type II epithelial cells from the lung of Syrian hamsters: isolation and metabolism. Exp Mol Pathol 27:152–166

Pour P, Birt D (1979) Spontaneous diseases of Syrian hamsters – their implications in toxicological research: facts, thoughts and suggestions. Prog Exp Tumor Res 24:145–156

Ranga V, Kleinerman J (1981) Lung injury and repair in the blotchy mouse. Effects of nitrogen dioxide inhalation. Am Rev Respir Dis 123:90–97

Reid LM (1980) Needs for animal models of human diseases of the respiratory system. Am J Pathol 101(Suppl 3):S89–S102

Rigdon RH, Corssen G (1963) Pulmonary lesions in dogs from methylcholanthrene. Arch Pathol Lab Med 75:323–331

Robinson FR (1976a) Naturally occurring neoplastic diseases. III. Hamster. In: Melby EC, Altman NH (eds) CRC Handbook of laboratory animal science, vol. 3. CRC Press, Cleveland, Ohio, pp 253–270

Robinson FR (1976b) Naturally occurring neoplastic diseases. V. Guinea pig. In: Melby EC, Altman NH (eds) CRC Handbook of laboratory animal science, vol. 3. CRC Press, Cleveland, Ohio, pp 275–278

Robinson FR, Casey HW, Weibel ER (1974) Animal model of disease. Oxygen toxicity. Animal model: oxygen toxicity in nonhuman primates. Am J Pathol 76:175–178

Robinson NE, Gillespie JR, Berry JD, Simpson A (1972) Lung compliance, lung volumes, and single-breath diffusing capacity in dogs. J Appl Physiol 33:808–812

Roe FJC (1966) The relevance and value of studies of lung tumours in laboratory animals in research on cancer of the human lung. In: Sever L (ed) Lung tumours in animals. Proceedings of the 3rd quadrennial conference on cancer. University of Perugia, Perugia, Italy, pp 101–126

Rosenbaum RM, Wittner M, Lenger M (1969) Mitochondrial and other ultrastructural changes in great alveolar cells of oxygen-adapted and poisoned rats. Lab Invest 20:516–528

Rossi GA, Hunninghake GW, Kawami O, Ferrans VJ, Hansen CT, Crystal RG (1982) "Motheaten" mice: an animal model with an inherited interstitial lung disease. Am Rev Respir Dis 125 (no 4, part 2):238 (Abstract)

Roth JA (1979) Use of the isolated perfused lung in biochemical toxicology. In: Hodgson E, Bend JR (eds) Reviews in biochemical toxicology, vol 1. Elsevier/North Holland, New York, pp 287–309

Roth RA (1981) Effect of pneumotoxicants on lactate dehydrogenase activity in airways of rats. Toxicol Appl Pharmacol 57:69–78

Saffiotti U, Cefis F, Kolb LH (1968) A method for the experimental induction of bronchogenic carcinoma. Cancer Res 28:104–124

Sahebjami H, Wirman JA (1981) Emphysema-like changes in the lungs of starved rats. Am Rev Respir Dis 124:619–624

Schreiber H, Nettesheim P, Lijinsky W, Richter CB, Walburg HE Jr (1972) Induction of lung cancer in germfree, specific-pathogen-free and infected rats by N-nitrosoheptamethyleneimine: enhancement by respiratory infection. J Natl Cancer Inst 49:1107–1114

Sheppard D, Wong WS, Uehara CF, Nadel JA, Boushey HA (1980) Lower threshold and greater bronchomotor responsiveness of asthmatic subjects to sulfur dioxide. Am Rev Respir Dis 122:873–878

Sikic BI, Collins JM, Mimnaugh CG, Gram TE (1978) Improved therapeutic index of bleomycin when administered by continuous infusion in mice. Cancer Treat Rep 62:2011–2017

Silver EH, Leith DE, Murphy SD (1981) Potentiation by triorthotolyl phosphate of acrylate ester-induced alterations in respiration. Toxicology 22:192–203

Skornik WA, Heiman R, Jaeger RJ (1981) Pulmonary mechanisms in guinea pigs: repeated measurements using a nonsurgical computerized method. Toxicol Appl Pharmacol 59:314–323

Slauson DO, Hahn FF (1980) Criteria for development of animal models of diseases of the respiratory system. The comparative approach in respiratory disease model development. Am J Pathol 101(Suppl 3):S103–S122

Smith JE (1976) Animal model of human disease. Inherited erythrocyte glutathione deficiency. Animal model: glutathione deficiency and partial gamma-glutamylcycsteine synthetase deficiency in sheep. Am J Pathol 82:233–235

Snider GL, Sherter CB, Koo KW, Karlinsky JB, Hayes JA, Franzblau C (1977) Respiratory mechanics in hamsters following treatment with endotracheal elastase or collagenase. J Appl Physiol 42:206–215

Snider GL, Celli BR, Goldstein RH, O'Brien JJ, Lucey LC (1978) Chronic interstitial pulmonary fibrosis produced in hamsters by endotracheal bleomycin. Am Rev Respir Dis 117:289–297

Stedham MA (1976) Naturally occurring neoplastic diseases. VI. Rabbit. In: Melby EC, Altman NH (eds) CRC Handbook of laboratory animal science, vol. 3. CRC Press, Cleveland, Ohio, pp 279–285

Streilein JW (1979) Hamster. In: Altman PL, Katz DD (eds) Inbred and genetically defined strains of laboratory animals, part 2. Hamster, guinea pig, rabbit, and chicken. Federation of American Societies for Experimental Biology, Bethesda, Maryland, pp 425–430 (Biological handbooks, vol 3)

Stuart BO (1976) Selection of animal models for evaluation of inhalation hazards in man. In: Aharonson EF, Ben-David A, Klingberg MA (eds) Air pollution and the lung. Wiley, New York, pp 268–292

Sylvester JT, Harabin AL, Peake MD, Frank RS (1980) Vasodilator and constructor responses to hypoxia in isolated pig lungs. J Appl Physiol 49:820–825

Takezawa W, Miller FJ, O'Neil JJ (1980) Single-breath diffusing capacity and lung volumes in small laboratory mammals. J Appl Physiol 48:1052–1059

Takino Y, Sugahara K, Horino I (1970) Two lines of guinea pigs sensitive and non-sensitive to chemical mediators and anaphylaxis. J Allergy Clin Immunol 47:247–261

Travis EL, Vojnovic B, Davies EE, Hirst DG (1979) A plethysmographic method for measuring function in locally irradiated mouse lung. Br J Radiol 52:67–74

Travis EL, Down JD, Holmes SJ, Hobson B (1980) Radiation pneumonitis and fibrosis in mouse lung assayed by respiratory frequency and histology. Radiat Res 84:133–143

Vesell ES, Lang CM, White WJ, Passananti GT, Hill RN, Clemens TL, Liu DK, Johnson WD (1976) Environmental and genetic factors affecting the response of laboratory animals to drugs. Fed Proc 35:1125–1132

Vinegar A, Sinnett EE, Leith DE (1979) Dynamic mechanisms determine functional residual capacity in mice, mus musculus. J Appl Physiol 46:867–871

Voelker DR, Snyder F (1979) Subcellular site and mechanism of synthesis of disaturated phosphatidylcholine in alveolar type II cell adenomas. J Biol Chem 254:8628–8633

Wagner JE, Manning PJ (eds) (1976) The biology of the Guinea pig. Academic, New York, pp 1–317

Wanner A, Mezey RJ, Reinhart ME, Eyre P (1979) Antigen induced bronchospasm in conscious sheep. J Appl Physiol 47:917–922

Watanabe S, Frank R (1975) Lung volumes, mechanics, and single-breath diffusing capacity in anesthetized cats. J Appl Physiol 38:1148–1152

Watanabe S, Frank R, Yokoyama E (1973) Acute effects of ozone on lungs of cats. I. Functional. Am Rev Resp Dis 108:1141–1151

Wehner AP, Stuart BO, Sanders CL (1979) Inhalation studies with Syrian golden hamsters. Prog Exp Tumor Res 24:177–198

Weisbroth SH, Flatt RE, Kraus AL (eds) (1974) The biology of the laboratory rabbit. Academic, New York, pp 1–496

Weiss KD, Weiss HS (1976) Increased lung compliance in mice exposed to sulfur dioxide. Res Commun Chem Pathol Pharmacol 13:133–136

Wilson AF, Fairshter RD, Gillespie JR, Hackney J (1976) Evaluation of abnormal lung function. Ann Rev Pharmacol Toxicol 16:465–486

Wong KL, Alarie Y (1982) A method for repeated evaluation of pulmonary performance in unanesthetized, unrestrained guinea pigs and its application to detect effects of sulfuric acid mist inhalation. Toxicol Appl Pharmacol 63:72–90

Wykle RL, Malone B, Snyder F (1977) Biosynthesis of dipalmitoyl-SN-glycero-3-phosphocholine by adenoma alveolar type II cells. Arch Biochem Biophys 181:249–256

Wykle RL, Malone B, Blank ML, Synder F (1980) Biosynthesis of pulmonary surfactant: comparison of 1-palmitoyl-SN-glycero-3-phosphocholine and palmitate as precursors of dipalmitoyl-SN-glycero-3-phosphocholine in adenoma alveolar type II cells. Arch Biochem Biophys 199:526–537

Young S, Hallowes RC (1973) Tumours of the mammary gland. In: Turusov VSM (ed) Pathology of tumours in laboratory animals. I. Tumours of the rat, part 1. International Agency for Research on Cancer, Lyon, France, pp 31–74

CHAPTER 5

Epidemiologic Studies in Human Populations

MARGARET R. BECKLAKE

A. Introduction

This volume addresses the general principles of inhalational toxicology. It emphasizes the range of responses that can be measured in animals and in humans after exposure to inhaled particles and vapors. Chapters dealing with exposure techniques and methods of measurement (by no means all of which can be applied to humans) provide a thorough review of up-to-date information.

The orientation of this chapter is different because it deals with a discipline and an approach to scientific study, not only with its techniques and methods of measurement. The chapter is offered to complete the inventory of methods available to assess the toxic effects of inhaled materials which this volume seeks to cover. It aims to sensitize readers who are not epidemiologists to the powerful contribution epidemiologic studies can make in this field; obviously, it cannot serve as a recipe book on how to do such studies. For a concise and clear description of the approach and methods of epidemiology in relation to occupational lung disease, the reader may consult McDONALD et al. (1982), and for a more complete discussion of the principles of epidemiology, one of the standard texts is recommended (ABRAMSON 1979; LILIENFELD and LILIENFELD 1981; MacMAHON and PUGH 1970). A recent volume specifically addresses the approach to diseases related to occupational exposure (MONSON 1980).

B. Scope

Epidemiology has been described as the study of the distribution of disease in human populations and of the factors which influence its distribution; this definition is in conformity with the Greek origins of the word: *epi* (concerning), *demos* (people), and *logos* (discussion). In epidemiologic studies therefore, an individual is regarded in the context of a population of like individuals appropriately selected. As in other branches of medicine, knowledge comes from where and why diseases (in this context poisonings) occur and of their mechanisms. Only epidemiology can address the former; together with pathology and physiology it may also address the latter.

Toxicology encompasses the full range of toxic effects both in respect to time (from immediate to delayed, measured in months, years, or decades) and severity (from changes at the level of the cell, the organ, and the organism, and ranging from accommodation and adaptation to failure and death). While in toxicology emphasis is on the role of the external agent (and in the present volume on inhaled materials), response is nevertheless also determined by certain host characteristics. Thus MCDONALD (1981) reminds us of "the evolutionary and ecological concepts of adaption whereby man has inherited and acquired resistance, often of a high order, to a wide range of potentially harmful agents and circumstances." Epidemiologic studies in human populations can be used to address the full range of effects in time and in severity, as well as the role of human susceptibility. What can be measured is limited by the tools available.

For inhaled materials, the lung may be the target organ or the organ of entry into the body. In this chapter, as in this volume, the emphasis will be on those inhaled materials for which the lung is the target organ. The epidemiologic approach, however, is equally applicable to the assessment of toxic effects of inhaled agents which enter via the lung and have their effects elsewhere.

Inhaled materials may be in the form of fumes/vapors or in the form of particles/fibers (Table 1). Broadly speaking, the time course for detectable nonmalignant human response to exposure is shorter for the former than the latter (particularly for higher doses); in addition, the responses to exposure to fumes/vapors are primarily in airways. By contrast, the responses to exposure to particles/fibers tend to be delayed longer and to be primarily in lung parenchyma and pleura. These comments refer to inorganic materials; organic materials as well as some inorganic materials (BROOKS 1977) are also capable of evoking reactions mediated and/or amplified through the immune system, affecting primarily the airways (asthma) and/or the parenchyma (extrinsic allergic alveolitis). Thus, host characteristics may play an important part in mediating the response. In addition, malignant as well as nonmalignant responses to inhaled materials may occur; here the time course is seldom measured in less than decades, even though exposure may have been for relatively brief periods. Not only can epidemiologic studies in human populations be used to assess all these types of toxic effects, but they can also be used to study the variety of personal characteristics (or host factors) which collectively make up an individual's susceptibility to such toxic effects.

Table 1. Time course of human responses[a] to inhaled materials[b]

Physical state of agents	Immediate (minutes, hours, or days)	Delayed (weeks, months, or years)
Fumes/vapors	Usually higher dose	Usually lower dose
Particles/fibers	If present, probably nonspecific	Response usually related to exposure dose, and probably related to dose delivered at target site

[a] Nonmalignant
[b] Refers to inorganic materials; organic materials, besides evoking nonspecific effects, are also capable of evoking reactions mediated and amplified though the immune system

C. Uses of Epidemiology in the General Assessment of the Toxic Effects of Inhaled Materials

Given the varied potential of the epidemiologic approach, what are its uses in addressing the issues implicit in the title of this section of the present volume? Information on the distribution of abnormality/toxic effects/disease within populations may:

1. Permit the *identification* of toxic effects hitherto unrecognized, as well as the *detection* of recognized toxic effects in populations not previously thought to be at risk.
2. Provide the basis for *assessing the extent and severity* of a problem (how many subjects are affected and how severely?) as well as *assessing trends* (is the problem increasing or diminishing?).
3. Taken together with data from other disciplines, *elucidate its etiology*; in the present context the most important aspect of etiology is an exploration of the dose relationship of response to exposure.
4. Provide the basis *for developing and evaluating preventive and control strategies.*

The second, third, and fourth issues are general; the first specific to the assessment of environmental agents, included in which are inhaled materials. Thus though, in general, epidemiologic studies consider both host and environmental factors, the issues implicit under the title "toxic effects" call for emphasis on the latter, whatever the objective and/or design of the study.

D. Exposure

The usefulness of studies in human populations to assess the toxic effects of inhaled materials is directly related to the success with which the harmful agent and/or exposure variable can be measured. How may this be done?

Ideally, what is wanted is as precise an assessment as possible in line with the general principles of toxicology, i. e., a measurement of the amount of the agent or agents under study delivered to the target organ (in the present context the respiratory tract and/or lung parenchyma and/or pleura) and retained for the period necessary to evoke a response. In the case of gaseous materials, this is probably very close to the amount of the agent or agents inhaled minus the amount exhaled during the period of exposure. However, in the case of particulate material, a number of factors (discussed in detail elsewhere in this volume) influence penetration and deposition, such as aerodynamic behavior of the particles as well as their physical and chemical characteristics, in addition to the air exchange profile (including rate and depth of breathing, nose/mouth breathing, and whether the subject is exercising). Host characteristics such as age (WACHTLOVA et al. 1981) and lung geometry (GREEN et al. 1974) may also be important. Much of the inhaled particulate material in the respirable range is exhaled in the same breath; in addition, a considerable amount of what is deposited in conducting airways is cleared over the immediate short term (measured in hours or days) by the mucociliary esclator; material deposited on the nonciliated epithelium is cleared over the less immediate short term, probably in several phases, measured in half-times of weeks or perhaps months (LIPPMANN et al. 1980). What is not cleared accumulates, free or in macrophages. The long-term effects of accumulated dust relate to its biologic potency. The contribution to human response of whatever amount of the agent is cleared in the immediate and not so immediate short term will also of course depend on its chemical and biologic properties. For instance, in the case of relatively inert dusts such as coal or iron, the effect of dust retained in the short term relative to the effect of what is retained in the long term is likely to be minimal, at least as far as the lung parenchyma is concerned, and probably, though less certainly, as far as the airways are concerned (MORGAN (1978). In the case of a biologically active dust such as asbestos, the possibility must be entertained that even what is retained in the short term might also contribute to the process or processes which eventually lead to the development, for example, of overt lung cancer.

The elements necessary to describe exposure include its character, its duration, and its intensity (Table 2). In practice, for particulate materials, it is seldom possible to construct an index of exposure which reflects anything more than duration and/or levels and, given the efficiency of clearance (see the previous paragraph), this must clearly be a very poor reflection of what is retained. Nevertheless, for many occupations and even using the simplest indices of exposure such as years of exposure, exposure–response relationships have been demonstrable (BEADLE 1970; BECKLAKE 1976).

For gaseous materials, indirect assessment of absorption by the target organ can often be made from analysis of excretion products, an approach used widely in the field of toxicology and beyond the scope of this chapter. However, for a

Table 2. Elements in the exposure variable

Element	Descriptor
Character	Particulate, gaseous Physical properties such as size distribution (respirable/nonrespirable), median mass, and dimensional characteristics [a] Chemical composition Biologic properties
Duration	Time exposed (net and gross) Time elapsed since first exposure Modifiers to the above include adjustments for shift, overtime, and vacations
Intensity	Place of residence, occupation, job title, job description Modifiers to the above include: 1. Environmental measurements by area or personal sampling; 2. Activity level (assessed by estimated minute volume for job or daily activities); 3. Time weighting 4. Measurement of agent in biologic material, e.g., saliva, urine, skin 5. Measurement of agent in human tissue, e.g., hair, biopsy, and autopsy material

[a] LE BOUFFANT (1980)

few agents which may directly affect the lung, a similar approach has been used, e. g., the measurement of urinary fluorides as an indicator of exposure in studies of the acute respiratory effects of potroom exposure in aluminium smelters (G. B. FIELD and M. SMITH 1973, Pulmonary Function in Aluminum Smelters, unpublished report).

Whatever the nature of the inhaled material under study, the measurement used to describe exposure is a compromise between the possible and the desirable, the compromise being reached in light of the study objectives. For instance, in etiologic research, particularly examining exposure–response relationships, relative exposure of one group or subpopulation in relation to another is usually more important than absolute levels of exposure (and can be more readily achieved, even using area sampling). For case-referent studies aimed at establishing the relationship between asbestos exposure and mesothelioma, historical information on plant, industry, and occupation has proved an adequate measure (McDONALD et al. 1970). By contrast, a study of the reasons for variation between individuals in response to what appears to be comparable overall exposure would require greater precision in the exposure measurement, e. g., the use of personal samplers or electron microscopy of tissues, as in the study of mesothelioma (McDONALD et al. 1982), while for research upon which environmental controls are to be based, the most precise measurements of exposure/pollution levels possible should be used, based on techniques which can subsequently be incorporated into ongoing environmental monitoring (SIMPSON 1979).

E. Epidemiologic Studies in Human Populations

I. Definitions, Some Basic Concepts, and the General Assessment of a Problem

Epidemiology has been described as the science of head-counting and vital statistics as the bookkeeping of public health. Epidemiology depends on the recording of facts about the individuals within a defined group or population and/or about events which occur in their lives, and it is "in the essence of epidemiology that observed facts and occurrences are related wherever possible to the appropriate denominator" (McDONALD 1981). Though recording the facts and events may be relatively simple, defining and counting the appropriate population may often be much more difficult. When their occurrence in time is unimportant, these facts and events may be described as proportions or percentages i.e. as *prevalence* rates related to a given point or period in time, and as *incidence* rates when related to their appearance rate over a defined period of time. Prevalence rates also represent the summation of incidence rates over periods of time, modified by the duration of the disease in question (LILIENFELD and LILIENFELD 1981). Incidence rates are used to describe birth and death, two major incidents in human life, as well as many lesser incidents such as the acute infective childhood and adult illnesses, whereas prevalence rates are used to describe chronic ill health or good health. When the events studied relate to the death of an individual, the term mortality study is also used; when related to facts about his or her health status in life, the term used is morbidity study. The former is usually more appropriate for diseases which kill in short periods (for example, many cancers), the latter for a great variety of other acute and chronic conditions.

The word survey, often used in relation to epidemiologic studies, merits definition. To those unfamilar with the epidemiologic approach, it generally conjures up the indiscriminate gathering of data on large numbers of subjects at their place or residence or at their place of work, often by simplified techniques which to the clinical eye provide at best an incomplete description. How, the clinician asks, can the epidemiologist seriously consider diagnosing chronic bronchitis on the basis of an affirmative answer to questions, posed baldly and without elaboration, and as vague as "do you usually cough?" and "do you cough like this for 3 months in the year?" Why, the respiratory physiologist asks, does the epidemiologist seem to think that the performance of the lung can be completely described by the volume of air expelled by the lung in 1 s during a forced expiration (FEV_1)?

By contrast, to an epidemiologist (ABRAMSON 1979, p 5), the term survey means "an investigation which information is systematically gathered, but in which the experimental method is not used" (see also Sect. F. II). It is perhaps the equivalent of a clinical case description, with the case being not one person but a defined population. As clinical case descriptions become part of a hospital's records, so survey reports become part of the records of the health of a community. As will be seen later, if appropriately planned, they merit the term descriptive research; they may also address etiologic questions.

II. The Elements of a Planned Study

It has been said that an epidemiologic study is a group (the study team) studying a group (the target population). This emphasizes the point that epidemiologic studies are invariably interdisciplinary; the more effective the interdisciplinary collaboration, the better the study. In planning an epidemiologic study, (or equally in evaluating the results of a study already completed), four questions should be asked: "why? (the objectives); how? (the design); who? (the population); and what? (the methods of measurement). Most important of these is the first, what MCDONALD (1981) calls the "fundamental ingredient of any scientific endeavour," namely, "an attainable objective or answerable question clearly and unambiguously defined". He also recommends as a useful discipline asking the subsidiary question "and what will I do with the answer?" Obviously, using the answers at the clinical or public health level is often not within the scope of the researcher planning the study. Consultation with potential users of the information is thus an important step in framing the question. Alternatively, if the study is being planned by the potential user (not an epidemiologist), prior consultation with an epidemiologist or biostatistician may ensure better methodology. Continued consultation undoubtedly ensures the most successful outcome. It must, of course, be added that the presently perceived usefulness of information, though important, is not the only criteria for judging the value of a study. An equally valid scientific endeavour is to explain, and explanatory information invariably turns out to be useful in a practical sense.

Comment on how to read critically and evaluate the report of an epidemiologic study is also in order, an exercise most of us carry out more often than we do the exercise of planning and executing a study. This is also based on the same series of questions (how, who, what, and often also when in relation to why). In this light the conclusions and/or inferences drawn by the investigator can be judged, taking into account potential sources of bias, perceived, considered, and dealt with or not by the investigator, as well as those perceived by the reader and/or critic. Always we are advised by HILL (1977, p 294), to ask: "is there any other way of explaining the set of facts before us?"

The criteria for internal and external validity, proposed by CAMPBELL and STANLEY (1966) for use in educational research, are applicable in the present context. Internal validity reflects the quality of the study, external validity is generalizability. Relevant to internal validity are the following:

1. History: sometimes called the cohort or temporal effect (refers to the changing circumstances between observations); for instance income, nutrition, smoking, and drinking have all increased over the past decades, while environmental pollution has decreased. This included what McDONALD (1981) refers to as the process of regression: the worst, he says, tends to improve, the best to deteriorate. Controls are used when pollution is bad; mechanization on the other hand may increase respirable dust levels.
2. Maturation (or aging): subjects grow older, undergo more environmental assaults with time, to some of which they may become more resistant, to others more susceptible.
3. Testing: undergoing a test may affect the results of the same test repeated or those of another test. For instance, diagnosis based on questionnaire responses, e. g., byssinosis, may be affected if the questionnaire is being answered for the second time; the same is true for the results of what appear to be more objective tests such as those of lung function, even if the time since the last test runs into months (STEBBINGS 1971).
4. Instrumentation: including calibration as well as reading procedures.
5. Statistical regression (regression to the mean): this phenomenon, inherent in all pairs of measurement over time, is the consequence of chance (OLDHAM 1968), and describes the fact that due to measurement error low measurements tend to be higher when repeated, high lower. The tendency can be countered by design, e. g., the use of three as opposed to two consecutive measurements to describe trend (BLOMQUIST 1977), or in analysis (OLDHAM 1968).
6. Selection bias into subgroups compared; for instance, long-service workers have by definition a greater resistance to the assaults of a given environment than those who left after less exposure, the "healthy worker effect" (FOX and COLLIER 1976; MONSON 1980, p 117). This leads to an underestimate of exposure-related health problems.
7. Differential loss of subjects from comparison groups affecting ascertainment of response as well as of subjects at risk: thus labor turnover rates are the consequence of many factors, economic and social, which must inevitably affect the risk of, as well as the detection of the toxic effects of inhaled material in workplaces.

External validity refers to the extent to which results are generalizable; if the same observations were made in another group of subjects, would the results and conclusions be the same? Relevant to external validity are the interaction of both selection bias and differential losses in relation to the exposure index used as well as factors relating to interactions of the circumstance of testing or examining with the subject's own responsiveness. Generalizability however to other workforces must always be guarded; as FIELD (1981) points out any workforce must be regarded as "a biased sample of the general population and inhomogeneous within itself."

F. Design

Choice of study design (how) can be made once objectives (why) are defined. Several design options can usually be considered, the selection being the best compromise which the investigator can achieve between the ideal and the practical. Cost–benefit considerations operate in the minds of most investigators in terms of money as well as time, interest span, and the chances of sustaining the quality of data collection. Other practical constraints are matters such as source and quality of existing data, available documentation on target population, etc. Thus, many who at the beginning of the computer era might have opted for testing whole populations rather than sampling, now prefer fewer observations of better quality on more carefully selected subjects. Indeed the adage, small is beautiful, often applies. There are two major groups of study design which can be used for epidemiologic studies in human populations: (a) experimental and quasiexperimental designs; and (b) surveys (nonexperimental designs) which may be analytic or descriptive.

I. Experimental Designs

Experiments are described as "investigations in which the researcher wishing to study the effects of exposure to (or deprivation of) a defined factor, himself decides what subjects will be exposed to, or deprived of the factor" (ABRAMSON 1979, p 4). If the exposed and nonexposed are compared, then the study is a controlled experiment, if exposure and nonexposure is determined by chance, the study is a randomized control trial; if objectivity is enhanced by the observer not knowing which subjects were exposed and which not, the study is a blind experiment; if the subjects also are unaware of whether they are exposed or not, a double-blind experiment.

This type of study which has been used extensively in evaluation research, particularly of treatments in humans, cannot be used (except in a very limited way, e. g., laboratory response studies) in the general assessment of the toxic effects of inhaled materials for the obvious reasons that the investigator may not have (for ethical or practical reasons) the power to control exposures. There may also be other limitations, such as no nonexposed subjects to study, or if there are, no certainty that exposed and nonexposed were comparable to start with. Studies which fall short of the controlled experiment have been called quasiexperimental (CAMPBELL and STANLEY 1966). Included under this term are time series (before and after), and multiple time series designs, designs using nonequivalent control groups and what is called patched-up design, the aim of which is to control those sources of error most likely to crop up in a given situation. Several of these designs have high internal validity, and are favorably reviewed by WEISS (1972) in the context of program evaluation. As pointed out by McDONALD (1981), designs of this sort lend themselves well to the real world of hospitals, clinics, factories, and mines where not only is the experimental design difficult or impossible to apply, but where the degree of rigidity required, for instance in subject selection, may be so great that it lacks external validity, i. e., generalizability. In recommending their use in the context of evaluation of preventive measures used in relation to workplace and other exposures, he points out that such evaluation studies also test the validity of the concepts of causation and disease mechanism on which the control program is based.

Finally, circumstances may arise in the natural course of events which make it possible to observe the effects of, for instance, a given exposure; these are sometimes called natural experiments or experiments of opportunity. In fact, they are not experiments, but surveys. Examples are the detonation of the atomic bomb over Hiroshima (COBB et al. 1959) and the recent eruption of Mount St. Helens (MERCHANT et al. 1982).

II. Nonexperimental Designs

Surveys (i. e., studies in which neither the experimental nor the quasiexperimental method is used) may be analytic or descriptive. Analytic surveys seek "to study the determinative process" (ABRAMSON 1979) and are usually planned around etiologic hypotheses. In the present context, they address issues of cause and effect such as dose–response, and indirectly threshold levels when subjects with low exposure and/or no exposure are included (SIMPSON 1979). By contrast, descriptive surveys have, as their name implies, the objective of describing a situation, e. g., the distribution of a disease or abnormality in a population in relation to certain characteristics such as occupation and location as well as personal characteristics such as age and sex. They should give a "balanced picture of a situation at a point in time or at intervals along the way" (McDONALD 1981). Often, such surveys are required to service decisions in the field of public health related to planning, resource management, and research priorities. For instance, a health authority may wish to know whether there is evidence of an occupational disease in a given plant prior to instituting a surveillance program. If appropriately planned, however, with suitable incorporation of the exposure variable into the design, such a study becomes analytic in purpose and may also contribute information as to whether distribution of abnormality/disease within the workforce is dose-related to exposure. Thus as ABRAMSON (1979) points out, the distinction between the descriptive and analytic surveys is not always clear and a single survey may combine both purposes. The bulk of published epidemiologic studies assessing the toxic effects of inhaled materials, falls into this category (MONSON 1980).

G. Types of Survey

Surveys are of three main types: longitudinal, cross-sectional, and case-referent (or case-control). Longitudinal surveys provide information about the individu-

Table 3. Contrasting arguments in longitudinal and case-referent studies [a]

	Effect	
	Present	Absent
Exposure to the agent		
Present	A	B
Absent	C	D

[a] Longitudinal studies argue from exposure to agent (or suspected agent) to effect of the agent, i.e., horizontally across the table; thus, the occurrence of the effect in exposed $A/(A+B)$ is compared with its occurrence in the nonexposed $C/(C+D)$. Case-referent studies argue from effect (or suspected effect) of the agent to exposure, i.e., vertically down the table; the occurrence of exposure in those demonstrating the effect $A/(A+C)$ is compared with its occurrence in those not demonstrating the effect $B/(B+D)$

als under study at more than one point in time. The term cohort study has also been used to describe the gathering of such information on a particular group (or cohort) of individuals (MacMahon and Pugh 1970). The particular group may be defined by birth date (e. g., birth cohort of 1900–1909) as is often the case in mortality studies. In addition, the terms retrospective and prospective have also been applied to cohort studies to describe the occurrence of the events under study relative to the investigator's place in time; in the former, information about the events studied usually comes from existing records and follow-up is to the study date, while in the latter, this information is gathered by the investigator from the start time of the study (MacMahon and Pugh 1970). Longitudinal surveys are most suitable for recording the incidence of clearly defined events (such as acute illnesses, accidents, and death) which occur with fair frequency. By contrast, cross-sectional surveys, also called prevalence surveys, provide information about the individuals under study at a given point or given period in time; they are more readily applied to description of chronic ailments or slowly developed abnormalities, for instance, the radiologic indicators of dust disease in an exposed population.

Case-referent (case-control) studies contrast with both longitudinal and cross-sectional studies in that they argue not from exposure to effect, but from recognizable effect to exposure, past or present (Table 3). This type of survey is particularly applicable when the effect studied is a rare outcome with a long latent period. As pointed out by McDonald (1981), "this approach is a simple one derived from the traditions of clinical medicine and everyday life; events are examined and interpreted against other comparable experience." A recent development is the use of the case-referent approach to the analysis of a cohort study; this approach has proved powerful in mortality studies of certain exposed populations (McDONALD et al. 1980), and offers promise in identifying personal characteristics which place an individual at risk for inhaled materials (BECKLAKE et al. 1983).

While the choice of type of survey to be used is primarily dependent on the nature of the effect to be examined (acute or chronic, sudden or slow, rare or common), the strengths and weaknesses of the different survey types also merit consideration. Thus, as McDONALD (1981) points out, longitudinal surveys, though they cannot achieve the internal validity of the experimental design, do nevertheless have strength comparable to the quasiexperimental time-series design. Ideally, the population (or populations) should be defined (and examined) before exposure, follow-up should be complete, and classification by exposure (exposed/nonexposed, high/low) should be such that comparisons are not biased. In practice, populations are often defined against payroll or union records at a certain date (thus, excluding the sick and the dead); follow-up is seldom complete with loss to view more likely to affect the numerator than the denominator; classification by exposure is often confounded by age, i.e., high indices of exposure can only be accumulated in older subjects, and age is often correlated with other etiologic factors. All these shortcomings tend to bias in favor of underestimating the occurrence of disease. The extent to which these various threats to internal validity can be overcome is a measure of the ingenuity of the investigator as well as of the quality of the study.

These potential shortcomings of longitudinal surveys all usually apply very much more to cross-sectional studies. However, the most important bias in this type of study is due to confining the observations to those who have survived the exposure long enough to remain in the workforce or exposure group under study. Criteria for definition of the study population may exaggerate this effect (e.g., if only subjects with, for example at least 5 years exposure are included) and need to be taken into account in interpreting the results. McDONALD (1981) concludes that the only way of dealing with this shortcoming is to identify "those who by rights should have been included and examine a representative sample of them." He adds an encouraging note in relation to one of the classic earlier cross-sectional studies (DREESEN et al. 1938). This study was important since it was the basis for establishing the first threshold value for asbestos and as he remarked, "the results had considerable value for even an imperfect survey is better than none." Cross-sectional studies are often all that is possible.

A basic advantage of case-referent studies is their economy of time and effort; basic weaknesses include difficulty in selection of appropriate controls and the potential bias which knowledge of the hypothesis under study may introduce in the selection of cases, in the information gathered from cases or their families and to a lesser extent from their controls, as well as in the information supplied by observers, e.g., pathologic diagnosis. Furthermore, in both longitudinal and cross-sectional surveys, information on the subjects and/or case ascertainment is carried out after the population has been defined, a strength in design not shared by the case-referent study. This can be countered by careful selection of cases if possible, registered in ignorance of the causal hypothesis under study, as well as by precise definition of criteria for diagnosis.

H. Population

Decision as to who should be studied is made in the same way as decisions are made on the questions of how to carry out the study (the design) and what to study (the methods of measurement); the choice hinges on what subjects are most appropriate for the objectives of the study. This choice may have been implicit in the choice of subject matter and definition of objectives, e. g., health issues in a given workforce. In analytic studies, the investigator, in order to consider several possibilities, may need to gather information about size, age distribution, and exposure in several populations before making the choice. Other issues include choice of the reference or nonexposed population, whether sampling is to be used and in some cases sample size.

Issues related to the basis of comparison in analytic surveys, in particular in cohort studies, are discussed with great lucidity by MCDONALD (1981). He emphasizes that since these surveys copy the logic of the experimental model, internal comparison, i. e., comparison of subgroups within the cohort divided by exposure, is the first approach. This gets around the problem of the selective forces by which the workforce or target population was built up from members of the general population, and assumes that once in the workforce there was random allocation with respect to exposure. This may not be so; for instance, in the coal pits of the United Kingdom, face workers who tend to have the heaviest exposure also have fewer days of incapacity than surface workers, suggesting that they are fitter (LIDDELL 1973). Other problems with internal comparison include the fact that logical subdivisions by exposure grouping often result in unbalanced numbers of subjects per group while logical balancing of numbers may blur the exposure differences.

The investigator may thus be led to make external comparisons. This occurs particularly in relation to mortality studies where data on the nonexposed populations can be obtained from national statistics. Since these are based on the general population, and include the sick, disabled, and unemployed, health experience, including death rates, is liable to be less good (GOLDSMITH 1975). Indeed, standardized mortality rates for most working populations are below 1, even for diseases which are probably work related, reflecting again the healthy worker effect. Special studies can be carried out to assess this source of bias in particular populations (VINNI and HAKAMA 1980; PETERSEN and ATTFIELD 1981). Other selection factors affecting working groups include differences in the level and quality of medical care, as well as the health requirements upon which certain workforces are selected. In mortality studies, many investigators offer both internal and external comparisons. In morbidity studies, data for external comparison seldom if ever exist, and if the study calls for greater certainty about lack of exposure to the agent under study in the reference group than can be provided by classification within the workforce, the best approach may be to identify a comparable workforce elsewhere for study. For instance, in a study to examine the health effects of exposure to red cedar dust, workers in cedar sawmills were compared with workers doing similar jobs in non-cedar sawmills (CHAN-YEUNG et al. 1978).

In case-referent studies, clearly definition of the first (i. e., precisely what defines a case) and selection of the second (what sampling framework will be used) are the essential elements. Some of the issues have been discussed earlier in this section. McDonald (1981) emphasizes two differences between cases and the general population which are relevant to selection of referents: (a) factors related to the cause of the disease; and (b) selective factors leading to their registration. Matching should be done for the second, but not the first, and he warns against overmatching. As he points out, it is rarely possible to match beyond three simple factors, of which sex and age are two, the third factor should therefore be how the case came to light (e. g., hospital, autopsy, or clinical service). Selecting the source of the referent group is more important than selecting referents within it (MacMahon and Pugh 1970, p 250).

Issues related to sampling and sample size, both extremely important in the planning of a study, are beyond the scope of this chapter, but there are excellent reference texts to be consulted, (MacMahon and Pugh 1970). In prevalence studies of exposed populations, the total population is generally studied if it is not too large and within the scope and resources of the investigator; larger populations require a sampling strategy which should be random or systematic, but not haphazard. For other sampling strategies, the reader should consult an appropriate text. Suffice it to repeat the advice of the experienced that easily acquired types of information such as age, sex, and job history should be obtained about the entire target population and more intensive information about one or more samples (Abramson 1979, p 44). Thus, the first step in a research program to assess the effects of occupational exposure to chrysotile in the Québec asbestos mines and mills was a census to register anyone who had ever worked in the industry for 1 month or more since it started in the 1890's, a total of approximately 30,000 individuals, and to record simple facts about age and duration of employment (McDonald et al. 1972).

For certain types of study a minimal sample size is necessary. This applies to mortality studies where a realistic appraisal should be made of the potential number of deaths for study which the target population will generate. Likewise, for studies in which the response to be measured is a continuous variable (e. g., a longitudinal study of lung function in exposed workers or cross-sectional studies comparing exposed and nonexposed) similarly realistic calculations can be made about the size of the effect of interest (Berry 1974). In practice, these decisions are usually empirical, based on resources and time, and they should conform to the rule: as many as possible and as few as necessary, which, though formulated in relation to the number of study variables (Abramson 1979, p 68), is equally applicable to sample size. In a sense this reflects the scepticism sometimes expressed for sample size calculation, for instance, by Miettenen (1975), who suggests that the only crucial decision is whether the sample size should be 0 (i. e., the study should not be done) or not 0 (i. e., the study should be done), a decision based not on a mathematical calculation, but on what he calls the "utility of the study, i. e. the resultant of its yield of information and its cost."

J. Variables

The term "variable" is defined as a characteristic, measurement of which is to be incorporated into the study (Table 4). What is to be measured requires both con-

Table 4. Some examples of conceptual and operational definitions of study variables

Variable	Definition	
	Conceptual	Operational
Obesity	Corpulence[a]	Measured weight (clothed without shoes) in relation to ideal weight[b]
Bronchitis	Chronic mucus hypersecretion[c]	Answers yes to the question[d]: do you usually cough up sputum?
Potman	Worker exposed to pot fumes in an aluminum foundry	Worker currently in one of several defined occupations (potman, helper) who has been employed for at least 10 years, at least half of which have been in the present occupation
Cumulative exposure index	Reflects level and duration of exposure to a given agent	Sum of product of average environmental levels (known or estimated) associated with a given job title and period of employment in that job, cumulated for a worker over all the jobs the worker ever held in a particular plant or industry[e]

[a] *The Shorter Oxford English Dictionary,* 3rd ed (1965)
[b] *Metropolitan Life Insurance Tables* (1959)
[c] Fletcher and Peto (1977)
[d] ATS-DLD standardized respiratory questionnaire (Ferris 1978)
[e] For example, as described by Gibbs and Lachance (1972) for use in the Québec chrysotile asbestos mining industry

ceptual and operational definition; the former describes as carefully as possible the characteristic the investigator wishes to measure, a definition often comparable to that found in medical or other dictionaries, the latter specifies by what means it will be measured (Abramson 1979).

Variables are usually designated as independent (or stimulus) and dependent (or response), and the objective is to determine whether there is an association or relationship of the second to the first. Other terms used to describe the independent variable (or variables) are "explanatory", "predictive", and in the present context, the "exposure" variable. In addition, there are characteristics which may obscure associations because they are associated with both independent and dependent variables (confounding variables) and those associated with either one or the other (moderator variables).

All variables require precise definition, however they are to be used in the analysis of the material. For instance, the examples cited in Table 4 include variables used for classification or selection, e. g., the definition of a potman (G. B. Field and Smith 1973, Pulmonary Function in Aluminum Smelters, unpublished report); an independent variable, e. g., cumulative exposure index (Gibbs and Lachance 1972); a response variable, e. g., bronchitis (McDonald et al. 1974); and a moderator variable, e. g., obesity which may modify lung function (Ghezzo 1983).

For morbidity studies which include measurements or tests, there are certain general rules for their selection. Thus the methods used for measurement should:

1. Be a valid measurement of the characteristic to be studied.
2. Be sensitive (i. e., be able to detect a certain minimal level of change, acute or chronic), as well as specific (i. e., be able to distinguish the abnormal from the normal); they should also be able to detect trends.
3. Be simple to administer, perform, and analyze (note that automation and dedicated computers may facilitate and standardize both administration and analysis of a test).
4. Be repeatable, i. e., be as independent as possible of outside noise; in the present context this refers to sources of variation other than the one under study.
5. Have few contraindications: (e. g., exercise testing which may not be carried out with impunity in older subjects in whom there is an increased risk of acute myocardial infarction); this is, however, generally an unimportant issue when dealing with a working and therefore relatively healthy population.

K. Measurement

I. Health Measurements

Measurement constitutes the basis of all scientific studies; what is to be measured can be thought of as the signal, and anything that reduces the precision of the measurement as *noise*. It is hardly necessary to point out that there is a certain amount of variation inherent in all measurement and results on the same individual on different occasions will not be the same. This variation may be due to the instrument, the observer, or the subject, and to their interactions. The first two of these sources of variation always constitute noise and should always be reduced to a minimum, the third may or may not, depending on the study objectives. If it does, every effort should be made to reduce it also to a minimum. A common misconception about epidemiologic studies is that large numbers of subjects make up for imprecision of measurement which can therefore be more than in the clinical context. The reality is quite the contrary; the number of subjects required is a function of the imprecision which is cumulative over the number of subjects studied. Precision should therefore be greater if possible, not less than in the clinical context.

There are three methods in common use for the measurement of respiratory health status in morbidity studies to assess the toxic effects of inhaled materials: the respiratory symptom questionnaire, the chest radiograph, and respiratory function tests. A preliminary to their use in any study should include an assessment of the relative contribution of the sources of variation already listed (instrument, observer, subject) under the particular circumstances of the study in question, and in relation to its objectives, i. e., to assess signal : noise ratios. This information allows the investigator to take the necessary steps to reduce noise as much as possible.

A standardized respiratory symptom questionnaire was first developed by the Medical Research Council in Britain with instructions for use, including the method of posing and following up the questions and training of interviewers.

More recently, it has been adapted for use in North America (FERRIS 1978) and the American Thoracie Society, Division of Lung Diseases (ATS-DLD) questionnaire is now not only generally accepted, but is very widely used; this enhances the comparability of information obtained in different studies and in different workforces on, for instance, smoking habits and the symptoms of bronchitis. If extra questions are required for particular studies (and they usually are), they are best added at the end of the questionnaire; if not, they should be added in such a way as to preserve its flow, particularly if comparability with published data is an objective. Even apparently small changes may affect the way questions are perceived and answers given (ABRAMSON 1979, pp 125–129). Self-administered questionnaires are easier and cheaper, given a certain educational level in the respondents, while administered questionnaires if done by a skilled interviewer can often elicit more information even when conducted by phone (SIEMIATYCKI 1979), though skepticism has been expressed that they do little more than add error due to the interviewer (ABRAMSON 1979, p 126). Postal questionnaires generally produce a low response rate. Variability attributable to instrument and observer respectively can be reduced by use of standardized questionnaires and one trained observer; if more than one is used, efforts must be made to promote its administration in as comparable a fashion as possible (ABRAMSON 1979; BOEHLECKE and MERCHANT 1981).

For the chest radiograph, variability may also be due to instrument and subject and attempts to standardize these factors are part of the training of any good radiologic technician in the clinical as well as in the epidemiologic context. Perhaps the most important source of variability for this form of measurement however, is in the observer. This source of variability has been addressed by the development of a standardized approach with clear instructions for the systematic reading for different abnormalities and the use of standard reference films (INTERNATIONAL LABOUR OFFICE 1980). Other features of the system include the participation of several readers reading independently; this permits an appreciation of variation between readers (OAKES et al. 1982) and is lost if only consensus readings are considered which tend on the whole to be influenced toward the highest reading. This standardized approach was first used in a study of approximately 9,000 films on Québec chrysotile asbestos workers (ROSSITER et al. 1972) and is now generally used in epidemiologic studies (WEILL and JONES 1975). Even so, variation between observers may be considerable; in one study using an earlier version of the ILO classification, it ranged from 12% to 42% abnormal films read by 4 observers in a series of 270 films (EYSSEN 1980); nor was it less, ranging from 18% to 45%, in a similar study comparing the 1980 version with the earlier version (OAKES et al. 1983). Readers may also be categorized according to their performance in training sessions developed to improve uniformity of reading for diagnostic purposes (FELSON et al. 1975; MORGAN et al. 1973). The use of nonmedically trained personnel has also been shown to be feasible, provided that the films are also read for diagnostic purposes by a suitably qualified physician (COPLAND et al. 1981).

For lung functions which are measured on a continuous scale, the signal to noise ratio is not only useful conceptually, but is also susceptible to direct measurement (BECKLAKE et al. 1975). Its quantitation should ideally form part of the prepara-

Table 5. Some sources of variation in lung function measurements [a]

Variation	Source
Within individual	1. Instrument [b]: within and between instruments 2. Observer [b]: administering and reading the tests 3. Subject [c]: cooperation, posture, learning effect, endocrine-induced variation
Between individuals	1. All above sources of differences within each individual 2. Host factors [d]: age, size, sex, race, other genetic characteristics and previous and present health habits, e.g., cigarettes, exercise 3. Environmental [e]: residence and income level, household, (e.g., family smoking, cooking sources), occupation (personal, family)
Between populations	1. All above sources of differences within and between individuals 2. Selection factors influencing original entry into the study population [f] 3. Past and present health status influencing whether or not a subject can continue to remain in a given population [f]

[a] Most data refer to FCV and/or FEV_1
[b] FERRIS (1978); BECKLAKE and PERMUTT (1979)
[c] STEBBINGS (1971); GUBERAN et al. (1969); GLINDMEYER et al. (1981); PHAM et al. (1981); HANKINSON and BOEHLECKE (1981)
[d] STEBBINGS (1971); HIGGINS and KELLER (1973)
[e] STEBBINGS (1971); MONSON (1980)
[f] FOX and COLLIER (1976); MONSON (1980, p 117)

tory work for any field study. The concept can be addressed by considering all sources of variation, within each individual, between individuals, and between populations (Table 5), which may arise, and then in the context of a given study identifying which constitute signal and which noise.

As already pointed out, whatever the objective of the study, whatever the measurement, variation within each individual due to the instrument is noise and must be kept to the minimum possible. In the context of lung function measurements, the general rules for the scientific method apply such as calibration of instruments using external measuring systems as well as cross-calibration of instruments. Several devices exist for providing a calibration signal external to the instrument (FERRIS 1978; GLINDMEYER et al. 1980); in addition, internal electronic calibration signals are provided in most modern electronic equipment. Differences between instruments may also pose a threat to the internal (FERRIS et al. 1973) and external (GRAHAM et al. 1981) validity of a study, and there is an increasing literature pointing to the need for cross-calibration if more than one instrument is used (OLDHAM et al. 1979).

Clearly also variation within each individual due to observer differences always constitutes noise and must be kept to a minimum. Again, in the context of lung function tests, observer effects are of two types, those related to the administration of the test, and those related to the reading of tests (DUCIC et al. 1975). The former relate to the success with which the subject comprehends what is asked and how hard he or she tries, and their influence is well recognized by those who run clinical lung function laboratories (AMERICAN TORACIC SOCIETY 1979). It is countered by technician training: few can have passed by a lung function laboratory without hearing the insistent call to "blow, blow, blow,...more...more, you can do better." Fortunately, the influence of subject effort, while not inconsiderable in some tests such as maximum inspiratory and expiratory pressures (BLACK and HYATT 1969), is much less in others such as the maximum forced expiratory flow rates below approximately 70% of forced vital capacity (FVC), for reasons related to the inherent mechanical properties of the respiratory system (BATES et al. 1971, pp 34–37). Nevertheless, subject effort as well as comprehension account for more variability between subjects than is often recognized (LEECH et al. 1983). Variation in the reading, even of spirometer tracings, has been recognized as a source of error in clinical laboratories for some time (SNIDER et al. 1967); and more recently a variation between readers has also been documented for measurements of greater complexity (BECKLAKE et al. 1975; DUCIC et al. 1975; ZECK et al. 1981). Automated procedures and analysis do not always get around this problem, and the "black box" itself many under- or over-read.

In addition to instrument and observer variation, subjects themselves vary from one measurement to the next, variation which might be called physiologic or ecologic in that it represents the ongoing adaptation of the individual to various changes in his or her internal and/or external milieu. Some of these sources of variation are known (see Table 3) and there are likely others not yet identified. If the objective of an epidemiologic study is to evaluate the effects of exposure to an inhaled agent in the short term, e. g., shift effects of work in cotton mills or in the potrooms of aluminum smelters, the other factors which influence short-term variation should be taken into account in planning the study. For instance, an acute but small decrease in FVC and FEV_1 in response to exposure late in a morning shift might be evident only as a failure to show the usual circadian rise in these measurements (HETZEL and CLARK 1980; STEBBINGS 1971). For assessing effects in the long term, i. e., over months and years, different algorithms have been examined by different investigators for reproducibility, e. g., best or mean of three trials, best or mean of five trials, mean of three tests of five trials, etc. In practical terms, what was sought is a balance between a sufficient number of trials at any one session to overcome the learning effect and not so many as to induce fatigue or boredom. With the publication of the Epidemiology Standardization project (FERRIS 1978) the investigator is provided with carefully considered guidelines for all commonly used tests which should become standard practice, unless for reasons specific to a particular study these need to be modified.

In epidemiologic studies to examine the toxic effects of inhaled materials, comparison of populations with different exposures will usually provide the basis on which the investigator addresses the question to be answered. Ideally, he or she seeks to compare populations similar in all factors that affect the lung function measurement under scrutiny except exposure. In fact, given populations with the appropriate differences in exposure, an effort must be then made to deal with all the other sources of variations between individuals populations (see Table 5), which might exaggerate or minimize the differences otherwise attributed to the consequences of exposure. Strategies for dealing with these sources of variation include: (a) matching (subject selection); (b) partitioning the data into cells; (c) use of the factors as covariates in some form of analysis of variance; and (d) standardization of observed values against an expected value, based on comparisons internal or external to the study. The first and second are rarely practical unless the target population is very large, so most investigators adopt the third or the fourth. These issues are further discussed elsewhere (BOEHLECKE and MERCHANT 1981; GHEZZO 1982).

In conclusion, reliability in measurement is clearly an objective in any scientific study and enhancing it is clearly part of preparatory work for any field study. The wise investigator will, if possible, measure it directly in the context of a given study, and include in his or her report information about differences between apparatus, technicians, and readers, depending on which is applicable, in addition to an assessment of potential biases due to the systematic operation of these sources of variation across study groups. There is, however, another side to the question. While, on the one hand, attention to the details of measurement must continue to remain an issue (GRAHAM 1981), on the other hand, there is, as has been pointed out by ELINSON (1972), "a danger in studies of reliability of permitting the perfect to become the enemy of the good." ABRAMSON (1979) therefore urges that the measurement of a phenomenon should not be given up simply because there is some degree of unreliability. Achieving the balance marks the good investigator.

II. Measurements Underlying the Exposure Variable

The importance of the exposure variable, already alluded to, cannot be overemphasized, yet it is frequently only scantily defined in workplace studies (BAUMGARTEN and OSEASOHN 1980). As indicated earlier in Table 2, elements in its measurement include quality, duration, and intensity. In McDONALD's view (1981) failure to specify exposure, except in terms of duration, is the most serious weakness in occupational epidemiology and, while recognizing the inherent difficulties, he blames investigators themselves for a certain amount of defeatism. For this type of measurement, it is not so much the perfect that is the enemy of the good but that no measurement at all is the enemy of "better-than-nothing," and he urges that every effort should therefore be made to incorporate some assessment of intensity, even a largely subjective one, provided this is done blind to the outcome. The industrial hygienist is an invaluable partner if not an essential member of the investigative team in this regard. Indices based on measurement of the agent in human tissues have been mentioned (see also Table 2).

In dealing with acute effects, the relevant exposure is current or recent, not past, and this can often be measured directly. Furthermore, the experimental approach with simulation in the laboratory, e. g., in cases of occupational asthma (PEPYS and HUTCHCROFT 1975) opened the way to studies in the workplace with direct measurement of the relevant environmental levels (BROOKS 1977; NEWMAN-TAYLOR 1980).

In dealing with chronic effects, however, the relevant exposures are almost certainly those which occurred in the past, often the remote past. Not only were they not usually measured, but it is difficult even to conceptualize the appropriate measurement, other than to say it should be that which most closely predicts health outcome, i. e., the measurement which gives the highest exposure–response relationship. By implication, this might well be different for different types of health effect. For instance, particles in the respirable size range may be responsible for silicosis and the other pneumoconioses, whereas larger particles may be responsible for industrial bronchitis (MORGAN 1978; COPES et al. 1984). There is also evidence to suggest that the asbestos fibers responsible for pulmonary fibrosis are on the average of greater diameter than those responsible for cancer (WAGNER 1980). In practice, as is so often the case, the investigator has really no choice but to adopt empirical solutions. The simplest approach is to classify subjects into exposure groups, e. g., low, medium, and high, using other criteria (usually a combination of job title, task, and location) and then provide in addition descriptive information on the range of environmental levels covered by the terms low, medium, and high.

Another approach used with increasing frequency in recent years is based on the development of a *cumulative exposure index* for each subject studied, reflecting his or her personal exposure experience. This type of index takes into account plant production and engineering history and any available past measurements, supplemented if necessary with descriptive information of past conditions provided by long-service workers, if possible, obtained without collusion between them. These impressions can then be related to current environmental measurements to permit a grading of dustiness. Environmental information of this sort can, in turn, be linked to job titles by year and so to the worker's employment record, permitting the calculation of an index of cumulative exposure (GIBBS and LACHANCE 1972).

Potential inaccuracies in this type of assessment are numerous and include the following: job titles on payrolls tend to describe remuneration, not the place of work and/or task executed; job change may not be recorded if pay is not affected; dust counts are often made to assist engineering housekeeping (i. e., to check a poor valve or identify a malfunctioning fan) rather than to assess air quality (HAMMAD et al. 1981); methods used are chosen to comply with regulation (e. g., the change from particle to fiber count as a measure of asbestos exposure in the early 1970s) and, unless the two techniques continue in parallel, it becomes difficult to link the present with the past. Despite these inaccuracies, which undoubtedly lead to misrepresentation of an individual's past exposure, cumulative exposure indices of one sort or another invariably provide a reasonable basis for classifying individuals into the more or less exposed relative to one another. Their main disadvantage is in failing to separate duration and intensity which can be seriously misleading.

Attempts have also been made to assess the influence of modifiers of the exposure level (see Table 2), such as the activity level of a job and weighting the index to take into account estimated residence time of dust in the lung. For instance, in Québec asbestos miners and mill workers, ROSSITER et al. (1972) showed some, though inconsistent, effects of these modifiers on the relationship between X-ray readings and cumulative exposure, while COPES et al. (1984) found a time weighting to relate to indices of airway abnormality, and peaks of exposure to pleural abnormality read on the chest radiograph.

Cumulative exposure indices tend to reflect the working conditions of the past when controls were minimal and pollution heavy (GIBBS and LACHANCE 1972); under more modern conditions it may not be possible to show dose relationships when this type of exposure index is used (BECKLAKE et al. 1982). Strategies for assessing exposure in the future may well therefore have to be different, for instance, the development of the exposure zone concept in which zones are identified for work similarity as well as exposure and environmental similarity. Exposures are then directly measured in a sample of the workforce in any given zone (CORN 1981). Likewise, ingenuity in sampling, e. g., personal samplers which are responsive to variable breathing patterns, may also offer some promise in the future (KUCHARSKI 1980).

L. Analysis and Inference

The mathematical treatment of the data in any study is directed towards two ends, description and analysis; both are carried out in light of the stated objectives of the study, and follow naturally from the design chosen. In other words, the approach to this phase of a study is inherent in its planning. In the present context, namely epidemiologic studies to assess the toxic effects of inhaled materials, analysis is invariably directed towards looking for associations (or their absence) between mortality and/or morbidity and the exposure variable, and interpreting the meaning of any such associations.

A general strategy for a descriptive analysis is that it should record in logical sequence the sequential phases of the study. Thus, the target population, the sample selected (if sampling is used), and the numbers contacted and examined as well as the number for whom valid data are available must all be given, as well as reasons for the shortfall in each successive step, and any other information available about the missing subjects. Next comes the presentation of characteristics of the subjects studied, including frequency distribution of study variables. The cautious approach is recommended, examining the variables first separately, then in pairs, and then in sets of three or more using simple methods such as cross-tabulation to reveal associations (ABRAMSON 1979, p 180). An early phase in the analysis should be the exploration of associations between the dependent variables particular to the study and what ABRAMSON (1979) calls the "universal" variables, namely, age, sex, race; in the context of lung functions, this also includes size descriptors such as height and weight. Next to consider is the distribution of confounding, potentially confounding, and modifying variables in relation to the exposure variable. This leads into the further analysis of the nature of the associations between exposure and the dependent variables chosen for study using the statistical techniques of multivariate analysis, techniques which require statistical expertise (ABRAMSON 1979, p 182; MONSON 1980) and for which the appropriate statistical texts should be consulted.

Interpretation of the significance (medical, not statistical) of associations (or lack of them) is the key issue in analytic surveys, in particular, those concerned with the toxic effects of inhaled materials. Answers to some or all of the following questions about association (ABRAMSON 1979, p 190) assist the investigator in interpretation: actual or artificial, i. e., due to technical factors? how strong? how likely to have occurred by chance? how consistent? influence of confounding factors? and finally causal? For a detailed discussion of the criteria for interpretation, the reader should consult other texts such as HILL (1977) and MONSON (1980, pp 93–97).

Inferences based on the interpretation of the results of the analysis (including consideration of any demonstrated associations) must be made in light of the extent to which the execution of the study fell short of the ideal (it always does) and of what was planned (it usually does) and of how such shortcomings may have biased the findings or reduced their sensitivity. In brief, the questions to answer are: could any associations with exposure shown have been due to bias, or could the lack of association have been due to imprecision? Bias may have been introduced in selection, in observation, or in confounding (MONSON 1980, p 97). Most other potential shortcomings have been already discussed; see comments on internal and external validity in Sect. E. II, as well as the all-important issue implicit in Hill's question (1977): "is there any other way of explaining the set of facts before us?" Consideration of these factors is an essential in the preparation of any report as well as in its external evaluation; in general, the more complete the consideration of these factors, the better the report.

M. Uses of Epidemiologic Studies in the General Assessment of Toxic Effects of Inhaled Agents

I. Identification

This refers to the identification of new or unrecognized toxic effects due to agents not known to be associated with effects, as well as the detection of recognized toxic effects in populations not previously thought to be at risk. Failure to demonstrate effects may also at times be useful. In the past, previously unrecognized toxic effects, if sufficiently unusual in clinical experience, have been detected by shrewd clinical observation. For instance, when C. A. Sleggs, a community physician practicing in the asbestos mining district of the Northwest Cape, South Africa, referred a series of over 30 pleural tumors to a surgeon, P. Marchand, whose biopsy/surgical material was handled by a single pathologist, J.C. Wagner, the clustering of cases unusual in the experience of all three led to the first report suggesting an association between this tumor and asbestos exposure (SLEGGS et al. 1961). Subsequently, a more systematic study of the problem on a worldwide basis, as reviewed by McDONALD and McDONALD (1977) has amply confirmed the association, now generally accepted as causal (see Sect. M. II for a discussion of criteria for judging whether an association is causal). Another example was the occurrence of 20 cases of nasal cancer in furniture workers from High Wycombe, a town in Buckinghamshire, England. This association was sufficiently unusual in the clinical experience of Hadfield and MacBeth (otolaryngologists working respectively in High Wycombe and Oxford) to alert them to the potential association of cancer and occupation, an association also subsequently confirmed not only for this exposure (the epidemic in the Buckinghamshire woodworkers may now be on the decline), but also in association with the occupations of leather work and shoe manufacture (ACHESON 1976). Angiosarcoma in relation to exposure to polyvinylchloride manufacture is another example of an association originally recognized by alert clinical observation (CREECH and JOHNSON 1974). Indeed, the view has been expressed that there is no substitute for astute clinical observation and the best surveillance system would be one which permitted rapid informal communication of clinical concerns for scientific evaluation (McDONALD and HARRINGTON 1981).

Hitherto unrecognized toxic effects are also usually readily recognized if the time course between exposure and response is relatively short and a sufficiently large number is affected, even if the manifestations suggest a common illness. An example was the outbreak of an acute respiratory illness in 210 members of a workforce of approximately 2000, manufacturing synthetic rubber tires, after introduction of new materials into the tire carcass stock formulation (DoPICO et al. 1975). In this outbreak, the exact identity of the volatile materials thought to be responsible was not established. Another approach, applicable when morbidity information is available on large workforces, is to investigate illness patterns of occupational groups by cluster analysis (STILLE 1980). For smaller workforces, a matched pair approach has been used (KRAMER et al. 1978).

On the other hand, for diseases which are relatively common in the general population, and for which the incubation period between exposure and clinical manifestation is long (decades or more), the identification of an increased risk in association with exposure is much less likely to occur if left simply and solely to chance. This is so for most cancers and for chronic lung diseases such as bronchitis and emphysema. Mortality attributable to the former and probably to the latter of these groups of diseases continues to rise in industrialized countries (DIVISION of LUNG DISEASES 1980), as does the exposure of their citizens to environmental pollution. Insofar as exposure to environmental agents represents an avoidable risk for lung cancer (DOLL and PETO 1981), large-scale surveillance programs of an ongoing nature have been developed to discern and subsequently investigate any such associations (BROSS et al. 1978; SIEMIATYCKI et al. 1981). The next few years should see an evaluation of such programs; their justification is the need to bypass the time-consuming agent-by-agent study of potential hazards; their weakness is the rapidity with which new materials are being introduced into the workplace so that today's cancers may well reflect workplace exposures to combinations of agents no longer in use. No systematic ongoing effort to determine the role of workplace exposures in what appears to be a rising prevalence of chronic obstructive lung disease (DIVISION of LUNG DISEASES 1980) has as yet been described despite the now general recognition of the entity of "industrial bronchitis" (MORGAN 1978).

The demonstration of (or failure to demonstrate) the presence of toxic effects of inhaled materials in populations thought (or not thought) to be at risk or in workforces not previously examined is often regarded more as a service function than as research. Thus, such studies (which simply ask the question: is there a health hazard in a given workforce?) are frequently called for to provide a basis for making decisions in the public health field, decisions relating to issues such as environmental controls, distribution of resources, and priorities. Such questions, obviously important for workers and management in the plant itself, may also have wider implications. Indeed, insofar as the answer is generalizable, the results may contribute to the overall picture of dose–response relationships which form the scientific basis for establishing environmental control levels (ACHESON and GARDNER 1981). For instance, no radiologic abnormality of an asbestotic nature will be expected in the workforce of a relatively new plant utilizing asbestos in which the environmental levels, monitored since its inception, indicate compliance with current threshold limit values (TLVs). If there is evidence of radiologic abnormality, it must be assumed that the proposed TVLs do not protect human health, or that the workforce concerned was unduly susceptible because of host and/or other environmental factors, or that the environmental measurements made in conformity with the maintenance of control levels do not adequately reflect the elements in the exposure relevant to the production of the abnormality or disease in question. The latter might be due to size or chemical characteristics of the toxic material or to the presence of other agents or cofactors in the plant processes and/or air. Note that a TLV (or any other proposed norm) is no more, no less, than the expression of a hypothesis that, if human exposure is confined to the stated levels, then human health will be protected. The hypothesis stands so long as there is no evidence upon which to question it.

II. Etiologic Studies

In the present context this consists primarily in exploring the relationships between exposures and responses. Studies with this objective in mind form by far the bulk of published research under the heading of the general assessment of the toxicity of inhaled materials, and clearly no more than a few of the very large number of publications can be cited. The choice is arbitrary, preference being given to those which incorporate an unusual and/or useful feature in technique; otherwise the examples cited deal with asbestos exposure in the Québec chrysotile asbestos mines and mills, health effects of exposure to which was the subject of a comprehensive research program carried out by a large team of which the author was a member (McDONALD et al. 1974; McDONALD 1981).

The first approach to the general assessment of the toxicity of an agent is invariably a descriptive survey of mortality and/or morbidity (depending on the expected effects) in a workforce exposed to the agent under study. If there is doubt about its toxicity, comparison of exposure (definite) with no exposure (also definite) is desirable; if its toxicity is already well recognized, as was the case for chrysotile asbestos when the Québec studies were started, then internal comparisons can be made to examine for exposure–response relationships.

Several types of study were carried out in this research program the objective of which was, as already indicated, to assess the health consequences of exposure to asbestos in the Québec chrysotile mines and mills (McDONALD et al. 1974). The first step, also already alluded to, was the preparation of a census of all past and present workers (approximately 30,000) together with their recorded work histories. Within the complete workforce so defined, different target populations were identified for a series of mortality and morbidity studies, designed to study the occurrence of the recognized serious health effects of asbestos exposure, e. g., fibrosis of the lungs and pleura as well as cancer of the lungs and pleura. Thus, a prevalence survey was carried out on an age-stratified random sample of approximately 1,000 of the approximately 6,000 current workers who were assessed by respiratory symptom questionnaire (MCDONALD et al. 1972), and lung function tests (BECKLAKE et al. 1972) for abnormalities suggesting pulmonary fibrosis. The prevalence studies on current workers were complemented by prospective measurements 7 years later, for which a relationship to cumulative exposure was no longer evident, probably owing to the changing exposure profile (BECKLAKE et al. 1982). Prevalence of radiologic abnormality was also assessed in approximately 9,000 films of past and present workers (ROSSITER et al. 1972), and mortality, in particular that due to lung cancer, studied in a birth cohort (1890–1920) of approximately 11,000 men (MCDONALD et al. 1971) with subsequent follow-up (MCDONALD et al. 1980). In all these studies, the independent or explanatory variable was a cumulative exposure index of the type described in Sect. K. II (GIBBS and LACHANCE 1972), and in all studies exposure–response relationships were demonstrated. Other aspects of the exposure–response relationships were also explored, e. g., the relationship of exposure to the progression of radiologic change (LIDDELL et al. 1977), the influence of exposure profile on abnormality (COPES et al. 1984), the effect of withdrawal from exposure (BECKLAKE et al. 1980), and the prognostic value of radiologic abnormality (LIDDELL and MCDONALD 1980). The prevalence of obstructive and restrictive function profiles was also examined (FOURNIER-MASSEY and BECKLAKE 1975) as well as the interrelationship of functional and radiologic change (BECKLAKE et al. 1970). In view of the very infrequent occurrence of malignant mesothelioma (approximately one per million in the general population) the approach chosen was a case-referent study based on ascertainment across Canada (MCDONALD et al. 1970), later extended to include the United States (MCDONALD and MCDONALD 1980).

While the scientific basis for the development of environmental standards is essentially whatever information is available on exposure–response relationships, studies which have as their specific objective the provision of information for this purpose tend to differ in emphasis. Thus, in such studies particular attention is given to the technology of the environmental measurements which service the exposure variable, in particular, sampling strategy as well as technique and accuracy, all of which may or will become incorporated into the definition of the proposed control levels (BERRY et al. 1979). Indeed, ACHESON and GARDNER (1981) point out that the introduction of more sensitive dust counting methods may have resulted in de facto improvements in hygiene standards without a change in TLV.

As in other fields of epidemiology, the question arises of whether demonstrated associations are causal. This requires a complete review of published information. Criteria for this assessment elaborated by HILL (1977) include consistency (are the findings similar in different populations studied by different observers and in different parts of the world?), strength (are the relationships strong or barely detectable?), specificity, time relationship (does exposure consistently precede the development of the disease in question?), dose–response, and biologic plausibility. Based on these criteria, asbestos now joins cigarettes as one of the recognized causal agents of lung cancer (MCDONALD 1980), and is one of 18 agents recognized by the INTERNATIONAL AGENCY for RESEARCH on CANCER (1979) as human carcinogens.

Finally, data collected in epidemiologic studies in exposed populations may also elucidate disease mechanisms. For instance, ZUSKIN et al. (1979) in a study of airway responsiveness in 59 workers processing polyester resins, were able to show that propanolol administered before the start of a shift exaggerated the changes observable at the end of the shift, while atropine abolished them. This suggested that the autonomic nervous system played a dominant role in mediating the response.

III. Evaluation

Preventive strategies are elaborated on the basis of what is known about the diseases in question, their etiology, and underlying mechanisms. In the present context where the diseases and/or abnormalities under consideration are known or believed to be due to the toxic effects of inhaled materials, the preventive strategies include:

1. Removal or neutralization of the toxic component of the material before human exposure occurs, an ideal solution if the toxic component is known (it usually is not) or can be neutralized without jeopardizing its commercial usefulness.
2. Control of exposure to levels known or believed to protect human health: the certainly safe level (i. e., no exposure) can often be realized by engineering methods (such as complete enclosure of the process to cut emissions to zero) or by substitution; if this is not possible the approach is to establish, monitor, and enforce environmental standards which are believed to protect human health (see Sect. M. I for comments on TLV).
3. Environmental and health surveillance usually accompany these strategies, in a sense as support mechanisms.

Epidemiologic studies in human populations provide the means for evaluating the effectiveness of all these control strategies. An example of evaluation of the implementation of the first strategy is given by the reports of IMBUS and SUH (1974) and MERCHANT et al. (1973) and refers to cotton processing. Laboratory studies had suggested that the toxic component of cotton dust was neutralized by steam washing prior to its further processing. Two studies were carried put looking respectively at the health effects following introduction on an experimental basis (MERCHANT et al. 1974) and discontinuation, prior to engineering changes (IMBUS and SUH 1974), of the process of steam washing. Though obviously neither was an experimental design (for instance, mills were not randomly selected and assigned for introduction or not of the steam washing process), these quasiexperimental designs which fall into the time series type of study have good internal validity, and though not multiple in the sense of including several plants studied in random order at irregular intervals, nevertheless provide convincing evidence in support of the preventive strategy.

Evaluation of the implementation of the second strategy is also straightforward if the toxic effects are acute. For example, it was hardly necessary to restudy the rubber tire plant in which a large number of workers had suffered acute respiratory illnesses once the new formulation process had been phased out, even though the putative agent (or agents) was not specifically identified (DoPICO et al. 1975). However, when the effects are only seen in the long term, evaluation is more difficult. For instance, one of the objectives of a 3-year prospective study carried out in 14 Lancashire cotton mills was to investigate the effectiveness of dust suppression equipment (MOLYNEUX and TOMBLESON 1970); information on prevalence of byssinosis at the outset and of incidence determined by reexamination at 6-month intervals of the approximately 1,500 operatives under study, together with information on the average dust levels in the different mills, led the authors to conclude that "dust control measures though they have produced considerable improvement are not now fully effective with present methods of production."

Another such evaluation was that of the effectiveness of the British Occupational Hygiene Society's hygiene standards for chrysotile (BERRY et al. 1979). The standard of 2 fibers/cm^3 had been proposed on the basis of prevalence studies involving approximately 300 workers with 10 years or more employment in an asbestos textile plant (BRITISH OCCUPATIONAL HYGIENE SOCIETY 1968). Using basal rales as the indicator of asbestosis, the authors proposed a standard which they estimated would control the incidence of this disease to less than 1% for an exposure of 2 fibers/cm^3 for a period of 50 years. Follow-up measurements including ex-workers showed a higher prevalence of rales than was observed previously at all exposure levels, leading the authors to conclude that "there is no room for complacency about the fiber/cm^3 standard" though they felt it was "impossible to state that the standard is inadequate."

N. Summary

1. Epidemiologic studies in human populations can be used to study the full range of responses in time (acute/chronic), in character (nonmalignant/malignant), and in severity (discomfort/adaptation/disease/disability/death) which may follow exposure to inhaled materials, whether they be gaseous or particulate.

2. Crucial to the success of such studies is the appropriate assessment of exposure, without which the value of the study is much diminished, however successful it may be in respect of its other elements, namely, objectives (why), design (how), population (who), and methods (what is to be measured and how it is to be measured).

3. While experimental designs are seldom appropriate in the context of assessment of the toxic effects of inhaled materials, quasiexperimental designs can often be effectively used. However, most studies fall into the category of survey, i.e., investigations in which information is systematically gathered, but in which the experimental method is not used. Surveys may be longitudinal, cross-sectional, or case-referent, and may be primarily explanatory in purpose, primarily descriptive, or as is usually the case, a combination.

4. The choice of population of study, and of the variables to be examined, together with the measurements underlying these variables, whether they describe health status of the subjects studied or their exposure, is made in light of the objectives of the study and usually represents the best compromise the investigator can achieve between the ideal and the practical.

5. Epidemiologic studies in human populations can be used: (a) to identify previously unrecognized toxic effects or identify the presence of toxic effects in populations not previously thought to be at risk; (b) to clarify etiology, primarily by examining dose–response relationships to exposure (this includes providing information for the formulation of preventive strategies such as setting TLV), and (c) to evaluate preventive strategies so formulated.

6. Further refinements in epidemiologic techniques (in particular, in design and in methodology of analysis) will obviously benefit studies designed to assess the toxic effects of inhaled materials. However, of particular importance in such studies is the assessment of exposure, more specifically of delivery of the agent to the target organ and its retention for a sufficient period to cause harmful effects. Thus, future research should be directed towards developing more appropriate and more precise ways of making such assessments.

Acknowledgments. The author would like to acknowledge with much appreciation the critical comments on this text by Professors J. C. McDonald and R. Oseasohn, respectively, Director, School of Occupational Health and Safety, and Chairman, Department of Epidemiology and Health, McGill University, Montreal, Québec. This work was supported by a grant from the Conseil de Recherche en Santé du Québec for studies in the working environment and health. The author is a Career Investigator, Medical Research Council of Canada.

References

Abramson JH (1979) Methods in community medicine, 2nd edn. Churchill Livingston, Edinburgh

Acheson ED (1976) Nasal cancer in the furniture and boot and shoe manufacturing industries. Prev Med 5:295–315

Acheson ED, Gardner MJ (1981) Exposure limits – the scientific criteria. In: McDonald JC (ed) Recent advances in occupational health. Churchill Livingstone, Edinburgh, pp 257–270

American Thoracic Society (1979) Snowbird workshop on standardisation of spirometry. Am Rev Respir Dis 119:831–838

Bates DV, Macklem PT, Christie RV (1971) Respiratory function in disease, 2nd edn. WB Sauncers Coy, Philadelphia

Baumgarten M, Oseasohn R (1980) Studies in occupational health: a critique. J Occup Med 22:171–176

Beadle DG (1970) The relationship between the amount of dust breathed and the development of radiological signs of silicosis: an epidemiologic study in South African goldminers. In: Walton WH (ed) Inhaled particles III. Unwin, London, pp 953–966

Becklake MR (1976) Asbestos-related diseases of the lungs and other organs: their epidemiology and implications for clinical practice. Am Rev Respir Dis 114:187–227

Becklake MR (1982) Asbestos-related diseases of the lungs and pleura: current clinical issues. Am Rev Respir Dis 126:187–194

Becklake MR, Permutt S (1979) Evaluation of tests of lung function for early detection of chronic obstructive lung disease. In: Macklem PT, Permutt S (eds) The lung in the transition between health and disease. Marcel Dekker, New York, pp 345–388

Becklake MR, Fournier-Massey FG, McDonald JC, Siemiatycki J, Rossiter CE (1970) Lung function in relation to chest radiographic changes in Quebec asbestos workers. Bull Physio-Pathol Respir 6:637–659

Becklake MR, Fournier-Massey G, Rossiter CE, McDonald JC (1972) Lung function in chrysotile asbestos mine and mill workers of Quebec. Arch Environ Health 24:401–409

Becklake MR, Leclerc M, Strobach H, Swift J (1975) The N closing volume test in population studies: sources of variation and reproducibility. Am Rev Respir Dis 111:141–147

Becklake MR, Thomas D, Liddell FDK, McDonald JC (1982) Follow-up respiratory measurements in Quebec chrysotile asbestos miners and millers. Scand J Work Environ Health 8(Suppl):105–110

Becklake MR, Toyota B, Stewart M, Hanson R, Hanley J (1983) Lung structure as a risk factor in adverse pulmonary responses to asbestos exposure: a casereferent study in Quebec chrysotile asbestos miners and millers. Am Rev Respir Dis (in press)

Berry G (1974) Longitudinal observations: their usefulness and limitations with special reference to the forced expiratory volume. Bull Physio-Pathol Respir 10:643–656

Berry G, Gilson JC, Holmes S, Lewinsohn HC, Roach SA (1979) Asbestosis: a study of dose-response relationships in an asbestos textile factory. Br J Ind Med 36:98–112

Black LF, Hyatt RE (1969) Maximal respiratory pressures: normal values and relationship to age and sex. Am Rev Respir Dis 99:696–702

Blomquist N (1977) On the relation between change and initial value. J Am Stat Assoc 72:746–749

Boehlecke BA, Merchant JA (1981) The use of pulmonary function testing and questionnaires as epidemiologic tools in the study of occupational lung disease. Chest 79/4 (Suppl):114S–122S

Brain JD, Valberg PA (1974) Models of lung retention based on ICRP Task Group Report. Arch Environ Health 28:1–11

British Occupational Health Society (1968) Hygiene standards for chrysotile asbestos dust. Ann Occup Hyg 11:47–69

Brooks SM (1977) Bronchial asthma of occupational origin: a review. Scand J Work Environ Health 3:53–72

Bross IDJ, Viadanna E, Houten L (1978) Occupational cancer in men exposed to dust and other environmental hazards. Arch Environ Health 33:300–307

Campbell DT, Stanley JC (1966) Experimental and quasi-experimental designs for research. Rand McNally and Coy, Chicago

Chan-Yeung M, Ashley MJ, Corey P, Willson G, Donken E, Grzybowski S (1978) A respiratory survey of cedar mill workers. I. Prevalence of symptoms and pulmonary function abnormality. J Occup Med 20:323–327

Cobb S, Miller M, Wald N (1959) On the estimation of the incubation period in malignant disease. J Chronic Dis 9:385–393

Copes RL, Thomas D, Becklake MR (1984) Temporal patterns of exposure and non-malignant pulmonary abnormality in Québec chrysotile workers. Arch Environ Health (in press)

Copland L, Burns J, Jacobsen M (1981) Classification of chest radiographs for epidemiological purposes by people not experienced in the radiology of pneumoconioses. Br J Ind Med 38:254–261

Corn M (1981) Strategies of air sampling. In: McDonald JC (ed) Recent advances in occupational health. Churchill Livingstone, Edinburgh, pp 199–210

Creech JL, Johnson MN (1974) Angiosarcoma of the liver in the manufacture of polyvinyl chloride. J Occup Med 16:150–151

Division of Lung Diseases, National Heart, Lung and Blood Institute (NHLBI) (1980) Report of a task force on the epidemiology of respiratory diseases. US Department of Health and Human Services, NIH Publication No 81–2019, Washington, DC

Doll R, Peto R (1981) The causes of cancer: quantitative estimates of avoidable risks of cancer in the United States today. J Natl Cancer Inst 66:1191–1308

DoPico GA, Rankin J, Chosy LW, Reddan WG, Barbee RA, Gee B, Dickie HA (1975) Respiratory tract disease from thermosetting resins: study of an outbreak in rubber tire workers. Ann Intern Med 83:177–184

Dreesen WC, Dallaville TI, Miller JW, Sayers RR (1938) A study of asbestosis in the asbestos textile industry. US Treasury Department: Public Health Service Bulletin 241, US Government Printing Office, Washington, DC

Ducic S, Swift J, Martin RR, Macklem PT (1975) Appraisal of a new test: between technician variation in the measurement of closing volume. Am Rev Respir Dis 112:621–627

Elinson J (1972) Methods of sociomedical research. In: Freeman HE, Levine S, Reeder LG (eds) Handbook of medical sociology, 2nd edn. Prentice-Hall, Englewood Cliffs, pp 483–500

Eyssen G (1980) Development of radiographic abnormality in chrysotile miners and millers. Chest 78/1 (Suppl):411–414

Felson B, Jacobsen G, Pendergrass EP, Linton O, Harrington J (1975) Viewbox seminar: a new teaching method for roentgenology. Radiology 116:75–78

Ferris BG Jr (1978) Epidemiology standardisation project. Am Rev Respir Dis 6(2):1–120

Ferris BG, Higgins ITT, Higgins M, Peters JM (1973) Chronic nonspecific respiratory disease in Berlin, New Hampshire, 1961 to 1967: a followup study. Am Rev Respir Dis 107:110–122

Field GB (1981) Worker surveys. In: Weill H, Turner-Warwick M (eds) Occupational lung diseases: research approaches and methods. Marcel Dekker, New York, pp 406–26

Fletcher CE, Peto R (1977) The natural history of chronic airflow obstruction. Br Med J 1:1645–1648

Fournier-Massey GF, Becklake MR (1975) Pulmonary function profiles in Quebec asbestos workers. Bull Physio-Pathol Respir 11:429–431

Fox AJ, Collier PF (1976) Low mortality rates in industrial cohort studies due to selection for work and survival in the industry. Br J Prev Soc Med 30:225–230

Ghezzo H (1983) Normalisation of lung function tests for epidemiologic studies. PhD Thesis, McGill University

Gibbs GW, Lachance M (1972) Dust exposure in the chrysotile asbestos mines and mills of Quebec. Arch Environ Health 24:189–197

Glindmeyer H, Anderson, ST, Kern RG, Hughes J (1980) A portable adjustable forced vital capacity simulator for routine spirometer calibration. Am Rev Respir Dis 121:599–603

Glindmeyer H, Diem J, Hughes J, Jones RN, Weill H (1981) Factors influencing the interpretation of FEV1 declines across the working shift. Chest 79/4 Suppl:71S–73S

Goldsmith JR (1975) What do we expect from an occupational cohort? J Occup Med 17:126–131

Graham WGB, O'Grady RV, Dubuc B (1981) Pulmonary function loss in Vermont granite workers: a long-term follow up and critical appraisal. Am Rev Respir Dis 123:25–28

Green M, Mead J, Turner JM (1974) Variability of maximum expiratory flow volume curves. J Appl Physiol 37:67–74

Guberan E, Williams MK, Walford J, Smith MM (1969) Circadian variation of FEV in shift workers. Br J Ind Med 26:121–125

Hammad Y, Corn M, Dharmarajan V (1981) Environmental characterisation. In: Weill H, Turner-Warwick M (eds) Occupational lung diseases: research approaches and methods. Marcel Dekker, New York, pp 291–372

Hankinson JL, Boehlecke BA (1981) Variability of spirometric pulmonary function studies. Am Rev Respir Dis 4(2):123–148

Hetzel MR, Clark TJH (1980) Comparison of normal and asthmatic circadian rhythms in peak expiratory flow rate. Thorax 35:732–738

Higgins MW, Keller JB (1973) Seven measures of ventilatory lung function: population values and comparison of their ability to discriminate between persons with and without chronic respiratory symptoms and disease, Tecumseh, Michigan. Am Rev Respir Dis 108:258–272

Hill AB (1977) A short textbook of medical statistics. Hodder and Stroughton, London

Imbus HR, Suh MW (1974) Steaming of cotton to prevent byssinosis: a plant study. Br J Ind Med 31:209–219

International Agency for Research on Cancer (1979) Chemicals and industrial processes associated with cancer in humans. IARC Monographs 1–20, Abstract, Lyon, pp 1–14

International Labour Office (1980) Guidelines for the use of the ILO international classification of radiographs of pneumoconioses, revised edition. Occupational Safety and Health Series No. 22, International Labour Office, Geneva

Kramer CG, Oh MG, Fulkeson JE, Hicks N, Imbus HR (1978) Health of workers exposed to 1,1,1-trichlorethelene: a matched pair study. Arch Environ Health 33:331–342

Kucharski R (1980) A personal dust sampler simulating variable human lung function. Br J Ind Med 37:194–196

Le Bouffant L (1980) Physics and chemistry of asbestos dust. In: Wagner JC (ed) Biological effects of mineral fibres, vol 1. IARC Scientific Publication No 30, Lyon, pp 15–33

Leech JA, Ghezzo H, Stevens D, Becklake MR (1983) Respiratory pressures and function in young adults. Am Rev Respir Dis 128:17–23

Liddell FDK (1973) Morbidity of British coal miners in 1961–1962. Br J Ind Med 30:1–14

Liddell FDK, McDonald JC (1980) Radiological findings as predictors of mortality in Quebec asbestos workers. Br J Ind Med 37:257–267

Liddell FDK, McDonald JC (1981) Survey design and analysis. In: McDonald JC (ed) Recent advances in occupational health. Churchill Livingstone, Edinburgh, pp 95–105

Liddell FDK, Eyssen G, Thomas D, McDonald JC (1977) Radiological changes over 20 years in relation to chrysotile exposure in Quebec. In: Walton WH (ed) Inhaled particles IV. Pergamon, Oxford, pp 799–812

Lilienfeld AM, Lilienfeld DE (1981) Foundations of epidemiology, 2nd edn. Oxford University Press, New York

Lippmann M, Yeates DB, Albert RE (1980) Deposition, retention and clearance of inhaled particles. Br J Ind Med 37:337–362

MacMahon B, Pugh TF (1970) Epidemiology: principles and methods. Little, Brown, Boston

McDonald AD, McDonald JC (1980) Malignant mesothelioma in North America. Cancer 46:1650–1656

McDonald AD, Harper A, El Attar OA, McDonald JC (1970) Epidemiology of primary malignant mesothelial tumours in Canada. Cancer 26:914–919

McDonald AD, McDonald JC, Pooley FD (1982) Mineral fibre content of the lung in mesothelial tumours in North America. Ann Occup Hyg 26:417–421

McDonald JC (1980) Asbestos and lung cancer: has the case been proven? Chest 78/2 Suppl:374–376

McDonald JC (1981) Epidemiology. In: Weill H, Turner-Warwick M (eds) Occupational lung diseases: research approach and methods. Marcel Dekker, New York, pp 373–404

McDonald JC, Harrington JM (1981) Early detection of occupational hazards. J Soc Occup Med 31:93–98

McDonald JC, McDonald AD (1977) Epidemiology of mesothelioma from estimated incidence. Prev Med 6:426–446

McDonald JC, McDonald AD, Gibbs GW, Siemiatycki J, Rossiter CE (1971) Mortality in the chrysotile asbestos mines and mills of Quebec. Arch Environ Health 22:677–681

McDonald JC, Becklake MR, Fournier-Massey G, Rossiter CE (1972) Respiratory symptoms in chrysotile asbestos mine and mill workers of Quebec. Arch Environ Health 24:358–363

McDonald JC, Becklake MR, Gibbs GW, McDonald AD, Rossiter CE (1974) The health of chrysotile asbestos mine and mill workers of Quebec. Arch Environ Health 28:61–68

McDonald JC, Liddell FDK, Gibbs GW, Eyssen GE, McDonald AD (1980) Dust exposure and mortality in chrysotile mining 1910–1975. Br J Ind Med 37:11–24

Merchant JA, Lumsden JC, Kilburn KH, Germino VH, Hamilton JD, Lynn WS, Byrd H, Baucom D (1973) Preprocessing cotton to prevent byssinosis. Br J Ind Med 30:237–247

Merchant JA, Baxter P, Bernstein R, McCawley M, Falk H, Stein G, Ing R, Attfield M (1982) Health implications of the Mount St. Helens eruption: epidemiological considerations. Ann Occup Hyg 26:911–919

Metropolitan Life Insurance Tables (1959) In: Diem K (ed) Documenta Geigy: Scientific Tables, 6th edn (1962). Geigy, Basle, p 624

Miettinen O (1975) Principles of epidemiology research. Course text, epidemiology 203bc and biostatistics 204d (1975–1976). Harvard School of Public Health

Molyneux MKB, Tombleson JBL (1970) An epidemiologic study of respiratory symptoms in Lancashire cotton mills, 1963–1966. Br J Ind Med 27:225–234

Monson RR (1980) Occupational epidemiology. CRC Press, Boca Raton, Florida

Morgan RH, Donner MW, Gayler BW, Margolies SI, Rao PS, Wheeler PS (1973) Decision processes and observer error in the diagnosis of pneumoconiosis by chest radiography. Am J Roentgenol Radium Ther Nucl Med 117:757–764

Morgan WKC (1978) Industrial bronchitis. Thorax 35:285–291

Morgan WKC, Seaton A (1975) Occupational lung diseases. WB Saunders Coy, Philadelphia

Newman-Taylor A (1980) Occupational asthma. Thorax 35:241–245

Oakes D, Douglas R, Knight K, Wusteman M, McDonald JC (1982) Respiratory effects of prolonged exposure to gypsum dust. Ann Occup Health 26:833–839

Oakes D, Gilson J, Sheers G, Springett VH, McDonald JC (1983) A comparison of the ILO/UC 1971 and 1980 classifications of radiographs (abstract). Scand J Work Environ Health 9:62

Oldham P (1968) Measurement in medicine: the interpretation of numerical data. English University Press, London, pp 142–152

Oldham HG, Bevan MM, McDermott M (1979) Comparison of the new Wright peak flow meter with the standard Wright peak flow meter. Thorax 34:304–309

Pepys J, Hutchcroft BJ (1975) Bronchial provocation tests in etiologic diagnosis and analysis of asthma. Am Rev Respir Dis 112:829–859

Petersen M, Attfield M (1981) Estimates of bias in a longitudinal coal study. J Occup Med 23:45–48

Pham QT, Mur JM, Gimenez M, Mastrangelo G, Henquel JC (1981) Variabilite des tests fonctionnels respiratoires sur period d'ovservation de neuf semaines. Rev Epidemiol Sante Publique 29:15–26

Rossiter CE, Bristol LJ, Cartier PH, Gilson JC, Grainger TR, Sluis-Cremer GK, McDonald JC (1972) Radiographic changes in chrysotile asbestos mine and mill workers in Quebec. Arch Environ Health 24:388–400

The Shorter Oxford English Dictionary, 3rd edn (1965) Little W, Fowler HW, Coulson J, Onions CT (eds) Clarendon, Oxford

Siemiatycki J (1979) A comparison of mail, telephone, and home interview strategies for household health surveys. Am J Public Health 69:238–245

Siemiatycki J, Day NE, Fabry J, Cooper JA (1981) Discovering carcinogens in the occupational environment: a novel epidemiologic approach. J Natl Cancer Inst 66:217–225

Simpson W (1979) Asbestos, vol 1. Final report of the advisory committee. Health and Safety Commission, Her Majesty's Stationery Office, London, pp 72–73

Sleggs CA, Marchand P, Wagner JC (1961) Diffuse mesothelioma in South Africa. S Afr Med J 35:28–34

Snider GL, Rieger RA, Demas T, Doctor L (1967) Variations in the measurements of spirograms. Am J Med Sci 126:679–684

Stebbings JH Jr (1971) Chronic respiratory disease among non-smokers in Hagerstown, Maryland. II. Problems in the estimation of pulmonary function values in epidemiological surveys. Environ Res 4:163–192

Stille WT (1980) Hazard detection by illness pattern similarities. Arch Environ Health 35:325–332

Vinni K, Hakoma (1980) Healthy worker effect in the Finnish population. Scand J Work Environ Health 37:180–184

Wachtlova M, Holusa R, Herget J, Vrtna L, Kysela B, Palacek V (1981) Pulmonary response to quartz dust in different periods of postnatal development of the rat. Eur J Respir Dis 62 (Suppl 113):189–190

Wagner JC (1980) Environmental and occupational exposure to natural mineral fibres. In: Wagner JC (ed) Biological effects of mineral fibres. International Agency for Research on Cancer, Lyon, no 30, pp 995–997

Weill H, Jones R (1975) The chest roentgenogram as an epidemiologic tool. Arch Environ Health 30:435–439

Weiss CH (1972) Evaluation research; methods of assessing program effectiveness. Prentice-Hall, Englewood Cliffs
Zeck PT, Solliday NH, Celic L, Cugell D (1981) Variability of the volume of isoflow. Chest 79:269–272
Zuskin E, Saric M, Bouhuys A (1979) Airway responsiveness in workers processing polyester resins. J Occup Med 21:825

CHAPTER 6

The Isolated Perfused Lung

A. B. FISHER

A. Perspective

I. Historical Developments

In isolated organ perfusion experiments, performed as early as the last century (BERNARD 1855; MARTIN 1883), the lungs were used mainly as a convenient and physiologic method to oxygenate the blood. As interest in lung function increased, the isolated perfused preparation was used to evaluate control of the pulmonary circulation (LOHR 1924) and pulmonary blood volume (DRINKER et al. 1926). BERRY and DALY (1931) studied pressure–flow relationships in the pulmonary artery of guinea pig, monkey, and dog lungs. A similar preparation was subsequently used by NISELL (1948) and by DUKE (1951) to study the effect of alveolar gas composition on alveolar vessels of cat lungs and by HUGHES et al. (1958) to study edema formation in rabbit lungs. By this time, the perfused lung preparation had reached a stage of development where it could be applied routinely (although perhaps not without difficulty) to studies of circulatory and ventilatory mechanics (ALLISON et al. 1961; LLOYD 1964; WEST et al. 1964; HAUGE 1968), pulmonary edema (LUNDE 1976), and pulmonary gas exchange (ROSENBERG and FORSTER 1960; NIDEN et al. 1962).

Parallel with these developments, the isolated perfused lung preparation was used for study of lung metabolism and lung metabolic function. The earliest observations are perhaps those of VERNEY and STARLING (1922) who reported that blood, after passing through the heart–lung preparation, lost the (undesired) effect of constricting the renal artery. Metabolic studies were carried out by EVANS et al. (1934) who showed that isolated lungs utilize glucose and produce lactate during perfusion. In 1953, GADDUM et al. showed that isolated cat lungs metabolize serotonin to inactive products. KOGA (1958) and LEVEY and GAST (1966) further evaluated pulmonary glycolytic activity and intermediary metabolism with isolated lungs from the rabbit and rat. HEINEMANN (1961) demonstrated lipoprotein lipase activity in the perfused rabbit lung. EISEMAN et al. (1964), HUGHES et al. (1969), and ALABASTER and BAKHLE (1970) further explored the pulmonary metabolism of vasomotor agents. WEBER and VISSCHER (1969) measured oxygen uptake of the isolated dog lung. ROSENBLOOM and BASS (1970) described a perfused rat lung system with advantages for the study of drug metabolism. During the past 10 years, an increasing number of perfusion systems have been described (NIEMEIER and BINGHAM 1972; GILLIS and IWASAWA 1972; LONGMORE et al. 1973; JUNOD 1973; O'NEIL and TIERNEY 1974; FISHER et al. 1974; RHOADES 1974; WATKINS and RANNELS 1979; CHIANG et al. 1979; MACDONALD and BOARDMAN 1980).

II. Lung Perfusion Systems

While most lung perfusion systems share common features, differences in techniques can be useful for specific situations. Allison et al. (1961) described a system for simultaneous perfusion of bronchial and pulmonary circulations. Several groups have described systems to perfuse isolated lobes as opposed to whole lung (West et al. 1964; Smith and Mitzner 1980); this approach is chiefly useful for study of lung function of large animals. Lungs for perfusion are generally removed from the thorax, but can be perfused in situ (Leary and Smith 1970; Watkins and Rannels 1979); the latter approach is less difficult technically, but the lung is then less effectively isolated. Gillis and Iwasawa (1972) and Tucker and Shertzer (1980) have described systems for split perfusion of right and left lungs from individual small laboratory animals. The rat lung is a convenient size for studies of lung metabolic function, and many of the published reports have utilized this preparation. Therefore, the techniques for isolation and perfusion of lungs that will be described are specifically oriented toward this species.

III. Merits of the Perfused Lung Preparation

The advantages and disadvantages of the isolated perfused lung preparation have recently been well summarized by Mehendale et al. (1981). The major advantage compared with other in vitro preparations for study of the lung is that functional and structural integrity of the organ is maintained. Thus, substrates can be delivered by the physiologic route, functional manipulation of the organ is possible, and possible cell – cell interactions are preserved. Further, tissue damage is relatively slight compared with slice or homogenization techniques. A major advantage compared with in vivo preparations is the control over physiologic parameters. Thus, one avoids the physiologic constraints that regulate lung function in the intact animal. Another major advantage for the isolated lung compared with the in vivo organ is the increased flexibility to use potentially toxic agents. The isolated lung can be directly exposed to concentrations of chemicals that might be lethal for the whole animal, and precious chemicals can be used in smaller amounts. A final advantage is that accurate chemical analysis and mass balance is generally easier to attain with use of the perfused organ than would be the case with the intact animal. This is especially true for the lung where the very large blood flow in relation to tissue mass makes accurate calculation of metabolic rates impossible in most situations.

The several disadvantages of the isolated organ system must also be kept in mind when choosing among the various preparations for study of the lung. The maintenance of normal structural integrity may impede some studies such as evaluation of intracellular enzyme activity. The known cellular heterogeneity of the lung (and perhaps more importantly, the changing cell population in response to lung toxicity) may markedly influence results and interpretation. Interactions between the lung and neurohumoral factors which may be important for some reactions are lost when the organ is studied in isolation. Finally, the relatively limited period during which isolated lungs maintain their integrity (generally less than 5 h) limits the type of study for which their use is appropriate.

B. Technique of Lung Perfusion

I. Introduction

There are two major differences between the lung and other organs that must be considered in designing a perfusion system. The most obvious is the large gas phase of the lung and the necessity to ventilate the lung in order to simulate normal physiologic conditions. The corollary of this is that, unlike other organs, the lung is not dependent on perfusion to maintain tissue oxygenation and remove CO_2 since these roles are quite efficiently accomplished through alveolar ventilation. A second major difference from other organs is the relatively vast normal blood flow in relation to tissue mass; the lung physiologically receives the entire cardiac output through a tissue mass that is less than 1% of body weight. The corollary of this is that measurement of arteriovenous difference across the lung for most metabolites is generally not possible.

II. Isolation of the Lung for Perfusion

The first variable in preparation of the isolated lung for perfusion is the method for killing the animal. Cervical dislocation is not suitable because the trauma frequently produces pulmonary edema while decapitation results in difficulty with subsequent cannulations. Inhalational anesthetics expose lungs directly to possible toxicity, although the agent will be removed during subsequent ventilation of the lung. Agents that can be used for anesthesia by the inhalation route include halothane (3%) or high CO_2 (approximately 80%). Sytemically administered anesthetics reach the lung in relatively high and possibly toxic concentrations through the pulmonary circulation before dispersal into the systemic arterial blood. Nevertheless, the use of a systemic anesthetic has been the usual choice. The anesthetic agent most commonly used for rats is pentobarbital by intraperitoneal injection in a dose of approximately 50–60 mg/kg. This route of anesthesia resulted in a subsequent concentration of pentobarbital in the recirculating perfusate of approximately $2 \times 10^{-6} M$ (RANNELS et al. 1982), a concentration that has not yet been demonstrated to alter lung metabolism.

The next step in preparation of the animal is to institute respiratory support in order to provide adequate blood oxygenation and to prevent lung collapse (atelectasis) during subsequent surgery. A tracheostomy is performed (a 15-gauge blunt needle is a satisfactory cannula for the rat) and the lungs are ventilated with a mechanical respirator (e. g., Model 680, Harvard Apparatus, Millis, Massachusetts). Collapse of lungs after thoracotomy is prevented with application of positive pressure at end expiration; this is accomplished most easily by placing the expiratory line from the respirator under water to a depth of approximately 2 cm. Rats are commonly ventilated at a frequency of 60 min^{-1} and 2 ml tidal volume (approximately 1 ml/100 g), a combination that approximates their normal minute ventilation.

Next, the lungs are cleared of their residual blood. This can be accomplished by cannulating a large abdominal vein (hepatic portal or inferior vena cava), and infusing the clearing medium (see Sect. B. V. 2). A large abdominal artery (aorta) is severed to decompress the circulation. An alternative method is to open the thorax and directly cannulate the pulmonary artery. The ribs should be fractured in the posterior lateral thoracic line to give wide exposure and to minimize the possibility of subsequent lung trauma. The heart is then transected and a cannula is inserted through the right ventricle. A rapid flow of perfusate as the cannula is passed through the ventricle will prevent air bubbles from entering the pulmonary circulation. The left atrium is cut or cannulated to permit free efflux of perfusate from the lung. Lungs should become uniformly pale as perfusion is started and become uniformly white within 2–3 min. Lungs cleared of blood by abdominal perfusion require pulmonary arterial catheterization as the next step. Lungs cleared of blood through abdominal perfusion generally have less residual blood than those perfused directly through the pulmonary artery; however, only rarely is the difference between the two techniques worth the additional effort. In either case, it is not possible to remove all of the hemoglobin from the lung during this relatively short period of perfusion. Lungs cleared by pulmonary artery perfusion were found to contain 18 ± 1.8 µl blood per lung which represented less than 5% of the original blood content of the lung (Cross et al. 1979). In our experience with this method for clearing lungs, pretreatment of animals with anticoagulant (e. g., heparin) does not facilitate washout of blood.

The lung can now be removed from the thorax using extreme care to prevent laceration of the lung tissue by the fractured ribs. Further, it is important to avoid touching lung tissue during removal since the mechanical trauma can result in local compression atelectasis and the later development of localized edema, possibly due to the localized release of prostaglandins or other mediators. Once the lungs are removed from the thorax, heart, esophagus, thymus, and other structures can be trimmed away. The lungs are hyperinflated with approximately 3–4 times the usual tidal volume (by blocking the expiratory port of the respirator) and then transferred to the perfusion chamber. The entire procedure for lung isolation from the start of surgery to placement in the chamber can be accomplished within 10 min without interruption of ventilation and with interruption of perfusion for no more than 5 s. However, the lungs readily tolerate short interruptions of ventilation or perfusion provided that they are not allowed to collapse and that air bubbles are not permitted to enter the pulmonary perfusion line.

III. Lung Perfusion Apparatus

Perfusion circuits can be classified as open-circuit (once-through) or recirculating systems. The once-through system permits a more direct assessment of the effect of the lung on perfusate composition, but requires much greater volumes of perfusate. An additional difficulty is that the arteriovenous differences in metabolite concentration are frequently small and difficult to measure. The recirculating perfusion system magnifies these small arterivenous differences by repeated passage through the lung.

An isolated lung perfusion system that is used in our laboratories will be described in considerable detail. The circuit consists of four identifiable components (Fig. 1). The first component is the air pump and associated equipment for ventilation. The second component is the perfusion circuit including a peristaltic

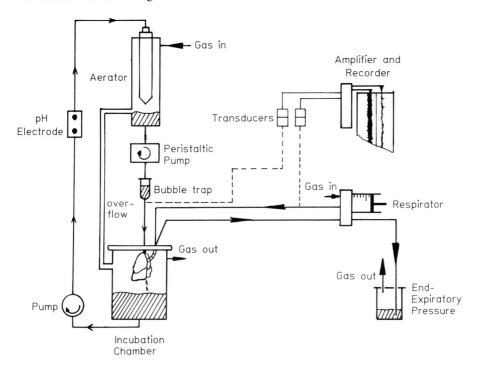

Fig. 1. Schematic diagram of a perfusion circuit for isolated rat lungs. Identifiable components are those for ventilation, perfusion, temperature control, and monitoring. The lungs are suspended from the incubation chamber lid by their tracheal and pulmonary artery cannulae in a water-jacketed incubation chamber. The chamber serves for temperature and humidity control and to collect the effluent perfusate from the left atrium. The perfusate is pumped to an aerator (consisting of an acrylic plastic rod which exposes a thin film of perfusion medium to gas) which is also water-jacketed to permit temperature control. From the aerator, the perfusate is pumped (using a peristaltic pump) through a bubble trap and into the pulmonary artery. The overflow tube of the aerator is for convenience in preventing excessive perfusate accumulation, to facilitate mixing of perfusate, and to provide a pathway for the aerating gas from the aerator to the incubation chamber. This latter arrangement ensures that the gas composition surrounding the lung is identical to the gas composition used for aeration of perfusate. Lungs are ventilated with a positive pressure respirator with appropriate end expiratory pressure to prevent lung collapse. Generally, the same gas mixture is used for ventilation and aeration of perfusate. Pressure transducers are used to monitor pressures for ventilation and perfusion; the sensing port for these transducers is placed as close to the lung as possible. Perfusate pH is monitored with electrodes in a flow-through cuvette. (Modified from BASSETT and FISHER 1976a)

pump and perfusate aerator. The third component is for monitoring and includes transducers for ventilation and perfusion pressure and a flow-through cuvette with pH electrodes. The perfusion components are connected with plastic tubing which should be a nontoxic (e. g., medical) grade. It is important to note that the tubing may absorb a variety of perfusate components which could desorb in subsequent experiments; therefore, tubing should be thoroughly cleaned or discarded after use. These three components will be described subsequently in more detail.

The fourth component of the perfusion apparatus is for temperature control since most isolated lung studies are carried out at 37 °C. In this system (Fig. 1), temperature is maintained by circulating water from a thermostatted bath through a water-jacketed glass or plastic incubation chamber in which the lungs are suspended. This incubation chamber further serves the purposes of collecting effluent perfusate from the left atrium and maintaining appropriate humidity and gas tensions at the lung surface. Temperature control is facilitated by water-jacketing the aerator-perfusate reservoir (Fig. 1). Alternatively, the temperature of the preparation can be controlled by placing the entire perfusion apparatus in a box in which air temperature is maintained by appropriate heating elements (RHOADES 1974). No matter what method is employed, the perfusate should be recirculated in the apparatus prior to the start of an experiment to permit equilibration of temperature, pH, and dissolved gases.

IV. Ventilation of the Lung

1. Volumes and Pressures

Isolated lungs are ventilated in order to simulate physiologic conditions and to prevent lung collapse. The energy for ventilation is supplied by a pump with the lungs passively following the externally generated pressure changes. Therefore, ventilation does not result in large metabolic changes in the lung tissue such as occur with a beating vs a nonbeating heart. Nevertheless, there may be some limited increase in lung intermediary metabolism and oxygen utilization as a consequence of lung ventilation (FARIDY and NAIMARK 1971). Furthermore, ventilation may modulate the synthesis and secretion of the alveolar surfactant (McCLENAHAN and URTNOWSKI 1967; OYARZUN and CLEMENTS 1978) and may influence the distribution of pulmonary capillary blood flow (MEAD and WHITTENBERGER 1964).

Two general approaches have been used to provide lung ventilation. The first uses a pump to push air into the trachea and has been called positive pressure ventilation. The second uses a pump to reduce the pressure in a chamber surrounding the lungs and has been called negative pressure ventilation. As a first impression, the latter may appear more physiologic. However, these methods are essentially equivalent when used with an isolated lung system. With either method, the pressure in the airway must exceed the pressure at the lung surface in order to produce lung inflation. For expiration to occur, airway pressure must exceed ambient pressure. Therefore, negative and positive pressure ventilation produce similar pressure gradients in the lungs during the respiratory cycle. This concept is easiest to understand if one thinks in terms of absolute pressures (Fig. 2). It can be readily appreciated that positive and negative pressure ventilation differ only by the direction of the pressure vector and by a very small absolute pressure. These differences have not been shown to have any physiologic significance. It must be appreciated that spontaneous and artificial ventilation in an intact animal do have different hemodynamic effects, but positive pressure and

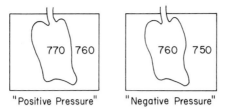

"Positive Pressure"   "Negative Pressure"

Fig. 2. Schematic representation contrasting the absolute pressures required to ventilate lungs by positive and by negative pressure. Positive pressure ventilation may be provided by a respirator at the trachea while negative pressure ventilation can be provided by decreasing the pressure surrounding the lung. Indicated are the approximate pressures in mmHg that would be required to inflate the lung to approximately 75% of its total capacity. Note that the pressure in the alveoli (inside the lung) in both cases exceeds the pressure in surrounding lung by 10 mmHg. As indicated by this analysis, ventilation of the isolated lung by either method is essentially equivalent

whole body negative pressure ventilation in the intact animal are essentially equivalent (MALONEY and WHITTENBERGER 1951; FISHER and HYDE 1969).

Ventilation of the isolated lung is accomplished most convienently with a respirator that produces a sine wave pattern of airflow. Reasonable ventilatory parameters for the rat lung are a frequency of 60 c/min, 2 ml volume per cycle, and an end expiratory pressure of 2 cmH$_2$O. This produces a peak inspiratory pressure of approximately 5–7 cmH$_2$O. Periodic hyperinflation of the lung (as already described) may be necessary to overcome microatelectasis.

2. Ventilating Gases

The composition of the gas used to ventilate the isolated lung will in turn determine gas composition in the alveolar space. CO_2 and O_2 are the major gases of physiologic concern. In the normal lung, alveolar gas tensions are $PCO_2 = 40$ mmHg and $PO_2 = 100$ mmHg. Alveolar PCO_2 needs to be maintained in the normal range in order to maintain perfusate and intracellular pH if a physiologic bicarbonate buffer system is used in the perfusion medium. In addition, CO_2 is a reactant in some metabolic processes, for example, fatty acid synthesis (LONGMORE et al. 1973), so that use of physiologic alveolar CO_2 levels may have biochemical relevance. Normal alveolar CO_2 is most easily maintained by including 5%–6% CO_2 (at sea level) in the ventilating gas. An alternative (but more complicated) approach is to add CO_2 to the perfusate and then regulate alveolar gas composition by balancing ventilation and perfusion.

The normal role of the lung in supplying oxygen for maintenance of peripheral tissue is eliminated in studies of the isolated perfused organ. However, the alveolus does represent a source of O_2 for the lung cells. It is important to note that the supply of oxygen in the airspaces is huge in relation to lung tissue mass and ventilation of the lung continually renews the alveolar oxygen. Since diffusion distances in the lung are short (and O_2 generally equilibrates across the cell layers), the internal PO_2 of cells of the alveolar septum should approximate alveolar PO_2. Because of this, intermediary metabolism and ATP content of the lung are not affected until the oxygen content of the ventilating gas is decreased to very low levels (below 1%) (FISHER et al. 1976; FISHER and DODIA 1981). Therefore, precise regulation of alveolar O_2 is generally unimportant with respect to bioenergetics of lung cells. Likewise, mixed-function oxidation (cytochrome P-450-linked) reactions are maintained at constant rate until similar low levels of alveolar PO_2 are attained (FISHER et al. 1979 b). However, oxygenases with lower oxygen affinity may exist in lung cells (and may in fact be amenable to study by this method). For example, the prolyl hydroxylase reaction for collagen synthesis has an apparent K_m in the perfused lung of approximately 5 mmHg PO_2 (ALPER et al. 1982). Therefore, the use of 15%–20% oxygen, corresponding to an approximate alveolar PO_2 of 100–150 mmHg, would appear most appropriate for routine perfused lung studies.

Based on these considerations, 5% CO_2 in air is an economical gas mixture that is adequate for routine lung perfusion. This provides (at sea level) approximate PO_2 141 mmHg and PCO_2 36 mmHg. One alternative gas mixture is 5% CO_2 in oxygen which entails the risk (so far undefined) of hyperoxic changes in lung cells (FISHER et al. 1979 a) although this risk is probably minimal during short-term perfusion. A filter in the gas line (e. g., Grade A disposable filter unit, Balston Incorporated, Lexington, Massachusetts) is useful to remove particulate contaminants from commercial gas mixtures. A gas washing bottle (e. g., Fisher–Milligan, Fisher Scientific Company, Pittsburgh, Pennsylvania) can also remove contaminants and in addition provides partial humidification of the ventilating gas.

V. Perfusion of the Lung

1. Volumes and Pressures

Open-circuit (once-through) perfusion requires approximately 1 liter perfusate per hour of rat lung perfusion. With recirculating systems, several factors influence the choice of perfusate volume. The first constraint, is physically to occupy the volume of the perfusion circuit. Larger perfusate volumes minimize the errors introduced by removing perfusate aliquots for analysis and dilute the concentration of potentially "toxic" metabolites released from the lung. On the other hand, smaller perfusate volumes result in more rapid equilibration between tissue and perfusate and maximize the ability to detect small changes in perfusate content of metabolites. The perfusate circuit described in Fig. 1 can satisfactorily accommodate perfusate volumes of 40–80 ml.

Lungs are perfused through the pulmonary artery and the effluent is allowed to drip from the transected left atrium into a collection vessel. This method is generally adequate for most metabolic studies unless precise measurements of pulmonary transit time are required. Alternatively, the left atrium can be cannulated for direct collection of venous effluent. The force for driving perfusate through the pulmonary artery can be supplied either by a hydrostatic pressure gradient or by a perfusion pump. The use of a hydrostatic gradient is simpler (and cheaper) and permits control over pulmonary perfusion pressure. Pump perfusion, on the other hand, permits control over perfusion flow rate. A peristaltic pump (e. g., Model 1210, Harvard Apparatus) is satisfactory.

The significance of the difference between the constant pressure and constant flow methods for perfusion can be evaluated by considering the response to an increasing pulmonary vascular resistance during a lung perfusion experiment. If this occurs, either pulmonary perfusion pressure must increase or perfusion flow rate must decrease. Conversely, either perfusion pressure or flow rate (but not both) can be maintained constant during a lung perfusion experiment. For investigation of lung metabolic function, maintenance of a constant flow rate facilitates calculation of metabolic rates and the interpretation of changes in perfusate concentrations. It should be noted that an increasing perfusion pressure (at constant flow) owing to increasing pulmonary vascular resistance indicates instability of the preparation and frequently results in pulmonary edema (see Sect. C. III). In these cases, it is preferable to discard the preparation rather than to manipulate the perfusion pressure to prevent edema.

The physiologic resting cardiac output (lung perfusion rate) for a normal rat is approximately 120 ml min^{-1} kg^{-1}. Perfusion at these flow rates with the isolated lung preparation results in a relatively high rate of failure due to lung edema. Perfusion at approximately one-half the physiologic rate (15 ml/min for a 250 g rat) results in relatively uniform perfusion of lung tissue, maintenance of normal tissue metabolism, and an acceptably low incidence of lung edema. The mean pulmonary artery perfusion pressure at this flow rate (measured with a fluid-filled manometer and "zeroed" to the top of the lung) is approximately 10 mmHg (approximately 14 cmH$_2$O). It should be noted that this flow rate is approximately 10 ml per gram lung weight, a very high rate with respect to metabolic requirements.

Lung perfusion is facilitated by inclusion in the perfusion circuit of a bubble trap to remove air bubbles which may inadvertently enter the perfusate line; their entry into the lung can result in rapid deterioration of the preparation. A filter to remove particulates facilitates prolonged perfusions (up to 5 h) although one is not necessary for shorter perfusion periods. A 0.45-μm pore size filter appears suitable. These filters remove denatured albumin, fibrin clots, bacteria, and other particulates which would otherwise by filtered by the lung.

In the perfusion circuit described, the bronchial circulation is not perfused by its normal physiologic route, i. e., the bronchial arteries. Previous studies have indicated that systemic blood supply to the lung is not needed, provided that the pulmonary circulation remains intact. The reason is that retrograde perfusion through bronchopulmonary anastomosis at the capillary and venous levels can maintain viability of the bronchial tissue (ELLIS et al. 1951; HUGHES et al. 1954). Some evidence for perfusion and viability of the bronchial tissue in the isolated lung preparation is the relatively brisk bronchoconstriction after addition of 5-hydroxytryptamine or other bronchomotor agents to the pulmonary perfusate (STEINBERG et al. 1975; and see Sect. C. V). An isolated lung preparation in which bronchial as well as pulmonary arteries are cannulated has been described for dog lungs (ALLISON et al. 1961), but not for lungs of rats and other small mammals.

2. Perfusion Media

Both natural (whole blood, plasma) as well as artificial media have been used for perfusion of the isolated lung. Whole blood has the inherent advantage of being a physiologic medium, but it is difficult to obtain and store, requires addition of

Table 1. Composition of Krebs–Ringer bicarbonate buffer

Compound	Concentration (mM)
NaCl	119
NaHCO$_3$	25
KCl	5.9
CaCl$_2$	1.3
Na$_2$HPO$_4$	1.8
MgSO$_4$	1.2

an anticoagulant to prevent clotting, has a relatively poorly defined composition, may release a variety of potentially toxic agents during the perfusion process, and has its own metabolic rate which may mask the intrinsic metabolic activity of the lung. Plasma is somewhat easier to handle and has little intrinsic metabolic activity. For most studies of lung metabolism, the choice of an artificial perfusate is appropriate.

The important properties of an artificial perfusion medium are related to its ionic composition, osmolality, and pH buffering capacity. Krebs–Ringer bicarbonate buffer solution (Table 1) is a simple solution that provides the basic requirements for a perfusion medium. The osmolality of this solution is approximately 300 mosmol/l, a normal physiologic level. Bicarbonate–carbonic acid functions as the pH buffer system; this bicarbonate concentration requires ventilation with 5% CO_2 in order to maintain perfusate pH in the approximately normal range of 7.35–7.45. Phosphate can be substituted for bicarbonate as a buffer (and CO_2 eliminated from the ventilating gas) although the perfusion medium is then somewhat less physiologic. Organic buffers (e. g., HEPES, N-2-hydroxyethylpiperazine-N'-2-ethanesulfonic acid, 10–20 mM) can be added for additional buffering capacity; in our experience, this is rarely necessary with the bicarbonate buffer system. Perfusate pH can be adjusted during perfusion by dropwise addition of dilute (0.1 M) HCl or NaOH.

Perfusion with Krebs solution alone results in limited stability of the isolated lung preparation (FISHER et al. 1980b). Stability can be improved by addition of a high molecular weight (nonpermeable) compound to increase the oncotic pressure of the perfusate. Albumin is the most common addition and its presence at a concentration of 30–50 g/l does protect the lung from the development of pulmonary edema (FISHER et al. 1980b). Albumin may function additionally by binding potentially toxic low molecular weight substances, by serving as a vehicle for lipid transport, and by exerting a nonspecific effect on the endothelial cell membranes (RENKIN 1962). However, these latter effects are probably not of major importance for lung stability since the presence of 0.1 g/l albumin does not delay the onset of edema (FISHER et al. 1980b). Bovine serum fraction V is a relatively inexpensive albumin preparation, but it is contaminated with fatty acids and other serum components. Partially purified albumin preparations with limited fatty acid contamination (CHEN 1967) should be used where precise control of perfusate composition is important. Other agents are available for use in special situations (synthetic plasma expanders). Dextran (average molecular weight 40,000–70,000), gelatin, and hydroxyethyl starch are examples of such agents, although their use to date in isolated lungs has been relatively infrequent (TUCKER and SHERTZER 1980). These macromolecules may cause release of histamine from tissues in some species (LORENZ et al. 1976). Another group of potentially useful compounds is the pluronic polyols (e. g., F-68 or F-108, Wyandotte Chemical, Corporation, Wyandotte, Michigan) that, in addition to their oncotic properties, may act as nonionic surfactants to stabilize medium components (MIYAUCHI et al. 1966). These agents have also been used infrequently for lung perfusion (BLOCK and SCHOEN 1981) and have the disadvantage of interfering with subsequent extraction and analysis of tissue metabolites.

Washed red blood cells (RHOADES 1974) or emulsions of perflouro chemicals (STEINBERG et al. 1979) have been added to the perfusion medium in some studies. In other organs, these particulates function for O_2 delivery (SLOVITER and KAMIMOTO 1967), but this function is unnecessary for the lung. Suggestions that viability of the lung in the presence of red cells is prolonged (NICOLAYSEN 1971) remain unconfirmed and the possible mechanism remains unexplained. Further, one group has suggested that heterogeneity of perfusion may be increased by the presence of erythrocytes in the perfusion medium (LINEHAN al. 1981).

The perfusion medium is the source of exogenous substrate for metabolism by the lung cells. Although lungs can be perfused in the absence of substrate added to the medium, addition of glucose delays the onset of edema (FISHER et al. 1980 b). Glucose is readily metabolized by the lung as a fuel for energy generation and can serve as a carbon source for synthesis of lipids, proteins, nucleoproteins, and other macromolecules (FISHER 1976 a, 1984). Saturation of the glucose utilization process in the lung requires approximately 10 mM glucose perfusate concentration (KERR et al. 1979). Lactate (or pyruvate) can adequately substitute for glucose as a carbon source to support a wide range of metabolic functions (FISHER et al. 1979 c, 1981; KERR et al. 1981). In order to simulate a physiologic perfusate, other substrates such as fatty acids (0.5 mM), mixed amino acids (0.5 g/l), glycerol (0.2 mM), and lactate (1 mM) may be added to the perfusion medium (RHOADES 1974; O'NEIL and TIERNEY 1974). The precise requirement for these substrates in maintaining normal tissue metabolism has not been adequately evaluated and their routine use appears to be unnecessary.

The requirement for serum hormones in maintenance of normal lung metabolism has, for the most part, not been evaluated adequately. The one exception is insulin, which has been studied widely because of its potential influence on intermediary metabolism. Studies with experimental diabetes (MORISHIGE et al. 1977; MOXLEY and LONGMORE 1977; FRICKE and LONGMORE 1979) have suggested that insulin has a role in lung metabolism. With perfused lungs from normal animals, the addition of insulin to the perfusate has been shown to increase the uptake of deoxyglucose (FRICKE and LONGMORE 1979) and (variably) to stimulate glycolytic activity (WEBER and VISSCHER 1969; STUBBS et al. 1977; KERR et al. 1979). The variability of insulin effect on glycolysis has not been adequately explained, but may reflect variations in the preperfusion hormonal state of the animal. In any event, the effect of insulin is generally of limited magnitude and the routine addition of insulin to the perfusate appears not to be necessary.

In summary, a basic medium suitable for long-term perfusion of the isolated lung is Krebs–Ringer bicarbonate buffer containing 5–10 mM glucose, 30–50 g/l bovine serum albumin, aerated with 5% CO_2 in air, and adjusted to pH 7.4. Additions to the basic medium are dictated by the experimental protocol.

3. Aeration of Perfusate

An aerator is not an essential component of the lung perfusion apparatus, but can be included in the perfusion circuit (see Fig. 1) so that perfusate gas tensions can be independently regulated. Aeration of perfusate with the same gas mixture used for lung ventilation assures the condition of no net gas exchange across the lung and essentially defines the tissue gas tensions. Alternatively, the perfusate can be gassed with 6% O_2 plus 6% CO_2 in N_2 to simulate normal mixed venous blood gas tensions. The aerator has the additional functions of being a convenient perfusate reservoir and of facilitating equilibration of perfusate in the preperfusion period. Bubble aerators are inconvenient to use with protein solutions because of frothing and protein denaturation. A simple aerator can be constructed by using a rod that admits the flow of a thin film of perfusate (see Fig. 1).

4. Efflux of Metabolites

The lung may modify the perfusate not only by uptake of substrate, but also through efflux of metabolites and other components from the tissue. Efflux of some metabolites has been used as a means to estimate metabolic rates of the tissue. The appearance of other metabolites in the perfusate (for example, prostaglandins) may influence lung function. In addition, loss of regulatory metabolites from lung cells may alter intrinsic lung metabolic activity, although this possibility has not yet been documented. For most metabolites, their rate of release from lung can be most readily documented with the recirculating perfusion system.

The most thoroughly studied of the metabolites appearing in the lung perfusate are lactate and its redox mate, pyruvate. They are generated in the tissue primarily through glycolysis, although amino acids, glycerol, and other carbon sources may contribute (LONGMORE and MOURNING 1976; RHOADES et al. 1978; KERR et al. 1979). Their presence in the perfusate presumably reflects passive diffusion from the lung cells, although the presence of a carrier-mediated process has not been excluded. Lactate and pyruvate are both organic acids that exist primarily in the ionized form at physiologic pH; their appearance in the perfusate represents a net increase in perfusate acidity. For normal rat lungs, production of lactate plus pyruvate is approximately 10 µmol/per gram wet tissue weight per hour.

The efflux of other metabolites has been less well studied. Ascorbic acid increases in the perfusate as a function of time, presumably reflecting passive efflux from the lung cells. The rate of efflux varies with species and also with tissue ascorbate content (ARAD et al. 1980). Perfusion of guinea pig lungs for 1 h may result in the loss of one-third of total lung ascorbate. Small quantities of thiobarbituric acid-reacting material have been detected in perfusate (BLOCK and CANNON 1980; STEINBERG et al. 1982; ALDRICH et al. 1983), presumably representing malondialdehyde arising from peroxidation of lung lipids. Prostaglandins (and perhaps other eicosanoids) are also produced during perfusion, the amount depending, among other things, on the extent of mechanical trauma to the tissue (PALMER et al. 1973; VOEKEL et al. 1981; SPLAWINSKI and GRYGLEWSKI 1981). Efflux of oxidized glutathione (GSSG) has also been demonstrated (NISHIKI et al. 1976), although the amount lost from normal lungs is very low (ARAD et al. 1980). CHIANG et al. (1979) have recently demonstrated the presence of a high molecular weight (greater than 12,000) inhibitor of proteolysis in the medium following lung perfusion.

Experimental manipulations that alter tissue concentrations of metabolites may modify the rate or pattern of metabolite efflux. Examples of such manipulations are the increased efflux of lactate with hypoxia (FISHER and DODIA 1981), increased efflux of GSSG (NISHIKI et al. 1976) and decreased efflux of ascorbic acid (ARAD et al. 1980) with hyperoxia, and increased efflux of malondialdehyde owing to paraquat (ALDRICH et al. 1983) or other generators of free radicals (STEINBERG et al. 1982).

C. Properties of the Perfused Lung

I. Monitors of Lung Stability

A wide variety of problems may arise during the course of lung perfusion. Collapse of the lung (atelectasis) may result from dislodging the tracheal cannula, a foreign body or mucous plug in the airway, failure to apply end expiratory pressure, kinking of airways owing to rotation of the lung in the chamber, or external compression of the lung. Lung overdistension can result from partial airway obstruction with air trapping or by an inadvertent increase of end expiratory pressure. Obstruction to perfusion can occur from air bubbles in the circulation, fibrin clots, foreign particles, or overdistension of lungs. The occurrence of one or more of these complications during lung perfusion can result in failure of the preparation, almost uniformly through the final common pathway, pulmonary edema (see Sect. C. III). Useful information concerning the physiologic state of the isolated perfused lung preparation and the adequacy of the various components of the circuit can be obtained by monitoring mechanical properties related to pulmonary ventilation and pulmonary perfusion and the perfusate pH.

1. Ventilation Pressure

An index of lung distension can be readily monitored by measuring the airway pressure with a strain gauge at a site close to the tracheal cannula. With a constant respiratory pattern and tidal volume, the pressure changes measured at the airway reflect the lung mechanical properties, i.e., airflow resistance and lung compliance (Fig. 3). A small increase in airway pressure may indicate the need for hyperinflation, while a progressive increase may reflect the imminent failure of the preparation.

2. Perfusion Pressure

In a similar manner, pulmonary artery pressure can be monitored during constant pulmonary perfusion in order to monitor possible changes in pulmonary vascular

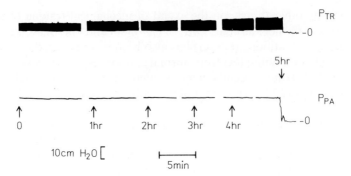

Fig. 3. Record of ventilation and perfusion pressures during a 5-h period of recirculating perfusion of the isolated rat lung. The tracings indicate approximate 5-min segments recorded at 1-h intervals during the perfusion. Zero time indicates the start of perfusion. Zero tracheal and pulmonary artery pressures are indicated at the end of perfusion. The zero level for the pulmonary artery pressure transducer was the top of the lungs. The pulmonary artery pressure is recorded as the mean pressure. The tracheal pressure tracing indicates the pressure changes during the respiratory cycle. Note the slightly positive end expiratory tracheal pressure. There is a slight increase in peak inspiratory pressure during the perfusion, perhaps suggesting the development of interstitial edema or alteration of lung surface forces. This figure should be contrasted with pressure recordings shown in Fig. 5. (Adapted from Fisher et al. 1980 b)

resistance (Fig. 3). Alternatively, perfusion pressure can be maintained constant (for example, by a hydrostatic pressure head) in which case flow rate measurement would reflect changing pulmonary vascular resistance. For reasons already stated, we prefer the constant flow system for studies of pulmonary metabolism. A progressively increasing perfusion pressure generally indicates deterioration of the preparation (see Sect. C. III). In our experience, the change in perfusion pressure provides an earlier indication than ventilation pressure of the eventual failure of perfusion.

Unlike ventilation pressure, the measurement of perfusion pressure requires a liquid-filled system and, therefore, the manometer must be "zeroed" in order to determine absolute pressures. (The top of the lung is a convenient point of zero reference.) In order to calculate absolute pulmonary vascular resistance, the resistance of the pulmonary arterial cannula and associated tubing must be taken into account. It is convenient to make this calibration at the end of the experiment when the perfused lung is cut away and the pressure required to produce constant flow though the cannula can be measured.

3. Perfusate pH

Perfusate pH can be monitored continuously using electrodes with a flow-through cuvette (e. g., the Bench Mark, Markson Science, Incorporated, Del Mar, California).

4. Lung Weight

Development of edema, a constant threat during lung perfusion, can be monitored by continuous measurement of lung weight. A relatively simple method is to suspend the lung (and attached cannulae) from a balance (STEINBERG et al. 1975); it is helpful to "tare" the tubing and other "nonlung" components beforehand. In our experience, measurement of lung weight gives little additional information over that obtained with monitors of lung mechanical properties.

5. Perfusate Gas Tensions

Monitoring of the tension of respiratory gases (PO_2, PCO_2) in the perfusate might be expected to provide information on the gas exchange function of the perfused lung preparation. However, in the absence of hemoglobin in the perfusate, O_2 and CO_2 behave essentially as inert gases and rapidly equilibrate between alveolar gas and perfusate during passage of perfusate through the lung. Even with hemoglobin present, the limited rate of O_2 utilization by lung will generally preclude major shifts in hemoglobin saturation during perfusion.

6. Metabolic Indices

The measurement of metabolic rates may provide the most sensitive index of organ viability, but available techniques are not readily adapted to study of the isolated lung. O_2 consumption is difficult to measure reliably with the isolated lung preparation (FISHER 1976 b). Glucose utilization and CO_2 production can be measured, but are difficult to monitor continuously. Pyridine nucleotide redox state (evaluated by surface fluorescence) has been tried as a monitor of intracellular metabolism, but is unreliable because of a low signal from the lung and artifacts of tissue movement (FISHER et al. 1976).

II. Lung Tissue Compartments

For proper assessment of some metabolic rates, it is important to evaluate the functional compartments of intracellular and extracellular spaces in the perfused lung. The relative size of these spaces is best defined in terms of their fluid content. Thus, the water content of the perfused lung (measured by the dry to wet weight difference) is approximately 83% of total wet weight (see Sect. C. III). The extracellular water space is approximately 35% of lung weight (FRICKE and LONGMORE 1979; CHIANG et al. 1979; KERR et al. 1981) and the intracellular space, therefore, comprises approximately 48% of lung weight or approximately 60% of the lung water. The relatively large extracellular compartment compared with other tissues largely reflects the great vascularity of the lung and must be considered in the interpretation of tissue concentrations based on measurements in the whole lung.

The extracellular water space of the lung can be measured from the distribution of a tracer compound that does not penetrate the cells. Suitable markers are radiolabeled inulin (FRICKE and LONGMORE 1979; CHIANG et al. 1979) or polyethylene glycol (KERR et al. 1981). Equilibration between the vascular and interstitial compartments of the rat lung may require more than 30 min (Fig. 4), presumably reflecting the permeability characteristics of the endothelial barrier as well as the distribution of the pulmonary perfusate (see Sect. C. IV).

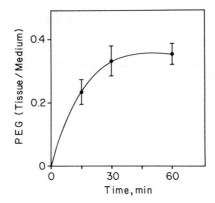

Fig. 4. Time course to equilibration of an extracellular indicator, polyethylene glycol (PEG), during perfusion of an isolated rat lung. The molecular weight of PEG was 4,000. The recirculating perfusate volume was 40 ml and the perfusion rate was 14 ml/min. PEG uptake is expressed as the ratio between tissue concentration (gram PEG per gram wet weight of lung) and concentration in the medium (g/ml) Note that approximately 30 min of perfusion was required to reach a plateau value. At equilibration, 35% of lung weight was represented by extracellular water. Results are mean ± standard error for four perfusions at each time point. (Modified from KERR et al. 1981)

III. Pulmonary Edema

The uncomplicated lung perfusion experiment is characterized by a lung which maintains a normal appearance and inflates and deflates uniformly. Tracheal and perfusion pressures remain constant (see Fig. 3). The ratio of dry to wet weight at the end of perfusion is approximately 0.17 (FRICKE and LONGMORE 1979; KERR et al. 1981). Although this dry to wet weight ratio is lower than seen with normal lungs in vivo, the decrease is due in large part to replacement of formed blood elements with liquid perfusion media.

In lung perfusion experiments destined to fail, a clearly different pattern emerges. Peak inspiratory ventilation pressure and mean perfusion pressure show progressive increases during perfusion (Fig. 5) accompanied by increasing wet weight of the lung. These changes indicate developing interstitial lung edema. The onset of alveolar edema is frequently a sudden event heralded by a rapid and large increase in ventilation pressure. Observation of the lung at this time indicates an enlarged, fluid-filled structure with translucent pulmonary parenchyma and frothy fluid at the tracheal cannula. The wet weight of the lung can increase more than threefold and the dry to wet weight ratio may decrease to 0.06.

The factors responsible for development of edema can be understood most readily by considering normal pathways of lung fluid formation (STAUB 1974; GUYTON et al. 1979). Capillary perfusion results in fluid filtration across the pulmonary capillary wall (lined by capillary endothelial cells) into the lung interstitium. The rate of fluid formation is governed by the Starling forces, namely the capillary hydrostatic and interstitial oncotic pressures opposed by the interstitial hydrostatic and capillary oncotic pressures. The effect of these forces will be in-

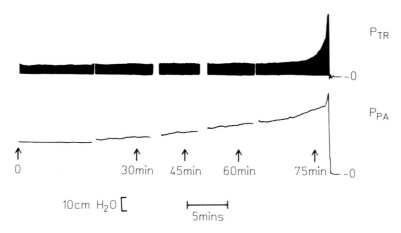

Fig. 5. Ventilation and perfusion pressures in an isolated rat lung perfused with Krebs bicarbonate buffer solution alone (no glucose or albumin present). The pressure tracings are presented as in Fig. 3. Note, however, that the segments of recorded pressure were obtained at approximately 15-min intervals. There is a progressive rise in mean perfusion pressure and a terminal rapid increase in ventilation pressure, indicating the abrupt onset of alveolar edema. (Adapted from FISHER et al. 1980 b)

fluenced by the permeability characteristics of the endothelial and epithelial barriers and by pulmonary lymphatic function. The endothelial barrier is relatively permeable to water and low molecular weight compounds and is somewhat permeable to albumin; consequently the endothelium is not a major barrier to movement of fluid from capillaries into the tissue. The interstitial fluid that is formed by filtration through the endothelium moves in response to the hydrostatic pressure gradient to the perivascular and peribronchial spaces, into the pulmonary lymphatics, and eventually returns to the general circulation. The normal alveolar epithelium is the major permeability barrier and prevents entry of interstitial fluid into the alveolar space (SCHNEEBERGER 1979). This barrier function may be facilitated by the alveolar surfactant which maintains a low surface tension in the alveolar space, thereby decreasing the net force tending to promote edema (GIL 1979; GUYTON 1979) and by the epithelial transport of H_2O (and electrolytes) from the alveolar space toward the interstitium (GOODMAN et al. 1982).

Some of the differences from the normal in vivo situation may help to explain the propensity of the isolated perfused lung for development of edema. The effects of altered mechanical (Starling) forces, that is hydrostatic and oncotic pressures, will be considered first. These alterations may affect the net balance of forces and thereby promote fluid accumulation in lungs and "hydrostatic" pulmonary edema. The process of isolating lungs appears generally to result in increased pulmonary vascular resistance so that perfusion at physiologic flow rates may result in elevated pulmonary capillary hydrostatic pressure. If this occurs on a regional rather than generalized basis, focal areas of edema may develop, resulting in a redistribution of perfusion, relative overperfusion of adjacent lung areas, and subsequent development of generalized edema. This sequence can be prevented by perfusion at less than physiologic flow rates, although the limitation to this approach is the resultant likelihood of inhomogeneous perfusion (see Sect. C. IV). Capillary hydrostatic pressure in the perfused preparation may also be increased by obstruction to the pulmonary venous outflow. This possibility can be minimized by wide excision of the left atrium in free flow systems or use of large-bore tubing for cannulation of the left atrium. A decrease in tissue hydrostatic pressure has an effect similar to that of elevated capillary hydrostatic pressure. The usual mechanism is overdistension of the lung, either by use of an excessively high end expiratory pressure or by ventilation with excessive tidal volume. Perfusate oncotic pressure is the other important Starling force in considering edema of the isolated lung. The oncotic pressure of the lung perfusate depends primarily on the presence of albumin or other macromolecules (see Sect. B. V. 2) and addition of albumin (approximately 30–50 g/l) to the perfusate protects against pulmonary edema (FISHER et al. 1980 b).

While mechanical factors are of decided importance, changes in function of the lymphatic system may also influence the onset of "hydrostatic" edema. Of necessity, the lymphatic vessels from the lung are transected during preparation of the isolated lung. Although lymphatic continuity is interrupted and their function might be impaired, the precise effects of this on lymphatic drainage are not clear.

The role of the barriers to fluid filtration is only slightly better understood, although clearly damage to the barriers can lead to "permeability" pulmonary edema. The integrity of the epithelial and endothelial barriers depends in part on the intrinsic metabolism of their constituent cells. Thus, in the absence of metabolizable substrate in the perfusate, alveolar edema in the isolated rat lung develops after approximately 60 min of perfusion at physiologic flow rates. The time to edema can be extended by about 50% if glucose is added to the perfusion medium and can be extended approximately fourfold with a complete nutritional medium (FISHER et al. 1980 b). There is some evidence that decreasing cellular ATP content may promote lung edema, presumably through alteration of permeability barriers (POSTLETHWAIT and YOUNG 1980). Cellular permeability barriers may also be altered through mechanical trauma to the lung or through toxic reactions occurring in the capillary space or lung tissue. However, the precise mechanisms responsible for integrity of these cellular barriers remain an important unresolved problem of lung cell physiology.

IV. Distribution of Pulmonary Perfusate

The pulmonary perfusate is delivered to the lung via the pulmonary artery and then dispersed through the pulmonary capillary circulation. At any given perfusion flow rate, the distribution of perfusate within the lung determines the transit time of a particular component and the duration of contact between this component and the lung cells. Thus, the relative distribution of the pulmonary perfusate is of major importance for the determination of lung metabolic properties and their responses to toxic challenge.

Several distinguishing characteristics of the pulmonary circulation must be appreciated to evaluate parameters affecting distribution of pulmonary perfusion. First, the lung has a vast capillary bed which can readily accommodate the entire cardiac output. The multiple channels result in an intrinsic potential for variable distribution of perfusion at the microscopic level. Second, the pulmonary circulation is a low pressure, high flow, low resistance system. As a consequence, relatively small changes in focal tissue parameters may result in considerable unevenness in the distribution of the pulmonary perfusate.

One of these focal influences is the effect of gravity which results in a vertical gradient of perfusion and can lead to hypoperfusion of the superior portions of the lung (WEST et al. 1964). This effect is relatively less important with the lungs of small mammals where the vertical distance is limited, but becomes increasingly important with increasing lung size. As an example of this effect, isolated rat lungs perfused at 14 ml/min showed 30% less perfusion per unit weight to the upper lobes as compared with lower lobes (BLOCK and FISHER 1977a). Another focal effect is mechanical trauma to the lung tissue which can promote atelectasis, compress capillaries, and result in a local limitation of perfusion. The tendency to uneven perfusion can be minimized by use of a flow rate sufficiently great to perfuse the major portion of the pulmonary capillary bed. However, complete uniformity of perfusion in the isolated lung is probably rarely acheived as indicated by the persistence of occasional red blood cells in the pulmonary capillaries on histologic examination at some time after the institution of perfusion. Although the use of even higher perfusate flow rate could theoretically improve distribution of perfusate, this approach is limited in practice by the increased tendency to lung edema.

Several methods are available to evaluate the distribution of perfusate at the gross level. Evaluation of the distribution of perfusate at the microscopic (capillary) level is considerably more difficult and available methods are not entirely satisfactory. Gross inhomogeneity of perfusion can frequently be appreciated by visual inspection of the perfused lung surface showing slow clearance of blood from one or more regions of the tissue. Uneven perfusion can be more easily appreciated by noting distribution of a dye (for example, carbon black or indocyanine green) added to the perfusate. Local distribution can be quantitated by radioactive counting of lung samples after infusion of radiolabeled microspheres which lodge in the pulmonary circulation (BLOCK and FISHER 1977a).

Compensation for the effects of inhomogeneity of perfusion in metabolic studies can be achieved in part by the simultaneous infusion of an intravascular tracer along with the test substance (RYAN et al. 1968; LINEHAN et al. 1981; RICKABY et al. 1981). This approach is applicable for "single-pass" experiments. If results are expressed in terms of the intravascular indicator, the measurement essentially gives a result based on perfused lung mass. However, if used to study a saturable process, this approach may fail to make adequate correction for large heterogeneity of flow. For recirculating experiments, the best approach appears to be careful monitoring of the physiologic state of the perfused lung preparation with appropriate action as the preparation deteriorates.

V. Viability of the Perfused Lung

The viability of the isolated perfused lung is of limited duration and failure of the preparation (generally by development of pulmonary edema) within 5 h can be virtually assured. One would predict a priori that subtle but progressive changes in the lung presage the phase of rapid deterioration. The nature of these factors remains incompletely understood. Nevertheless, during the stable phase of perfusion, many indices indicate that the preparation is metabolically intact and viable. As discussed previously, ventilation pressure, perfusion pressure, and lung weight remain constant for prolonged periods. Distribution of pulmonary perfusate, at least on the gross level, remains relatively uniform. Both bronchial and vascular smooth muscle show appropriate reactivity by reversible bronchoconstriction and vasoconstriction on exposure to appropriate agonists. For example, bronchoconstriction can be shown (in guinea pig lungs) with infusion of 5-hydroxy-tryptamine and vasoconstriction has been demonstrated with alveolar hypoxia and with infusion of angiotensin II (Nilsen and Hauge 1968; McMurtry et al. 1976). The vasoconstrictor responses are more readily elicited when lungs are perfused with blood and all smooth muscle responses require the presence of calcium (Steinberg et al. 1975; McMurtry et al. 1976).

Examination of tissue from the perfused lung with the light microscope shows normal histology at the alveolar septal level; although peribronchial and perivascular spaces are generally distended with fluid, this appears to represent a "sump" function of the spaces (Staub 1974) which apparently drain at slower rates in the isolated than in the intact lung. Electron micrographs of the lung parenchyma studied after 15–60 min of perfusion show intact cytoarchitecture and normal interstitial space (Bassett and Fisher 1976a; Fisher and Pietra 1981). Evaluation of lung metabolic function indicates linear rates of metabolism following the initial period for substrate equilibration in the lung cells. Further, the lung tissue is maintained in a normally highly energized state with a normal redox ratio (see Sect. D. I).

D. Metabolic Function of the Perfused Lung

The perfused lung preparation has been used to study a wide range of metabolic activities which can be divided into two broad categories: metabolic function that is required for maintenance of cellular integrity (including intermediary metabolism and the biosynthesis of macromolecules); and metabolism of hormones, biotransformation of drugs and other xenobiotics.

I. Intermediary Metabolism and Energy State

The isolated perfused lung oxidizes a wide range of carbon substrates, including glucose, lactate, glycerol, fatty acids, and amino acids (Bassett et al. 1981; Bassett and Fisher 1976a; Rhoades 1974; Wolfe et al. 1979). Under usual physiologic conditions, glucose probably serves as the major fuel (Shaw and Rhoades 1977). Hexoses are transported into lung cells by carrier-mediated facilitated diffusion (Fricke and Longmore 1979) while some lung cells may also have active sugar transport (Kerr et al. 1981). The rate of glucose utilization is half-maximal at a perfusate glucose concentration of approximately 3.5 mM; maximal glucose utilization for the control perfused lung is approximately 70 µmol/h per gram dry weight of tissue (Kerr et al. 1979).

The metabolic fate of glucose is indicated in Table 2. Approximately 50% of glucose is converted to lactate plus pyruvate, 25% is oxidized to CO_2, and 25%

Table 2. Metabolic properties of isolated rat lung perfused with artificial media (based on data from BASSETT and FISHER 1976a, b, c; FISHER 1978; FISHER and DODIA 1981)

Metabolism (μmol/h per gram dry weight)		Content (μmol per gram dry weight)		Ratios	
Glucose utilization	44	ATP	10.7	Lactate/pyruvate	10
Lactate production	33	ADP	1.2	ATP/ADP	8
Pyruvate production	3.3	AMP	0.4	Energy charge	0.92
CO_2 from glucose	53	CrP	2.2[a]		

[a] BUECHLER and RHOADES (1980)

is incorporated into tissue components such as lipids and proteins. The pentose shunt pathway of glucose metabolism is present and accounts for approximately 25% of the total CO_2 production and 12% of glucose utilization (BASSETT and FISHER 1976c). The ratio of lactate to pyruvate production, reflecting the redox state of the lung, is approximately 10. The response of metabolism to various inhibitors indicates that intermediary metabolism of the lung is regulated by the usual control processes (BASSETT and FISHER 1976a, b). Thus, the lung has a Pasteur effect (increased glycolysis with inhibition of oxidative metabolism) and shows appropriate changes in redox state with inhibitors or uncouplers of ATP synthesis. The intermediary metabolism of the perfused lung has recently been reviewed in detail (FISHER 1984).

Adenine nucleotides in the lung exist in a highly energized state with the major fraction of this pool in the form of ATP (Table 2). Creatine phosphate is present, but in limited quantities (BUECHLER and RHOADES 1980) and ATP therefore represents the major high energy store. The ATP, if distributed throughout the intracellular space, would be present at a mean intracellular concentration of approximately 5 mM, comparable to other tissues with moderate energy requirements, such as liver but lower than working tissues such as heart muscle. Although ATP is generated during glycolysis, oxidative metabolism is required to maintain the ATP stores of the perfused lung at normal levels (BASSETT and FISHER 1976a). However, as already noted, the lung cells are efficient in utilizing alveolar oxygen and tissue ATP levels are not affected significantly until alveolar O_2 is less than 1% (FISHER and DODIA 1981).

II. Biosynthesis

Perfused lungs show active biosynthesis and catabolism of carbohydrate, protein, and lipid components. Glucose can be converted to glycogen; however, the extent of this activity is limited. Glycogen stores in the adult lung are small, and this pool appears to be relatively stable, even in the face of increased glucose requirements (KERR et al. 1979). Nonspecific protein synthesis has been demonstrated by incorporation of precursor amino acids, such as phenylalanine, or incorporation of carbon from a labeled precursor such as glucose into the crude protein fraction (BASSETT and FISHER 1976a; WATKINS and RANNELS 1979). Synthesis of collagen by the perfused lung has been demonstrated by the incorporation of proline into lung collagen (ALPER et al. 1982). Approximately 10% of total protein synthesis, based on proline incorporation in the perfused lung, was directed toward collagen. Proteolysis has also been demonstrated in the perfused lung through liberation of radioactivity from prelabeled proteins (CHIANG et al. 1979).

Lipid biosynthesis has been extensively investigated in the perfused lung. All classes of lipids are synthesized, but synthesis of phosphatidylcholine, especially dipalmitoylphosphatidylcholine, predominates, reflecting the synthesis of the alveolar surfactant material (GODINEZ and LONGMORE 1973; JOHNSON et al. 1979). The precursors for synthesis of phosphatidylcholine include fatty acids, glycerol-3-phosphate, and choline. Fatty acids can be synthesized de novo in the lung (WANG and MENG 1974) or can be obtained exogenously from the perfusion medium. Glycerol phosphate is generated during glycolysis or by the phosphorylation of glycerol (FISHER and CHANDER 1982). Choline is derived predominantly from the circulation. The synthesis of phosphatidylglycerol has also been demonstrated in perfused rat lung (GODINEZ et al. 1975).

III. Metabolism of Hormones and Xenobiotics

The isolated perfused lung preparation has been shown to metabolize a variety of hormones and endogenous metabolites. Some of these activities have been localized to the pulmonary endothelium, but the cellular site of others remains unresolved. The endothelial compartment of perfused lungs actively accumulates 5-hydroxytryptamine (serotonin) and norepinephrine by a transcellular transport system and metabolizes them by monoamine oxidase to inactive products (FISHER et al. 1980a). By contrast, the converting enzyme for activation of angiotensin I by conversion to angiotensin II and for degradation of bradykinin is localized to the pulmonary endothelial surface (RYAN et al. 1968, 1970, 1976). Other pulmonary enzymatic activities that have been demonstrated in the perfused lung include lipoprotein lipase that catalyzes hydrolysis of circulating triglycerides (HEINEMANN 1961; PIETRA et al. 1976), carbonic anhydrase that catalyzes the dehydration of carbonic acid (CRANDALL and O'BRASKY 1978; EFFROS et al. 1978; KLOCKE 1978), and prostaglandin dehydrogenase that converts some prostaglandins to inactive products (PIPER et al. 1970; HOOK and GILLIS 1975; ANDERSEN and ELING 1976; KLEIN et al. 1978; BOURA and MURPHY 1979).

The perfused lung system has also been used to study metabolism of drugs and other foreign compounds. Degradative systems that are present include both A and B types of monoamine oxidase (BAKHLE and YOUDIN 1976), an amine N-oxidase (DEVEREAUX and FOUTS 1974), and the cytochrome P-450-linked mixed-function oxidase pathway of the endoplasmic reticulum. This latter pathway exhibits activity toward a broad range of substrates and catalyzes a spectrum of hydroxylation, demethylation, and other "detoxification" reactions. At least two different cytochromes of this class have been identified in the lung, one of which appears similar to the phenobarbital-inducible cytochrome P-450 of the liver (WOLF et al. 1980). The greatest specific activity of cytochrome P-450 is in bronchiolar Clara cells, although the cuboidal alveolar epithelial cell compartment may have more total activity since these cells are more numerous (DEVEREAUX et al. 1981). Although rates of drug metabolism for most substrates are considerably lower in the perfused lung than for the liver, the lung nevertheless represents one of the major extrahepatic sites for drug metabolism. Metabolism of a variety of compounds by the isolated perfused lung has been studied through chemical or radiochemical assay of effluent perfusate. Specific agents that are metabolized include methadone (ORTON et al. 1973), pentobarbital (LAW et al. 1974), aldrin (MEHENDALE and EL-BASSIOUNI 1975), benzo[a]pyrene (SMITH et al. 1978), nicotine (TURNER et al. 1975; MC GOVREN et al. 1976), lidocaine (POST et al. 1978), carbaryl (BLASE and LOOMES 1976), Δ ^{1}-tetrahydrocannabinol (WIDMAN et al. 1975), and a variety of steroids, including testosterone and cortisone (NICOLAS and KIM 1975; HARTIALA 1976). It has been noted that some activities present in lung microsomes preparations are not seen with perfused lungs (PHILPOT et al. 1977), illustrating the importance of the permeability barriers that prevent access of the substrate to the microsomal enzyme. The perfused lung has also been used to evaluate glucuronide conjugation of drug metabolites (AITIO 1976), although this pathway is not of major importance.

One reaction that is particularly well adapted to the perfused lung system is the O-demethylation of colorless p-nitroanisole to form yellow p-nitrophenol (ITAKURA et al. 1977). In the perfused rabbit lung, this reaction requires glucose or mitochondrial substrates for maximal activity (FISHER et al. 1981) and is inhibited by 50% when the alveolar PO_2 is reduced to about 0.3 mmHg or when CO/O_2 is about 0.5 (FISHER et al. 1979b). Thus, the perfused lung system is amenable to metabolic manipulation for study of its interaction with the respiratory gases.

E. Lung Toxicology

I. Exposure Regimens

Toxicologic effects in the isolated perfused lung system can be evaluated by either direct exposure of the perfused lung or exposure of the animal followed by subsequent isolation and perfusion of the lung. In the former approach, the agent under consideration can be added either to the perfusate or to the inspired gas and may be chosen to simulate physiologic conditions.

The major advantage of directly exposing lungs to toxins is the elimination of possible systemic influences of the agent that secondarily effect the lung. Another advantage is the possibility of using higher concentrations of agent than would otherwise be possible, thereby permitting evaluation of the entire spectrum of dose–response characteristics. The major limitation to this approach is the relatively limited duration for viability of the perfused lung preparation. Thus, agents that produce delayed effects (for example, fibrogenesis) would not be suitable for study by this method. Further, those agents that are only slowly accumulated by the tissue might result in a changing pattern of response during perfusion. Therefore, the rate of accumulation must be considered in the experimental design. For example, paraquat is accumulated from the perfusate against a concentration gradient by a process that takes hours to reach saturation (FORMAN et al. 1982). One possible approach to this problem is to use initially high perfusate concentrations so that toxic intracellular concentrations are attained relatively rapidly.

The potential distribution of the agent must also be considered in evaluation of response to a toxic agent. Delivery via the perfusate leads to immediate exposure of the pulmonary endothelium. Access to the interstitial or epithelial compartments will vary with the permeability of the endothelium for the particular agent under consideration. Although this will not be a major consideration for most low molecular weight toxins, macromolecules will equilibrate more slowly. The major determinant for distribution of volatile agents is the chemical reactivity of the toxin. Thus, the highly reactive gases NO_2 or O_3 interact predominantly with the proximal airway mucosa while less reactive agents (e. g., O_2) are distributed more evenly throughout the alveolar septum.

The other strategy in using isolated lungs to study toxic response is to pretreat the animal at some time before isolated lung perfusion is carried out. This approach has the disadvantages of potential secondary effects on the lung owing to systemic effects of the toxic agent and the limited dose of agent that can be administered. On the other hand, this approach does permit the evaluation of the chronic effects of a particular toxic agent. In the final analysis, the two approaches are complementary.

II. Pulmonary Responses to Hyperoxia

Damage to the lungs is known to be the major organ toxicity when animals breathe oxygen in concentrations between 0.5 and 2 atm absolute (FISHER 1980). Higher concentrations lead primarily to central nervous system (CNS) effects, manifested by convulsions and paralysis. The CNS manifestations have a secondary effect upon the lungs. Consequently, the isolated lung perfusion system presents advantages for the evaluation of the direct effects (unrelated to the CNS) of high partial pressures of oxygen upon lung metabolism. On the other hand, oxygen breathing at 1 atm requires one or more days for pulmonary effects to develop. Consequently, studies designed to evaluate the metabolic effects of oxygen at 1 atm are best carried out with in vivo exposure.

1. Exposure of Isolated Lungs to Hyperbaric Oxygen

In order to produce a severe hyperoxic stress during a relatively limited time, isolated rat lungs were exposed to oxygen at 5 atm absolute (BASSETT and FISHER 1979). This required modification of the lung perfusion apparatus to permit perfusion of the isolated lungs in a hyperbaric pressure chamber. The major modification was to divert the perfusate through ports in the chamber wall to the outside of the chamber to permit access to perfusate samples and to decrease the hazard of fire by placing the perfusion pump motor outside the oxygen atmosphere.

Exposure of isolated lungs to hyperbaric oxygen resulted in a rapid effect on lung metabolism. The major change was a 55% increase in the rate of glucose metabolism associated with marked stimulation of the pentose phosphate cycle. There was a slight decrease in the lactate : pyruvate ratio, indicating an oxidation of cellular pyridine nucleotides. Glutathione efflux from the lung increased, suggesting an increase in the rate of glutathione oxidation (NISHIKI et al. 1976). These results indicate an increase in the rate of oxidation of cellular components during exposure to hyperoxia associated with an increase in the rate of generation of reducing equivalents (NADPH) for detoxification of oxygen-derived radicals and their oxidation products.

2. Exposure to Hyperoxia In Vivo

The effects of hyperoxia on metabolism of the isolated perfused lung have also been studied following exposure of intact rats to elevated partial pressures of oxygen. Lungs were subsequently removed from rats and evaluated for their ability to remove 5-hydroxytryptamine from the recirculating perfusate, a reasonably sensitive index of pulmonary endothelial cell function (FISHER et al. 1980a). These studies showed a significant depression in clearance of 5-hydroxytryptamine after 18 h of oxygen exposure (BLOCK and FISHER 1977a). The effect of oxygen on the lungs was accelerated if animals were vitamin E deficient or were exposed to oxygen at 4 atm absolute (BLOCK and FISHER 1977b). Pretreatment of rats with superoxide dismutase partially protected against the decrease in 5-hydroxytryptamine clearance (BLOCK and FISHER 1977c). The use of this regime permitted evaluation of the pulmonary effects of oxygen over a time period that would not have been possible by directly exposing lungs to elevated PO_2.

F. Conclusions

The isolated perfused lung preparation has been developed as an important tool in modern physiologic, pharmacologic, and toxicologic research. Compared with other organs, the lung system presents some unique challenges that have been largely overcome through the rigorous application of physiologic principals. It is now possible routinely to perfuse isolated lungs for relatively long periods and the technique complements the use of in vivo and isolated cell preparations to provide a strong basis for evaluation of the effects of toxins in the lung.

Acknowledgments. I thank my collaborators through the years who performed many of the isolated perfused lung experiments described in this chapter. These collaborators include Drs. Harry Steinberg, Edward Block, Norio Itakura, Janet Kerr, Ilan Arad, and Thomas Aldrich. Special thanks are due to Dr. David Bassett who was largely responsible for the initial development and characterization of the preparation and to Mr. Chandra Dodia who has become the bulwark of our lung perfusion program. I thank Mrs. Mary Pili for her unfailing secretarial support. This chapter was written during the tenure of an Established Investigatorship award from the American Heart Association.

References

Aitio A (1976) Glucuronide conjugation in the lung. Agents Actions 6:531–533
Alabaster VA, Bakhle YS (1970) Removal of 5-hydroxytryptamine in the pulmonary circulation of rat isolated lungs. Br J Pharmacol 40:468–482
Aldrich TK, Fisher AB, Cadenas E, Chance B (1983) Evidence for lipid peroxidation by paraquat in the perfused rat lung. J Lab Clin Med 101:66–73
Allison PR, deBurgh Daly I, Waaler BA (1961) Bronchial circulation and pulmonary vasomotor nerve responses in isolated perfused lungs. J Physiol 157:462–474
Alper R, Kerr JS, Kefalides NA, Fisher AB (1982) Relation between alveolar PO_2 and collagen biosynthesis in the perfused rat lung. J Lab Clin Med 99:442–450
Andersen MW, Eling TE (1976) Prostaglandin removal and metabolism by isolated perfused rat lung. Prostaglandins 11:645–676

Arad ID, Forman HJ, Fisher AB (1980) Ascorbate efflux from guinea pig and rat lungs: Effect of starvation and O_2 exposure. J Lab Clin Med 96:673–681

Bakhle YS, Youdin MBH (1976) Metabolism of phenylethylamine in rat isolated perfused lung: evidence for monoamine oxidase "Type B" in lung. Br J Pharmacol 56:125–127

Bassett DJP, Fisher AB (1976a) Metabolic response to carbon monoxide by isolated rat lungs. Am J Physiol 230:658–663

Bassett DJP, Fisher AB (1976b) Stimulation of rat lung metabolism with 2, 4-dinitrophenol and phenazine methosulfate. Am J Physiol 231:898–902

Bassett DJP, Fisher AB (1976c) Pentose cycle activity of the isolated perfused rat lung. Am J Physiol 231:1527–1532

Bassett DJP, Fisher AB (1979) Glucose metabolism in rat lung during exposure to hyperbaric O_2. J Appl Physiol 46:943–949

Bassett DJP, Hamosh M, Hamosh P, Rabinowitz J (1981) Pathways of palmitate metabolism in the isolated rat lung. Exp Lung Res 2:37–47

Bernard C (1855) Sur le mechanisme de la formation du sucre dans la foie. CR Seances Acad Sci 41:461

Berry JL, deBurgh Daly I (1931) The relation between the pulmonary and bronchial vascular systems. Proc R Soc Lond 109:319–336

Blase BW, Loomes TA (1976) The uptake and metabolism of Carbaryl by isolated perfused rabbit lung. Toxicol Appl Pharmacol 37:481–490

Block ER, Cannon JK (1980) Paraquat induced lipid peroxidation in isolated perfused rat lungs. Am Rev Respir Dis 121 (part 2):147 (abstract)

Block ER, Fisher AB (1977a) Depression of serotonin clearance by rat lungs during oxygen exposure. J Appl. Physiol 42:33–38

Block ER, Fisher AB (1977b) Effect of hyperbaric oxygen exposure on pulmonary clearance of 5-hydrocytryptamine. J Appl Physiol 43:254–257

Block ER, Fisher AB (1977c) Prevention of hyperoxic-induced depression of pulmonary serotonin clearance by pretreatment with superoxide dismutase. Am Rev Respir Dis 116:441–447

Block ER, Schoen FJ (1981) Effect of alpha naphthylthiourea on uptake of 5-hydroxytryptamine from the pulmonary circulation. Am Rev Respir Dis 123:69–73

Boura ALA, Murphy RD (1979) The influence of drugs and other factors on inactivation of prostaglandin E_2 by the rat isolated perfused lung. Clin Exp Pharmacol Physiol 6:381–191

Buechler KF, Rhoades RA (1980) Fatty acid synthesis in the perfused rat lung. Biochim Biophys Acta 619:186–195

Chen RF (1967) Removal of fatty acids from serum albumin by charcoal treatment. J Biol Chem 242:173–181

Chiang MJ, Whitney P Jr, Massaro D (1979) Protein metabolism in lung: use of isolated perfused lung to study protein degradation. J Appl Physiol 47:72–78

Crandall ED, O'Brasky JE (1978) Direct evidence for participation of rat lung carbonic anhydrase in CO_2 reactions. J Clin Invest 62:618–622

Cross CE, Watanabe TT, Hasegawa GK, Goralnick GN, Roertgen KE, Kaizu T, Reiser KM, Gorin AB, Last JA (1979) Biochemical assays in lung homogenates: artifacts caused by trapped blood after perfusion. Toxicol Appl Pharmacol 48:99–109

Devereux TR, Fouts JR (1974) N-oxidation and demethylation of N,N-dimethylaniline by rabbit liver and lung microsomes, Effects of age and metals. Chem Biol Interac 8:91–105

Devereux TR, Serabit-Singh CJ, Slaughter SR, Wolf RM, Philpot RM, Fouts JR (1981) Identification of cytochrome P-450 isozymes in non-ciliated bronchiolar epithelial (Clara) and alveolar type II cells isolated from rabbit lung. Exp Lung Res 2:221–230

Drinker CK, Churchill ED, Ferry RM (1926) The volume of blood in the heart and lungs. Am J Physiol 77:590–624

Duke HN (1951) Pulmonary vaso-motor responses of isolated perfused cat lungs to anoxia and hypercapnia. J Exp Physiol 36:75

Effros RM, Chang RSY, Silverman P (1978) Acceleration of plasma biocarbonate conversion to carbon dioxide by pulmonary carbonic anhydrase. Science 199:427–429

Eiseman B, Bryant L, Waltuch T (1964) Metabolism of vasomotor agents by the isolated perfused lung. J Thorac Cardiovasc Surg 48:798–806

Ellis FH Jr, Grinley H, Edwards JE (1951) The bronchial arteries – experimental occlusion. Surgery 30:810–826

Evans CL, Hsu FY, Kosaka T (1934) Utilization of blood sugar and formation of lactic acid by lungs. J Physiol 82:41–61

Faridy EE, Naimark A (1971) Effect of distension on metabolism of excised dog lung. J Appl Physiol 31:31–37

Fisher AB (1976a) Normal and pathologic biochemistry of the lung. Environ Health Perspect 16:3–9

Fisher AB (1976b) Oxygen utilization and energy production. In: Crystal R (ed) Biochemical basis of lung function. Dekker, New York, PP 75–104

Fisher AB (1978) Energy status of the rat lung after exposure to elevated PO_2. J Appl Physiol 45:56–59

Fisher AB (1980) Oxygen therapy: side effects and toxicity. Am Rev Respir Dis 122:61–69

Fisher AB (1984) Intermediary metabolism of the lung. Environ Health Perspect 55: 149–133

Fisher AB, Chander A (1982) Glycerol kinase activity and glycerol metabolism of rat granular pneumocytes in primary culture. Biochim Biophys Acta 711:128–133

Fisher AB, Dodia C (1981) The lung as a model for evaluation of critical intracellular PO_2 and PCO. Am J Physiol 247:E47–E50

Fisher AB, Hyde RW (1969) Decrease of diffusing capacity and pulmonary blood flow during passive lung inflation. J Appl Physiol 27:157–163

Fisher AB, Pietra GG (1981) Comparison of serotonin uptake from the alveolar and capillary spaces of isolated rat lung. Am Rev Respir Dis 123:74–78

Fisher AB, Steinberg H, Bassett D (1974) Energy utilization by the lung. Am J Med 57:437–446

Fisher AB, Furia L, Chance B (1976) Evaluation of redox state of the isolated perfused rat lung. Am J Physiol 230:1198–1204

Fisher AB, Bassett DJP, Forman HJ (1979a) Oxygen toxicity of the lung: biochemical aspects. In: Fishman A, Renkin E (eds) Pulmonary edema. Am Physiol Soc, Bethesda, pp 207–216

Fisher AB, Itakura N, Dodia C, Thurman G (1979b) Relationship between alveolar PO_2 and the rate of p-nitroanisole o-demethylation by the cytochrome P-450 pathway in isolated rabbit lungs. J Clin Invest 64:770–774

Fisher AB, Steinberg H, Dodia C (1979c) Reversal of 2-deoxyglucose inhibition of serotonin uptake in isolated guinea pig lung. J Appl Physiol 46:447–450

Fisher AB, Block ER, Pietra GG (1980a) Environmental influences on uptake of serotonin and other amines. Environ Health Perspect 35:191–198

Fisher AB, Dodia C, Linask J (1980b) Perfusate composition and edema formation in isolated rat lungs. Exp Lung Res 1:13–22

Fisher AB, Itakura N, Dodia C, Thurman RG (1981) Pulmonary mixed-function oxidation: stimulation by glucose and the effects of metabolic inhibitors. Biochem Pharmacol 30:379–383

Forman HJ, Aldrich TK, Fisher AB (1982) Differential paraquat uptake and redox kinetics of rat granular pneumocytes and alveolar macrophages. J Pharmacol Exp Ther 221: 428–433

Fricke RF, Longmore WJ (1979) Effects of insulin and diabetes on 2-deoxy-D-glucose uptake by the isolated perfused rat lung. J Biol Chem 254:5092–5098

Gaddum JH, Hebb CO, Silver A, Swan AAB (1953) 5-Hydroxytryptamine: pharmacological action and destruction in perfused lungs. QJ Exp Physiol 38:225–262

Gil J (1979) Influence of surface forces on pulmonary circulation. In: Fishman AP, Renkin EM (eds) Pulmonary edema. Am Physiol Soc, Bethesda, pp 53–64

Gillis CN, Iwasawa I (1972) Technique for measurement of norepinephrine and 5-hydroxytryptamine uptake by rabbit lung. J Appl Physiol 33:404–408

Godinez RI, Longmore WJ (1973) Use of the isolated perfused rat lung in studies on lung lipid metabolism. J Lipid Res 14:138–144

Godinez RI, Sanders RL, Longmore WJ (1975) Phosphatidylglycerol in rat lung. I. Identification as a metabolically active phospholipid in isolated perfused rat lung. Biochemistry 14:830–834

Goodman BE, Fleischer RS, Crandall ED (1982) Effects of metabolic inhibitors on dome formation by cultured alveolar epithelial cells. Fed Proc 41:1245

Guyton AC, Parker JC, Taylor AE, Jackson TE, Moffatt DS (1979) Factors governing water movement in the lung. In: Fishman AP, Renkin EM (eds) Pulmonary edema. Am Physiol Soc, Bethesda, pp 65–78

Hartiala J (1976) Steroid metabolism in adult lung. Agents Actions 6:522–526

Hauge A (1968) Conditions concerning the pressor response to ventilation hypoxia in isolated perfused rat lungs. Acta Physiol Scand 72:33–44

Heinemann (1961) Free fatty acid production by rabbit lung tissue in vitro. Am J Physiol 201:607–610

Hook R, Gillis CN (1975) The removal and metabolism of prostaglandin E_1 by rabbit lung. Prostaglandins 9:193–201

Hughes FA, Kehne JH, Fox JR (1954) Reimplantation and transplantation of pulmonary tissue in dogs. Surgery 36:1101–1108

Hughes J, May AJ, Widdicome JG (1958) Mechanical factors in the formation of oedema in perfused rabbit lungs. J Physiol 142:292–305

Hughes J, Gillis CN, Bloom FE (1969) Uptake and disposition of norepinephrine in perfused rat lungs. J Pharmacol Exp Ther 169:237–248

Itakura N, Fisher AB, Thurman RG (1977) Cytochrome P-450 linked p-nitroanisole o-demethylation in the perfused lung. J Appl Physiol 43:238–245

Johnson RG, Lugg MA, Nicholas TE (1979) Uptake of [^{14}C]choline and incorporation into lung phospholipid by the isolated perfused rat lung. Lipids 14:555–558

Junod AF (1973) Uptake, metabolism and effux of [^{14}C]-5-hydroxytryptamine in isolated perfused rat lungs. J Pharm Exp Ther 183:341–355

Kerr JS, Baker NJ, Bassett DJP, Fisher AB (1979) Effect of perfusate glucose concentration on rat lung glycolysis. Am J Physiol 236:E229–233

Kerr JS, Fisher AB, Kleinzeller A (1981) Transport of glucose analogues in rat lung. Am J Physiol 241:E191–E195

Klein LS, Fisher AB, Soltoff S, Coburn RF (1978) Effect of O_2 exposure on pulmonary metabolism of prostaglandin E_2. Am Rev Respir Dis 118:622–625

Klocke RA (1978) Catalysis of CO_2 reactions by lung carbonic anhydrase. J Appl Physiol 44:882–888

Koga H (1958) Studies on the function of isolated perfused mammalian lung. Kumamoto Med J 11:1–11

Law FCP, Eling TE, Bend JR, Fouts JR (1974) Metabolism of xenobiotics by the isolated perfused lung. Drug Metab Dispos 2:433–442

Leary WP, Smith U (1970) In situ perfusion of the isolated rat lung. Life Sci 9:1321–1326

Levey S, Gast R (1966) Isolated perfused rat lung preparation. J Appl Physiol 21:313–316

Linehan JH, Dawson CA, Wagner-Weber VM (1981) Prostaglandin E_1 uptake by isolated cat lungs perfused with physiological salt solution. J Appl Physiol 50:428–434

Lloyd TC (1964) Effect of alveolar hypoxia on pulmonary vascular resistance. J Appl Physiol 19:1086–1094

Lohr HZ (1924) Untersuchungen zur Physiologie und Pharmakologie der Lunge. Z Gesamte Exp Med 39:67–130

Longmore WJ, Mourning JT (1976) Lactate production in the isolated perfused rat lung. Am J Physiol 231:351–354

Longmore WJ, Niethe CN, Sprinkle DJ, Godinez RI (1973) Effect of CO_2 concentration on phospholipid metabolism in the isolated perfused lung. J Lipid Res 14:145–151

Lorenz W, Doenicke A, Messmer K, Reimann H-J, Therman M, Lann W, Berr J, Schmal A, Dormann P, Regenfuss P, Hamelman H (1976) Histamine release in human subjects by modified gelatin (haemaccel) and dextran: an explanation for anaphylactoid reactions observed under clinical conditions? Br J Anesth 48:151–165

Lunde PKM (1976) The influence of perfusate composition on edema development in isolated perfused rabbit lungs. Thesis, Universitetsforlaget, Oslo

MacDonald CM, Boardman LE (1980) An isolated rat lung perfusion system for use in tobacco smoke studies. J Pharmacol Methods 3:103–113

Maloney JV, Whittenberger JL (1951) Clinical implications of pressures used in the body respirator. Am J Med Sci 221:425–430

Martin H (1883) The direct influence of gradual variations of temperature upon the rate of beat of the dog's heart. Philos Trans R Soc Lond 174:663

McClenahan JB, Urtnowski A (1967) Effect of ventilation on surfactant and its turnover rate. J Appl Physiol 23:215–220

McGovren JP, Lubawy WC, Kostenbauder HB (1976) Uptake and metabolism of nicotine by the isolated perfused rabbit lung. J Pharmacol Exp Ther 199:198–207

McMurtry IF, Davidson AB, Reeves JT, Grover RF (1976) Inhibition of hypoxic pulmonary vasoconstriction by calcium antagonists in isolated rat lungs. Circ Res 38:99–104

Mead J, Whittenberger JL (1964) Lung inflation and hemodynamics. In: Fenn WO, Rahn H (eds) Handbook of physiology respiration, section 2, vol I. Am Physiol Soc, Washington DC, pp 477–486

Mehendale HM, El-Bassiouni EA (1975) Uptake and disposition of aldrin and dieldrin by isolated perfused rabbit lung. Drug Metab Dispos 3:543–556

Mehendale HM, Angevine LS, Ohmiya YO (1981) The isolated perfused lung – a critical evaluation. Toxicology 21:1–36

Miyauchi Y, Inone T, Paton BC (1966) Adjunctive use of a surface-active agent in extra corporeal circulation. Circulation 33 [Suppl I]:71–77

Morishige WK, Uetake CA, Greenwood FC, Akaka J (1977) Pulmonary insulin responsitivity: in vitro effects of insulin on the diabetic rat lung and specific insulin binding to lung receptors in normal rats. Endocrinology 100:1710–1722

Moxley MA, Longmore WJ (1977) Effect of experimental diabetes and insulin on lipid metabolism in the isolated perfused rat lung. Biochim Biophys Acta 488:218–244

Nicholas TE, Kim PA (1975) The metabolism of ^{3}H-cortisol by the isolated perfused rat and guinea pig lungs. Steroids 25:387–402

Nicolaysen G (1971) Perfusate qualities and spontaneous edema formation in an isolated perfused lung preparation. Acta Physiol Scand 83:563–570

Niden AH, Mittman C, Burrows D (1962) Pulmonary diffusion in the dog lung. J Appl Physiol 17:885–892

Niemeier RW, Bingham E (1972) An isolated perfused lung preparation for metabolic studies. Life Sci 11:807–820

Nilsen KH, Hauge A (1968) Effects of temperature changes on the pressor response to acute alveolar hypoxia in isolated rat lungs. Acta Physiol Scand 73:111–120

Nisell O (1948) Effects of oxygen and CO_2 on the circulation of isolated and perfused lungs of the cat. Acta Physiol Scand 15:121–127

Nishiki K, Jamieson D, Oshino N, Chance B (1976) Oxygen toxicity in the perfused rat liver and lung under hyperbaric conditions. Biochem J 160:343–355

O'Neil JJ, Tierney DF (1974) Rat lung metabolism: glucose utilization by isolated perfused lungs and tissue slices. Am J Physiol 226:867–873

Orton TC, Anderson MW, Pickett RD, Eling TE, Fouts JR (1973) Xenobiotic accumulation and metabolism by isolated perfused rabbit lungs. J Pharmacol Exp Ther 186:482–497

Oyarzun MJ, Clements JA (1978) Control of lung surfactant by ventilation, adrenergic mediators, and prostaglandins in the rabbit. Am Rev Respir Dis 117:879–891

Palmer MA, Piper PJ, Vane JR (1973) Release of rabbit aorta contracting substance (RCS) and prostaglandins induced by chemical or mechanical stimulation of guinea-pigs lungs. Br J Pharmacol 49:226–242

Philpot RM, Anderson MW, Eling TE (1977) Uptake, accumulation and metabolism of chemicals by the lung. In: Bakhle YS, Vane JR (eds) Metabolic functions of the lung. M. Dekker, New York, pp 123–171

Pietra GG, Spagnoli LG, Capuzzi DM, Sparks CE, Fishman AP, Marsh JB (1976) Metabolism of ^{125}I-labelled lipoproteins by the isolated rat lung. J Cell Biol 70:33–46

Piper PJ, Vane JR, Wyllie JH (1970) Inactivation of prostaglandins by the lungs. Nature 225:600–604

Post C, Andersson RGG, Ryrfeldt A, Nilsson E (1978) Transport and binding of lidocaine by lung slices and perfused lung of rats. Acta Pharmacol Toxicol 43:156–163

Postlethwait EM, Young SL (1980) Alteration of rat lung adenine nucleotide content after pulmonary edema. Lung 157:165–177

Rannels DE, Roake GM, Watkins CA (1982) Additive effects of pentobarbital and halothane to inhibit synthesis of lung proteins. Anesthesiology 57:87–93

Renkin EM (1962) Techniques of vascular perfusion. In: Nastuk WL (ed) Physical techniques in biological research. Academic, New York, pp 107–136

Rhoades RA (1974) Net uptake of glucose, glycerol, and fatty acids by the isolated perfused rat lung. Am J Physiol 326:144–149

Rhoades RA, Shaw ME, Eskew ML, Wali S (1978) Lactate metabolism in perfused rat lung. Am J Physiol 235:E619–623

Rickaby DA, Linehan JH, Bronikowski TA, Dawson CA (1981) Kinetics of serotonin uptake in the dog lung. J Appl Physiol 51:405–414

Rosenberg E, Forster RE (1960) Changes in diffusing capacity of isolated cat lungs with blood pressure and flow. J Appl Physiol 15:883–892

Rosenbloom PM, Bass AD (1970) A lung perfusion preparation for the study of drug metabolism. J Appl Physiol 29:138–144

Ryan JW, Roblero J, Stewart JM (1968) Inactivation of bradykinin in the pulmonary circulation. Biochem J 110:796–797

Ryan JW, Stewart JM, Leary WP, Ledingham JG (1970) Metabolism of angiotensin I in the pulmonary circulation. Biochem J 120:221–223

Ryan U, Ryan JW, Whitaker C, Chui A (1976) Localization of angiotensin converting enzyme (kininase II). Tissue Cell 8:125–145

Schneeberger EE (1979) Barrier function of intercellular junctions in adult and fetal lungs. In: Fishman AP, Renkin EM (eds) Pulmonary edema. Am Physiol Soc, Bethesda, pp 21–38

Shaw ME, Rhoades RA (1977) Substrate metabolism in the perfused lung: response to changes in circulating glucose and palmitate levels. Lipids 12:930–935

Sloviter HA, Kamimoto T (1967) Erythrocyte substitute for perfusion of brain. Nature 216:458–460

Smith BR, Philpot RM, Bend JR (1978) Metabolism of benzo [a]-pyrene by the isolated perfused rabbit lung. Drug Metab Dispos 6:425–431

Smith JC, Mitzner W (1980) Analysis of pulmonary vascular interdependence in excised dog lobes. J Appl Physiol 48:450–467

Splawinski JS, Gryglewski RJ (1981) Release of prostacyclin by the lung. Clin Respir Physiol 17:553–569

Staub NC (1974) Pulmonary edema. Physiol Rev 54:678–811

Steinberg H, Bassett DJP, Fisher AB (1975) Depression of pulmonary 5-hydroxytryptamine uptake by metabolic inhibitors. Am J Physiol 228:1298–1303

Steinberg H, Fisher AB, Sloviter HA (1979) Accelerated removal of platelets during perfusion of isolated lungs with perfluoroerythrocyte substitute. Proc Soc Exp Biol Med 162:179–182

Steinberg H, Greenwald RA, Sciubba J, Das DK (1982) The effect of oxygen-derived free radicals on pulmonary endothelial cell function in the isolated perfused rat lung. Exp Lung Res 3:163–173

Stubbs WA, Morgan I, Lloyd B, Alberti KBMM (1977) The effect of insulin on lung metabolism in the rat. Clin Endocrinol 7:181–184

Tucker LD II, Shertzer HG (1980) Split lung perfusion: a new method to test the effects of chemical agents on pulmonary metabolism. Toxicol Appl Pharmacol 55:353

Turner DM, Amnitage AK, Briant RH, Dollery CT (1975) Metabolism of nicotine by the isolated perfused dog lung. Xenobiotics 5:539–551

Verney EB, Starling EH (1922) On secretion by the isolated kidney. J Physiol 56:355–358

Voekel NF, Gerber JG, McMurtry IF, Nies AS, Reeves JT (1981) Release of vasodilator prostaglandin PGI$_2$ from isolated rat lung during vasoconstriction. Circ Res 48:207–213

Wang MC, Meng HC (1974) Synthesis of phospholipids and phospholipid fatty acids by isolated perfused rat lung. Lipids 9:63–67

Watkins CA, Rannels DE (1979) In situ perfusion of rat lungs: stability and effects of oxygen tension. J Appl Physiol 47:325–239

Weber KC, Visscher MB (1969) Metabolism of the isolated canine lung. Am J Physiol 217:1044–1052

West JB, Dollery CT, Naimark A (1964) Distribution of blood flow in isolated lung: relation to vascular and alveolar pressures. J Appl Physiol 19:713–724

Widman M, Nordquist M, Dollery CT, Briant RH (1975) Metabolism of Δ^1-tetrahydrocannabinol by the isolated perfused dog lung. Comparison with in vitro liver metabolism. J Pharm Pharmacol 27:842–848

Wolf CR, Slaughter SR, Marciniszyn JP, Philpot RM (1980) Purification and structural comparison of pulmonary and hepatic cytochrome P-450 from rabbits. Biochim Biophys Acta 624:409–419

Wolfe RR, Hochachka PW, Trelstad RL, Burke JF (1979) Lactate metabolism in perfused rat lung. Am J Physiol 236:E276–282

CHAPTER 7

Pulmonary Cell and Tissue Cultures

B. T. SMITH

A. Introduction

The lung is a complex organ and the eventual understanding of physiologic or pathologic changes at the cellular and molecular level requires that we understand how individual cell types interact with their environment. In this chapter various in vitro systems are reviewed which have been developed for pulmonary cells and tissues and their individual strengths and weaknesses are considered.

B. Lung Cell and Tissue Culture Systems

I. Strengths and Weaknesses

A variety of approaches are available to maintain and/or grow pulmonary cells and tissues in vitro. No single technique adequately represents functions of lung cells as they occur in vivo. An understanding of the strengths and weaknesses of the various models available is central to selecting the model most appropriate to the hypotheses being tested. Often, use of more than one model can enhance the value of the observations made.

As a general rule, errors of interpretation made with in vitro systems tend to be of the Type Two variety. Failure to observe a given cellular activity or response in vitro is more often a commentary on the quality of the system than on the real world. In contrast, observation of a given cellular response or function in vitro can be taken as strong evidence that such behavior is, at least potentially, expressed in vivo.

1. Pure Cultures of Individual Cell Types

The availability of pure cultures of individual lung cell types has provided a powerful approach to understanding their composition, their biochemical activity, and control mechanisms which act directly upon them. On the other hand, the experimental methods tend to be somewhat tedious and complex, and the risk of damage to the cells during isolation is relatively high (see for instance FINKEL-STEIN and MAVIS 1979). Such damage may not only reduce yields (or prevent successful isolation entirely), but it also introduces a serious concern: that only a particular subpopulation of the cell type of interest is selected by the process used, such that its behavior in vitro, even if respresentative of its behavior in vivo, may not be typical of the population at large. Historically, the commonest procedure for isolating a single cell population has depended simply on growing an initially complex population of cells under conditions which favor propagation of a single cell type. With continued culturing, the hardier, favored cell type overgrows other cell types, resulting in a relatively homogeneous population. This approach has been used for many years to isolate mesenchymal "fibroblastic" cell cultures from a variety of tissues. A similar approach has been used successfully to isolate transformed lung cells (LIEBER et al. 1976), since such cells have a selective growth advantage over nontransformed cells (SPORN and TODARO 1980). Such approaches are relatively simple and gentle, but a considerable number of cell generations must occur before adequate purity and yield of cells is achieved. A considerable loss of phenotypic expression may result from in vitro aging (DIGLIO and KIKKAWA 1977; TANSWELL and SMITH 1981). Indeed, the very large body of work relating in vitro to in vivo aging (CRISTOFALO et al. 1979) has traditionally utilized human fetal lung fibroblasts (HAYFLICK 1965).

A second approach is to isolate cells by physical characteristics, most commonly size or density, although other characteristics such as electrical charge, magnetic properties after ingestion of iron particles by phagocytic cells, etc., have been used. Such approaches, when optimized, often provide relatively large yields of cells which can be studied acutely after isolation or maintained in short-term primary culture, thus obviating problems in interpretation which accrue to cells which are propagated for longer periods of time. On the other hand, while purities in excess of 90% are often attained, minor contamination by other cell types can be of importance in interpreting certain types of data, such as determining whether an observed metabolic activity might be conferred on a population by the contaminating cell type. On occasion, if populations of the contaminating cell type can be prepared, it is possible to add known, increasing numbers to the cell population of interest, establish a dose–response curve for the contaminating cell type, and extrapolate back to zero contamination.

Clonal isolation techniques are the most powerful means of obtaining homogeneous populations of cells. By a variety of strategies (REID 1979), a single cell is isolated and grown into a cell population all descended from the same progenitor. Such techniques are tedious and time-consuming and assume that the cell type of interest can be propagated in vitro. A large number of population doublings must occur before a population of sufficient size to characterize and study is obtained. This greatly increases the risk of loss of expression of differentiated features. Furthermore, the major requirement for successful clonal isolation is extensive doubling capacity, a characteristic which may not be shared by the entire population of interest. For example, alveolar type II cells have been clonally isolated from adult rat (DOUGLAS and KAIGHN 1974) and human fetal (TANSWELL and SMITH 1981) lung, thus representing readily dividing cell populations. In contrast, alveolar type II cells isolated by density gradient centrifugation techniques from the rat (MASON et al. 1977) or rabbit (KIKKAWA and YONEDA 1974) can be maintained in primary culture, but show no potential for cell division (MASON and DOBBS 1980; DIGLIO and KIKKAWA 1977).

2. Isolated Cells in Heterogeneous Systems

These systems generally utilize dispersed populations of cells which are maintained in short-term culture with little or no attempt to reduce the number of different cell types which make up the population. Depending upon the technique of culture maintenance, there may be little growth, or quite vigorous growth for a limited period of time. Subculturing is seldom undertaken, since overgrowth of a single, hardy cell type will usually occur with time. These techniques provide relatively fresh cells with a limited in vitro age, decreasing the risk of loss of differentiated capacity. Again, it must be remembered that the techniques used for cell dispersal (usually enzymatic) may only release a subpopulation of one or more of the cell types making up the culture or, similarly, only certain subpopulations may survive the procedure.

In view of the heterogeneity of such cultures, it is difficult to ascribe observed metabolic activity to a given cell type. Use of such cultures for biochemical studies can be greatly enhanced with autoradiographic or cytochemical techniques. The heterogeneity also provides potential strengths, however, in that the cells can selectively recombine with either homologous (DOUGLAS et al. 1980) or heterologous (INDO and WILSON 1976; TANSWELL and SMITH 1981) cells in ways which may more closely mimic their in vivo environment. Such recombination may be beneficial either in terms of the substrate provided for cell adhesion (DOUGLAS et al. 1980; GEPPERT et al. 1980) or in terms of soluble molecules from adjacent cells altering the microenvironment (SMITH 1978).

3. Organ Cultures

These systems use intact fragments of tissue maintained in nutrient media of varying degrees of complexity. Such approaches are generally relatively straightforward. The cells comprising the tissue are exposed to much less manipulation and a normal microenvironment is maintained by virtue of normal cellular relationships.

The major disadvantage of organ culture approaches is the loss of the normal means of cell nutrition, which can no longer occur via the vasculature, but must occur via diffusion. Thus, concentration gradients for nutrients, waste products, and dissolved gases occur. Problems can be partially corrected by using very small explant fragments (usually 0.5–1 mm) and, at times by manipulating gradients to facilitate diffusion.

II. Pure Cultures of Individual Cell Types

1. Fibroblasts

Lung fibroblasts have been widely studied in the past two decades (HAYFLICK and MOORHEAD 1961), but investigations have largely focused on these cells as diploid human cell strains (HAYFLICK 1965; CRISTOFALO et al. 1979) rather than as specific lung cells. More recently, however, several lines of evidence have suggested that pulmonary fibroblasts have many features that distinguish them from fibroblasts isolated from other organs. Such features include glucocorticoid metabolism and effects (SMITH and GIROUD 1975), population kinetics (SCHNEIDER et al. 1977), glycosaminoglycan production (SJOBERG and FRANSSON 1977), collagen synthesis (BRADLEY et al. 1980), nutritional requirements (HAM 1980), and production of lung-specific peptides which mediate hormonal effects on pulmonary epithelial maturation (SMITH 1979). The latter observation is reminiscent of the classical observations of GROBSTEIN (1967) that morphogenesis of the pulmonary epithelium is dependent on the adjacent mesenchyme, in an organ-specific fashion. In this light, it must be remembered that mesenchyme from varying regions of the developing lung convey different, specific information to the adjacent epithelium (WESSELS 1970). Thus, mass populations of lung fibroblasts are likely composed of multiple subpopulations which may have different functional and anatomic specificities (for a discussion of this point, see BRADLEY et al. 1980).

Two primary methods for isolating mass cultures of pulmonary fibroblasts have been used: explant techniques and differential adhesion. In the former technique, small pieces of lung tissue (~ 1 mm^3) are placed in an appropriate culture vessel and outgrowth of cells is allowed to occur. Since outgrowth is dependent upon the anchoring surface provided by the culture flask, it must be ensured that the explants do not float off the surface, either by maintaining the explant in a single drop of medium for the first 12–24 h until cell outgrowth anchors the fragment, or by anchoring the explant under a submerged coverslip (BRADLEY et al. 1980). An initial outgrowth of epithelioid cells often occurs, but is soon followed by an extensive outgrowth of fibroblastic cells. The initial epithelioid outgrowth is either lifted off the surface by the subsequent outgrowth and lost in subsequent medium changes or rapidly overgrown and lost with subculturing. Once sufficient outgrowth has occurred, the initial explants can be removed from the flask mechanically and the fibroblasts subcultivated by standard techniques. It is important that subcultivation not be attempted onto too large a surface area, since below a certain cell density growth is very slow or nonexistent. This may reflect dependence for growth upon substances produced by the fibroblasts themselves (ATKISON et al. 1980; CLEMMONS et al. 1981; ATKISON and BALA 1981). Split ratios of 1 : 2 to 1 : 4 seem most useful.

Greater yields can often be achieved using enzymatic dispersal of lung tissue followed by differential adherence. Finely minced lung tissue is readily dispersed into individual cells with 0.1–0.5% trypsin in a divalent cation-free buffer (e. g., phosphate-buffered saline) at 37 °C on a magnetic stirrer. A single 10- to 30-min enzyme treatment will completely disperse fetal tissue, while numerous sequential treatments may be required to obtain maximal yields from more mature lung. In some cases, yields can be improved by adding DNase (to free cells trapped in a sticky matrix of DNA released from damaged cells) or chicken serum (which, unlike mammalian sera, does not contain trypsin inhibitors to block the enzyme activity). The dispersed cells are harvested by aspiration after allowing undigested tissue to settle to the bottom of the digestion flask and the trypsin activity is quickly stopped by addition of mammalian (e. g., bovine) serum or by lowering the temperature. After one or more washes of the cell harvest, usually with the tissue culture medium to be used, the cells can be counted, studied for viability, and implanted in appropriate culture vessels. Again, observance of a minimum inoculum density (about 10^5 cells/cm^2) enhances subsequent growth. The cells are then incubated under appropriate conditions (37 °C under 5% CO$_2$) for 30 min to 2 h, at which time a significant proportion of the fibroblasts will have attached to the flask, while most other cell types will not yet have done so (SMITH and GIROUD 1975). The flasks are now vigorously agitated and the medium and unattached cells are removed by aspiration and replaced with fresh medium. While occasional contaminating cell types remain, they are rapidly overgrown by the fibroblasts and lost in subsequent passages. DAVIS et al. (1979) have reported successful culture of fibroblasts obtained by pulmonary lavage in human subjects. This opens the way for study of connective tissue cells from normal subjects and patients with a variety of lung diseases.

2. Macrophages

The pulmonary alveolar macrophage is a readily accessible lung cell type. It is easily recovered via bronchoalveolar lavage from animals (SODERLAND and NAUM 1973; NAUM 1975; LIN et al. 1975). The recent advent of fiber optic bronchoscopy has made it possible to obtain and culture human alveolar macrophages (LEFFINGWELL and LOW 1975; CRYSTAL et al. 1976; HUNNINGHAKE et al. 1980). Although derived from bone marrow, alveolar macrophages show certain functional differences from macrophages isolated from other tissues, including adaptation to the relatively high alveolar PO_2 (SIMON et al. 1977). The functions of alveolar macrophages include clearing debris and bacteria constantly deposited in the lung by ventilation (HARRIS et al. 1970), metabolism of certain carcinogens (CANTRELL et al. 1973; HARRIS et al. 1978), complement synthesis (COLE et al. 1980), and production and secretion of chemoattractant signals to recruit inflammatory cells.

Although originally thought to be a terminally differentiated cell (VAN FURTH 1970), it is now clear that at least a subpopulation of alveolar macrophages possess the ability to divide extensively (LIN et al. 1975; NAUM 1975). In a typical procedure, the lungs are lavaged with sterile phosphate-buffered saline and the cells recovered by centrifugation. The cell pellet is resuspended in tissue culture medium for plating. Homologous serum may be advantageous: HUNNINGHAKE et al. (1980) have successfully cultured human alveolar macrophages in RPMI-1640 medium supplemented with 20% heat-inactivated human AB serum. Nonadherent cells (lymphocytes, etc.) are rinsed away by a medium change after 1–2 h. NAUM et al. (1979) report that if healthy young animals (mice) are used, up to 98% of viable cells recovered by lavage will be adherent mononuclear phagocytes. Their rapid identification as macrophages can be accomplished by staining for nonspecific esterase (TUCKER et al. 1977). If desired, clonal populations can be isolated in soft agar (LIN et al. 1975). The growth of alveolar macrophages in vitro can be considerably enhanced by the use of conditioned medium from a variety of cell lines, such as BHK (baby hamster kidney) cells (NAUM 1975). Such media contain "pulmonary macrophage growth factor," a 68,000-daltons acidic polypeptide (NAUM et al. 1979).

3. Endothelial Cells

The pulmonary endothelial cell has been recognized as the single most important cell to regulate serum concentrations of various vasoactive agents (VANE 1969). Biochemical differences in vascular beds from different anatomic locations within the lung (COX 1980) as well as different properties observed for pulmonary artery endothelial cells, as opposed to pulmonary venous endothelial cells (JOHNSON 1980), have led to the development of a variety of techniques to culture pulmonary endothelial cells from different anatomic sites within the lung.

Ryan et al. (1978b) used calf hearts with attached great vessels freshly obtained at the time of slaughter. The pulmonary artery is ligated at the heart, removed, and washed with Puck's saline containing antibiotics in three times the normal concentration. The artery segments are then filled with a solution containing 0.25% collagenase, suspended in a beaker of buffered saline, and incubated at low speed in a shaking water bath for 25 min at 37 °C. The resulting cells are recovered by centrifugation, suspended in medium 199 with 30% fetal bovine serum and grown in culture flasks. With serial subcultivation by standard techniques, such cells have been maintained for over 60 passages (Ryan et al. 1978b). Subsequently, this technique has been modified to isolate cells by gently scraping the inverted pulmonary artery segments with a scalpel blade, the cells are then shaken into medium 199 with 10% fetal bovine serum and plated into standard tissue culture flasks (Ryan et al. 1980a, b). When these cultures were in log phase, the monolayer was scraped with a rubber policeman, passed through a 30-gauge neddle to break up clumps and seeded onto a suspension of polyacrylamide beads (Bio-Carriers, Bio-Rad Laboratories, Richmond, California) maintained in a standard roller bottle system. In this system, the cells divide readily and can be "subcultured" simply by subdividing the bead suspension and adding additional medium and fresh beads.

Johnson (1980) applied a similar collagenase dispersal technique to the one described to major human pulmonary arteries and veins. She also used 10% homologous serum (human Type O+), in addition to 20% fetal bovine serum to maintain the resultant cells. Pulmonary artery endothelial cells showed very much greater ability to metabolize vasoactive agents than did endothelial cells from pulmonary veins.

Habliston et al. (1979) used a reverse perfusion technique (pulmonary vein to pulmonary artery) with 0.5% collagenase to isolate endothelial cells from the lungs of rabbits. Endothelial cells were successfully cultured from the effluent and had structural features of endothelial cells from the pulmonary microvasculature. However, these workers could not be sure that at least some of the cells did not arise from the major branches of the pulmonary artery. An alternative approach for obtaining endothelial cells from the microvasculature of various tissues is that of Folkman et al. (1979). After enzyme digestion of tissues, capillary segments are isolated by sequential filtration and placed in culture. Occasional contaminating pericytes are mechanically destroyed under a dissecting microscope. Parshley et al. (1979) have reported successful clonal isolation of endothelial cells from a mixed cell population of adult rat lung cells which had been maintained in culture for more than 3 years.

Endothelial cells can be reliably identified in culture by, in addition to their typical pavement-like morphology, assays for factor VIII antigen (Jaffe et al. 1973), demonstration of the presence of angiotensin-converting enzyme (Ryan et al. 1978a), and by ultrastructural appearance (Smith and Ryan 1972).

Vascular endothelial cell growth in vitro can be enhanced by a variety of substances, including tumor-conditioned medium (Folkman and Cotran 1976), medium conditioned by differentiated adipocytes (Castellot et al. 1980), and plasma-derived serum (Dickinson and Slakey 1980). In addition to responding to a number of growth-stimulating agents, vascular endothelial cells also produce a growth factor which is active on smooth muscle, as well as other, cells (GAJDUSEK et al. 1980). Since pulmonary endothelial cells are the first cell type to show an adverse response to oxidant injury, studies of the effects of hyperoxia on these cells in vitro are of considerable interest (BOWMAN et al. 1981; CUMMISKEY et al. 1981). Finally, evidence that endothelial cells mediate the effects of vasoactive agents on pulmonary vascular tone in vivo (CHAND and ALTURA 1981) suggests that studies of interactions between endothelial cells and smooth muscle cells in vitro will be of considerable value.

4. Smooth Muscle Cells

Several toxins lead to pulmonary hypertension associated with hyperplasia of medial smooth muscle and extension of smooth muscle into regions of the pulmonary circulation not normally muscularized (MEYRICK and REID 1979). Thus, in vitro study of pulmonary vascular smooth muscle cells might be expected to provide important clues in understanding these changes. While pulmonary smooth muscle cells seem not to have been previously isolated and studied, methods have been developed to isolate smooth muscle cells from various large and medium-sized arteries. These should be readily applicable to the larger ramifications of the pulmonary vascular tree.

Ross (1971) first described the culture of smooth muscle cells. The method requires large vessels, since the intimal and adventitial portions are first stripped away, followed by explant cultures of the remaining media. Most workers grown such cells in a standard medium with 10% fetal bovine serum. An outgrowth of cells readily emerges which can be subcultured and fairly readily grown to confluence. The cells have an elongated, spindle-shaped appearance similar to fibroblasts. However, unlike fibroblasts, upon reaching confluence, their growth does not cease, but continues, at a slower rate, with piling up, or multilayering, which leads to a typical "hill and valley" appearance of the cultures (SALCEDO and FRANZBLAU 1981). They continue to produce connective tissue components for rather long periods of time and profound hormonal effects on this process have been noted (BELDEKAS et al. 1981). The cells can be unequivocally identified by electron microscopy by their characteristic contractile elements and, particularly, by the presence of dense bodies (CHAMLEY-CAMPBELL et al. 1979). Growth of human smooth muscle cells from punch biopsies has recently been described (ESKIN et al. 1981).

Methods for culturing smooth muscle cells from smaller vessels are not presently available. A possible approach might be developed from the technique of HABLISTON et al. (1979) for isolation of endothelial cells by enzyme perfusion of the lung. Endothelial cells were contaminated by occasional smooth muscle cells, which were removed by changing the culture medium 2 h after implantation. Thus, the 2-h supernatant media might provide good starting material for the culture of this "contaminating" cell type.

5. Pericytes

The neomuscularization of pulmonary vessels already referred to (MEYRICK and REID 1979) is thought to involve "differentiation" of pericytes into smooth muscle cells. If such a process could be induced in vitro, then studies of this process and means to prevent or reverse it could be undertaken. Again, means to culture pericytes are not described in the literature. However, B. R. Zetter (1981, personal communication) has had preliminary success in culturing pericytes from nonpulmonary tissue using the capillary segment technique described (FOLKMAN et al. 1979).

6. Airway Epithelial Cells

The airway epithelium is the first pulmonary cell layer to be exposed to exogenous toxic agents which are carried into the lung in the inspired air. Availability of cultured airway epithelial cells can be expected to be of major importance in defining the biologic response to a wide variety of noxious agents. Despite this urgent need, progress in developing in vitro systems for airway epithelial cells (as opposed to organ culture systems, see Sect. B. IV) has been slow, perhaps reflecting the difficulty encountered in maintaining many types of differentiated epithelia in vitro (DANES 1980). A description of bronchial epithelial cell types and their characteristics in vivo has recently been published (REID and JONES 1979).

GOLDMAN and BASEMAN (1980a) described a method to isolate and culture epithelial cells from the hamster trachea. Tracheal rings, opened at the membranous portion, are stirred in a 0.01% thermolysin solution. Subsequently, GOLDMAN and BASEMAN (1980b) have demonstrated that these cells synthesize and secrete mucous glycoproteins apparently identical to those produced by tracheal explants.

STONER et al. (1980a) have successfully prepared epithelial cell cultures from human bronchi. Explant cultures are prepared in an enriched medium (CMRL-1066) to which is added insulin, hydorcortisone and pyruvic acid, and 10% fetal bovine serum. As with many types of explant, small epithelial outgrowths are the first to appear. As soon as they are seen, the explant is transferred to a second dish to start a new culture, and any fibroblastic outgrowth is mechanically removed. The cells were maintained in primary culture for prolonged periods. While ciliary activity was observed in some cells for as long as 6 months, most "differentiated" to keratin-producing squamous epithelium. Other biochemical products noted include mucopolysaccharides, fibronectin, and type IV collagen (STONER et al. 1981). In contrast, fibroblasts derived from these explants produced only types I and III collagen (STONER et al. 1980a). Subsequently, STONER et al. (1980b) have shown that addition of putrescine to the culture medium of the explants provides a selective growth advantage to the epithelial cells.

7. Alveolar Type I Cells

The alveolar type I cell is a very attenuated cell across which gas exchange is thought to take place. Although only 15% of alveolar cells are type I cells, together they cover over 90% of the alveolar surface area. A common form of pulmonary injury is damage to this cell type (WITSCHI 1976). Since type I cells are thought to be terminally differentiated and incapable of growth in vivo, it is unlikely that they can be grown in vitro. However, their isolation and maintenance (as opposed to growth) could facilitate study of mechanisms of toxic effects on this cell type, as well as elucidation of proposed interactions between these cells and pulmonary connective tissue (BRODY et al. 1981). PICCIANO and ROSENBAUM (1978) have described in detail a method to isolate a cell population from the adult rabbit lung which is enriched (70%) with respect to type I cells. Type I cells isolated by this technique can be identified by ultrastructure and by the appearance of surface blebs following exposure to cytochalasin-D (ROSENBAUM and PICCIANO 1978).

8. Alveolar Type II Cells

The alveolar type II cell has attracted considerable interest from cell biologists in view of its major function to produce the pulmonary surfactant. Less attention has been focused on the other major role for the alveolar type II cell: its function as the stem cell of the alveolus. As noted previously, many toxic injuries damage the type I cell which is sloughed off the alveolar basement membrane. Repair ensues by proliferation of type II cells, some of which transform morphologically into type I cells, while others remain as surfactant-producing type II cells (ADAMSON and BOWDEN 1975).

Perhaps the commonest approach to the culture of alveolar type II cells has been to purify large numbers of these cells from populations of individual lung cells dispersed by enzymatic techniques. Here it must be remembered that exposure to such enzymes causes internal damage to a variety of enzyme systems (FINKELSTEIN and MAVIS 1979), although recovery can likely occur during subsequent maintenance in vitro. KIKKAWA and YONEDA (1974) isolated type II cells from adult rabbits. The lungs were cleared of blood by perfusion and the macrophage population was reduced by lavage. They were then chopped and incubated in 0.5% trypsin in a solution containing barium sulfate. The latter is ingested by macrophages, facilitating their separation from type II cells by centrifugation techniques. The resulting cell suspension was filtered through nylon mesh, layered above a Ficoll solution (density 1.047), Pharmacia, Uppsala, Sweden, and spun at 3.750 rpm for 1 h. In addition to electron microscopy, rapid identification of type II cells was accomplished by using a modified Papanicolaou stain, the surfactant-containing lamellar bodies appearing as small blue intracytoplasmic inclusions. Each procedure typically yields about 15×10^6 type II cells of about 80%–90% purity (KIKKAWA and YONEDA 1974). The cells can be maintained in primary culture, although no proliferation is seen. Attachment efficiency (about 10%) is best in 10% fetal bovine serum (DIGLIO and KIKKAWA 1977). The cells maintain ultrastructural features of type II cells for 3–5 days in culture, after which they lose specific markers and spread out. DIGLIO and KIKKAWA (1977) have speculated that this might respresent "maturation" to type I cells. Early cultures have been extensively studied with respect to surfactant-associated phospholipid synthesis (ROONEY et al. 1977; SMITH and KIKKAWA 1978, 1979; F. B. SMITH et al. 1980).

MASON et al. (1977) isolated alveolar type II cells from the lungs of rats. The lungs were perfused with calcium and magnesium-free buffer, then lavaged to remove part of the macrophage population. The lungs were then instilled, via the airways, with fluorocarbon–albumin emulsion and left at 37 °C for 20 min, again so the macrophages would ingest this dense material. Following this, they were instilled for 10 min with a trypsin (3%, recrystallized bovine trypsin) solution followed by trypsin inhibitor. They were then minced and shaken for 10 min in a 37 °C water bath to free the already loosened cells. After filtering, the cells were layered over a discontinuous gradient of albumin, densities 1.040 and 1.080 and spun at 315 g. Type II cells were recovered from the band between 1.040 and 1.080. The average yield was $8-20 \times 10^6$ per rat, with 60%–67% purity. Again, in addition to ultrastructure, rapid identification was accomplished using the fluorescent dye phosphine 3R, which relatively specifically stains the lamellar bodies (MASON et al. 1977). Subsequently, application of centrifugal elutriation following the technique already described increased the purity to 86% (GREEN-LEAF et al. 1979). These cells have been maintained in primary culture and studied with respect to phospholipid synthesis (BATENBURG et al. 1978; MASON and DOBBS 1980; POST et al. 1980a, b; BATENBURG et al. 1981). They have been shown to secrete surfactant-associated phospholipid in response to a calcium ionophore and to β-adrenergic agonists (DOBBS and MASON 1978, 1979). Response to the latter agent, however, was only observed after the procedure was modified to replace trypsin with elastase, perhaps reflecting trypsin damage to β-adrenergic receptors (DOBBS and MASON 1979). GEPPERT et al. (1980) showed that cells isolated by this technique maintained better structural preservation if cultured on floating collagen membranes, as opposed to standard plastic tissue culture flasks.

While these methods resulted in large populations of cells which could be studied shortly after isolation, the cells isolated by these techniques show no ability to divide. In contrast, type II cells have been clonally isolated, a method totally dependent upon extensive growth. DOUGLAS and KAIGHN (1974) dispersed adult rat lung tissue into individual cells enzymatically and plated the cells at low cell density in Petri dishes. Once individual cells had grown into small, delimited populations, these populations were isolated from the remaining cells by encircling them with a glass cloning cylinder coated with silicone grease. Clones could then be individually trypsinized and subcultured. One of these (L2) was identified as type II in nature by ultrastructural techniques. These cells retain specific biochemical and morphological characteristics for many passages (DOUGLAS et al. 1976), although dedifferentiation occurs eventually (SCHMIDT-SOMMERFELD and BORER 1979). These cells have been studied for thyroid hormone binding sites (WILSON et al. 1979), for prostaglandin production (TAYLOR et al. 1979), and have been shown to possess aryl hydrocarbon hydroxylase activity (TEEL and DOUGLAS 1980). TANSWELL and SMITH (1980a) cloned type II cells from the human fetal lung. Unlike the cloning cylinder method, they used a multiple well approach, attempting to seed individual cells in single wells. They observed a dependence for growth of type II cells at such low cell densities upon fibroblasts or fibroblast-conditioned medium. These cells showed some morphological changes after 8–10 passages, but retained differentiated biochemical characteristics for at least 20 passages (TANSWELL and SMITH 1980a). These cells have been used to demonstrate that glucocorticoid effects on developing pulmonary epithelium are mediated by the mesenchyme (SMITH 1978, 1979), to study secreted glycosaminoglycans (SAHU et al. 1980), and to examine oxidant effects (TANSWELL and SMITH 1979). It has also been observed that serum from rabbits undergoing postpneumonectomy lung regeneration will stimulate the growth of these cells (B. T. SMITH et al. 1980).

Recently, SEVANIAN et al. (1981) have reported a method to isolate large numbers of rabbit fetal alveolar type II cells. The cells are grown on a Gelfoam sponge (Upjohn, Kalamazoo, Michigan) and type II cells reaggregate into spherical structures (DOUGLAS et al. 1976, see Sect. B. III. 2). After 5–7 days, when reaggregation had occurred, the Gelfoam was dissolved with collagenase and the spheres separated at unit gravity from the remaining single cells (primarily fibroblasts). The aggregates were transferred into culture flasks where they formed monolayers and showed some ability to divide. Interestingly, the biochemical composition of these cells was less differentiated than in the organotypic system or if they were recombined with fibroblasts (SEVANIAN et al. 1981). FINKELSTEIN et al. (1981) have recently presented a preliminary report indicating that alveolar type II cells can be isolated by laser flow cytometry using the fluorescent dye phosphine 3R (MASON et al. 1977).

Since alveolar type II cells isolated by these techniques either will not grow or show varying degrees of loss of phenotypic expression with continued growth, attempts have been made to culture various transformed cells which retain, to a variable degree, features of differentiated type II cells. Their transformed nature bestows upon them virtually unlimited growth potential (LIEBER et al. 1976; SMITH 1977).

One approach has been to use adenoma tissues induced in mouse lung with urethane. Mice are given four daily injections of urethane (1 mg/g) and 8 months later the lungs are removed and found to contain multiple adenomas with the morphological appearance of alveolar type II cells. The adenomas can be dissected and studied for short-term incubations in balanced salt solution or for longer terms in medium 199. They have been extensively used for studies of surfactant-associated phospholipid synthesis (WYKLE et al. 1977, 1980; VOELKER and SNYDER 1979).

LIEBER et al. (1976) isolated a continuous cell line (A549) from a human pulmonary carcinoma. The cells were found to have morphological and biochemical features of alveolar type II cells even after 1,000 cell generations in vitro. While there is some disagreement in the literature (MASON and WILLIAMS 1980), most workers have found that these cells have a phospholipid profile similar to that of untransformed type II cells (SMITH 1976; ROONEY et al. 1977; NARDONE and ANDREWS 1979). The cells have been used to study the synthesis and secretion of surfactant phospholipids (SMITH 1976; NARDONE and ANDREWS 1979) and to study regulation of these processes by cyclic AMP (NILES and MAKARSKI 1979).

9. Mesothelial Cells

JAURAND et al. (1981) have recently reported a technique to culture rat pleural mesothelial cells. Cells are isolated simply by scraping the parietal pleura and grown in NCTC 109 medium with 10% fetal bovine serum. The cells grew in monolayers with a morphology similar to cultured endothelial cells and could be subcultured for at least 18 passages. These cells should be especially useful for studying asbestos-induced changes (CHAMBERLAIN and BROWN 1978).

III. Isolated Cells in Heterogeneous Systems

1. Primary Mixed Monolayer Cultures

SMITH et al. (1974a) used primary mixed monolayer cultures of fetal rabbit lung. Cells identified in the cultures included fibroblasts, endothelial cells, and alveolar type II cells. Interestingly, the latter were invariably found growing on top of bundles of fibroblasts. Such cultures were used to study hormonal regulation of surfactant-associated phospholipid synthesis (presumably by the type II cell subpopulation) (SMITH et al. 1974a, 1975; SMITH and TORDAY 1974; TORDAY et al. 1975). More recently, it has been shown that the hormone responsiveness of fetal type II cells is dependent upon (indeed, mediated by) fetal lung fibroblasts (SMITH 1978). INDO and WILSON (1976) used similar cultures derived from fetal mouse lung to study epithelial–mesenchymal interactions in more detail.

2. Organotypic Cultures on Gelfoam

DOUGLAS and TEEL (1976) reported that monodisperse fetal rat lung cells would recombine in an organotypic fashion in vitro. Lung cells were dispersed with collagenase and trypsin, in the presence of chicken serum. They were then pelleted and the pellet incubated for 1 h at 37 °C. The cells were then inoculated at high density onto Gelfoam sponges, which provide a three-dimensional surface for reaggregation. After several days, the type II cells form spherical structures, whose polarity is indicated by their secretion of lamellar bodies into the interior of the spheres. Around the spheres and in the interstices of the Gelfoam were observed many fibroblasts. The biochemistry of these cells has been extensively studied (ENGLE et al. 1980), and similar cultures have been prepared from human fetal lungs (STRATTON et al. 1978; DOUGLAS et al. 1980). As already noted, SEVANIAN et al. (1981) have used this system as starting material for isolating type II cell monolayers.

3. Organotypic Cultures on Pigskin

YOSHIDA et al. (1980) have grown organotypic cultures on the dermal surface of sterile pigskin. Lung explants from near term fetal mice were placed on this surface which was suspended above a reservoir of medium, bathing the explants by wick action. Cells from the explants migrated into the pigskin and formed ductular structures with structural and enzymic markers of bronchial epithelium and, between the ductular structures were found cells with the features of alveolar type II cells.

IV. Organ Cultures

1. Parenchyma: Fetal Lung

Organ (explant) cultures have long been used in the study of the embryonic and fetal development of the lung. SOROKIN (1961) showed that the mammalian fetal lung would continue to mature in organ culture. Recently, such cultures have been used to study hormonal regulation of development in the fetal rat (ADAMSON and BOWDEN 1975; PYSHER et al. 1977) and human (EKELUND et al. 1975) lung, as well as to examine the synthesis of macromolecules (HUSSAIN et al. 1978), and the development of neuroepithelial bodies (SONSTEGARD et al. 1979). Perhaps the best-documented method for fetal lung organ culture is that reported by GROSS et al. (1978), in which 19-day fetal rat lungs were chopped into 0.6- to 1.0-mm cubes with a McIlwain tissue chopper (Brinkmann Instruments, Westbury, New York). Twenty such cubes were placed on a Metricel filter (Gelman Instruments, Ann Arbor, Michigan) over a 25-cm^2 stainless steel grid elevated 4 mm above the surface of a 35-mm tissue culture dish. The dish contained 5.5 ml culture medium, just enough to reach the undersurface of the grid and nourish the explants by capillary action through the filter. Acceptable results were obtained with serum free F-12 or MB 752/1 medium. The cultures were maintained at 37 °C and optimal results were obtained with a gas phase of 95% O_2/5% CO_2. Subsequently, the method has been modified whereby the explants are placed directly on the culture dish and, after 2 h to allow them to attach, the dishes are placed on a rocking platform cycling at 3c/min such that the explants are alternately exposed to medium and the gas phase (GROSS et al. 1979). Such cultures show excellent preservation of ultrastructure and biochemical function for up to 96 h (GROSS et al. 1978, 1979), but for longer periods require fetal bovine serum in the medium and, nevertheless, show some decrease in the size of airspaces. Such cultures have been extensively studied with respect to regulation of phospholipid production (GROSS et al. 1979, 1980a, b; GROSS and ROONEY 1977; MANISCALCO et al. 1979; ROONEY et al. 1980).

2. Parenchyma: Adult Lung

Adult lung has been particularly difficult to maintain in organ culture because airspaces collapse and normal structure and function are rapidly lost (DAVIS 1967; TROWELL 1959). An initial attempt to solve this problem was made by HACKNEY et al. (1967) who inflated rabbit lung with warm fluid agar. This not only provided structural support, but also allowed very thin sections to be made and cultured, allowing their microscopic study during culture. Nevertheless, the explants began to deteriorate after 5 days. GUERRERO et al. (1977) prepared similar cultures maintained in Rose chambers (as were those of HACKNEY et al. 1967), but provided a continuous flow of medium through the chamber and added a second chamber to serve as an air reservoir. The explants could be maintained for up to 1 month. MCATEER and HEGRE (1978) reported a similar continuous flow method using somewhat more complex equipment. The most successful method to date has been that of ROSE and YAJIMA (1977). A relatively simple medium (minimum essential medium) was used and supplemented with 9% fetal bovine serum. Lung fragments were placed on collagen-coated coverslips and covered with a sheet of cellulose (molecular weight cutoff 70,000). This unit was then placed in a Rose chamber equipped for continuous flow of medium from a nutrient medium reservoir. A total of 400 ml medium was used for 12 such chambers and circulated with a pulse pressure of 1–2 mmHg. The medium in the reservoir was replaced every 4–5 days. The cultures could be continuously monitored by phase contrast microscopy. Excellent preservation of structure was shown for 75 days, including continued ciliary activity and macrophage mobility (ROSE and YAJIMA 1977). For shorter-term studies, good results have been achieved with standard explants of human lung on Gelfoam sponges (Stoner 1980) and rat lung on stainless steel grids (Weinhold et al. 1979).

3. Airways

Airway organ cultures have been frequently studied, most often by the method of Trowell (1959). For example, Coles and Reid (1978) prepared 10×1-mm explants of human bronchial mucosa from surgical pneumonectomy specimens. These cultures have been used to study glycoconjugate secretion by incubation with labeled glucosamine. Recently, Coles and Reid (1981) have described a two-period incubation technique whereby secreted material can be studied under baseline and experimental conditions, each explant serving as its own control. Trump et al. (1980) have described a similar technique for the culture of human and bovine bronchi. Using an enriched medium (CMRL-1066 supplemented with cortisol, insulin, and 5% fetal bovine serum), explants could be maintained for as long as 1 year. Submerged cultures have also been used. For example, Marchok et al. (1975) cultured 2×6-mm explants from the tracheas of vitamin A-deficient rats in serum-free MB 752/1 medium in 5% CO_2 in air. The cultures were maintained for up to 3 weeks. Reversal of morphological and biochemical features of vitamin A deficiency was shown by in vitro exposure to retinyl acetate (Clark et al. 1980). Such treatment has also been shown to reverse the effects of asbestos on hamster trachea in vitro (Mossman et al. 1980). Williams and Gallagher (1978) described an improved method for the culture of porcine trachea. The airways were filled with warm agar and sectioned with a specially devised cutting apparatus into 0.5- to 1-mm tracheal rings. These were placed in Leighton tubes in minimum essential medium with 20% fetal bovine serum and 0.5% lactalbumin hydrolysate. The tubes were rotated at 12 r/h to provide alternate exposure to the medium and to the gas phase. The gas phase was not described, and was presumably air. With medium changes every 3–5 days, 0.5-mm-thick explants showed normal morphology after 3 months and normal ciliary motility. In contrast, 1-mm-thick rings showed ciliostasis after 2–3 weeks.

4. Pulmonary Vasculature

Methods for the organ culture of the pulmonary vasculature have not been described. However, B. Meyrick, P. Davies, and L. Reid (personal communication) have used lung slices from mature rats maintained in short-term (several hours) culture in minimum essential medium without added serum in a gas phase of 95% O_2/5% CO_2. By morphometric techniques, reactivity (vasoconstriction) of vessel segments at various levels of the pulmonary circulation has been demonstrated in response to epinephrine.

C. Summary and Future Directions

From the foregoing, it can be seen that explant cultures for the study of virtually every tissue component of the mammalian lung and cell cultures for the study of a large number of their component cells are already available. These systems can significantly enhance our understanding of pulmonary pathophysiology. It is critical, however, to match the system carefully to the hypothesis being tested.

References

Adamson IYR, Bowden DH (1975) Reaction of cultured adult and fetal lung to predniso-lone and thyroxine. Arch Pathol 99:80–85

Atkison PR, Bala RM (1981) Partial characterization of a mitogenic factor with somatomedin-like activity produced by culture WI-38 human fibroblasts. J Cell Physiol 107:317–327

Atkison PR, Weidman ER, Bhaumick B, Bala RM (1980) Release of somatomedin-like ac-tivity by cultured WI-38 human fibroblasts. Endocrinology 106:2006–2012

Batenburg JJ, Longmore WJ, VanGolde LMG (1978) The synthesis of phosphatidylcho-line by adult rat lung alveolar Type II epithelial cells in primary culture. Biochim Bio-phys Acta 529:160–170

Batenburg JJ, Post M, VanGolde LMG (1981) Synthesis of surfactant lipids: studies with Type II alveolar cells isolated from adult rabbit lung. Prog Respir Res 15:1–19

Beldekas JC, Smith B, Gerstenfeld LC, Sonenshein GE, Franzblau C (1981) Effects of es-tradiol on the biosynthesis of collagen in cultured bovine aortic smooth muscle cells. Biochemistry 20:2162–2167

Bowman CM, Harada RN, DeLong S, Vatter AE, Repine JE (1981) Hyperoxia damages endothelial cells in tissue culture. Pediatr Res 15:715 (Abstract)

Bradley KH, Kawanami O, Ferrans VJ, Crystal RG (1980) The fibroblast of human lung alveolar structures: A differentiated cell with a major role in lung structure and func-tion. Methods Cell Biol 21:37–64

Brody AR, Soler P, Basset F, Haschek WM, Witschi H (1981) Epithelial-mesenchymal as-sociations of cells in human pulmonary fibrosis and in BHT-oxygen induced fibrosis in mice. Exp Lung Res 2:207–220

Cantrell ET, Warr GA, Martin RR (1973) Induction of aryl hydrocarbon hydroxylase in alveolar macrophages by cigarette smoking. J Clin Invest 52:1881–1884

Castellot JJ, Karnovsky MJ, Spiegelman BM (1980) Potent stimulation of vascular endo-thelial cell growth by differentiated 3T3 adipocytes. Proc Natl Acad Sci USA 77:6007–6011

Chamberlain M, Brown RC (1978) The cytotoxic effects of asbestos and other mineral dust in tissue culture cell lines. Br J Exp Pathol 59:183–189

Chamley-Campbell J, Campbell GR, Ross R (1979) The smooth muscle cell in culture. Physiol Rev 59:1–61

Chand N, Altura BM (1981) Acetylcholine and bradykinin relax intrapulmonary arteries by acting on endothelial cells: Role in lung vascular diseases. Science 213:1376–1379

Clark JN, Klein-Szanto AJP, Stephenson KB, Marchok AC (1980) Reestablishment of a mucociliary epithelium in tracheal organ cultures exposed to retinyl acetate: a biochem-ical and morphometric study. Eur J Cell Biol 21:261–268

Clemmons DR, Underwood LE, VanWyk JJ (1981) Hormonal control of immunoreactive Somatomedin production by cultured human fibroblasts. J Clin Invest 67:10–19

Cole FS, Matthews WJ, Marino JT, Gash DJ, Colten HR (1980) Control of complement synthesis and secretion in bronchoalveolar and peritoneal macrophages. J Immunol 125:1120–1124

Coles SJ, Reid L (1978) Glycoprotein secretion in vitro by human airway: Normal and chronic bronchitis. Exp Mol Pathol 29:326–341

Coles SJ, Reid L (1981) Inhibition of glycoconjugate secretion by colchicine and cytochalasin B. Cell Tissue Res 214:107–118

Cox RH (1980) Differences in chemical content of pulmonary arteries from extralobar and intralobar sites. IRCS Med Sci 8:401–402

Cristofalo VJ, Wallace JM, Rosner BA (1979) Glucocorticoid enhancement of proliferative activity in WI38 cells. In: Sato GH, Ross R (eds) Hormones and cell culture, Cold Spring Harbor conferences on cell proliferation, vol 6. Cold Spring Harbor, pp 875–887

Crystal RG, Fulmer JD, Roberts WC, Moss ML, Line BR, Reynolds HY (1976) Idiopathic pulmonary fibrosis. Ann Intern Med 85:769–788

Cummiskey JM, Yu G, Krumpe PE, Wong S (1981) The effect of chronic hyperoxia on angiotensin converting enzyme activity in pulmonary artery endothelial cells in vitro. Clin Res 29:67 (abstract)

Danes BS (1980) In vitro epithelia and birth defects. Liss, New York

Davis GS, Moehring JM, Absher PM, Brody AR, Kelley J, Low RB, Green GM (1979) Isolation and characterization of fibroblasts obtained by pulmonary lavage of human subjects. In Vitro 15:612–623

Davis JMT (1967) The structure of guinea-pig lung maintained in organ culture. Br J Exp Pathol 48:371–378

Dickinson ES, Slakey LL (1980) Plasma-derived serum as a selective agent to obtain endothelial cell cultures from swine aorta. In Vitro 16:227–228

Diglio CA, Kikkawa Y (1977) The Type II epithelial cells of the lung. IV. Adaptation and behavior of isolated Type II cells in culture. Lab Invest 37:622–631

Dobbs LG, Mason RJ (1978) Stimulation of secretion of disaturated phosphatidylcholine from isolated alveolar Type II cells by 12-O-tetradecanoyl-13-phorbol acetate. Am Rev Respir Dis 118:705–713

Dobbs LG, Mason RJ (1979) Pulmonary alveolar Type II cells isolated from rats. Release of phosphatidylcholine in response to beta-adrenergic stimulation. J Clin Invest 63:378–387

Douglas WHJ, Kaighn ME (1974) Clonal isolation of differentiated rat lung cells. In Vitro 10:230–237

Douglas WHJ, Teel RW (1976) An organotypic in vitro model system for studying pulmonary surfactant production by Type II alveolar pneumonocytes. Am Rev Respir Dis 113:1723–1728

Douglas WHJ, DelVecchio P, Teel RW, Jones RM, Farrell PM (1976) Culture of Type II alveolar lung cells. In: Bouhuys A (ed) Lung cells in disease. North Holland Biomedical, New York, pp 53–68

Douglas WHJ, Sanders RL, Hitchcock KR (1980) Maintenance of human and rat pulmonary Type II cells in an organotypic culture system. Methods Cell Biol 21:79–94

Ekelund L, Arvidson G, Astedt B (1975) Cortisol-induced accumulation of phospholipids in organ culture of human fetal lung. Scand J Clin Lab Invest 35:419–423

Engle MJ, Sanders RL, Douglas WHJ (1980) Type II alveolar cells in organotypic culture. A model system for the study of surfactant synthesis. Biochim Biophys Acta 617:225–236

Eskin SG, Sybers HD, Lester JW, Navarro LT, Gotto AM, DeBakey ME (1981) Human smooth muscle cells cultured from atherosclerotic plaques and uninvolved vessel wall. In Vitro 17:713–718

Finkelstein JN, Mavis RD (1979) Biochemical evidence for internal proteolytic damage during isolation of type II alveolar epithelial cells. Lung 156:243–254

Finkelstein JN, Leary JF, Notter RH, Shapiro DL (1981) Isolation of alveolar Type II cells with a laser flow cytometer. Pediatr Res 15:719 (abstract)

Folkman J, Cotran RS (1976) Relation of vascular proliferation to tumour growth. Int Rev Exp Pathol 16:207–248

Folkman J, Haudenschild CC, Zetter BR (1979) Long-term culture of capillary endothelial cells. Proc Natl Acad Sci USA 76:5217–5221

Gajdusek C, DiCorleto P, Ross R, Schwartz SM (1980) An endothelial-derived growth factor. J Cell Biol 85:467–472

Geppert EF, Williams MC, Mason RJ (1980) Primary culture of rat alveolar Type II cells on floating collagen membranes. Exp Cell Res 128:363–374

Goldman WE, Baseman JB (1980a) Selective isolation and culture of a proliferating epithelial cell population from the hamster trachea. In Vitro 16:313–319

Goldman WE, Baseman JB (1980 b) Glycoprotein secretion by cultured hamster trachea epithelial cells: a model system for in vitro studies of mucus synthesis. In Vitro 16:320–329

Greenleaf RD, Mason RJ, Williams MC (1979) Isolation of alveolar Type II cells by centrifugal elutriation. In Vitro 15:673–684

Grobstein C (1954) Tissue interactions in the morphogenesis of mouse embryonic rudiments in vitro. In: Rudnick D (ed) Aspects of synthesis and order in growth. Princeton University Press, Princeton, pp 233–267

Grobstein C (1967) Mechanisms of organogenetic tissue interaction. Natl Cancer Inst Monogr 26:279–299

Gross I, Rooney SA (1977) Aminophylline stimulates the incorporation of choline into phospholipid in explants of fetal rat lung in organ culture. Biochim Biophys Acta 488:263–269

Gross I, Walker Smith GJ, Maniscalco WM, Czajka MR, Wilson CM, Rooney SA (1978) An organ culture model for study of biochemical development of fetal rat lung. J Appl Physiol 45:355–362

Gross I, Wilson CM, Ingleson LD, Brehier A, Rooney SA (1979) The influence of hormones on the biochemical development of fetal rat lung in organ culture. I. Estrogen. Biochim Biophys Acta 575:375–383

Gross I, Walker Smith GJ, Wilson CM, Maniscalco WM, Ingelson LD, Brehier A, Rooney SA (1980 a) The influence of hormones on the biochemical development of fetal rat lung in organ culture. II. Insulin. Pediatr Res 14:834–838

Gross I, Wilson CM, Ingelson LD, Brehier A, Rooney SA (1980 b) Fetal lung in organ culture. III. Comparison of dexamethasone, thyroxine, and methylxanthines. J Appl Physiol 48:872–877

Guerrero RR, Rounds DE, Booher J (1977) An improved organ culture method for adult mammalian lung. In Vitro 13:517–523

Habliston DL, Whitaker C, Hart MA, Ryan US, Ryan JW (1979) Isolation and culture of endothelial cells from the lungs of small animals. Am Rev Respir Dis 119:853–868

Hackney JD, Bils RF, Takahashi Y, Rounds DE, Collier CR (1967) Organotypic culture of mammalian lung. Studies on morphology, ultrastructure, and surfactant. Am Rev Respir Dis 95:871–872

Ham RG (1980) Dermal fibroblasts. Methods Cell Biol 21:255–276

Harris CC, Hsu IC, Stoner GD, Trump BF, Selkirk JK (1978) Human pulmonary alveolar macrophages metabolise benzo[a]pyrene to proximate and ultimate mutagens. Nature 272:633–634

Harris JO, Swenson EW, Johnson JE (1970) Human alveolar macrophages: comparison of phagocytic ability, glucose utilization, and ultrastructure in smokers and non-smokers. J Clin Invest 49:2086–2096

Hayflick L (1965) The limited in vitro lifespan of human diploid cell strains. Exp Cell Res 37:614–636

Hayflick L, Moorhead PS (1961) The serial cultivation of human diploid cell strains. Exp Cell Res 25:585–621

Hunninghake GW, Gadek JE, Szapiel SV, Strumpf IJ, Kawanami O, Ferrans VJ, Keogh BA, Crystal RG (1980) The human alveolar macrophage. Methods Cell Biol 21:95–112

Hussain MZ, Belton JC, Bhatnagar RS (1978) Macromolecular synthesis in organ cultures of neonatal rat lung. In Vitro 14:740–745

Indo K, Wilson RB (1976) Cell interactions between epithelial and mesenchymal components in primary sheets of fetal rat lung cells, and the effects of 3-methylcholanthrene treatment. JNCI 57:1333–1339

Jaffe EA, Nachman RL, Becker CG, Minick CR (1973) Culture of human endothelial cells derived from umbilical veins. Identification by morphologic and immunologic criteria. J Clin Invest 52:2745–2756

Jaurand MC, Bernaudin JF, Renier A, Kaplan H, Bignon J (1981) Rat pleural mesothelial cells in culture. In Vitro 17:98–106

Johnson AR (1980) Human pulmonary endothelial cells in culture. Activities of cells from arteries and cells from veins. J Clin Invest 65:841–850

Kikkawa Y, Yoneda K (1974) The Type II epithelial cell of the lung. I. Method of isolation. Lab Invest 30:76–84

Leffingwell CM, Low RB (1975) Protein biosynthesis by the pulmonary alveolar macrophage. Am Rev Respir Dis 112:349–359

Lieber M, Smith BT, Szakal A, Nelson-Rees W, Todaro G (1976) A continuous tumour-cell line from a human lung carcinoma with properties of Type II alveolar epithelial cells. Int J Cancer 17:62–70

Lin HS, Kuhn C, Kuo TT (1975) Clonal growth of hamster free alveolar cells in soft agar. J Exp Med 142:877–886

Maniscalco WM, Wilson CM, Gross I (1979) Influence of aminophylline and cyclic AMP on glycogen metabolism in fetal rat lung in organ culture. Pediatr Res 13:1319–1322

Marchok AC, Cone MV, Nettesheim P (1975) Induction of squamous metaplasia and hypersecretory activity in tracheal organ cultures. Lab Invest 33:451–460

Mason RJ, Dobbs LG (1980) Synthesis of phosphatidylcholine and phosphatidylglycerol by alveolar Type II cells in primary culture. J Biol Chem 255:5101–5107

Mason RJ, Williams MC (1980) Phospholipid composition and ultrastructure of A549 cells and other cultured pulmonary epithelial cells of presumed Type II cell origin. Biochim Biophys Acta 617:36–50

Mason RJ, Williams MC, Greenleaf RD, Clements JA (1977) Isolation and properties of Type II alveolar cells from rat lung. Am Rev Respir Dis 115:1015–1026

McAteer JA, Hegre OD (1978) A continuous-flow method of organ culture. In Vitro 14:795–803

Meyrick B, Reid L (1979) Development of pulmonary arterial changes in rats fed Crotolaria spectabilis. Am J Pathol 94:37–50

Mossman BT, Craighead JE, MacPherson BV (1980) Asbestos-induced epithelial changes in organ cultures of hamster trachea: inhibition by retinyl methyl ether. Science 207:311–313

Nardone LL, Andrews SB (1979) Cell line A549 as a model of the Type II pneumocyte. Phospholipid biosynthesis from native and organometallic precursors. Biochim Biophys Acta 573:276–295

Naum Y (1975) Growth of pulmonary alveolar macrophages in vitro: responses to media conditioned by lung cell lines. Cytobios 14:211–216

Naum Y, Chang CM, Houck JC (1979) Pulmonary macrophage growth factor. Inflammation 3:253–260

Niles RM, Makarski JS (1979) Regulation of phosphatidylcholine metabolism by cyclic AMP in model alveolar Type II cell line. J Biol Chem 254:4324–4326

Parshley MS, Cerreta JM, Mandl I, Fierer JA, Turino GM (1979) Characteristics of a clone of endothelial cells derived from a line of normal adult rat lung cells. In Vitro 15:709–722

Picciano P, Rosenbaum RM (1978) The Type I alveolar lining cells of the mammalian lung. I. Isolation and enrichment from dissociated adult rabbit lung. Am J Pathol 90:99–122

Post M, Batenburg JJ, Schuurmans EAJM, VanGolde LMG (1980a) Phospholipid-transfer activity in Type II cells isolated from adult rat lung. Biochim Biophys Acta 620:317–321

Post M, Batenburg JJ, VanGolde LMG (1980b) Effects of cortisol and thyroxine on phosphatidylcholine and phosphatidylglycerol synthesis by adult rat lung alveolar Type II cells in primary culture. Biochim Biophys Acta 618:308–317

Pysher TJ, Konrad KD, Reed GB (1977) Effects of hydrocortisone and pilocarpine on fetal rat lung explants. Lab Invest 37:588–594

Reid LCM (1979) Cloning. Methods Enzymol 58:152–164

Reid L, Jones R (1979) Bronchial mucosal cells. Fed Proc 38:191–196

Rooney SA, Nardone LL, Shapiro DL, Motoyama EK, Gobran L, Zaehringer N (1977) The phospholipids of rabbit Type II alveolar epithelial cells: comparison with lung lavage, lung tissue, alveolar macrophages, and a human alveolar tumour line. Lipids 12:438–442

Rooney SA, Ingleson LD, Wilson CM, Gross I (1980) Insulin antagonism of dexamethasone-induced stimulation of cholinephosphate cytidylyltransferase in fetal rat lung in organ culture. Lung 158:151–155

Rose GG, Yajima T (1977) Fetal mouse lung in circumfusion system cultures. In Vitro 13:749–768

Rosenbaum RM, Picciano P (1978) The Type I alveolar lining cells of the mammalian lung. II. In vitro identification via the cell surface and ultrastructure of isolated cells from adult rabbit lung. Am J Pathol 90:123–144

Ross R (1971) The smooth muscle cell. II. Growth of smooth muscle in culture and formation of elastic fibers. J Cell Biol 50:172–186

Ryan JW, Chung A, Martin LC, Ryan US (1978a) New substrates for the radioassay of angiotensin converting enzyme of endothelial cells in culture. Tissue Cell 10:555–562

Ryan US, Clements E, Habliston D, Ryan JW (1978b) Isolation and culture of pulmonary artery endothelial cells. Tissue Cell 10:535–554

Ryan US, Mortara M, Whitaker C (1980a) Methods for microcarrier culture of bovine pulmonary artery endothelial cells avoiding the use of enzymes. Tissue Cell 12:619–635

Ryan US, Schultz DR, DelVecchio PJ, Ryan JW (1980b) Endothelial cells of bovine pulmonary artery lack receptors for C3b and for the Fc portion of immunoglobulin G. Science 208:748–749

Sahu SC, Tanswell AK, Lynn WS (1980) Isolation and characterization of glycosaminoglycans secreted by human foetal lung Type II pneumocytes in culture. J Cell Sci 42:183–188

Salcedo LL, Franzblau C (1981) Collagen synthesis and accumulation in long-term rabbit aortic smooth muscle cell cultures. In Vitro 17:114–120

Schmidt-Sommerfeld E, Borer RC (1979) Biochemical characterization of clonally isolated and continuously cultured Type II cells from adult rat lung. Am Rev Respir Dis 120:1145–1148

Schneider EL, Mitsui Y, Au KS, Shorr S (1977) Tissue-specific differences in cultured human diploid fibroblasts. Exp Cell Res 108:1–6

Sevanian A, Kaplan SA, Barrett CT (1981) Phospholipid synthesis in fetal lung organotypic cultures and isolated Type II pneumocytes. Biochim Biophys Acta 664:498–512

Simon LM, Robin ED, Phillips JR, Acevedo J, Apline SG, Theodore J (1977) Enzymatic basis for bioenergetic differences of alveolar versus peritoneal macrophages. J Clin Invest 59:443–448

Sjoberg I, Fransson L (1977) Synthesis of glycosaminoglycans by human embryonic lung fibroblasts. Biochem J 167:383–392

Smith BT (1976) A continuous tumour line with functions of the alveolar Type II cell. Clin Res 24:693 (abstract)

Smith BT (1977) Cell line A549. A model system for the study of alveolar Type II cell function. Am Rev Respir Dis 115:285–293

Smith BT (1978) Fibroblast-pneumonocyte factor: Intercellular mediator of glucocorticoid effect on fetal lung. In: Stern L, Oh W, Friis-Hansen B (eds) Neonatal intensive care, vol II. Masson, New York, pp 25–32

Smith BT (1979) Lung maturation in the fetal rat: acceleration by the injection of fibroblast-pneumonocyte factor. Science 204:1094–1095

Smith BT, Giroud CJP (1975) Effects of cortisol on serially propogated fibroblast cell cultures derived from the rabbit fetal lung and skin. Can J Physiol Pharmacol 53:1037–1041

Smith BT, Torday JS (1974) Factors affecting lecithin synthesis by fetal lung cells in culture. Pediatr Res 8:848–851

Smith BT, Torday JS, Giroud CJP (1974a) Evidence for different gestation dependent effects of cortisol on cultured fetal lung cells. J Clin Invest 53:1518–1526

Smith BT, Torday JS, Giroud CJP (1974b) The growth promoting effect of cortisol on human fetal lung cells. Steroids 22:515–524

Smith BT, Giroud CJP, Robert M, Avery ME (1975) Insulin antagonism of cortisol action on lecithin synthesis by cultured fetal lung cells. J Pediatr 87:953–955

Smith BT, Galaugher W, Thurlbeck WM (1980) Serum from pneumonectomized rabbits stimulates alveolar Type II cell proliferation in vitro. Am Rev Respir Dis 121:701–707

Smith FB, Kikkawa Y (1978) The Type II epithelial cells of the lung. III. Lecithin synthesis: a comparison with pulmonary macrophages. Lab Invest 38:45–51

Smith FB, Kikkawa Y (1979) The Type II epithelial cells of the lung. V. Synthesis of phosphatidylglycerol in isolated Type II cells and pulmonary alveolar macrophages. Lab Invest 40:172–177

Smith FB, Kikkawa Y, Diglio CA, Dalen RC (1980) The Type II epithelial cells of the lung. VI. Incorporation of 3H-choline and 3H-palmitate into lipids of cultured Type II cells. Lab Invest 42:296–301

Smith U, Ryan JW (1972) Substructural features of pulmonary endothelial caveolae. Tissue Cell 4:49–54

Soderland SC, Naum Y (1973) Growth of pulmonary alveolar macrophages in vitro. Nature 245:150–152

Sonstegard K, Wong V, Cutz E (1979) Neuro-epithelial bodies in organ cultures of fetal rabbit lungs. Ultrastructural characteristics and effects of drugs. Cell Tissue Res 199:159–170

Sorokin S (1961) A study of development in organ cultures of mammalian lungs. Dev Biol 3:60–83

Sporn MB, Todaro GJ (1980) Autocrine secretion and malignant transformation of cells. N Engl Med 303:878–880

Stoner GD (1980) Explant culture of human peripheral lung. Methods Cell Biol 21:65–77

Stoner GD, Harris CC, Myers GA, Trump BF, Connor RD (1980a) Putrescine stimulates growth of human bronchial epithelial cells in primary culture. In Vitro 16:399–406

Stoner GD, Katoh Y, Foidart J-M, Myers GA, Harris CC (1980b) Identification and culture of human bronchial epithelial cells. Methods Cell Biol 21:15–w35

Stoner GD, Katoh Y, Foidart JM, Trump BF, Steinert PM, Harris CC (1981) Cultured human bronchial epithelial cells: blood group antigens, keratin, collagens, and fibronectin. In Vitro 17:577–587

Stratton CJ, Douglas WHJ, McAteer JA (1978) The surfactant system of human fetal lung organotypic cultures: ultrastructural preservation by a lipid-carbohydrate retention method. Anat Rec 192:481–492

Tanswell AK, Smith BT (1979) Human fetal lung Type II pneumonocytes in monolayer cell culture: the influence of oxidant stress, cortisol environment, and soluble fibroblast factors. Pediatr Res 13:1097–1100

Tanswell AK, Smith BT (1980a) Cultured pulmonary epithelial cells: clonal isolation of human fetal alveolar type II cells. In: Danes BS (ed). In vitro epithelia and birth defects. Liss, New York, pp 249–259

Tanswell AK, Smith BT (1980b) Influence of oxygen tension and cortisol environment upon growth and cortisone conversion to cortisol by cultured human fetal lung fibroblasts. Biol Neonate 37:32–38

Taylor L, Polgar P, McAteer JA, Douglas WHJ (1979) Prostaglandin production by Type II alveolar epithelial cells. Biochim Biophys Acta 572:502–509

Teel RW, Douglas WHJ (1980) Aryl hydrocarbon hydroxylase activity in type II alveolar lung cells. Experientia 36:107

Torday JS, Smith BT, Giroud CJP (1975) The rabbit fetal lung as a glucocorticoid target tissue. Endocrinology 96:1462–1467

Trowell OA (1959) The culture of mature organs in a synthetic medium. Exp Cell Res 16:118–136

Trump BF, Resau J, Barrett LA (1980) Methods of organ culture for human bronchus. Methods Cell Biol 21:1–14

Tucker SB, Pierre RV, Jordon RE (1977) Rapid identification of monocytes in a mixed mononuclear cell preparation. J Immunol Methods 14:267–269

Vane JR (1969) The release and fate of vasoactive hormones in the circulation. Br J Pharmacol 35:209–242

VanFurth R (1970) The origin and turnover of promonocytes, monocytes and macrophages in mice. In: VanFurth R (ed) Mononuclear phagocytes. Blackwell, Oxford, pp
151–172
Voelker DR, Snyder F (1979) Subcellular site and mechanism of synthesis of disaturated
phosphatidylcholine in alveolar Type II cell adenomas. J Biol Chem 254:8628–8633
Weinhold PA, Burkel WE, Fischer TV, Kahn RH (1979) Adult rat lung in organ culture:
maintenance of histotypic structure and ability to synthesize phospholipid. In Vitro
15:1023–1031
Wessels NK (1970) Mammalian lung development: interactions in formation and morpho-
genesis of tracheal buds. J Exp Zool 175:455–460
Williams PP, Gallagher JE (1978) Preparation and long-term culture of porcine tracheal
and lung organ cultures by alternate exposure to gaseous and liquid medium phase. In
Vitro 14:686–696
Wilson M, Hitchcock KR, Douglas WHJ, Delellis RA (1979) Hormones and the lung. II.
Immunohistochemical localization of thyroid hormone binding in Type II pulmonary
epithelial cells clonally-derived from adult rat lung. Anat Rec 195:611–620
Witschi H (1976) Proliferation of Type II alveolar cells: a review of common responses in
toxic lung injury. Toxicology 5:267–289
Wykle RL, Malone B, Snyder F (1977) Biosynthesis of dipalmitoyl-sn-glycero-3-phos-
phocholine by adenoma alveolar Type II cells. Arch Biochem Biophys 181:249–256
Wykle RL, Malone B, Blank ML, Snyder F (1980) Biosynthesis of pulmonary surfactant:
comparison of 1-palmitoyl-sn-glycero-3-phsphocholine and palmitate as precursors of
dipalmitoyl-sn-glycero-3-phosphocholine in adenoma alveolar Type II cells. Arch Biochem Biophys 199:526–537
Yoshida Y, Hilborn V, Hassett C, Melfi P, Byers MJ, Freeman AE (1980) Characterization
of mouse fetal lung cells cultured on a pigskin substrate. In Vitro 16:433–445

CHAPTER 8

Bronchoalveolar Lavage

J. D. Brain and Barbara D. Beck

A. Introduction

After filling all or part of the lungs with saline via the airways, the fluid can be withdrawn. The recovered saline contains both cells and molecules harvested from airway and alveolar lining fluids. Thus, bronchoalveolar lavage (BAL) is a way to biopsy the extensive surfaces of the respiratory tract. This is both an advantage and a limitation. Sampling problems, so often characteristic of light and electron microscopy, do not occur since all of the surface in a lobe or lung is sampled. The average response of the entire lung can easily be described. On the other hand, as with many pulmonary function tests such as FEV_1, there is little or no information regarding the particular area injured. One should also note that BAL is a convenient way to recover macrophages and other cells for further in vitro studies. Thus, BAL is often a first step to studies of in vitro phagocytosis, chemotaxis, or mediator release. As will be evident from the rest of this chapter, there is little doubt that BAL has joined the armamentarium of analytic techniques available to the inhalation toxicologist.

BAL was first performed in dogs by Winternitz and Smith (1919) in an attempt to prevent the development of pneumonia from instilled virulent pneumococci. Early reports of BAL in humans described its therapeutic use to remove excess secretions in chronic bronchitis (Vicente 1928) or alveolar proteinosis (Ramirez 1967). Studies in animals used BAL to remove radioactive materials, such as ^{144}Ce particles. These studies suggested that BAL could be used to treat humans accidentally exposed to radioactive aerosols (Silbaugh et al. 1975; Pfleger et al. 1972).

The use of lung lavage to recover macrophages was first described by Gersing and Schumacher (1955), and has been used extensively since (LaBelle and Brieger 1960, 1961; Myrvik et al. 1961). Brain and Frank (1968a, b, 1973) attempted to make the technique more sensitive and reproducible by utilizing multiple lung washings and by identifying and controlling factors influencing macrophage yields.

During the last decade, BAL has been used increasingly to assess lung injury. BAL has been employed to discriminate among toxic agents such as metal salts or mineral dusts (Henderson et al. 1979a, b; Beck et al. 1982a). Key issues in the application of BAL to inhalation toxicology are the specificity and sensitivity of the procedure. What is the smallest amount of dust that causes a measurable response? More important, what is the ability of BAL to discriminate among dusts of varying toxicities and different resulting lesions? To what extent does

BAL have predictive value? Can one examine acute events and describe long-term irreversible chronic changes?

BAL has been used to diagnose disease and monitor the effectiveness of therapy in individuals with suspected interstitial lung disease (Hunninghake et al. 1979). BAL has also been useful in the study of disease mechanisms. The role of polymorphonuclear neutrophils (PMNs) in toxic lung injury (Shasby et al. 1981) has been explored. Thus, BAL has emerged as a useful tool in inhalation toxicology and an important complement to histopathologic analysis and pulmonary function in both animal and human studies.

In this chapter, we evaluate the use of BAL as a technique for evaluating the responses to inhaled particles and gases. We discuss methodological issues as well as specific cellular and biochemical parameters and their relevance to lung injury. We describe to what extent BAL discriminates among toxic agents and how it helps identify specific types of pulmonary lesions. The use of BAL to elucidate mechanisms of lung injury will also be considered.

B. Techniques of Lung Lavage

BAL is initiated by cannulating the trachea or by inserting a catheter through the trachea and wedging it in a bronchus. After instilling a wash solution, the lavage fluid is withdrawn by negative pressure. Excised lungs, whole lungs in situ, or parts of lungs in situ, can be lavaged. The lavage procedure for excised lungs is as follows: after dissecting the lungs free of other tissues, the trachea is cannulated with polyethylene tubing. Repeated (six or more) lavages with saline are recommended. Each wash takes approximately 1 min. During the washing procedure, the excised lungs are suspended in physiologic saline to eliminate hydrostatic gradients which might lead to uneven filling (Brain and Frank 1968a, 1973).

More frequently, lungs are washed in situ since the possibility of causing leaks in the lungs is thereby reduced. Following exsanguination, the neck is opened and the trachea cannulated. The chest wall or diaphragm should be opened to allow the lungs to empty themselves of as much air as possible. Washes are then carried out as described. The wash solution can be a balanced salt solution (Hook 1978; Myrvik et al. 1961) or physiologic saline (Brain and Corkery 1977; Henderson et al. 1979a, b; Low et al. 1978). The elimination of divalent cations (Ca^{2+} and Mg^{2+}), from the wash solution will result in a much greater yield of free cells from alveolar surfaces (Brain and Frank 1973; Morgan et al. 1980). Wash volumes in small animals are usually about 5 ml per gram lung (Brain 1971). Since the wash volume in these cases is large, all of the lung is washed uniformly.

Lungs of living animals may also be lavaged. This is convenient in large animals such as calves or dogs, although even small animals can be lavaged in vivo (Mauderly 1977). Following topical anesthesia of the upper airways, a cuffed endotracheal tube is introduced through the larynx and placed in the left or right bronchus or even in smaller airways. The cuff is then inflated to create a tight seal. The lung is freed of gas, if desired, by ventilating the lung with pure oxygen for 15–20 min, producing a low lung volume by making the airway pressures negative (approximately -5 cm H_2O) and then occluding the airway. After a few minutes, the remaining oxygen will be absorbed. It is possible to lavage a lobe or lung without removing the gas, and so frequently this step is eliminated. The intubated lung or lobe may then be lavaged while the remaining parenchyma meets the ventilatory demands of the animal. Recoveries of injected saline may be lower in animals possessing considerable collateral ventilation (i. e., dog). Instilled saline not recovered will be absorbed into the capillaries. Animals will tolerate the procedure better if the left lung or individual lobes are lavaged, since the right lung comprises about 60% of the total lung tissue.

Smaller subdivisions of the lung may be lavaged by using smaller caliber endotracheal tubes; tubes without inflatable cuffs may be simply wedged in an appropriately sized airway. Since only a small percentage of the total alveoli are washed, if injury or disease is nonuniformly distributed in the lungs, then BAL of different lung segments can yield different results.

Similar procedures have been used to lavage lungs in human subjects and also to remove unwanted cells and secretions from small airways and parenchyma. With the advent of flexible fiberoptic bronchoscopy (SACKNER 1975), access to the lower respiratory tract has become relatively easy and nontraumatic. Segmental lobes can be lavaged to obtain cytopathologic material and bacteriologic specimens. Typically, a fiberoptic bronchoscope is introduced following premedication with atropine, meperidine, or diazepam, and topical anesthesia of the respiratory tract with a 2% lidocaine spray. Sterile saline can then be instilled and recovered through a bronchoscope placed in a pulmonary segment. The lavage procedure may be repeated several times. BAL in humans generally uses volumes ranging from 100 to 1,000 ml (Low et al. 1978; REYNOLDS et al. 1977; BURNS et al. 1983). Depending on wash number, recovery of wash volume can be as low as 28% (MERRILL et al. 1982; DAVIES et al. 1982).

To obtain quantitatively consistent recoveries of macrophages, it is necessary to control all aspects of the harvesting procedure. BRAIN and FRANK (1968a) examined the effects of freeing the lungs of gas, of the length of the postmortem delay time, wash volume, leakage, pathologic changes, and of the number of washes. Another paper reported the effects of age, sex, lung weight, and body weight on the number of free cells recovered (BRAIN and FRANK 1968b). Additional observations (BRAIN and FRANK 1973) dealt with the effects of divalent cations, wash osmolarity and temperature, and duration of the washing cycle. Mechanical factors are also involved in the recovery of free cells from the alveolar surface and airways. Massage of the excised lungs or of the chest wall when the lungs are washed in situ increases macrophage recovery.

Of major importance in both animal and human studies is the number of washes which usually range from 2 to 12. Washout patterns of cells and molecules (expressed as a percentage of total recovered in each individual wash) usually differ from dilution models in which the contents are completely mixed with the initial lavage solution and then partially removed and diluted by subsequent lavages. There are fewer alveolar macrophages recovered in the first wash than in subsequent washes in humans and rodents (DAVIS et al. 1982; BECK et al. 1982a; BRAIN 1970) owing to cell adhesiveness and the need to remove divalent cations from alveolar surfaces (BRAIN and FRANK 1973). The lysosomal enzyme, β-N-acetylglucosaminidase (BECK et al. 1982a; SKOZA et al. 1983) and ascorbic acid (SKOZA et al. 1983) yield a washout pattern in rodents that resembles a dilution model. This indicates that these molecules are more easily removed from alveolar surfaces. In contrast, the washout pattern of potassium and carbohydrate in humans is delayed (Davis et al. 1982), suggesting that these molecules reside in a different compartment from ascorbic acid and glucosaminidase or that they are more tightly adsorbed to alveolar components. Washout patterns are also affected by lung injury; for example, albumin is washed out of the lung more readily from quartz-treated hamsters than from control hamsters (Beck et al. 1982a). This suggests that injury alters the fraction of albumin present in different compartments. Washout patterns may also reflect differences in anatomic location. In humans, IgA, an immunoglobulin produced by the airway epithelium, washes out more rapidly than IgG, which is present both in the airway epithelium and in the alveoli (Merrill et al. 1982). Analysis of washout patterns may help determine the source of cells and molecules recovered by lung lavage.

One can follow the time course of injury or disease progression by repeating the lavage procedure at periodic therapeutic intervals. BAL has been done serially in humans (Strumpf et al. 1981), dogs (Fahey et al. 1982), primates (Cohen and Batra 1980), and sheep (Begin et al. 1981a). The use of serial BAL in a single individual can help delineate changes caused by continued exposure to particles or gases, disease progression, or the use of therapeutic interventions. The BAL procedure is not without consequences. In dogs (Cohen and Batra 1980) and hamsters (Henderson et al. 1979b), BAL elicits increased PMNs in the lungs. BAL also stimulates phospholipid synthesis in hamsters (Henderson and Hackett 1978). In sheep and humans, BAL produces a transient hypoxemia (Begin et al. 1981a; Burns et al. 1983). However, these effects are relatively minor and short-lived. Furthermore, controlling the temperature of the wash fluid and using supplemental oxygen during the procedure (Burns et al. 1983) can reduce these effects.

C. Composition of BAL

I. Cells

1. Macrophages

BAL represents the main technique for obtaining alveolar macrophages. These cells are important since their migratory patterns and phagocytic behavior are pivotal events affecting the outcome of the interaction between injurious particles from the environment and a responding host. Macrophages also influence the length of time inhaled toxic and carcinogenic particles are retained in the respiratory tract. Thus, macrophages influence the dose to sensitive sites. The number and activity of macrophages and the speed of in situ phagocytosis influence the extent of particle penetration and retention since noningested particles have a greater probability of breaching epithelial barriers. These large phagocytic cells are also the primary defenders of the lungs against bacteria and other microorganisms (Brain et al. 1978; Hocking and Golde 1979a, b; Green et al. 1977) and help maintain the sterility of the lung. They regulate the proliferative response of lymphocytes (Pennline and Herscowitz 1981) and secrete chemotactic factors for PMNs and other phagocytic cells (Gadek et al. 1980; Lugano et al. 1982;

NATHAN et al. 1980; LEJEUNE and VERCAMMEN-GRANDJEAN 1979). Pulmonary macrophages release lysosomal hydrolases, and secrete inflammatory mediators such as leukotrienes and prostaglandins (O'FLAHERTY 1982; GOETZL 1980). BRAIN (1984) provides a discussion of the function of pulmonary macrophages and their participation in pathogenesis.

Variation in macrophage numbers and function can reflect lung injury and may be relevant to pathogenesis. A reduction in macrophage numbers or in macrophage phagocytic ability may increase the integrated dose of toxic particles and enhance susceptibility to infection (KIM et al. 1976; GARDNER and GRAHAM 1977). Increases in macrophage numbers may also have negative consequences by increasing the burden of active oxygen species, proteases, or fibrogenesis-stimulating factors (HOCKING and GOLDE 1979 a, b; REISER and LAST 1979; ALLISON 1977).

2. PMNs

PMNs usually represent less than 5% of the total cells in BAL from humans (HUNNINGHAKE et al. 1979) and animals (BECK et al. 1982 a, b). Following particle instillation, the number of PMNs can increase dramatically (BECK et al. 1982 a, b). The ability to mobilize PMNs to infected or injured sites is certainly of major importance in antimicrobial defenses and wound healing. However, the influx of PMNs in these circumstances may also have some adverse effects. Increased PMNs in extravascular compartments can increase vascular permeability (WEDMORE and WILLIAMS 1981); PMNs also release active oxygen species and neutral proteases (WEISSMAN et al. 1980), which play a role in some disorders such as adult respiratory distress syndrome (RINALDO and ROGERS 1982) and emphysema (SLOAN et al. 1981). The evidence from BAL studies implicating PMNs in disease processes is described in Sect. E.

3. Lymphocytes

Under normal conditions, lymphocytes represent less than 15% of the total cells recovered in BAL in most species, including humans (HUNNINGHAKE et al. 1979), guinea pig (DAUBER et al. 1982), and rat (THRALL et al. 1981). Increased lymphocyte numbers in BAL reflect immunologic alterations which may be involved in hypersensitivity reactions. For example, the increased antibody secretion by B-cells observed with primates immunized with nebulized antigen (KELLER et al. 1982) could result in immune complex deposition and subsequent activation of complement and infiltration of inflammatory cells (PEARSON et al. 1980). Increased helper T-lymphocytes observed in humans with sarcoid (KATZ et al. 1978) and in rats after bleomycin treatment (THRALL et al. 1981) could result in increased B-cell proliferation (HUNNINGHAKE et al. 1981). Lymphocytes may also participate in the release of fibrogenesis-stimulating factors (SPIELVOGEL et al. 1978; JOHNSON and ZIFF 1976), and macrophage-activating factors (FOWLES et al. 1973).

4. Red Blood Cells

Red blood cells are rarely present in BAL from normal humans or animals (BECK et al. 1982 a; HUNNINGHAKE et al. 1979). The presence of red blood cells recovered indicates rupture of capillaries and bleeding into alveolar spaces. Their presence is a reflection of hemorrhage and serious acute injury.

II. Small Molecules

Although most analyses of BAL have focused on cells and proteins, detection of small molecules can provide useful information. Ascorbic acid is present in BAL of normal rats, whereas glutathione is absent (Snyder et al. 1983). Ascorbic acid may play a role in protection against oxidants such as oxygen, ozone, or nitrogen dioxide. The presence of K^+ in BAL from humans can indicate cell damage or enhanced permeability of alveolar capillary membranes. It can also reflect lavage-induced injury (Davis et al. 1982). Cyclic AMP (Lemaire et al. 1981) and prosta-glandin E_2-like activity (Begin et al. 1981a) have been found in BAL of sheep. The significance of extracellular cyclic AMP is unclear since this molecule does not readily cross biologic membranes and thus may have little effect on other cells. Prostaglandin E_2 constricts intrapulmonary blood vessels (Kadowitz et al. 1981) and enhances vascular permeability (O'Flaherty 1982).

III. Macromolecules

1. Proteins

Many studies of lung injury have described changes in the quantity and type of protein in BAL. We now describe some frequently used protein indicators, their likely sources, and their relevance to disease.

a) Albumin

Albumin is primarily a serum protein whose presence in BAL is due to passage across endothelial and epithelial barriers. Albumin is usually the most abundant protein in BAL (Bell et al. 1981; Merrill et al. 1982). Elevated albumin levels indicate pulmonary edema, a common manifestation of acute pulmonary injury (Beck et al. 1982a, b; Chichester et al. 1981). Albumin levels are also used as a denominator for other serum proteins such as immunoglobulins or complement (Hunninghake et al. 1979; Low et al. 1978). This approach may not always be reliable since it assumes that other proteins diffuse across the air–blood barrier to the same extent as albumin in both normal and diseased states.

b) Immunoglobulins and Complement Proteins

Immunoglobulins, IgG and secretory IgA, are present in the BAL of humans (Rey-nolds and Newhall 1974; Merrill et al. 1980; Bell et al. 1981), rabbits (Stan-kus and Salvaggio 1981), and rats (Rylander et al. 1980). In normal conditions, IgG is derived mainly from serum (Hunninghake et al. 1979); IgA is mainly se-creted from cell in the airway epithelium. IgM is either absent (Low et al. 1978) or present at low levels (Bell et al. 1981) in BAL of humans under normal con-ditions. Its high molecular weight ($> 10^6$) limits its passage across the air–blood barrier. The paucity of IgM suggests relatively little local production. When pres-ent in human BAL during immediate hypersensitivity reactions, it probably comes from serum.

The complement proteins C3, C4, C5, and C6, have been described in BAL of humans and nonhuman primates (ROBERTSON et al. 1976; REYNOLDS and NEWBALL 1974; BELL et al. 1981; KOLB et al. 1981). Complement proteins may be derived from serum or synthesized locally by alveolar macrophages (NATHAN et al. 1980). Activated complement is a potent inflammatory mediator and critical in the recruitment of PMNs to the lung during bacterial infections in mice (LARSEN et al. 1982). It is also involved in alveolar macrophage recruitment in rats exposed to asbestos (WARHEIT et al. 1983).

c) Cytoplasmic Enzymes

The release of cytoplasmic enzymes into the extracellular supernatant of BAL has been used as a measure of cell damage and lysis. Lactate dehydrogenase (LD), which is involved in energy metabolism, has been assayed in BAL of hamsters (BECK et al. 1981, 1982a; HENDERSON et al. 1979a, b), rats (MOORES et al. 1981; ROTH 1981), and mice (FORKERT et al. 1982). Increased extracellular LD in BAL is a nonspecific measure of cell injury and death. However, LD isoenzyme patterns can help to discriminate among different types of injury and among different putative sources (BECK et al. 1983a; HENDERSON et al. 1978a). BECK et al. (1983) have evaluated a range of pneumotoxicants and observed that different agents produced different isoenzyme patterns. They also showed that different possible sources such as serum, type II cells, endothelial cells, macrophages, and PMNs had distinct LD patterns. They then were able to associate different toxicants with damage done to specific lung constituents.

Figure 1a presents graphically the percentage of each LD isoenzyme from serum or from lung lavage fluid of Syrian golden hamsters exposed to 100% O_2 for 96 h. The distribution of the five LD isoenzymes is similar and consistent with the hypothesis that oxygen toxicity caused damage to the air–blood barrier. Serum LD and other serum proteins leaked into alveolar spaces and were subsequently recovered by lavage.

In Fig. 1b, the LD pattern is shown for: (a) supernatant from BAL recovered from hamsters exposed to iron oxide aerosol; and (b) hamster peritoneal PMNs. The LD patterns shown in Fig. 1b are markedly different from those seen in Fig. 1a. For example, there is little LD1 ($< 3\%$), but a great deal of LD5 ($\sim 60\%$). The similarity in pattern suggests that the LD could be coming from PMNs. Macrophages have a similar LD composition, so they also may be a source.

Glucose-6-phosphate dehydrogenase (G6PD), glutathione reductase, and peroxidase have been measured in BAL of animals (HENDERSON 1979a, b; DENICOLA et al. 1981). These enzymes are elevated in lung homogenates in response to oxidant injury (WITSCHI 1977). Increases of these enzymes in BAL can be due to either: (a) increased leakage from damaged or dead cells; or (b) the similar leakage from cells where G6PD, peroxidase, and reductase levels are elevated.

d) Membrane Enzymes

Alkaline phosphatase, a plasma membrane-associated enzyme, can be found in BAL from rabbits (REASOR et al. 1978). Isoenzyme patterns demonstrate that it is lung derived, possibly from type II cells (DIAUGUSTINE 1974). Alkaline phosphatase could be a useful marker for type II cell injury, especially since it is present at much lower levels in alveolar macrophages.

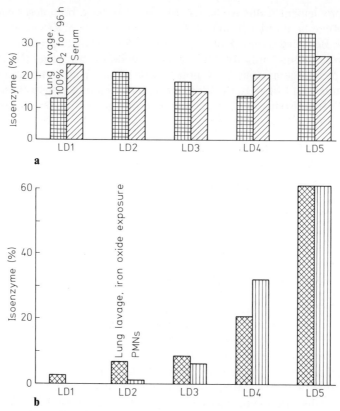

Fig. 1. a Comparison of LD isoenzyme patterns from hamster serum and from lung lavage fluid of hamsters exposed to 100% O_2 for 96 h. BECK et al. (1983 a) **b** Comparison of LD isoenzyme patterns from hamster peritoneal PMNs and from lung lavage fluid of hamsters exposed to 3.75 mg iron oxide per 100 g body weight. BECK et al. 1983 a)

e) Acid Hydrolases

Acid hydrolases are lysosomal enzymes that are released from cells during phagocytosis, cell injury, or cell death (WEISSMAN et al. 1980; NATHAN et al. 1980). PMNs (WEISSMAN et al. 1980), macrophages, and type II cells (HOOK 1978) all contain acid hydrolases. These enzymes facilitate microbial killing and digestion as well as degradation of damaged tissue during wound healing. Excessive release of these enzymes may elicit unwanted proteolysis from cathepsins or membrane destruction by phospholipases. Some of the commonly measured lysosomal hydrolases are β-N-acetylglucosaminidase, β-D-glucuronidase, and acid phosphatase.

f) Neutral Proteases

The balance between proteases and antiproteases in the lung is critical. Unchecked proteolytic activity may lead to the development of emphysema as shown in both human and animal models (SNIDER 1981, 1983; KARLINSKY and SNIDER 1978). Degradation of elastin by proteolytic enzymes is a key event in enlargement of alveolar spaces and loss of lung elasticity. Elastase has been assayed in BAL from hamsters (HENDERSON et al. 1978 b), rats (PADMANABHAN et al. 1982), and humans (JANOFF et al. 1983), as an indicator of increased proteolysis, and thus of an elevated risk of emphysema. Elastase is secreted by both PMNs (OHLSSON and OLSSON 1974) and macrophages (HINMAN et al. 1980), although levels are much higher in PMNs. Elastase in BAL in humans is derived from both macrophages and PMNs (JANOFF et al. 1983). Increased degradation of collagen by collagenase, may play a role in connective tissue turnover. Extracellular collagenase is found in BAL from humans with idiopathic pulmonary fibrosis (GADEK et al. 1979 a) and coal worker's pneumoconiosis (SABLONNIERE et al. 1983). It is important to remember that the protease in BAL may not accurately reflect protease levels in the pulmonary interstitium where susceptible connective tissue is found.

g) Antiproteases

Since uncontrolled degradation of pulmonary connective tissue would be detrimental, the lungs have developed an effective antiprotease system for protection (reviewed in SNIDER 1983). The main antiprotease in the lung is α-1-antiprotease (Pi) which is derived from serum. Local production by alveolar macrophages (WHITE et al. 1981) is another possible source. Reduced active α-1-antiprotease levels, which occur in genetically deficient individuals (ERIKSSON 1965) or in cigarette smokers (GADEK et al. 1979 b), are signs of increased risk for emphysema. α-2-Macroglobulin, another serum antiprotease, is either present at low levels or absent from human BAL (GADEK et al. 1981; Low et al. 1978). Its high molecular weight ($> 10^6$) limits its passage across the epithelium. However, α-2-macroglobulin can be synthesized by macrophages (WHITE et al. 1981). The slow release of active elastase from elastase–α-2-macroglobulin complexes in macrophages (WHITE et al. 1981) suggests that this antiprotease could play an important role in the modulation of elastin breakdown.

h) Extracellular Matrix Proteins and Related Substances

BAL has been employed in the study of events in the interstitium by quantitating proteins from the extracellular matrix. Procollagen peptide, a substance that is cleared extracellularly from newly formed collagen, is present in BAL in humans (Low et al. 1983); it may be a good marker for fibrogenesis. Another marker for collagen metabolism, elevated hydroxyproline levels, is found in rats exposed to hyperoxia (RILEY 1983). Fibronectin (FN) is a serum opsonin and a cell surface protein involved in cell adherence, synthesis of collagen in cell culture, and other functions (HYNES and YAMADA 1982). FN fragments are chemotactic for fibroblasts (POSTLETHWAITE et al. 1981), suggesting that FN degradation can modulate the fibrotic process. FN is found in BAL from humans (VILLIGER et al. 1981) and monkeys (SCHOENBERGER et al. 1982). The high molecular weight of fibronectin limits its passage across the alveolar epithelium. Thus, its presence in BAL implicates local synthesis as the major source. The study of connective tissue proteins and their fragments in BAL or other body fluids (blood and urine) may provide a useful way to monitor the progression of fibrosis or emphysema.

i) Angiotensin Converting Enzyme

Angiotensin converting enzyme (ACE) converts angiotensin I to angiotensin II, a potent vasopressor. Pulmonary endothelial cells are rich in ACE activity (ORDETTI and CUSHMAN 1982). Pulmonary macrophages also synthesize ACE (HINMAN et al. 1979). Increased ACE levels in BAL may reflect endothelial injury, for example, with hyperoxia (SHASBY et al. 1981). Increased ACE levels can also be due to increased macrophage numbers and activation of macrophages. This appears to be true in patients with sarcoid (HINMAN et al. 1979). Increased ACE levels relative to albumin in BAL imply increased local synthesis by macrophages as a major source of ACE.

2. Lipids

Lipids in BAL has been studied in many species, including humans (LOW et al. 1978), rats (MARTIN et al. 1983), rabbits (CASARETT-BRUCE et al. 1981), and hamsters (SELGRADE et al. 1981; HENDERSON and HACKETT 1978). Most of the lipid represents pulmonary surfactant derived from secretion by type II cells. Increased phospholipid in BAL has been observed in several diseases, including alveolar lipoproteinosis in humans (RAMIREZ 1967), silicosis in rats (MARTIN et al. 1983), and radiation injury in dogs (HENDERSON et al. 1978c). Changes in surfactant levels may be due to alterations either in synthesis or in removal from alveoli. Loss of surfactant is due to alveolar–bronchiolar transport, local recycling, or ingestion by macrophages. Alterations in the chemical nature of surfactant, e. g., changes in degree of saturation of phospholipids or increases in lysophosphatide levels, frequently alter its surface tension properties and could result in alveolar instability (AKINO and OHNO 1981).

3. Carbohydrate

Carbohydrate in BAL may be present as free carbohydrate or in the form of glycoproteins. Carbohydrate levels and types have not been extensively investigated (LOW et al. 1978). Carbohydrate is present in lung connective tissue, e. g., as glycosaminoglycans (RENNARD et al. 1982), in serum as glycoproteins (BELL et al. 1981), and in mucus as sialic acid (LAST 1982). Analysis of carbohydrate in BAL may provide some information about lung injury. For example, elevated sialic acid in BAL of H_2SO_4-exposed rats (HENDERSON et al. 1981) may reflect upper airway irritation and increased mucus synthesis.

D. Relationship Between BAL and Pulmonary Pathology

Many reported changes in the numbers and types of cells recovered in BAL can be correlated with similar alterations seen in human lung tissue obtained by biopsy. Correlations between BAL and biopsy include: increased PMNs and macrophages in smokers (DAVIS et al. 1982; REYNOLDS and NEWBALL 1974; NIEWOEHNER et al. 1974); increased lymphocytes in sarcoid (HUNNINGHAKE and CRYSTAL 1981); and increased PMNs in idiopathic pulmonary fibrosis (HUNNINGHAKE et al. 1981). Alveolar proteinosis is characterized by increased lipoproteinaceous material both in BAL and in anatomic specimens (RAMIREZ-R 1967).

Experimental models of injury in animals have also demonstrated a close relationship between BAL and histopathologic changes. The extent of lung injury produced by different metal salts in hamsters was consistent with variations in cellular and biochemical changes in BAL (HENDERSON et al. 1974a, b). Guinea pigs exposed to NO_2 exhibited extensive edema consistent with increased protein levels in BAL (HENDERSON et al. 1981). Increased PMNs and macrophages in bleomycin-treated rats were observed both in BAL and in preparations of teased cell populations (KAELIN et al. 1983). Similar increases in PMNs and macrophages were observed in BAL and in lung sections of silica-exposed guinea pigs (LUGANO et al. 1982). However, discrepancies may occur. Highly localized injury may not be reflected in BAL, since the number of normal alveoli sampled may be many times larger than the number of injured alveoli. Differences may also occur between the time course of changes in BAL versus the time course of anatomic changes. For example, increased levels of enzymes in BAL caused by exposure of hamsters to cadmium occurred before similar increases seen in whole lung homogenates (HENDERSON et al. 1979a).

BAL may also inadequately reflect events taking place in the interstitium. Elastase-treated hamsters demonstrated elevated elastase levels in BAL shortly after treatment, but these levels declined rapidly at a time when extensive connective tissue remodelling was still occurring (STONE et al. 1977). Perhaps elastase was rapidly inactivated or cleared from the lungs after instillation. Alternatively, active elastase still present in the connective tissue may not be available to the lavage procedure.

E. The Use of BAL as a Bioassay Tool

Cytologic and biochemical changes in BAL can be used to evaluate the responses to inhaled aerosols and gases. Assays utilizing lavage can provide estimates of relative toxicity. They can also be used to characterize the lesions produced by a specific agent, to determine the role of modifying factors, and to evaluate the progression of disease.

Henderson and coworkers have quantitated cell populations and the extracellular levels of cytoplasmic and lysosomal enzymes in the BAL of hamsters exposed to metal salts of varying toxicities such as $CdCl_2$ and $CrCl_2$ (HENDERSON et al. 1979a, b) as well as to NO_2 (HENDERSON et al. 1981). LD, β-glucuronidase, and PMN numbers were useful measures of metal toxicity. Metals of high, moderate, and low toxicity could be distinguished. The parameters most elevated after NO_2 exposure were PMN numbers and the quantity of sialic acid, possibly from serum glycoproteins. The different pattern of biochemical and cytologic changes after metal salts as compared with NO_2 probably reflects the different histopathologic alterations produced by the two classes of agents. Cadmium salts produced a diffuse interstitial pneumonia, whereas NO_2 caused a multifocal terminal bronchiolitis. Changes in the composition of BAL following $CdCl_2$ treatment have also been studied in rats. Elevations in elastase (PADMANABHAN et al. 1982), lysyloxidase (an enzyme involved in collagen cross-linking; CHICHESTER et al. 1981) and PMN numbers (PADMANABHAN et al. 1982) were observed soon after $CdCl_2$ exposure. Responses to insoluble salts of Pb and Ni were studied by BINGHAM et al. (1972). The Ni-exposed animals had increased macrophage numbers and extensive tissue injury as demonstrated by histopathology. The Pb exposure caused a reduction in macrophage numbers, but no histopathologic evidence of injury was seen.

Increased phospholipids in BAL were observed in rabbits after exposure to nickel dust, but not after exposure to iron, cobalt, or chromium dust (Johansson et al. 1980; Casarett-Bruce et al. 1981). Ni increased lung weight whereas other dusts did not. This suggests that phospholipid levels in BAL might be correlated with toxicity. Increased phospholipids in BAL have also been observed with exposure to other toxic agents such as silica (Martin et al. 1983), asbestos (Tetley et al. 1977), and NO_2 (Selgrade et al. 1981). Decreased surfactant levels in BAL were observed after exposure of rats to gasoline vapors (LeMesurier et al. 1979) and to cigarette smoke (LeMesurier et al. 1981). The extent of the reduction in surfactant levels occurred before morphological evidence of injury, but was correlated with the eventual degeneration of type II cells.

Cellular and biochemical changes have been measured in BAL of hamsters after exposure to α-quartz, iron oxide, and aluminum oxide (Beck et al. 1982a). α-Quartz is a highly toxic, fibrogenic mineral dust, whereas aluminum oxide and iron oxide are both of low toxicity; 1 day after exposure, the levels of β-N-acetyl-glucosaminidase were significantly elevated by exposure to 0.75 and 3.75 mg doses of all three dusts (see Fig. 2). However, the response to α-quartz was greater than the response to the other two dusts, especially at the highest dose. α-Quartz

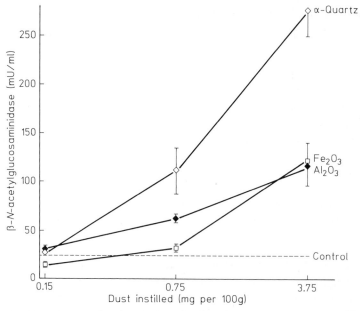

Fig. 2. Dose–response curve for β-N-acetylglucosaminidase. $P < 0.01$ for all points except 0.75 mg iron oxide and 0.15 mg aluminum oxide ($P < 0.05$) and 0.15 mg α-quartz (not significant). Beck et al. (1982a)

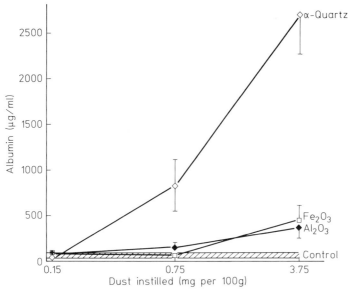

Fig. 3. Dose–response curve for albumin. $P < 0.01$ for all points except 0.75 mg aluminum oxide and all 0.15-mg samples (not significant). BECK et al. (1982a)

also elevated albumin levels in lavage fluid at both 0.75 and 3.75 mg doses as shown in Fig. 3. The highest dose caused a more than 40-fold increase above control levels. Aluminum oxide and iron oxide were also associated with an increase at 3.75 mg, but albumin levels distinguished between these relatively nontoxic dusts and the highly fibrogenic α-quartz.

Figure 4 illustrates that α-quartz also causes depressed macrophage function. The λ values shown are the fraction of radioactive gold colloid which was ingested 90 min after it had been instilled through the trachea. An essential aspect of bioassays like this is to compare the responses to dusts with other well-characterized standards. Both positive and negative controls should be used. The best calibrating materials would be those for which there is a considerable experience in humans. Then, the type and intensity of response for a new unknown dust could be compared with these standards.

Another feature of assays utilizing lung lavage is the time course of the response. Some agents will yield similar responses when examined soon after exposure. However, the more toxic material may frequently exhibit a more persistent elevation of cellular and enzymatic parameters than nontoxic controls. For example, there was a prolonged elevation in the numbers of macrophages and PMNs with quartz, but not with iron oxide. Figure 5 shows that PMN numbers in the lung lavage fluid were highest 4 days after exposure to α-quartz, although, after 2 weeks they still had not approached control levels. In contrast, PMN numbers in lung lavage fluid from iron oxide-exposed animals were highest 1 day after exposure; they subsequently declined, but were still higher than control values at 14 days.

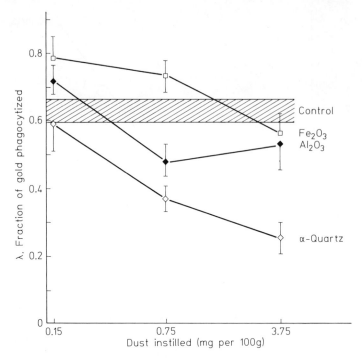

Fig. 4. Dose–response curve for λ assay 1 day after exposure to iron oxide, aluminum oxide, or α-quartz. The Wilcoxon rank sum test was used to compare experimental and saline only control subjects. $P < 0.01$ for 0.75 and 3.75 mg α-quartz, 0.75 mg aluminum oxide; $P < 0.05$ for 0.15 mg iron oxide. Beck et al. (1982a)

Figure 6 shows a somewhat different pattern for lactate dehydrogenase in lavage fluid. LD levels in lung lavage fluid were highest 1 day after exposure to both iron oxide and α-quartz. In time, LD levels declined significantly in the quartz-exposed animals and only slightly in the iron oxide-exposed animals. Nevertheless, the levels in the quartz-exposed animals remained higher than those in the iron oxide-exposed animals at all times. These effects were observed at relatively low levels of quartz compared with levels used in animal models of chronic silicosis.

Application of this system to dusts produced by the eruption of Mount St. Helens volcanic ash suggested that volcanic ash has low to moderate toxicity (Beck et al. 1981). It was concluded that adverse health effects in human populations are unlikely except with high or prolonged exposure. Surfactant levels in BAL in rats after quartz and Mount St. Helens volcanic ash exposure have been studied by Martin et al. (1983). Quartz causes a prolonged elevation in PMN numbers and surfactant levels. The effects were much less marked with volcanic ash than with quartz. These observations are consistent with histopathologic studies of lungs of exposed animals which demonstrated much greater fibrogenicity of α-quartz than of volcanic ash. These studies show the usefulness of BAL in providing a rapid evaluation of the toxicity of uncharacterized samples. Useful

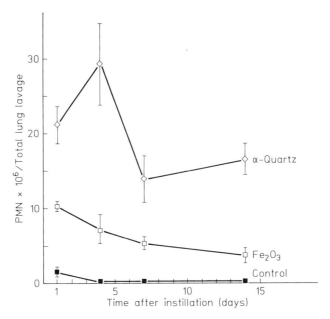

Fig. 5. Time course for PMNs. $P<0.01$ for 1 and 14 days α-quartz and 1 and 7 days iron oxide. $P<0.05$ for 4 and 7 days α-quartz and 14 days iron oxide. BECK et al. (1982a)

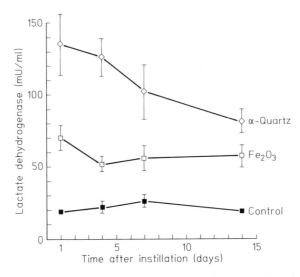

Fig. 6. Time course for LD in extracellular supernatant fraction of lung lavage fluid after exposure to 3.75 mg iron oxide or α-quartz per 100 g body weight. Student's t-test was used to compare experimental and saline only control subjects. $P<0.01$ for 1, 4, and 14 days α-quartz and for 1 day iron oxide; $P<0.05$ for 7 days α-quartz, and 4, 7, and 14 days iron oxide. BECK et al. (1982a)

results can be obtained even when chemical analyses and epidemiologic studies are not available or adequate for toxicity estimates.

BAL has been used in many other similar studies. The protein content of BAL from guinea pigs exposed to NO_2 (Selgrade et al. 1981) or ozone (Hu et al. 1982) has been studied in animals replete or deficient in vitamin C. Vitamin C deficiency enhances the toxicity of NO_2, but not O_3, suggesting different mechanisms of actions for the two oxidant gases. The elevation of protein in BAL is consistent with the presence of edema fluid observed histologically.

Extracellular LD levels in BAL of rats were elevated after exposure to a range of pulmonary toxicants including hyperoxia, monocrotaline, and paraquat (Roth 1981). LD is a more sensitive indicator of injury than total protein BAL. The hepatotoxin CCl_4 does not elevate LD in BAL which demonstrates the specificity of the technique for pulmonary effects. BAL provides a relatively simple tool for predicting toxicity and for studying mechanisms of injury. The development of more specific indicators such as connective tissue enzymes and LD isoenzymes, will permit more accurate estimates of toxicity, the identification of injured sites, and predictions of the types of lesions that may result.

F. BAL and Disease Progression

BAL has been used to follow the progression of disease in both animal models and in humans. As the natural history of respiratory disease is better understood, more accurate predictors of toxicity can be chosen. Changes in BAL from sheep given up to 15 monthly intratracheal instillations of asbestos have been described (Lemaire et al. 1981; Begin et al. 1981 a, b, 1983 a, b). These investigators were able to lavage the same animal sequentially and to obtain multiple biopsy samples. At 3 months, an increase in lymphocyte and macrophage numbers was seen (Begin et al. 1981 a, b). At 6 months, eosinophils and cyclic AMP levels in BAL were higher (Lemaire et al. 1981) than controls. At 12 months, serum proteins in BAL were elevated and the proliferative capacity of lymphocytes in BAL was lower (Begin et al. 1981 a, b). At 16 months, macrophages from asbestos-exposed sheep secreted more fibroblast-stimulating factor than control macrophages (Lemaire et al. 1983). Pulmonary function tests were normal until 12 months and abnormalities on chest X-rays consistent with fibrosis were not evident until 15 months after exposure (Begin et al. 1983 a). In sheep with fibrotic changes, an increased percentage of PMNs in BAL was observed (Begin et al. 1983 b). Macrophages and lymphocytes were more prominent during the initial stages of disease while PMNs contributed to later stages.

Changes in cell populations in BAL and their functions have been studied in guinea pigs exposed to quartz (Lugano et al. 1982; Dauber et al. 1982). Increased PMNs were observed shortly after quartz exposure; they remained elevated for up to 6 months. Shortly after exposure, macrophages isolated from BAL released factors that inhibited fibroblast proliferation. At 1.5 and 4 months, macrophages recovered from BAL released factors that stimulated fibroblast proliferation (Dauber et al. 1983). At these times, macrophages were also less adherent and motile than control macrophages (Dauber et al. 1982). These studies suggest that macrophage impairment may contribute to quartz-induced fibrosis.

Bleomycin is an anticancer drug with can cause pulmonary fibrosis in humans (CROOKE and BRADNER 1976), dogs (FAHEY et al. 1982), hamsters (SNIDER et al. 1978; TRYKA et al. 1982), rats (THRALL et al. 1979), and mice (ADAMSON and BOWDEN 1974). Increases in total macrophage, PMN, and lymphocyte numbers in BAL from dogs injected twice weekly with bleomycin were observed after 4 weeks of treatment, prior to the development of radiographic changes (FAHEY et al. 1982). Increased PMN numbers in BAL were observed up to 15 days after bleomycin treatment in hamsters (KAELIN et al. 1983; BECK et al. 1983b). A more transient increase in lymphocyte and macrophage numbers was also noted (KAELIN et al. 1983). In rats, PMN and lymphocyte numbers were higher for 14 days after exposure (THRALL et al. 1982). The percentage of T-cells in BAL was greater than that observed in blood or lymphoid tissue. There was also an increase in the relative contribution of suppressor T-cells (THRALL et al. 1982). In vitro lymphocytes secrete factors that stimulate collagen synthesis (JOHNSON and ZIFF 1976; SPIELVOGEL et al. 1978); lymphocytes could play a role in fibrogenesis. The significance of these early changes in BAL cell populations to pathogenesis is not clear. While PMNs do play a contributing role in oxygen toxicity (SHASBY et al. 1981), they may not produce similar effects with bleomycin. In fact, treatment of rats with anti-PMN serum results in increased collagen synthesis (THRALL et al. 1981), suggesting that PMNs may serve to reduce fibrogenesis with bleomycin. It has been reported that the increase in macrophage and PMNs in BAL was greater in hamsters treated with bleomycin than in hamsters treated with bleomycin followed by hyperoxia, a treatment which produced more extensive fibrosis over time than bleomycin alone (TRYKA et al. 1982; BECK et al. 1983b). It is clear from these studies and from those with silica and asbestos that macrophages and PMNs may have varied roles in different models of injury. Further characterization of the functional properties of these cells (e. g., release of fibrogenesis factors, degree of activation, extent of degranulation) will be useful in assessing how inflammatory cells influence the fibrogenic process.

G. BAL Assessments of Exposure to Toxic Agents

BAL can be used to assess past exposures to inhaled particles. The primary application of this approach has been in regard to asbestos fibers and asbestos bodies. Asbestos bodies in BAL are elevated in individuals with interstitial lung disease who have been exposed to asbestos when compared with unexposed individuals with lung diseases unrelated to asbestos exposure (DEVUYST et al. 1982; JAURAND et al. 1980). Asbestos bodies are also elevated, although to a lesser extent, in individuals with asbestos-induced pleural disease or malignant mesothelioma (DEVUYST et al. 1982). BAL is not a very sensitive technique for detecting occupational asbestos exposure since asbestos bodies are found in the lungs of almost all urban residents, even without evidence of occupational asbestos exposure (CHURG and WARNOCK 1977). The relationship among asbestos bodies in BAL, exposure levels, and time since last exposure must be further evaluated. The applicability of this approach to other exposures such as coal dust or silica should also be explored.

H. Conclusion

Experimental pathology has frequently advanced because of the addition of new diagnostic tools. During the last decade, BAL has emerged as a very useful tool in the assessment of lung injury. It is applicable both to animal models exposed to inhaled particles and gases in a laboratory and to humans encountering exposures to the same agents in occupational urban environments. Information can be gathered from BAL relating to the extent and type of lung injury, the magnitude of exposure, and the mechanisms involved in the responses seen. Needed are more extensive comparisons of injury as judged by other approaches with the results of BAL. It is also likely that other constituents of BAL can be quantified which will help make bioassays utilizing BAL more specific and sensitive.

References

Adamson IYR, Bowden DH (1974) The pathogenesis of bleomycin-induced pulmonary fibrosis in mice. Am J Pathol 77:185–198

Akino T, Ohno K (1981) Phospholipids of the lung in normal, toxic, and diseased states. CRC Crit Rev Toxicol 9:201–274

Allison AC (1977) Mechanism of macrophage damage in relation to the pathogenesis of some lung diseases. In: Brain JD, Proctor DF, Reid LM (eds) Respiratory defense mechanisms. Marcel Dekker, New York, pp 1075–1102

Beck BD, Brain JD, Bohannon DE (1981) The pulmonary toxicity of an ash sample from the Mt. St. Helens volcano. Exp Lung Res 2:289–301

Beck BD, Brain JD, Bohannon DE (1982a) An in vivo hamster bioassay to assess the toxicity of particulates for the lungs. Toxicol Appl Pharmacol 66:9–29

Beck BD, Brain JD, Bohannon DE (1982b) Are respirable combustion products from home heating stoves toxic to the lungs? Am Rev Respir Dis 125:156 (abstract)

Beck BD, Berson B, Feldman HA, Brain JD (1983a) Lactate dehydrogenase isoenzymes in hamster lung lavage fluid after lung injury. Toxicol Appl Pharmacol 71:59–71

Beck BD, Brain JD, Shera NS (1983b) Acute indicators of lung damage in hamsters exposed to bleomycin plus 70% O_2 or elastase. Am Rev Respir Dis 127:171 (abstract)

Begin R, Rola-Pleszczynski M, Sirois P, Masse S, Nadeau D, Bureau MA (1981a) Sequential analysis of the bronchoalveolar milieu in conscious sheep. J Appl Physiol 50:665–671

Begin R, Rola-Pleszczynski M, Sirois P, Lemaire I, Nadeau D, Bureau M-A, Masse S (1981b) Early lung events following low-dose asbestos exposure. Environ Res 26:392–401

Begin R, Rola-Pleszczynski M, Masse S, Lemaire I, Sirois P, Boctor M, Nadeau D, Drapeau G, Bureau MA (1983a) Asbestos-induced lung injury in the sheep model: the initial alveolitis. Environ Res 30:195–210

Begin R, Masse S, Rola-Pleszczynski M, Cantin A, Boileau R, Bisson G, Lamoureux G (1983b) Cellularity of lung biopsy and bronchoalveolar lavage in humans and sheep early asbestosis. Am Rev Respir Dis 127:168 (abstract)

Bell DY, Haseman JA, Spock A, McLennan G, Hook GER (1981) Plasma proteins of the bronchoalveolar surface of the lungs of smokers and nonsmokers. Am Rev Respir Dis 124:72–79

Bingham E, Barkley W, Zerwas M, Stemmer K, Taylor P (1972) Responses of alveolar macrophages to metals. Arch Environ Health 25:406–414

Brain JD (1970) Free cells in the lungs. Arch Intern Med 126:477–487

Brain JD (1971) The effects of increased particles on the number of alveolar macrophages. In: Walton WH (ed) Inhaled Particles III. Unwin Brothers, Old Woking, Surrey, pp 209–225

Brain JD (1985) Physiology and pathophysiology of pulmonary macrophages. In: Reichard SM, Filkins JP (eds) The reticuloendothelial system, vol 7B. Plenum, New York, pp 315–317

Brain JD, Corkery GC (1977) The effect of increased particles on the endocytosis of radiocolloids by pulmonary macrophages in vivo: Competitive and cytotoxic effects. In: Walton WH (ed) Inhaled particles IV. Pergamon, New York, pp 551–564

Brain JD, Frank NR (1968 a) Recovery of free cells from rat lungs by repeated washings. J Appl Physiol 25:63–69

Brain JD, Frank NR (1968 b) The relation of age to the numbers of lung free cells, lung weight, and body weight in rats. J Gerontol 23:58–62

Brain JD, Frank R (1973) Alveolar macrophage adhesion: wash electrolyte composition and free cell yield. J Appl Physiol 34:75–80

Brain JD, Golde DW, Green GM, Massaro DJ, Valberg PA, Ward PA, Werb Z (1978) Biologic potential of pulmonary macrophages. Am Rev Respir Dis 118:435–443

Burns DM, Shure D, Francoz R, Kalafer M, Harrell J, Witztum K, Moser KM (1983) The physiologic consequences of saline lobar lavage in healthy human adults. Am Rev Respir Dis 127:695–701

Casarett-Bruce M, Camner P, Curstedt T (1981) Changes in pulmonary lipid composition of rabbits exposed to nickel dust. Environ Res 26:353–362

Chichester CO, Palmer KC, Hayes JA, Kagan HM (1981) Lung lysyl oxidase and prolyl hydroxylase: Increases induced by cadmium chloride inhalation and the effect of beta-aminopropionitrile in rats. Am Rev Respir Dis 124:709–713

Churg A, Warnock M (1977) Correlation of quantitative asbestos body counts and occupation in urban patients. Arch Pathol Lab Med 101:629–634

Cohen AB, Batra GK (1980) Bronchoscopy and lung lavage induced bilateral pulmonary neutrophil influx and blood leukocytosis in dogs and monkeys. Am Rev Respir Dis 122:239–247

Crooke ST, Bradner WT (1976) Bleomycin, a review. J Med 7:333–428

Dauber JH, Rossman MD, Daniele RP (1982) Pulmonary fibrosis: Bronchoalveolar cell types and impaired function of alveolar macrophages in experimental silicosis. Environ Res 27:226–236

Dauber JH, Lugano EM, Jimenez SA, Daniele RP (1983) Regulation of lung fibroblast proliferation by alveolar macrophages in experimental silicosis. Am Rev Respir Dis 127:162 (abstract)

Davis GS, Giancola MS, Costanza MC, Low RB (1982) Analyses of sequential bronchoalveolar lavage samples from healthy human volunteers. Am Rev Respir Dis 126:611–616

Denicola DB, Rebar AH, Henderson RF (1981) Early damage indicators in the lung. V. Biochemical and cytological response to NO_2 inhalation. Toxicol Appl Pharmacol 60:301–312

De Vuyst P, Jedwab J, Dumortier P, Vandermoten G, Vande Weyer R, Yernault JC (1982) Asbestos bodies in bronchoalveolar lavage. Am Rev Respir Dis 126:972–976

Di Augustine RP (1974) Lung concentric laminar organelle. Hydrolase activity and compositional analysis. J Biol Chem 249:584–593

Eriksson S (1965) Studies in alpha-1 deficiency. Acta Med Scand 117 [Suppl 432]:1–85

Fahey PJ, Utell MJ, Mayewski RJ, Wandtke JD, Hyde RW (1982) Early diagnosis of bleomycin pulmonary toxicity using bronchoalveolar lavage in dogs. Am Rev Respir Dis 126:126–130

Forkert PG, Custer EM, Alpert AJ, Ansari GAS, Reynolds ES (1982) Lactate dehydrogenase activity in mouse lung following 1,1-dichloroethylene: Index of airway injury. Exp Lung Res 4:67–77

Fowles RE, Fajardo IM, Leibowitch JL, David JR (1973) The enhancement of macrophage bacteriostasis by products of activated lymphocytes. J Exp Med 138:952–964

Gadek JE, Kelman JA, Gells G, Weinberger SE, Horwitz AL, Reynolds HY, Fulmer JD, Crystal RG (1979 a) Collagenase in the lower respiratory tract of patients with idiopathic pulmonary fibrosis. N Engl J Med 301:737–742

Gadek JE, Fells GA, Crystal RG (1979 b) Cigarette smoking induces functional antiprotease deficiency in the lower respiratory tract of humans. Science 206:1315–1316

Gadek JE, Hunninghake GW, Zimmerman RL, Crystal RG (1980) Regulation of the release of alveolar macrophage-derived neutrophil chemotactic factor. Am Rev Respir Dis 121:723–733

Gadek JE, Fells GA, Zimmerman RL, Rennard SI, Crystal RG (1981) Antielastases of the human alveolar structures. Implications for the protease-antiprotease theory of emphysema. J Clin Invest 68:889–898

Gardner DE, Graham JA (1977) Increased pulmonary disease mediated through altered bacterial defenses. In: Sanders CL, Schneider RP, Dagle GE, Ragan HE (eds) Pulmonary macrophages and epithelial cells. Technical Information Center, Springfield, VA, pp 1–21

Gersing R, Schumacher H (1955) Experimentelle Untersuchungen über die Staubphagozytose. Beitr Silikoseforsch 25:31–34

Goetzl EJ (1980) Mediators of immediate hypersensitivity derived from arachidonic acid. N Engl J Med 303:822–825

Green GM, Jakab GJ, Low RB, Davis GS (1977) Defense mechanisms of the respiratory membrane. Am Rev Respir Dis 115:479–514

Henderson RF, Hackett NA (1978) Effect of pulmonary lavage on lung lecithin synthesis in the Syrian hamster. Biochem Med 20:98–106

Henderson RF, Damon EG, Henderson TR (1978 a) Early damage indicators in the lung. I. Lactate dehydrogenase activity in the airways. Toxicol Appl Pharmacol 44:291–297

Henderson RF, Rebar AH, Pickrell JA, Brownstein DG, Muhle H (1978 b) The use of pulmonary lavage fluid as an indicator of lung damage: Effect of species, age and method of lavage on baseline values. ITRI Annual Report 1977–1978, LF-60. National Technical Information Service, Springfield, VA, pp 339–345

Henderson RF, Muggenburg BA, Mauderly JL, Tuttle WA (1978 c) Early damage indicators in the lung. II. Time sequence of protein accumulation and lipid loss in the airways of beagle dogs with beta irradiation of the lung. Radiation Res 76:145–158

Henderson RF, Rebar AH, Pickrell JA, Newton GJ (1979 a) Early damage indicators in the lung. III. Biochemical and cytological response of the lung to inhaled metal salts. Toxicol Appl Pharmacol 50:123–136

Henderson RF, Rebar AH, Denicola DB (1979 b) Early damage indicators in the lung. IV. Biochemical and cytological response of the lung to lavage with metal salts. Toxicol Appl Pharmacol 51:129–135

Henderson RF, Gray RH, Hahn FF (1981) Acute inhalation toxicity of sulfuric acid mist in the presence and absence of respirable particles. Lovelace Inhalation Toxicology Research Institute, Annual Report, LMF-84. National Technical Information Service, Springfield, VA, pp 466–469

Hinman LJ, Stevens C, Matthay RA, Gee JBL (1980) Elastase and lysozyme activities in human alveolar macrophages. Am Rev Respir Dis 121:263–271

Hinman LM, Stevens C, Matthay RA, Gee JBL (1979) Angiotensin convertase activities in human alveolar macrophages: effects of cigarette smoking and sarcoidosis. Science 205:202–203

Hocking WG, Golde DW (1979 a) The pulmonary-alveolar macrophage, part 1. N Engl J Med 301:580–587

Hocking WG, Golde DW (1979 b) The pulmonary-alveolar macrophage, part 2. N Engl J Med 301:639–645

Hook GER (1978) Extracellular hydrolases of the lung. Biochemistry 17:520–528

Hu PC, Miller FJ, Daniels MJ, Hatch GE, Graham JA, Gardner DE, Selgrade MK (1982) Protein accumulation in lung lavage fluid following ozone exposure. Environ Res 29:377–388

Hunninghake GW, Crystal RG (1981) Mechanisms of hypergammaglobulinemia in pulmonary sarcoidosis: Site of increased antibody production and role of T-lymphocytes. J Clin Invest 67:86–92

Hunninghake GW, Gadek JE, Kawanami O, Ferrans VJ, Crystal RG (1979) Inflammatory and immune processes in the human lung in health and disease: evaluation by bronchoalveolar lavage. Am J Pathol 97:149–206

Hunninghake GW, Kawanami O, Ferrans VJ, Young RC Jr., Roberts WC, Crystal RG (1981) Characterization of inflammatory and immune effector cells in the lung parenchyma of patients with interstitial lung disease. Am Rev Respir Dis 123:407–412

Hynes RO, Yamada KM (1982) Fibronectins: Multifunctional modular glycoproteins. J Cell Biol 95:369–377

Janoff A, Raju L, Dearing R (1983) Levels of elastase activity in bronchoalveolar lavage fluids of healthy smokers and nonsmokers. Am Rev Respir Dis 127:540–544

Jaurand MC, Gaudichet A, Atassi K, Sebastien P, Bignon J (1980) Relationship between the number of asbestos fibres and the cellular and enzymatic content of bronchoalveolar fluid in asbestos exposed subjects. Bull Eur Physiopathol Resp 16:595–606

Johansson A, Lundborg M, Hellstrom P-A, Camner P, Keyser TR, Kirton SE, Natusch DFS (1980) Effect of iron, cobalt, and chromium dust on rabbit alveolar macrophages: A comparison with the effects of nickel dust. Environ Res 21:165–176

Johnson RL, Ziff M (1976) Lymphokine stimulation of collagen accumulation. J Clin Invest 58:240–252

Kadowitz PJ, Gruetter CA, Spannhake EW, Hyman AL (1981) Pulmonary vascular responses to prostaglandins. Fed Proc 40:1991–1996

Kaelin RM, Center DM, Bernardo J, Grant M, Snider GL (1983) The role of macrophage-derived chemoattractant activities in the early inflammatory events of bleomycin-induced pulmonary injury. Am Rev Respir Dis 128:132–137

Karlinsky JB, Snider GL (1978) Animal models of emphysema. Am Rev Respir Dis 117:1109–1133

Katz P, Haynes BF, Fauci AS (1978) Alteration of T-lymphocyte subpopulations in sarcoidosis. Clin Immunol Immunopathol 10:350–354

Keller RH, Calvanico NJ, Stevens JO (1982) Hypersensitivity pneumonitis in non-human primates. I. Studies on the relationship of immunoregulation and disease activity. J Immunol 128:116–122

Kim M, Goldstein E, Lewis JP, Lippert W, Warshauer D (1976) Murine pulmonary alveolar macrophages: Rates of bacterial ingestion, inactivation, and destruction. J Infect Dis 133:310–319

Kolb WP, Kolb LM, Wetsel RA, Rogers W, Shaw JO (1981) Quantitation and stability of complement (C5) in bronchoalveolar lavage fluids obtained from nonhuman primates. Am Rev Respir Dis 123:226–231

LaBelle CW, Brieger H (1960) The fate of inhaled particles in the early post-exposure period. Arch Environ Health 1:432–437

LaBelle CW, Brieger H (1961) Patterns and mechanisms in the elimination of dust from the lung. In: Davies CN (ed) Inhaled particles and vapors. Pergamon, London, pp 356–368

Larsen GL, Mitchell BC, Harper TB, Henson PM (1982) The pulmonary response of C5 sufficient and deficient mice to Pseudomonas aeruginosa. Am Rev Respir Dis 126:306–311

Last JA (1982) Mucus production and the ciliary escalator. In: Witschi H, Nettesheim P (eds) Mechanisms in respiratory toxicology, vol I. CRC Press, Boca Raton, Fl, pp 247–268

Lejeune FJ, Vercammen-Grandjean A (1979) Secretory activity of macrophages in relation to cytotoxicity and modulation of cell function. In: Dingle JT, Jacques PJ, Shaw IH (eds) Lysosomes in biology and pathology. North Holland, New York, pp 425–446

Lemaire I, Sirois P, Rola-Pleszczynski M, Masse S, Begin R (1981) Early biochemical reactions in the lung of sheep exposed to asbestos: evidence for cyclic AMP accumulation in bronchoalveolar lavage fluids. Lung 159:323–332

Lemaire I, Rola-Pleszczynski M, Begin R (1983) Asbestos exposure enhances the release of fibroblast growth factor by sheep alveolar macrophages. J Reticuloendothel Soc 33:275–285

Le Mesurier SM, Stewart BW, O'Connell PJ, Lykke AWJ (1979) Pulmonary responses to atmospheric pollutants. II. Effect of petrol vapour inhalation on secretion of pulmonary surfactant. Pathology 11:81–87

Le Mesurier SM, Stewart BW, Lykke AWJ (1981) Injury to Type-2 pneumocytes in rats exposed to cigarette smoke. Environ Res 24:207–217

Low RB, Davis GS, Giancola MS (1978) Biochemical analyses of bronchoalveolar lavage fluids of normal healthy volunteers. Am Rev Respir Dis 118:863–876

Lugano EM, Dauber JH, Daniele RP (1982) Acute experimental silicosis: Lung morphology, histology, and macrophage chemotaxin secretion. Am J Pathol 109:27–36

Marom Z, Weinberg KS, Fanburg BL (1980) Effect of bleomycin on collagenolytic activity of the rat alveolar macrophage. Am Rev Respir Dis 121:859–867

Martin TR, Chi EY, Covert DS, Hodson WA, Kessler DE, Moore WE, Altman LC, Butler J (1983) Comparative effects of inhaled volcanic ash and quartz in rats. Am Rev Respir Dis 128:144–152

Mauderly JL (1977) Bronchopulmonary lavage of small laboratory animals. Lab Animal Sci 27:255–261

Merrill WW, Goodenberger D, Strober W, Matthay RA, Naegel GP, Reynolds HY (1980) Free secretory component and other proteins in human lung lavage. Am Rev Respir Dis 122:156–161

Merrill W, O'Hearn E, Rankin J, Naegel G, Matthay RA, Reynolds HY (1982) Kinetic analysis of respiratory tract proteins recovered during a sequential lavage protocol. Am Rev Respir Dis 126:617–620

Morgan A, Moores SR, Holmes A, Evans JC, Evans NH, Black A (1980) The effect of quartz, administered by intratracheal instillation, on the rat lung. I. The cellular response. Environ Res 22:1–22

Moores SR, Black A, Evans JC, Evans N, Holmes A, Morgan A (1981) The effect of quartz administered by intratracheal instillation on the rat lung. II. The short-term biochemical response. Environ Res 24:275–285

Myrvik QN, Leake ES, Fariss B (1961) Studies on pulmonary alveolar macrophages from the normal rabbit: A technique to procure them in a high state of purity. J Immunol 86:128–132

Nathan CF, Murray HW, Cohn ZA (1980) The macrophage as an effector cell. N Engl J Med 303:622–626

Niewoehner DE, Kleinerman J, Rice DB (1974) Pathologic changes in the peripheral airways of young cigarette smokers. N Engl J Med 291:755–758

O'Flaherty JT (1982) Biology of disease: Lipid mediators of inflammation and allergy. Lab Invest 47:314–329

Ohlsson K, Olsson I (1974) The neutral proteases of human granulocytes: Isolation and partial characterization of granulocyte elastase. Eur J Biochem 42:519

Ordetti MA, Cushman DW (1982) Enzymes of the renin-angiotensin system and their inhibitors. Annu Rev Biochem 51:283–308

Padmanabhan RV, Gudapaty SR, Liener IE, Hoidal JR (1982) Elastolytic activity in the lungs of rats exposed to cadmium aerosolization. Environ Res 29:90–96

Pearson DJ, Mentnech MS, Gamble M, Taylor G, Green FHY (1980) Acute pulmonary injury induced by immune complexes. Exp Lung Res 1:323–334

Pennline KJ, Herscowitz HB (1981) Dual role for alveolar macrophages in humoral and cell-mediated immune responses: Evidence for suppressor and enhancing functions. J Reticuloendothel Soc 30:205–217

Pfleger RC, Muggenburg BA, Sesline DH, Harvey JW, Cuddihy RG, McClellan RO (1972) The removal of inhaled $^{144}CeCl_3$ from beagle dogs. I. Unilateral bronchopulmonary lavage with a DTPA solution. Health Phys 23:595–603

Postlethwaite AE, Keski-Oja J, Balian G, Kang AH (1981) Induction of fibroblast chemotaxis by fibronectin: Localization of the chemotactic region to a 140,000-molecular weight non-gelatin-binding fragment. J Exp Med 153:494–499

Ramirez-R J (1967) Pulmonary alveolar proteinosis. Treatment by massive bronchopulmonary lavage. Arch Intern Med 119:147

Reasor MJ, Nadeau D, Hook GER (1978) Extracellular alkaline phosphatase in the rabbit lung. Lung 155:321–335

Reiser KM, Last JA (1979) Silicosis and fibrogenesis: Fact and artifact. Toxicology 13:51–72

Rennard SI, Ferrano VJ, Bradley KH, Crystal RG (1982) Lung connective tissue. In: Witschi H, Nettesheim P (eds) Mechanisms in respiratory toxicology, vol II. CRC Press, Boca Raton, Fl, pp 115–153

Reynolds HY, Newball HH (1974) Analysis of proteins and respiratory cells obtained from human lungs by bronchial lavage. J Lab Clin Med 84:559–573

Reynolds HY, Fulmer JD, Kazmierowski JA, Roberts WC, Frank MM, Crystal RG (1977) Analysis of cellular and protein content of bronchoalveolar lavage fluid from patients with idiopathic pulmonary fibrosis and chronic hypersensitivity pneumonitis. J Clin Invest 59:165–175

Riley DJ, Chae CU, Guss HN, Kerr JS (1983) Degradation of lung collagen produced by oxygen toxicity in the rat: Assessment by hydroxyproline levels in lavage fluid. Am Rev Respir Dis 127:284 (abstract)

Rinaldo JE, Rogers RM (1982) Adult respiratory-distress syndrome. N Engl J Med 306:900–909

Robertson J, Caldwell JR, Castle JR, Waldman RH (1976) Evidence for the presence of components of the alternative (properdin) pathway of complement activation in respiratory secretion. J Immunol 117:900–903

Rola-Pleszczynski M, Sirois P, Begin R (1981) Cellular and humoral components of bronchoalveolar lavage in the sheep. Lung 159:91–99

Roth RA (1981) Effect of pneumotoxicants on lactate dehydrogenase activity in airways of rats. Toxicol Appl Pharmacol 57:69–78

Rylander R, Mattsky I, Snella MC (1980) Airway immune response after exposure to inhaled endotoxin. Bull Eur Physiopathol Resp 16:501–509

Sablonniere B, Scharfman A, Lafitte JJ, Laine A, Aerts C, Hayem A (1983) Enzymatic activities of bronchoalveolar lavages in coal workers pneumononiosis. Lung 161:219–228

Sackner MA (1975) Bronchofiberscopy. Am Rev Respir Dis 111:62–88

Schoenberger CI, Bitterman PB, Rennard SI, Fukuda Y, Ferrans VJ, Crystal RG (1982) Role of fibronectin and alveolar macrophage derived fibroblast growth factor in experimental pulmonary fibrosis. Am Rev Respir Dis 125:217 (abstract)

Schuyler MR, LaCuyetunia ST (1981) Accessory cell function of rabbit alveolar macrophages. Am Rev Respir Dis 123:53–57

Selgrade MK, Mole ML, Miller FJ, Hatch GE, Gardner DE, Hu PC (1981) Effect of NO_2 inhalation and vitamin C deficiency on protein and lipid accumulation in the lung. Environ Res 26:422–437

Shasby DM, Shasby SS, Bowman CM, Fox RB, Harada RM, Tate RM, Repine JE (1981) Angiotensin converting enzyme concentrations in the lung lavage of normal rabbits and rabbits treated with nitrogen mustard exposed to hyperoxia. Am Rev Respir Dis 124:202–203

Silbaugh SA, Felicetti SA, Muggenburg BA, Boecker BB (1975) Multiple bronchopulmonary lavages for the removal of [144]Ce in fused clay particles from beagle dog lungs. Health Phys 29:81–88

Skoza L, Snyder A, Kikkawa Y (1983) Ascorbic acid in bronchoalveolar wash. Lung 161:99–109

Sloan B, Abrams WR, Meranze DR, Kimbel P, Weinbaum G (1981) Emphysema induced in vitro and in vivo in dogs by a purified elastase from homologous leukocytes. Am Rev Respir Dis 124:295–301

Snider GL (1981) The pathogenesis of emphysema – twenty years of progress. Am Rev Respir Dis 123:321–324

Snider GL (1983) Emphysema, Clin Chest Med, vol 4/3. Saunders, Philadelphia

Snider GL, Celli BR, Goldstein RH, O'Brien JJ, Lucey EC (1978) Chronic interstitial pulmonary fibrosis in hamsters by endotracheal bleomycin. Am Rev Respir Dis 117:289–297

Snyder A, Skoza L, Kikkawa Y (1983) Comparative removal of ascorbic acid and other airway substances by sequential bronchoalveolar lavages. Lung 161:111–121

Spielvogel RL, Kersey JH, Goltz RW (1978) Mononuclear cell stimulation of fibroblast collagen synthesis. Clin Exp Dermatol 3:25–30

Stahl WR (1967) Scaling of respiratory variables in mammals. J Appl Physiol 22:453–460

Stankus RP, Salvaggio JE (1981) Bronchopulmonary humoral and cellular enhancement in experimental silicosis. J Reticuloendothel Soc 29:153–161

Stone PJ, Pereira W Jr, Biles D, Snider GL, Kagan HM, Franzblau C (1977) Studies on the fate of pancreatic elastase in the hamster lung: ^{14}C-guanidinated elastase. Am Rev Respir Dis 116:49–55

Strumpf IJ, Feld MK, Cornelius MJ, Keogh BA, Crystal RG (1981) Safety of fiberoptic bronchoalveolar lavage in evaluation of interstitial lung disease. Chest 80:268–271

Sykes SE, Morgan A, Evans JC, Evans N, Holmes A, Moores SR (1982) Use of an in vivo test system to investigate the acute and sub-acute responses of the rat lung to mineral dusts. Ann Occup Hyg 26:593–605

Tetley TD, Richards RJ, Harwood JL (1977) Changes in pulmonary surfactant and phosphatidylcholine metabolism in rats exposed to chrysotile asbestos dust. Biochem J 166:323–329

Thrall RS, McCormick JR, Jack RM, McReynolds RA, Ward PA (1979) Bleomycin-induced pulmonary fibrosis in the rat. Inhibition with indomethacin. Am Rev Respir Dis 95:117–127

Thrall RS, Phan SH, McCormick JR, Ward PA (1981) The development of bleomycin-induced pulmonary fibrosis in neutrophil depleted and complement depleted rats. Am J Pathol 105:76–81

Tryka AF, Skornik WA, Godleski JJ, Brain JD (1982) Potentiation of bleomycin-induced lung injury by exposure to 70% oxygen. Am Rev Respir Dis 126:1074–1079

Vicente G (1928) Sobre una technica simplificade en la terapeutica intrapulmonar. Rev Progr Clin 26:487–492

Villiger B, Broekelmann T, Kelley D, Heymach GJ III, McDonald JA (1981) Bronchoalveolar fibronectin in smokers and nonsmokers. Am Rev Respir Dis 124:652–654

Warheit DB, George G, Hill LH, Brody AR (1983) Inhaled asbestos fibers activate complement-depleted chemotactic factors for macrophages on alveolar surfaces. Am Rev Respir Dis 127:167 (abstract)

Wedmore CV, Williams TV (1981) Control of vascular permeability by polymorphonuclear leukocytes in inflammation. Nature 289:646–650

Weissman G, Smolin JE, Korchak HM (1980) Release of inflammatory mediators from stimulated neutrophils. N Engl J Med 303:27–39

White R, Habicht GS, Godfrey HP, Janoff A, Barton E, Fox C (1981 a) Secretion of elastase and alpha-2-macroglobulin by cultured murine peritoneal macrophages: studies on their interaction. J Lab Clin Med 97:718–729

White R, Lee D, Habicht GS, Janoff A (1981 b) Secretion of alpha$_1$-proteinase inhibitor by cultured rat alveolar macrophages. Am Rev Respir Dis 123:447–449

Winternitz MC, Smith GH (1919) Intratracheal pulmonary irrigation. In: Contributions to medical and biological research dedicated to Sir William Osler II, Hoeker, New York, p 1255

Witschi HP (1977) Environmental agents altering lung biochemistry. Fed Proc 36:1631–1634

Morphologic Techniques

CHAPTER 9

Morphological Methods for Gross and Microscopic Pathology

D. L. Dungworth, W. S. Tyler, and C. E. Plopper

A. Introduction

The size and structural complexity of the respiratory tract and the diversity of its responses to inhaled toxicants make the task of thorough morphological examination a challenging one. A variety of morphological techniques is available. Each method has advantages and disadvantages. None can provide the basis for answering all questions regarding the nature and pathogenesis of observed effects. Choice of appropriate methods therefore depends on the aims of a particular study. Methods to be used are also determined, as will become evident, by the topographic distribution of lesions in the respiratory tract and by the nature of the lesions. The final modifying influences in selection of methods are feasibility and cost.

B. Routine Examination

The gross examination is mainly to map the topographic distribution of detectable abnormalities and provide the basis for selection of appropriate fixation and sampling techniques for further investigations. Careful examination of the entire respiratory tract from external nares to distal lung is essential. In large animals such as dogs or monkeys, preliminary information on sites of damage will sometimes be available from radiographic or ultrasound examinations. Unless otherwise stated, examinations are carried out in animals killed by injection of sodium pentobarbital, either intraperitoneally in small animals such as rodents or intravenously in dogs and other large animals. Other than where fixation is to be by vascular perfusion, the animal should not be exsanguinated and the chest should not be opened until cardiac arrest has occurred.

I. Nasopharyngeal Region

1. Gross Examination

Production of nasal tumors by a variety of compounds, particularly formaldehyde, has focused attention on the need for detailed examination of the upper respiratory tract. Before this is done, the prosector should become familiar with the anatomy of the region (Schreider and Raabe 1981 a). In laboratory rodents, the nasal sinuses and conchae can be examined by removing the nasal bones and part of the frontal bones with forceps or by sagittal section. Unless there is gross deformity or nasal exudate, however, detailed examination is better left to histopathology. In larger animals such as the dog and monkey, dissection is necessary. For the dog, after the skin, eyes, and brain have been removed, the nasal conchae and frontal sinuses are exposed by removing the nasal and frontal bones with bone forceps. The ventral concha (maxilloturbinate) can be excised with scissors and the ethmoidal conchae further exposed by a sagittal saw cut lateral to the nasal septum. The septum is removed by scalpel and sampling of the ethmoidal conchae (ethmoturbinates) for microscopic examination is made from the cavity opposite to the one sectioned by sawing. In the monkey, which has a shorter, less complex nasal cavity, a parasagittal section is made by a saw cut, and the contra-lateral cavity is exposed by removal of the nasal septum. The superior nasal con-cha and portions of the septal mucosa and mucosa covering the lateral wall (in-cluding the inferior nasal concha) can be dissected free, flattened, and used for light microscopy (LM), scanning electron microscopy (SEM), and transmission electron microscopy (TEM).

2. Fixation

Nasopharyngeal structures in small laboratory animals are usually fixed whole, either in neutral buffered formalin if there is to be no electron microscopy (EM), or in one of the glutaraldehyde–formaldehyde fixatives suitable for EM, as de-scribed in Sect. B. II. 2. a for immersion fixation of epithelium of large airways. To ensure adequate penetration of fixative into recesses of the nasal passages, the nasal cavity is gently flushed with 10–15 ml fixative from a syringe fitted with a needle which is inserted approximately 0.5 cm into the caudal opening of the nasopharynx (Young 1981). Blocks of any abnormal tissues and representative portions of nasal, pharyngeal and laryngeal structures need to be taken from larger animals for immersion in fixative.

Fixation for detailed ultrastructural evaluation in rodents is achieved by vascular perfusion (Popp and Martin 1981). A catheter is inserted through the left ventricle into the ascending aorta of an anesthetized rat. Before fixation, the vessels are flushed for 1 min with 10% dextran 40 in 0.9% sodium chloride at a pressure of 110 cm fluid. Fixation is by Karnovsky's fixative in cacodylate buffer at a flow rate of about 20 ml/min under 110 cm pressure to a total volume of 250 ml fixative. The nasal cavity still needs to be flushed to remove adherent mucus and allow SEM of cell surfaces. This is done with 20 ml physiologic saline or 0.1 M cacodylate buffer containing 1 mg/ml hyaluronidase. Analogous vascular per-fusion could be used for larger laboratory animals.

3. Sampling for Microscopic Examination

The nasal cavity of rodents is examined by a standardized set of transverse sec-tions after decalcification. The fixed upper jaw and nasal region are decalcified in formic acid–sodium citrate (Young 1981) or 10% EDTA (Popp and Martin 1981). After decalcification, transverse cuts are made with a razor blade using pa-latine structures as reference points. A satisfactory method (J. A. Popp, personal communication) is to invert the skull so it rests on the plane of the nasofrontal bones. Four vertical cross sections are then made: (a) rostral to the incisor teeth; (b) 1 mm caudal to the free tip of the incisor teeth; (c) through the middle of the

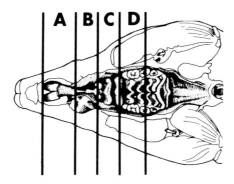

Fig. 1. Ventral aspect of the hard palate region of the rat, showing reference lines for cutting standardized cross sections of the nasal cavity. (Courtesy of Dr. J. A. Popp, Chemical Industry Institute of Toxicology Research Triangle Park, North Carolina)

second palatine ridge; and (d) through the middle of the molar teeth (Fig. 1). The resulting four blocks are embedded with the rostral face down. An alternative set of blocks is described by YOUNG (1981).

Blocks from proximal and distal regions of nasal sinuses and conchae (turbinates) and the pharynx and larynx need to be selected from dissections in large animals, as well as from any observed lesions. The sampling is needed to cover both the variations in deposition/retention of inhaled substances and the differences in epithelial covering. The importance of the latter is that more detailed study is needed of the relative sensitivities to damage of the several types of epithelium of the nasal cavity, e. g., with respect to variations in amounts of monooxygenases within epithelial cells (DAHL et al. 1982).

4. Microscopic Examination

Samples are examined in much the same fashion as described for pulmonary parenchyma in Sect. B. II. 4.

II. Tracheobronchial Tree and Pulmonary Parenchyma

1. Gross Examination

The trachea and lungs are carefully exposed after the diaphragm is punctured and the sternum removed. Search is made for abnormalities of the pleural cavity and its parietal and visceral surfaces (e. g., hemorrhage, edema, exudate, adhesions). At this point, a decision has to be made whether to fix the lung in situ, either by one or both of intratracheal infusion and intravascular perfusion, or to remove the trachea, lungs, and heart from the chest cavity. In general, the more obivously the lungs are affected the more necessary it is to remove them from the chest cavity for careful gross examination. Conversely, where changes are minimal it is often convenient to fix the lungs in situ. The best practical approach in most instances is to remove lungs from the chest cavity in initial studies and consider in situ fixation for special aspects of any follow-up investigations.

The lungs and heart are removed after transecting the trachea several rings distal to the larynx. Cannulation of the trachea prior to removal aids subsequent intratracheal infusion of fixative and prevents contamination with blood. The surfaces of the lungs are examined for signs of abnormalities (e. g., edema, hemorrhage, atelectasis, consolidation, scarring, possible tumor nodules). The partially collapsed state of the excised lung results in an exaggerated appearance of small lesions that sometimes cannot be detected in the inflated state. The weight of the lungs can be obtained after tying off major vessels and dissecting away the heart and mediastinum. The extent to which the major airways and vessels of large lungs need be opened depends on the amount of gross damage. If major intrapulmonary airways are opened, portions of lung should be retained for intrabronchial fixation. Subgross examination of surface or cut sections of lung by dissecting microscope is occasionally useful. It is more commonly an adjunct to special procedures for studies of airways or vessels which will be described in Sects. C. II and III.

2. Fixation

Important criteria for determining choice of fixation are production of least artifact, reproducibility, simplicity, and cost. To these should be added logistics of experimental design which dictate whether tissues will be processed without delay or whether a period of storage prior to processing is unavoidable. This is because fixatives such as glutaraldehyde, which provide excellent short-term ultrastructural preservation, are not satisfactory for long-term storage. For good EM observations and storage, glutaraldehyde–formaldehyde fixatives are required.

The main objective with respect to production of least artifact is to retain as closely as possible the in vivo appearance of the tissues immediately preceding death. With pulmonary tissue, in addition to the usual fixation artifacts that have to be avoided (e. g., shrinkage, swelling, mechanical distortion, changes in cellular organelles), there is the need to prepare lung for microscopic examination so as to try to retain correct relationships and configurations of airspaces, interstitium, and exudate or other abnormal components. The method best fitting the set of requirements for each specific study must be chosen.

The two major variables to be considered in fixation of lung are the fixative fluid and its mode of usage. For routine purposes, the choices are limited. Methods will be considered according to the mode of fixation since this has more influence on the procedure than the type of fixative.

a) Fixation by Immersion

Fixation by immersion of small blocks of lung in various fluids is the simplest and most common routine procedure. When dealing with pulmonary lesions in which the emphasis is on nonaerated tissue (e. g., atelectasis, edema, exudative processes, neoplastic masses), this it the best method. Neutral buffered formalin is the usual fixative for LM. For combined histologic and ultrastructural examinations, formaldehyde–glutaraldehyde fixatives are preferable (GLAUERT 1974). A suitable formula is 4% formaldehyde (paraformaldehyde) and 1% glutaraldehyde in 200 mosmol phosphate buffer (McDOWELL and TRUMP 1976).

Whereas hypertonic fixatives (approximately 550 mosmol) are needed for fixation by diffusion through tissue blocks, fixatives should be in the isotonic range for ultrastructural studies of epithelial surfaces such as of trachea and bronchi which are brought into immediate contact with large volumes of fluid by immersion or infusion. A suitable fixative is 2.5% glutaraldehyde in 0.05 *M* cacodylate buffer (360 mosmol) and pH 7.4 (MATHIEU et al. 1978). We prefer however to use modified Karnovsky's glutaraldehyde–formaldehyde fixative in cacodylate buffer (NOWELL and TYLER 1971) adjusted to 360 mosmol and pH 7.4 by further dilution with water. This is a better long-term storage fluid. The best osmolarity of fixative for preservation of the epithelium of large airways is not the same as for deep lung parenchyma. Fixatives used for immersion can be varied according to special stains to be used for LM or to enhance certain features such as the use of Zenkerformol for evaluation of proteinaceous exudates.

b) Fixation by Airway Infusion

Fixation of lungs for routine examination is best done by infusion into the airways. It is essential for recognition and interpretation of subtle lesions, but not recommended when there are severe lesions as mentioned in Sect. B. II. 2. a.

A disadvantage of airway infusion is that translocation of fluid exudates and nonadherent cells and particles can occur and some interstitial spaces are widened slightly (edema artifact). Exacting structural–functional analyses requiring maintenance of air–blood compartments as close to physiologic conditions as feasible, are better performed in perfusion-fixed lungs (BACHOFEN et al. 1982) or rapidly frozen lungs (MAZZONE et al. 1980). Detailed examination of pulmonary vasculature is also better done on perfusion-fixed lungs.

Initially, as developed for humans, lungs were excised and infused with formalin at a fluid pressure of 30 cm or more (HEARD 1958, HEARD et al. 1967). Since then, a variety of fixatives, fixative pressures, and excised versus in situ locations have been used in experimental animals. The first choice confronting the investigator is whether to fix the lungs in the thoracic cavity or remove, examine, and then fix. The most straightforward method is to cannulate the trachea and fix the lungs in situ after puncturing the diaphragm and removing the sternum. This has the advantage of lessening the chances of pleural leaks and keeps the conformation of the expanded lungs the same as the thoracic cavity. It helps prevent loss of blood from pulmonary vessels owing to compression by the fixative pressure. HAYATDAVOUDI et al. (1980) found that lungs of rats fixed in situ by infusion of 2% glutaraldehyde at 20 cm pressure were more inflated when blood was circulating through the pulmonary vascular bed at the start of infusion than when the rats had been exsanguinated before infusion began.

Infusion of excised lungs is acceptable if more thorough gross examination is required than can be done in situ (more likely with larger animals), if it is not feasible to retain the carcass overnight during fixation under pressure, or where one lung is to be subjected to a different type of analysis. Ligation of pulmonary vessels prior to removal of lungs from the thorax will retain blood in the vessels.

The second choice is of fixative solution. Neutral buffered formalin is acceptable for routine LM and would suffice for survey purposes. For definitive studies, however, a fixative for LM and EM examination is essential. Detailed considerations of fixatives for TEM are addressed by GLAUERT (1974) and for SEM by NOWELL and PAWLEY (1980). Principal variations are the nature and concentration of the fixatve agent or agents, the nature of the buffer, the osmolarity of the complete fixative and the vehicle, and the presence of added electrolytes and/or nonelectrolytes. The pH of 7.2–7.4 and fixative at room temperature are generally accepted. As far as fixative is concerned, the choice for initial fixative is between glutaraldehyde or a glutaraldehyde–formaldehyde mixture. Pure formaldehyde derived from paraformaldehyde should be used. Glutaraldehyde in concentrations of 2%–2.5% is commonly used in either phosphate or cacodylate buffer. With phosphate buffer, the final concentration should not exceed 0.1 M otherwise granular artifacts are produced on postfixation with osmium tetroxide (GIL and WEIBEL 1968; HENDRIKS and EESTERMANS 1982). Sodium cacodylate has the advantage of keeping the lung resilient enough so it is better able to return to its original state after the deformation associated with cutting. It also is preferable for storage purposes. The disadvantage of cacodylate is that it is toxic (WEAKLEY 1977), as is the piperazine-N–N'-bis-2-ethanolsulfonic acid (PIPES) buffer used for retention of membrane lipids (SCHIFF and GENNARO 1979).

Osmolarity of both fixative agent and vehicle are important (MATHIEU et al. 1978; LEE et al. 1982). Fixation by isotonic fixative consisting of 2.5% glutaraldehyde in 0.05 M cacodylate buffer (total osmolarity 360 mosmol) has been reported to give optimum results for alveolar fixation when a range of hypertonic glutaraldehyde fixatives was compared using morphometric techniques (MATHIEU et al. 1978). This does provide good preservation of tracheobronchial epithelium. For best preservation of bronchiolar and alveolar structures, however, we find diluted Karnovsky's fixative (SCHNEEBERGER-KEELEY and KARNOVSKY 1968; NOWELL and TYLER 1971) to be the best all round fixative. The stock solution is paraformaldehyde, 50 g/l; 50% glutaraldehyde solution, 100 ml/l; calcium chloride, 0,5 g/l; cacodylic acid (Na salt), 32 g/l. This can be stored at 4 °C for several months. Before use, the fixative is diluted to give a final osmolarity of 550 mosmol: 1 part stock fixative, 3.5 parts sodium-cacodylate solution (32 g/l), and 1 part distilled water. It is filtered after adjusting the pH to 7.2–7.4 with 1.0 M HCl. Room temperature is suitable for most species, but those with sensitive airways (e.g., guinea pigs) infuse better with fixative at body temperature. This fixative has the advantage of also being an excellent storage fluid at room temperature.

The final parameter to be selected is the infusion pressure, usually measured by the height of fixative in the reservoir above the level of liquid in the bath in which the lung is supported (excised) or above the hilus of the lung (in situ). Pressures of 15–30 cm have been used for rodents and 25–30 cm or more for larger animals. HAYATDAVOUDI et al. (1980) investigated in normal rats the effects of varying fixatives, pressure, rate of infusion, and location of lungs (in situ or excised) on the degree of inflation of intratracheally infused lungs. They found with glutaraldehyde that limiting the flow rate of fixative by use of long tubing and a narrow stub adapter in the tracheostomy opening led to reduced inflation. This emphasizes the need for short tubing and adapters of as wide a gauge as possible (14 or 15). With the low resistance tubing, fixative pressure of 20 cm produced inflation to approximately 84% of total lung capacity as measured previously by gas dilution techniques. A pressure of 30 cm gave slightly higher inflation. The degree of inflation with formaldehyde did not vary significantly with tubing resistance and was similar to glutaraldehyde through the low resistance tubing. Their findings also confirmed that the degree of inflation was not influenced by prior degassing.

Adequate inflation of normal rat lungs can be obtained at 20 cm fluid pressure as already described. The focus of toxicologic studies is on damaged lungs, however, therefore we prefer to standardize the pressure at 30 cm because the additional hydrostatic pressure is necessary for consistent inflation of lungs with the range of lesions commonly encountered. Our experience with species larger than laboratory rodents has shown that 20 cm pressure is insufficient for complete filling. We have found that a pressure of 30 cm also properly inflates lungs of species ranging in size from rabbits to horses. Based on evaluation by TEM, this pressure does not cause tearing or rupture of tissues, even in small laboratory animals.

To summarize, a good standard method is to infuse lungs via the trachea with modified Karnovsky's fixative at 30 cm fluid pressure using short, large-bore tubing, adapters, and cannulas. For combined morphological and morphometric studies in rodents, lungs may be fixed either in situ or after excision with pulmonary vessels ligated. Indications for one procedure versus the other were discussed previously in this section. In larger animals, it is usually more convenient to ligate the pulmonary vessels, excise the lungs, and place them in a bath of fixative. We have used pumps to provide the constant reservoir height of fixative while minimizing the volume of fixative used for lungs of large animals such as horses. Marriott bottles are convenient for dogs, monkeys, and similar sized animals. Fixation of lungs from a large number of animals with multiple adaptors attached to a manifold connected to a single reservoir might seem simpler and less time consuming than use of individual reservoirs and connectors. In practice it is less satisfactory, however, because it results in incomplete filling caused by reduced pressure and flow rate of fixative. Although fixation appears complete within 1 h when using glutaraldehyde or its mixtures, we maintain fixative pressure overnight before tying off the trachea for volume estimation by liquid displacement (SCHERLE 1970). The additional fixation under pressure helps in maintenance of fixed volume by ensuring adequate fixation of pulmonary connective tissues. Tissues for TEM which have been fixed by glutaraldehyde or glutaraldehyde–formaldehyde are routinely postfixed in 1% osmium tetroxide.

3. Sampling for Microscopic Examination

Judicious sampling of tissue for microscopic examination is of paramount importance in both morphological and morphometric evaluation of the respiratory tract. Sampling must be widespread and precise in anatomic location. The number of large blocks taken for examination by LM and SEM will vary according to experimental aims. In all instances, however, the number must be sufficient to sample sites known or suspected to be affected differently.

For routine evaluations, proximal trachea and the tracheobronchial bifurcation are the minimal sites of extrapulmonary airways to be evaluated in animals of all sizes. Notice needs to be taken of differences in tracheal mucosa between dorsal and ventral regions and between cartilaginous and intercartilaginous portions (SCHWARTZ et al. 1976; MELLICK et al. 1977).

Sampling of lung tissue needs to take into account the airway orientation of many lesions caused by inhaled irritants, and possible gradients of damage in craniocaudal, dorsoventral, and hilar–peripheral axes. Various planes of sectioning can be used. For routine morphological assessment of rodent lungs, we prefer sections along the axes of major airways as shown for the right lung in Fig. 2. These provide best qualitative assessment of the distribution of lesions with respect to airways. This is particularly important for effective interpretation of centriacinar lesions such as produced by ozone (SCHWARTZ et al. 1976) and many other inhaled materials (GROSS et al. 1966). The sagittal section of the left lung is convenient for assessing craniocaudal and dorsoventral gradients, but is not as effective for following airway pattern of lesions because airways are more often cut obliquely. Sagittal sections are useful for some types of evaluation of normal lung. LANGSTON et al. (1979) investigated the proportion of parenchyma to non-parenchyma in human lungs of diverse sizes and found the midsagittal slice or the central two slices satisfactorily represented the overall lung with respect to those parameters. Similar sampling of damaged lungs would only be effective if the lesions were distributed evenly throughout the lungs.

The alternative method of making transverse sections of the left lung at intervals, as also shown in Fig. 2, has advantages for some studies because it provides transverse sections of large and small airways, as well as longitudinal sections

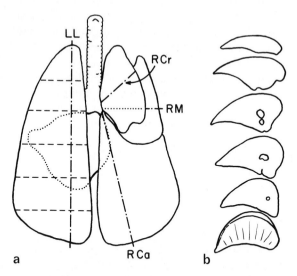

a   R Ca   b

Fig. 2. a Outline of the dorsal aspect of a rat's lung, illustrating various vertical planes of section for sampling tissue. Sections of the right lung marked by *dashed-dotted lines* are along the axes of major airways. Sections of the left lung marked by *dashed lines* contain cross sections of airways and vessels of various sizes as well as longitudinal sections of terminal airways and alveolar ducts. (*LL* left lung; *RCr* right cranial lobe; *RM* right middle lobe; *RCa* right caudal lobe; outline of the accessory lobe is indicated by the *dotted line*). **b** Caudal surfaces of slices of the left lung obtained by vertical cuts marked by *dashed lines* in **a**

through junctions of terminal airways and alveolar ducts. The transverse sections of the left lung from rats are also useful for determination of parenchyma and nonparenchyma (LUM 1981). Using a dissecting microscope for evaluations of sections from either normal or ozone-affected lung floating in fixative, the section 55% of the distance along the craniocaudal axis was found to be representative of the entire lung. These blocks are useful for LM, but much less so for SEM. Most information in a single study can therefore be obtained by sectioning the right lung along the axes of airways for qualitative and certain quantitative evaluations, and by sectioning the left lung transversely for additional morphometric evaluation.

More care in sampling is required for lungs of larger animals because of the bulk of tissue to be surveyed and the greater chance of there being regional variations in response. To minimize sampling errors, parenchymal sites covering the three main anatomic axes and alveoli served by either few or many airway generations should be chosen. For routine qualitative evaluation, seven standardized sampling sites from the right lung of a dog are illustrated in Fig. 3. If both lungs are available, they should both be sampled.

Precise comparison of lungs from animals of different treatment groups, and the search for subtle lesions, requires morphometric evaluation. For the canine lung, we are currently sectioning horizontally in the dorsal plane as shown in Fig. 4 and taking random samples from each layer using the template method of

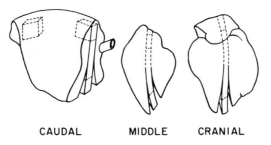

CAUDAL   MIDDLE   CRANIAL

Fig. 3. Outline of lateral view of major lobes of a dog's right lung, indicating seven sampling sites for comprehensive qualitative evaluation

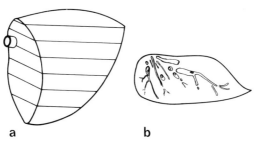

a   b

Fig. 4. a Schematic outline of lateral view of left caudal lobe of a dog's lung, showing sections in the dorsal plane providing slices suitable for combined morphological and morphometric evaluations. **b** Outline of slice immediately ventral to level of mainstem bronchus

THURLBECK (1967). For routine morphology, one block per slice is sufficient. The number of blocks per slice needed for morphometry depends on the required confidence level. Further information on morphometric approaches is provided in Chap. 10. Slices in the dorsal plane are especially useful for SEM because many airways are sectioned longitudinally. The longitudinal or oblique sections examined by LM also provide good appreciation of the distribution of lesions relative to airways.

4. Microscopic Examination

The extensiveness of microscopic evaluation varies according to the objectives of a study. The large numbers of animals needed for most routine studies, coupled with the necessity for multiple samples of lung as discussed previously, mean that LM of paraffin-embedded tissues must be the principal mode of evaluation. The search for subtle effects, or the complete description of lesions once they have been recognized, however, requires examination of a significant number of lungs by correlated LM, SEM, and TEM. This is best accomplished by taking complementary blocks of tissue from the same sampling site, embedding one in plastic suitable for large 1-µm sections and processing the other for SEM. The surface and sectioned views are then compared for interpretation.

The advantage of SEM, particularly for a surface-dominated structure like the lung, is that relatively large specimens can be examined at a wide range of magnification and with greater depth of field than any other optical system. The advantage of large 1-µm plastic-embedded sections is that they provide optimal resolution for LM. There are two main choices of embedding material, glycol methacrylate and epoxy resin. Glycol methacrylate is suitable if TEM evaluation is not required and enables the use of many water-soluble stains. Epoxy resins should be used when LM is to be followed by TEM of precisely defined and selected anatomic sites. This deliberate selection of pulmonary parenchyma for TEM, as described in Sect. B. II. 4. c should be the norm for all ultrastructural evaluations of pulmonary lesions.

a) Light Microscopy

Thorough examination by LM of sections cut from vacuum-embedded paraffin blocks is the backbone of routine morphological evaluation. Glycol methacrylate is replacing paraffin as the embedding medium in laboratories where the better resolution of 1-µm sections is constantly required. Both embedding methods permit the use of a large variety of special stains (LUNA 1968; THOMPSON 1974; CLARK 1981). Sections 1 µm in thickness cut from large, partly polymerized epoxy resin blocks are the essential link between LM and TEM as mentioned previously. Although SEM has largely replaced thick paraffin-embedded sections for three-dimensional observations of fine pulmonary structure, thick sections of lung are still useful for studying interrelationships of components of alveolar septa, e. g., connective tissue fibers, capillaries, and alveolar pores (KLEINERMAN and COWDREY 1964). Their main use has been for investigations of human emphysema (PUMP 1974).

b) Scanning Electron Microscopy

Large blocks of tissue, approximately $12 \times 12 \times 4$ mm can conveniently be prepared for SEM. Blocks are cut so that airways are sectioned longitudinally as described in Sect. II. 3, dehydrated in graded ethanol, and then dried by the critical point method using CO_2 (ANDERSON 1951; NOWELL et al. 1972). Considerable shrinkage occurs during these procedures, but it is uniform and distortion is uncommon when appropriate techniques are correctly used. The dried tissue blocks are attached to labeled standard SEM stubs with conductive paste which is allowed to dry thoroughly before coating with gold in a sputter coater or with carbon followed by gold–palladium in a high vacuum device (BRUMMER et al. 1975). The tissues are stored in a dessicator before and after examination in the SEM. Frequently, it is helpful to dissect the dried blocks under a dissecting microscope for better exposure of airways or other selected sites. The tissues are then recoated and reexamined by SEM. Dissecting lungs in the SEM using micromanipulators is possible, but not a routine procedure (PAWLEY and NOWELL 1973).

The limitation of SEM to the examination of surfaces is not a major problem in lung because of its very large surface area. Although mucus and other surface coats are removed by infusion of fixative through airways, they can be examined in lungs fixed by vascular perfusion or rapid freezing followed by freeze drying or freeze substitution and critical point drying (NOWELL and TYLER 1971). Internal aspects of tissues and cells can be studied using tissues which have been embedded and sectioned (WINBORN and GUERRERO 1974) or fractured after dehydration (HUMPHREYS et al. 1974) or after drying (FLOOD 1975).

There are occasions when critical lesions are identified by SEM, but are not frequent enough for random sectioning to reveal them. Though not a routine procedure, areas of interest identified on the SEM micrograph can be located on the block using an optical dissecting microscope, dissected out by razor blade, and orientated in the appropriate plane for sectioning and processing for LM and TEM (BRUMMER et al. 1975). For this series of examinations, the tissue is best osmicated before processing for SEM. Most tissues embed well since the media readily penetrate the freshly cut surfaces, but sectioning is slightly more difficult because of the metallic conductive coating. Cytologic preservation is adequate for most purposes, but of lower quality than in tissue prepared specifically for TEM.

c) Transmission Electron Microscopy

The very small size of the sample examined by TEM, combined with the focal nature of many pulmonary lesions and the frequency with which they have a specific localization within the pulmonary acinus, make it essential to know the exact anatomic location from which the sample was taken. This has long been recognized for inhalation toxicology of substances such as ozone (PLOPPER et al. 1973; STEPHENS and EVANS 1973). The recent finding by GIL and McNIFF (1982) that the lesions produced in lungs of rabbits by intravenous injection of ethchlorvynol are principally in alveolar corner capillaries reemphasizes the need for precise localization of samples. TEM of diced 1-mm cubes does not meet this need.

There are three methods for deliberate selection of tissue to be examined by TEM. The oldest is based on the technique used by GRIMLEY (1965). Large blocks of epoxy-embedded tissue are sectioned in a heavy duty microtome of the type used for cutting metal or bone. Alternate sections 30 and 10 µm in thickness are cut. Specific lesions or areas are identified by LM of the 10-µm sections. This facilitates localization and dissection of the same or similar features from the adjacent 30-µm section. The selected portion of the 30-µm section is cemented to the block of a BEEM capsule and ultrathin sections cut (PLOPPER et al. 1973). This method has the advantage of enabling TEM of the identical tissue observed by LM in the 30-µm section, although the resolution with LM is poor.

Less tedious and time-consuming techniques rely on examination by LM of 1-µm sections from partially polymerized, epoxy-embedded blocks with 8×12 mm surfaces. Polymerization is allowed to proceed for 8 h and the plastic is tested for appropriate hardness. If insufficient for cutting of good sections on a Sorval JB-4 (du Pont de Nemours and Company, Wilmington, Delaware) or equivalent microtome, polymerization is continued at 2-h increments until satisfactory hardness is achieved. After identifying the desired region in the 1-µm section, that portion of the large block is selected for ultrathin sectioning. This is done either by the "mesa" technique in which surrounding tissue is removed (LOWRIE and TYLER 1973), or by cutting the selected piece from the large block and cementing it to a block from a BEEM capsule (PLOPPER et al. 1983a). In either case, the epoxy resin needs to be fully polymerized before ultrathin sectioning. The advantage of the "mesa" method is easier maintenance of topographic relationships between the selected site and remainder of tissue in the block. The block dissection is usually preferable because it makes cutting on the ultramicrotome simpler, especially for sites from the periphery of the large block. It also allows sectioning of small blocks from more than one location on the same face. An alternate approach is the selection of areas by microdissection after osmium fixation, dehydration, and clearing (STEPHENS and EVANS 1973). This method provides high contrast to facilitate dissection, but since it is done on tissues in unpolymerized epoxy resins care must be taken to avoid contamination of personnel and equipment.

C. Special Methods

Special methods are required to provide information not obtainable by routine procedures. In this context, routine refers to the standard methods described in the previous section which are used for assessment of possible toxic effects from inhaled materials. Special methods usually have more limited focus and greater complexity, but they are an essential part of pathogenetic studies. Since special methods of fixation, processing, and examination are largely interdependent, they will be categorized for convenience according to the major purposes they serve.

I. Subgross Survey of Large Lungs

1. Whole Lung Macrosections

The technique of preparing 500-µm-thick whole sections of human lungs and mounting them on paper was developed by GOUGH and WENTWORTH (1960) for their studies of emphysema. Detection of minimal degrees of emphysema in lung slices was found to be enhanced after impregnation with barium sulfate (HEARD 1960). Subsequent modification included more rapid processing of paper-mounted sections (WHIMSTER 1969) and permanent mounting of the macrosections by laminating with plastic film (CÔTÉ et al. 1963; KORY et al. 1966).

2. Fixation Followed by Air Drying

A variety of formalin vapor and formalin–steam techniques have been used to prepare dry macroscopic specimens, as reviewed by PÄÄKKÖ (1981). These have no practical place in experimental studies.

II. Morphology and Morphometry of Airways

1. Corrosion Casts

Corrosion casts provide the most direct and effective approach to establishing the geometry of airways in normal or diseased states. They have been used principally to derive mathematical models for the mechanical properties of normal airways (HORSFIELD et al. 1971, 1982) and for the behavior of inspired gases and particulates (PHALEN et al. 1973, 1978; RAABE et al. 1976; SCHREIDER and RAABE 1980, 1981 b). Corrosion casts have also been used in the study of airway disease (HORSFIELD et al. 1966) and emphysema (PUMP 1973).

Two main types of casting material are used, silicone rubber and polyester resins. The technique for using silicone rubber was developed by PHALEN et al. (1973). Its advantage is the production of an accurate replica of airways (SCHREIDER and RAABE 1981 b) whose flexibility facilitates trimming and measurement of features such as dimensions and branching angles. Polyester resins are used as described by TOMPSETT (1956) or with minor modifications (HORSFIELD and CUMMING 1976).

Details of casts referred to previously are examined by dissecting microscope. For finer resolution of replicas of internal surface structures, whether of airways or vessels, microcorrosion casts can be examined by SEM. HODDE and NOWELL (1980) have analyzed the various techniques for preparing microcorrosion casts for SEM and presented the advantages of using polyester (methacrylate) resins rather than rubber compounds for this purpose.

2. Bronchography

Although bronchography is mainly used for clinical diagnosis, tantalum bronchography has been used as an aid in studying the structure of human peripheral airways and acini (GAMSU et al. 1971 a, b) and for validating the accuracy of airway casts in rats (YEH et al. 1975).

3. Airway Microdissection

This method has many of the advantages of airway casting, such as the potential for measuring airway branching angles and dimensions, but also avoids the major disadvantage of casts – the loss of tissue through digestion. Dissection is easiest on lungs fixed by airway infusion as discussed previously. After trachea and primary bronchi have been sectioned longitudinally, the lung lobes to be dissected

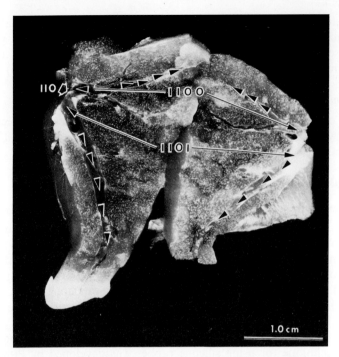

Fig. 5. Right cranial lobe of rabbit's lung after microdissection to expose the lobar bronchus (IIO), and its two major branches (IIOI and IIOO). The axial pathways (indicated by *rows of arrowheads*) of both of the branches are split longitudinally

are removed at the hilus. Using a high resolution stereomicroscope, fine scissors, and scalpels, the lobe is dissected longitudinally down the axial pathway of the lobar bronchus and its first large intrapulmonary branch. The largest number of airway generations can be exposed in most species by making the plane of section through the midline of the airway and roughly parallel to the costal surface of the lobe. This results in two halves as illustrated in Fig. 5. Complementary halves of the airways can then be numbered, the branching patterns recorded, and then selected tissues processed for LM, SEM, or TEM. The numbering pattern used is the binary system of PHALEN et al. (1973). Figure 6 illustrates the system for rabbit airways. The trachea is numbered I. The larger of the two branches from it, the right main bronchus, is numbered II. The smaller branch, the left main bronchus, is numbered IO. The bronchus to the right cranial lobe is numbered IIO. This system allows each airway generation to have its own unique number, which also gives its branching history.

Comparison of side branch (minor daughter) diameter from silicone rubber casts and dissections of rabbit cranial lobes has shown little difference in measurements of the same airway generation. Branching patterns differ between lobes (cranial versus caudal) of the same species and between the same lobe in different species. Marked differences in epithelial population distribution within the airway tree are found between the same lobe of different species, i.e., cranial lobes of rabbit and sheep, and between different lobes in the same species, i.e., cranial

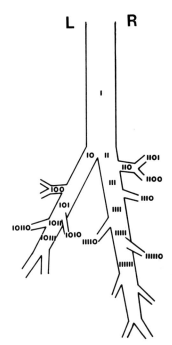

Fig. 6. Diagram of binary numbering system for the tracheobronchial tree of the rabbit Trachea (*I*), right primary bronchus (*II*), left primary bronchus (*IO*), right cranial lobar bronchus (*IIO*), and its intrapulmonary branches (*IIOI, IIOO*)

and caudal lobes of the sheep (PLOPPER et al. 1983 a, b; MARIASSY and PLOPPER 1983). The dissection approach to the morphological examination of pulmonary airways provides airway tissue specimens of precise definition in terms of branching history, generation number, and anatomic position within regions of the lung and within specific segments. Because precise sampling is possible, studies of airway epithelium can be performed which compare: (a) different generations in the same pathway; (b) bifurcation points and the airway segments between them; (c) terminal airways of short and long pathway lengths and large and small number of branchings; (d) terminal airways of different regions of same lobe (cranial versus caudal; dorsal versus ventral); (e) same generation in different lobes; and (f) same generation from animal to animal and species to species. While measurement of minor daughter openings appears reliable, dissections will not replace casts for such measurements as axial pathway lengths and diameters, branching angles, and total numbers of airways of a given generation.

III. Vascular Pattern

1. Vascular Injection

Examination of thin slices of lungs in which arterial and venous systems were injected with latex of different colors was used in studies of the comparative subgross pulmonary anatomy of a variety of mammals (MCLAUGHLIN et al. 1961, 1966). Vascular injection techniques currently are used as adjuncts to histologic examinations. They serve to differentiate arterial and venous systems, particularly at the microvascular level, and also enable contrast radiography to demonstrate overall vascular pattern. A method used extensively by L. Reid and her associates (DAVIES and REID 1970; MEYRICK and REID 1979, 1982) is based on the technique described by SHORT (1956). For rats, a barium sulfate and gelatin mixture at 60 °C is perfused through the pulmonary artery at a pressure of 100 cm H_2O. Lungs are subsequently inflated by intratracheal infusion of 2.5% buffered glutaraldehyde at a pressure of 23 cm H_2O (MEYRICK and REID 1982). This technique fills arteries down to about 15 μm in external diameter and the contrast medium does not cross the capillary bed. Arteriograms can be taken and the tissue sampled for qualitative and quantitative LM. The same technique applies to larger lungs such as those of humans, but adequate distension of the lung requires intratracheal infusion of fixative at a pressure of about 36 cm H_2O (RABINOVITCH and REID 1981).

An alternative technique for distinguishing arterial and venous sides of the capillary bed for histologic studies is the injection of gelatin mixed with chrome yellow dye into the pulmonary artery and with Monastral blue dye into the pulmonary vein (MICHEL 1982). The pulmonary capillary network can be contrasted for survey purposes by the examination of frozen sections of lungs injected with a mixture of india ink and gelatin (REID and HEARD 1962), but detailed evaluations of capillaries require morphometric approaches described elsewhere in this volume.

2. Vascular Casts

Corrosion casts of the pulmonary vascular tree have not been as widely used as those of the bronchial tree, although their advantages in providing three-dimensional data apply equally. References to the methods can be obtained from the work of HORSFIELD (1978).

IV. Structure of Pulmonary Vessels and Alveolar Walls

Where the focus of attention is on the structure of pulmonary vessels, the rigorous definition of the ultrastructure of alveolar walls, or both, fixation by vascular perfusion is preferable. This becomes paramount for most precise morphometry of these structures.

The closer one wants to approach the actual in vivo state, the more exacting become the methods both for preparing pulmonary tissue and for determining the nature and magnitude of processing artifacts. The advantages and disadvantages of various fixatives used for vascular perfusion by E. R. Weibel and his colleagues have been reevaluated recently (BACHOFEN et al. 1982). Their findings were based on the use of isolated, perfused rabbit lungs inflated by air at constant volume of 60% of total lung capacity. Perfusate flow rate, outflow pressure, pulmonary arterial pressure, transpulmonary pressure, and heart–lung weight were continuously recorded. Basically they found that, of various fixatives or combinations tested, best results from combined physiologic and practical standpoints were obtained with hypertonic glutaraldehyde (510 mosmol) followed in turn by isotonic osmium tetroxide and uranyl acetate. Isotonic glutaraldehyde solution (350 mosmol) was not suitable. All solutions contained 3% dextran T-70.

Where absolute morphometric measurements are not so critical, the technique of vascular perfusion can be simplified, either by perfusing vessels while maintaining steady intrapulmonary air pressure and without monitoring physiologic variables (HAIES et al. 1981) or by combined vascular perfusion and intratracheal instillation of fluid fixative. The latter is particularly useful for studies of pulmonary vessels. Histologic examination is carried out in lungs after vascular injection of a radiopaque barium sulfate and gelatin mixture, as described in Sect. C.III.1. This method is unsuitable for ultrastructural examination (MEYRICK and REID 1979). For ultrastructural observations, therefore, lungs are fixed by simultaneous injection of 2.5% glutaraldehyde in cacodylate buffer, total osmolarity 430 mosmol, into the pulmonary trunk and trachea at pressures of 100 and 23 cm H_2O, respectively. As used in rats, animals over 8 days of age have the pulmonary veins ligated at the hilus before fixation begins (MEYRICK and REID 1982). This causes blood to be cleared from arteries and accumulate in veins, thus aiding in distinguishing these two types of vessels.

Osmium vapor fixation through the airways combined with fixation by vascular perfusion provides highly effective demonstration of the alveolar lining layer (CALLAS 1982). Osmium vapor was used to inflate degassed lungs of rats. Pulmonary vessels were perfused serially with hypertonic glutaraldehyde, osmium tetroxide, and uranyl acetate. This was followed by perfusion with a graded series of ethanol solutions to enhance the reaction of the osmium tetroxide vapor and saturated lecithin in the surface lining layer.

V. Cryotechniques for Analysis of Structure and Function

Rapid freeze methods provide opportunities to obtain information concerning pulmonary morphology uncompromised by use of chemical fixatives. They are also required for microchemical elemental analyses of diffusible substances and cytochemical and immunologic procedures requiring the maximum number of undenatured active cell sites.

1. Morphological Studies Following Rapid Freezing

Chemical fixation by either the airways or vessels alters the physiologic properties of those tissues while they fix and are converted from flexible to rigid structures. The physical change causes alterations of resistance, flow, and pressures in the system by which the fixative is administered, which in turn influences pressures in adjacent interrelated structures. The overall results are slight changes in structural relationships as well as translocations of surface coats, fluids, and cells in the system or systems being perfused or infused. As discussed in Sect. C, precise control of pressures and flow rates can minimize these artifacts. For morphological studies in which these alterations and translocations are unacceptable, rapidly freezing lungs of anesthetized animals provides a narrow zone of tissue suitable for LM (STAUB and STOREY 1962), SEM (NOWELL and TYLER 1971; HOOK et al. 1980), and TEM (MAZZONE et al. 1979).

It is important to note that methods using rapid freezing followed by freeze substitution in substituting fluids without fixative resulted in more shrinkage than when substituting fluids containing fixatives were used (MAZZONE et al. 1980). In the latter case, shrinkage was the same as that from intravascular perfusion of the same fixative. Freeze drying of rapidly frozen lung in SEM results in less shrinkage than any of these procedures (HOOK et al. 1980) and provides opportunities to study nonvolatile substances in the pulmonary fluids. Morphometric studies must either consider this shrinkage or be performed on the frozen hydrated tissue. In general, however, rapidly frozen lungs are not suitable for widespread sampling necessary for morphometry of pulmonary parenchyma as a whole (WEIBEL et al. 1982).

Gross amounts of water and blood in lungs can be determined by a combination of gravimetric and tracer techniques (HUCHON et al. 1981). At the LM level, rapid freeze methods have been used to determine the localization of alveolar and interstitial fluids (PLOPPER et al. 1973) and capillary hematocrit (GLAZIER et al. 1969). At the ultrastructural level, the numbers and sizes of pinocytotic vesicles and "thoroughfare channels", factors which relate to transcapillary transport, can be determined in endothelium (MAZZONE and KORNBLAU 1981).

A major morphological application of rapid freezing is for study of surface structures revealed by freeze fracture or freeze fracture followed by freeze etching. Recent examples of use of the techniques are in studies of alveolar lining layer (MANABE 1979), lamellar bodies in alveolar type II cells (SCHULZ et al. 1980), mode of secretion of the Clara cell (YONEDA and BIRK 1981), intercellular junctions of tracheal epithelium as affected by ether anesthesia (INOUE and RICHARDSON 1979) or organ culture (CARSON et al. 1980), and intercellular junctions of the air–blood barrier (SCHNEEBERGER 1979) and alveolar epithelium (BARTELS et al. 1980; YONEDA 1982). A combination of freeze fracture and cytochemistry has been used by PINTO DA SILVA et al. (1981) to study anionic binding sites and concanavalin A binding sites in human leukocytes and HeLa cells.

2. Elemental Microanalysis

Microchemical elemental analyses can be performed on individual cells, and in most cases on individual cell organelles or inclusions, using analytic electron microscopy. General reference to the subject is provided in the monograph edited by HREN et al. (1979). While not in current use for evaluation of nonparticulate inhaled toxicants, these methods have broad application to biologic problems and will eventually be useful for evaluating pulmonary toxicity. The application of one form of analytic electron microscopy in pathology, X-ray microanalysis, has been reviewed by GHADIALLY (1979).

The problems related to the application of these techniques is not one of instrument capability, but rather of tissue preparation (HALL 1979). Using X-ray microanalysis, under favorable conditions, it is possible to detect approximately 10^{-19} g of an element in a thin section, with a spatial resolution of 20–30 nm (HALL 1979). While electron energy loss spectrometry is much less well developed for biologic studies, it has the ability to detect and quantitate elements with atomic number less than 10 and is thus useful for elements like carbon. An example of its potential usefulness is the mapping of fluorine-labeled serotonin (COSTA et al. 1978). New methods of microanalysis using electron beam instruments are being developed at a rapid pace (BAZETT-JONES and OTTENSMEYER 1981; OTTENSMEYER 1982).

Rapid "quench" freezing followed by examining frozen hydrated or frozen dried tissue appears to be the most useful method of tissue preparation for studies of diffusible or bound elements which occur naturally in pulmonary cells or are introduced by pretreatment (HALL 1979). Both research and commercially manufactured attachments are available for SEM to permit introduction and examination of hydrated frozen tissues which can be followed by further processing in the microscope or its attachments as required for additional observations or analyses (PAWLEY and NORTON 1978). Cryosectioning kits are now available for several ultramicrotomes and with modifications (ZIEROLD 1982) are useful for cutting hydrated frozen thin sections which can be introduced into TEM or STEM and examined in either the hydrated or freeze dried state. The difficulties inherent in cryoultramicrotomy as a preparative method for X-ray microanalysis and methods for circumventing them have recently been reviewed by ROOMANS et al. (1982).

When applied to freeze dried sections cut from carefully frozen tissue these powerful analytic methods are useful in localizing and obtaining semiquantitative analyses of diffusible ions and compounds of elements such as Na, P, S, Cl, K, and Ca on the cellular level (LECHENE 1980; RICK et al. 1982).

3. Cytochemistry

The usefulness of analytic EM can be extended through cytochemical introduction of elements not normally found in the cells. While most current cytochemical methods use fixed tissue, it is anticipated that the use of thin frozen sections will prove especially useful where preservation of undenatured active cell sites is critical. The final reaction products of immunoperoxidase cytochemical procedures can be quantitated with energy dispersive X-ray analysis when gold is substituted for osmium in the final diaminobenzidine reaction product (SIEGESMUND et al. 1979). Gold in the final reaction product of an immunocytochemical technique also results from the use of protein A labeled with colloidal gold (ROTH et al. 1978).

The protein A–gold technique was used for immunocytochemical localization and quantification of various pancreatic enzymes, including elastase, by BENDAYAN et al. (1980). The method would be useful for detecting constituents of pulmonary cells, but quantification by X-ray analysis would be more direct than the morphometric method used by BENDAYAN and colleagues. X-ray microprobe analysis has been used to study metal binding capacity of intestinal mucus (COLEMAN and YOUNG 1979).

VI. Morphological Assessment of Cellular Function

Because of the diversity of pulmonary cells and their corresponding functions, characterization of biologic activities by specific cell type is more critical for studies of lung than for most other organs. Correlation of structural and functional changes at the cellular and subcellular levels will rely to a large extent on techniques of cytochemistry, immunocytochemistry, and autoradiography.

1. Cytochemistry and Histochemistry

Emphasis in this section is on cytochemical methods at the ultrastructural level because of the greater investigative precision these provide. A number of different pulmonary cell products have been identified using a variety of electron-opaque stains. Several laboratories have demonstrated the utility of heavy metal stains to accentuate alveolar and bronchiolar surface lining material. Ruthenium red has been used to label intracellular and extracellular carbohydrates in lung, with routine methods of tissue processing (VACCARO and BRODY 1979, 1981) or with processing to retain lipid–carbohydrates (STRATTON et al. 1980). Carbohydrate moieties in the acellular lining layer of alveolar airspaces have been defined with concanavalin A (ROTH 1973; NIR and PEASE 1976) and ruthenium red (DIERICHS and LINDNER 1979). Phospholipids have been demonstrated by tricomplex flocculation (ADAMSON and Bowden 1970; Dermer 1970; Gil 1972). Alcian blue (ROTHMAN 1969), which has not as yet been used at the ultrastructural level on lung tissue, may also prove useful for surface carbohydrate localization. Combinations of osmium tetroxide and zinc (BLÜMCKE et al. 1973) or sodium iodide (McNARY and EL-BERMANI 1970) have been used to identify phopholipids within lamellar bodies of granular pneumonocytes.

Spicer and his co-workers have developed heavy metal stains for characterizing complex carbohydrates at the ultrastructural level (SPICER and SCHULTE 1982; SPICER et al. 1981). Periodic acid–thiocarbohydrazide–silver proteinate is used to identify glycoproteins (THIERY 1967) and dialyzed iron is used to demonstrate acidic glycoproteins (WETZEL et al. 1966). Sulfated glycoproteins are stained with high iron diamine (SPICER et al. 1978; SANNES et al. 1979). These methods have been employed to characterize glycoproteins and glycosaminoglycans in airway epithelium of the rat (SPICER et al. 1980), submucosal glands of the rat (MOCHIZU-KI et al. 1982), and serous epithelial cells in submucosal glands of the pig (TUREK et al. 1982). Tannic acid in sequence with ferric chloride, uranyl acetate, or gold chloride may also prove useful for localizing respiratory mucins (SANNES et al. 1978).

These ultrastructural methods have not yet been used for studies of changes in mucus following toxic insult to the lung, but histochemistry of mucus at the LM level has been used for assessing changes in epithelial and glandular mucous cell populations caused by inhalation of a variety of toxic substances. Examples are the studies of tobacco smoke (JONES and REID 1978; GREIG et al. 1980), sulfur dioxide (SPICER et al. 1974; RANA et al. 1979), and carbon monoxide and nitrogen dioxide (RANA et al. 1979).

Cytochemical procedures for identifying sites of intracellular enzyme activity by EM have proven effective when applied to normal lung tissue. Microbodies, or peroxisomes, have been characterized in both type II pneumonocytes and Clara cells in a large number of species (PETRIK 1971; SCHNEEBERGER 1972; ACH-TERRATH and BLÜMCKE 1975; GOLDENBERG et al. 1978). This procedure depends on the reaction of the catalase within peroxisomes with 3′,3′-diaminobenzidine and hydrogen peroxide. Cyclic adenosine monophosphate (cAMP) phosphodiesterase has recently has been demonstrated on the plasma membrane of type II pneumonocytes (SINGER and ARIANO 1981).

Various other enzymes have also been studied in lung cells by ultrastructural cytochemistry: glucose-6-phosphatase, thiamine pyrophosphatase, alkaline phosphatase, acid phosphatase, esterase, aryl sulfatase B, and β-glucuronidase. Some of these enzymes have been characterized in Clara cells (CASTLEMAN et al. 1973; KUHN and CALLAWAY 1975; YONEDA 1978) and type II pneumonocytes (GOLDFISCHER et al. 1968; VATTER et al. 1968; CASTLEMAN et al. 1973). Carbonic anhydrase has been found not only in pulmonary endothelial cells, but also in type I and II pneumonocytes (SUGAI et al. 1981).

Histochemical studies by LM include: oxidative enzymes in alveolar tissue (TYLER and PEARSE 1965; TYLER et al. 1965; SOROKIN 1967) and bronchial glands (SOROKIN 1965; AZZOPARDI and THURLBECK 1968); lactic acid dehydrogenase (SHERWIN et al. 1967); and reductases identified with tetrazolium salts (ETHERTON et al. 1973a). There have been few applications of cytochemistry and histochemistry to inhalation toxicology thus far. Reactivities of two enzymes, acid phosphatase (CASTLEMAN et al. 1973) and lactic acid dehydrogenase (SHERWIN et al. 1967) have been shown to be modified by inhalation of oxidant air pollutants. Quantitative changes in two lysosomal enzymes, acid phosphatase and β-glucuronidase, in alveolar macrophages of rats exposed to ozone were measured by LM cytospectrophometry and the results correlated with impaired bactericidal capability (GOLDSTEIN et al. 1978).

2. Immunocytochemistry

Immunocytochemistry has been little used for assessment of toxic effects on lung tissue, but shows great promise. Many procedures have been codified (STERNBERGER 1979). Five aspects have been investigated in normal lung: the localization of cell surface receptors on pulmonary alveolar macrophages in situ (McKEEVER and SPICER 1979); the amount and distribution of the cytochrome P-450 monooxygenase system (DEES et al. 1980; SERABJIT SINGH et al. 1980; DEVEREUX et al. 1981); the antigenic components of the alveolar lining layer (BIGNON et al. 1976; WILLIAMS and BENSON 1981); distribution of immunoglobins within the respiratory tract (BRADLEY et al. 1976; ALLEY et al. 1980); and localization of serotonin in intrapulmonary neuroepithelial bodies (LAUWERYNS et al. 1982). These may yield significant new information when applied to toxicologic studies. The basic requirements are a substance of interest which is sufficiently antigenic to produce an antibody reaction in a different species and either the purified primary antisera or a monoclonal antibody prepared by the hybridoma technique. The reaction can be carried out either en bloc in fixed or fresh tissue or on paraffin-embedded or plastic-embedded sections. Fluorescein, rhodamine, or peroxidase labels can be used for assessing the reaction product by LM, and peroxidase, colloidal gold, or ferritin can be used for TEM.

The potential for using monoclonal antibodies as specific probes of functional alterations in damaged cells opens up exciting new possibilities in toxicologic research. KENNETT et al. (1980), KOHLER (1981), SPRINGER (1981), and READING (1982) provide an introduction to the rapidly expanding literature on the hybridoma technique and applications of the monoclonal antibodies it produces.

3. Autoradiography

Autoradiography has been employed to assess the intracellular and extracellular distribution of two general categories of radioisotopically labeled tracers: precursors of DNA (primarily thymidine) and precursors of secretory products from granular pneumonocytes, Clara cells, and mucous goblet cells.

The utility and hazards of evaluating lung cell proliferation using autoradiography have recently been throughly reviewed by KAUFFMAN (1980). With the appropriate use of pulse labeling with thymidine^{3}H or thymidine^{14}C, and counts of labeled cells, cells in metaphase, and labeled cells in metaphase, most aspects of pulmonary cell kinetics can be determined. Detailed aspects of autoradiography for cell kinetic studies are contained in Chap. 11.

To assess synthetic pathways, a wide range of radiolabeled substances have been applied to lung tissue. The vast majority of these studies have been directed toward determining the source and cellular pathways of pulmonary surfactant biosynthesis in type II pneumonocytes. The precursors used have included choline (CHEVALIER and COLLET 1972; SMITH et al. 1980; SAFFITZ et al. 1981), palmitic and other fatty acids (BUCKINGHAM et al. 1966; ASKIN and KUHN 1971; ADAMSON and BOWDEN 1973; SMITH and KIKKAWA 1979, SMITH et al. 1980), glycerol (FAULKNER 1969), cholesterol (DARRAH et al. 1971), leucine (MASSARO and MASSARO 1972; CHEVALIER and COLLET 1972), and galactose (CHEVALIER and COLLET 1972). Other work has focused on the Clara cell with palmitic acid (ETHERTON et al. 1973 b), leucine (PETRIK and COLLET 1974; EBERT et al. 1976), choline (PETRIK and COLLET 1974), acetate (PETRIK and COLLET 1974), glucosamine (EBERT et al. 1976), and galactose (PETRIK and COLLET 1974; EBERT et al. 1976). Mucus secretion by goblet cells has been studied with glucose (NEUTRA and LEBLOND 1966; MEYRICK and REID 1975) and threonine (MEYRICK and REID 1975).

The binding of toxic compounds to lung cells has also been determined with autoradiography. Two excellent examples are: the binding of ipomeanol, a substrate for the cytochrome P-450 monooxygenase system, to Clara cells in a number of species (BOYD 1977); and the binding of a carcinogen, N-nitrosodiethylamine to respiratory tract epithelium (REZNIK-SCHULLER and HAGUE 1981).

D. Conclusions

The methods for routine qualitative assessment of pulmonary damage from inhaled toxins are well established, although choice has to be made among several alternatives for fixation and sampling. Developments will occur in two major areas. One will be the increasing use of morphometry for quantification of structural abnormalities, which is especially important for the definition of subtle changes. The other will be the application of cytochemistry, immunocytochemistry, and electron probe analysis as crucial components of mechanistic studies.

Acknowledgments. The authors gratefully acknowledge the assistance of Jody Wall and Mary Whitehill in preparation of the manuscript.

References

Achterrath U, Blümcke S (1975) Electron-histochemical investigations on clara cells and type II pneumocytes of normal rat lungs. Pneumonologie 152:123–129

Adamson IYR, Bowden DH (1970) A cytochemical partition of phospholipid surfactant and mucopolysaccharide. Am J Pathol 61:359–368

Adamson IYR, Bowden DH (1973) The intracellular site of surfactant synthesis. Autoradiographic studies on murine and avian lung explants. Exp Mol Pathol 18:112–124

Alley MR, Wells PW, Smith WD, Gardiner AC (1980) The distribution of immunoglobulin in the respiratory tract of sheep. Vet Pathol 17:372–380

Anderson TF (1951) Techniques for the preservation of three-dimensional structure in preparing specimens for the electron microscope. Trans NY Acad Sci Ser II 13:130–134

Askin FB, Kuhn C (1971) The cellular origin of pulmonary surfactant. Lab Invest 25:260–268

Azzopardi A, Thurlbeck WM (1968) Oxidative enzyme pattern of the bronchial mucous glands. Am Rev Respir Dis 97:1038–1045

Bachofen H, Ammann A, Wangensteen D, Weibel ER (1982) Perfusion fixation of lungs for structure-function analysis: credits and limitations. J Appl Physiol 53:528–533

Bartels H, Oestern H-J, Voss-Wermbter G (1980) Communicating-occluding junction complexes in the alveolar epithelium. A freeze-fracture study. Am Rev Respir Dis 121:1017–1024

Bazett-Jones DP, Ottensmeyer DP (1981) Phosphorus distribution in the nucleosome. Science 211:160–170

Bendayan M, Roth J, Perrelet A, Orci L (1980) Quantitative immunocytochemical localization of pancreatic secretory proteins in subcellular compartments of the rat acinar cell. J Histochem Cytochem 28:149–160

Bignon J, Jaurand MC, Pinchon MC, Sapin C, Warnet JM (1976) Immunoelectron microscopic and immunochemical demonstrations of serum proteins in the alveolar lining material of the rat lung. Am Rev Respir Dis 113:109–120

Blümcke S, Kessler WD, Niedorf HR, Becker NH, Veith FJ (1973) Ultrastructure of lamellar bodies of type II pneumocytes after osmium-zinc impregnation. J Ultrastruc Res 42:417–433

Boyd M (1977) Evidence for the clara cell as a site of cytochrome P-450-dependent mixed-function oxidase activity in lung. Nature 269:713–715

Bradley PA, Bourne FJ, Brown PJ (1976) The respiratory tract immune system in the pig I. Distribution of immunoglobulin-containing cells in the respiratory tract mucosa. Vet Pathol 13:81–89

Brummer MEG, Lowrie PM, Tyler WS (1975) A technique for sequential examination of specific areas of large tissue blocks using SEM, LM and TEM. In: Johari O, Corvin I (eds) Scanning electron microscopy, vol I. IIT Research Institute, Chicago, pp 333–340

Buckingham S, Heinemann HO, Sommers SC, McNary WF (1966) Phospholipid synthesis in the large pulmonary alveolar cell. Its relation to lung surfactants. Am J Pathol 48:1027–1038

Callas G (1982) Osmium vapor fixation of pulmonary surfactant. Anat Rec 203:301–306

Carson JL, Collier AM, Hu SS (1980) Ultrastructural studies of hamster tracheal epithelium in vivo and in vitro. J Ultrastruc Res 70:70–78

Castleman WL, Dungworth DL, Tyler WS (1973) Cytochemically detected alterations of lung acid phosphatase reactivity following ozone exposure. Lab Invest 29:310–319

Chevalier G, Collet AJ (1972) In vivo incorporation of choline-^{3}H, leucine-^{3}H and galactose-^{3}H in alveolar type II pneumocytes in relation to surfactant synthesis. A quantitative radioautographic study in mouse by electron microscopy. Anat Rec 174:289–310

Clark G (ed) (1981) Staining procedures, fourth edn. Williams and Wilkins, Baltimore

Coleman JR, Young LB (1979) Metal binding by intestinal mucus. In: Johari O, Becker RD (eds) Scanning electron microscopy, vol II. SEM Inc., Chicago, pp 801–806

Costa JL, Joy DC, Maher DM, Kirk KL, Hui SW (1978) Fluorinated molecule as a tracer: difluoroserotonin in human platelets mapped by electron energy-loss spectroscopy. Science 200:537–539

Côté RA, Korthy AL, Kory RC (1963) Laminated lung macrosections: a new dimension in the study and teaching of pulmonary pathology. Dis Chest 43:1–7

Dahl AR, Hadley WM, Hahn FF, Benson JM, McClellan RO (1982) Cytochrome P-450-dependent monooxygenases in olfactory epithelium of dogs: possible role in tumorigenicity. Science 216:57–59

Darrah HK, Hedley-White J, Hedley-White ET (1971) Radioautography of cholesterol in lung. An assessment of different tissue processing techniques. J Cell Biol 49:345–361

Davies G, Reid L (1970) Growth of the alveoli and pulmonary arteries in childhood. Thorax 25:669–681

Dees JH, Coe LD, Yasukochi Y, Master BS (1980) Immunofluorescence of NADPH – cytochrome C (P-450) reductase in rat and minipig tissue injected with phenobarbital. Science 208:1473–1475

Dermer GB (1970) The fixation of pulmonary surfactant for electron microscopy II. Transport of surfactant through the air-blood barrier. J Ultrastruc Res 31:229–246

Devereux TR, Serabjit-Singh CJ, Slaughter SR, Wolf CR, Philpot RM, Fouts JR (1981) Identification of cytochrome P-450 isozymes in nonciliated bronchiolar epithelial (Clara) and alveolar type II cells isolated from rabbit lung. Exp Lung Res 2:221–230

Dierichs R, Lindner E (1979) Ultrahistochemical investigations of dog lung surfactant with ruthenium red and iodoplatinate reactions. Histochemistry 60:335–346

Ebert RV, Kronenberg RS, Terracio MJ (1976) Study of the surface secretion of the bronchiole using radioautography. Am Rev Respir Dis 114:567–573

Etherton JE, Conning DM, Jones GRN (1973a) The demonstration of mouse lung lactate-yellow tetrazolium reductase. Histochemie 33:287–290

Etherton JE, Conning DM, Corrin B (1973b) Autoradiographical and morphological evidence for apocrine secretion of dipalmitoyl lecithin in the terminal bronchiole of mouse lung. Am J Anat 138:11–36

Faulkner CS (1969) The role of the granular pneumocyte in surfactant metabolism. An autoradiographic study. Arch Pathol 87:521–525

Flood PR (1975) Dry-fracturing techniques for the study of soft internal biological tissues in the scanning electron microscope. In: Johari O, Corvin I (eds) Scanning electron microscopy, vol I. IIT Research Institute, Chicago, pp 287–294

Gamsu G, Thurlbeck WM, Macklem PT, Fraser RG (1971a) Peripheral bronchographic morphology in the normal human lung. Invest Radiol 6:161–170

Gamsu G, Thurlbeck WM, Macklem PT, Fraser RG (1971b) Roentgenographic appearance of the human pulmonary acinus. Invest Radiol 6:171–175

Ghadially FN (1979) Invited review. The technique and scope of electronprobe X-ray analysis in pathology. Pathology 11:95–110

Gil J (1972) Effect of tricomplex fixation on lung tissue. J Ultrastruc Res 40:122–131

Gil J, McNiff JM (1982) Early tissue damage in ethchlorvynol-induced alveolar edema in rabbit lung. Am Rev Respir Dis 126:701–707

Gil J, Weibel ER (1968) The role of buffers in lung fixation with glutaraldehyde and osmium tetroxide. J Ultrastruc Res 25:331–348

Glauert AM (1974) Fixation, dehydration and embedding of biological specimens. In: Glauert AM (ed) Practical methods in electron microscopy, vol 3. Elsevier, New York, p 1

Glazier JB, Hughes JMB, Maloney JE, West JB (1969) Measurements of capillary dimensions and blood volume in rapidly frozen lung. J Appl Physiol 26:65–76

Goldenberg H, Huttinger M, Kollner U, Kramar R, Pavelka M (1978) Catalase positive particles from pig lung. Biochemical preparations and morphological studies. Histochemistry 56:253–264

Goldfischer S, Kikkawa Y, Hoffman L (1968) The demonstration of acid hydrolase activities in the inclusion bodies of type II alveolar cells and other lysosomes in the rabbit lung. J Histochem Cytochem 16:102–109

Goldstein E, Bartlema HC, van der Ploeg M, van Duijn P, van der Stap JGMM, Lippert W (1978) Effect of ozone on lysosomal enzymes of alveolar macrophages engaged in phagocytosis and killing of inhaled staphylococcus aureus. J Infect Dis 138:299–311

Gough J, Wentworth JD (1960) Thin sections of entire organs mounted on paper. In: Harrison CV (ed) Recent advances in pathology, 7th edn. Churchill, London, p 80

Greig N, Ayers M, Jeffery PK (1980) The effect of indomethacin on the response of bronchial epithelium to tobacco smoke. J Pathol 132:1–9

Grimley PM (1965) Selection for electron microscopy of specific areas in large epoxy tissue sections. Stain Technol 40:259–263

Gross P, Pfitzer EA, Hatch TF (1966) Alveolar clearance: its relation to lesions of the respiratory bronchiole. Am Rev Respir Dis 94:10–19

Haies DM, Gil J, Weibel ER (1981) Morphometric study of rat lung cells I. Numerical and dimensional characteristics of parenchymal cell population. Am Rev Respir Dis 123:533–541

Hall TA (1979) Biological x-ray microanalysis. J Microsc 117:145–163

Hayatdavoudi G, Crapo JD, Miller FJ, O'Neil J (1980) Factors determining degree of inflation in intratracheally fixed rat lungs. J Appl Physiol 48:389–393

Heard BE (1958) A pathological study of emphysema of the lungs with chronic bronchitis. Thorax 13:136–149

Heard BE (1960) Pathology of pulmonary emphysema: methods of study. Am Rev Respir Dis 82:792–799

Heard BE, Esterly JR, Wootliff JS (1967) A modified apparatus for fixing lungs to study the pathology of emphysema. Am Rev Respir Dis 95:311–312

Hendriks HR, Eestermans IL (1982) Electron dense granules and the role of buffers: artefacts from fixation with glutaraldehyde and osmium tetroxide. J Microsc 126:161–168

Hodde KC, Nowell JA (1980) SEM of micro-corrosion casts. In: Becker RP, Johari O (eds) Scanning electron microscopy, vol II. SEM Inc., Chicago, pp 89–106

Hook G, Lai C, Bastacky J, Hayes T (1980) Conductive coatings studied on inflated lung in the frozen-hydrated and freeze dried states. In: Johari O, Becker RP (eds) Scanning electron microscopy, vol IV. SEM Inc., Chicago, pp 27–32

Horsfield K (1978) Morphometry of the small pulmonary arteries in man. Circ Res 42:593–597

Horsfield K, Cumming G (1976) Morphology of the bronchial tree in the dog. Respir Physiol 26:173–182

Horsfield K, Cumming G, Hicken P (1966) A morphologic study of airway disease using bronchial glands. Am Rev Respir Dis 93:900–906

Horsfield K, Dart G, Olson DE, Filley GF, Cumming G (1971) Models of the human bronchial tree. J Appl Physiol 31:207–217

Horsfield K, Kemp W, Phillips S (1982) An asymmetrical model of the airways of the dog lung. J Appl Physiol 52:21–26

Hren JJ, Goldstein JI, Joy DC (eds) (1979) Introduction of analytical electron microscopy. Plenum, New York

Huchon GJ, Hopewell PC, Murray JF (1981) Interactions between permeability and hydrostatic pressure in perfused dogs' lung. J Appl Physiol 50:905–911

Humphreys WJ, Spurlock BO, Johnson JS (1974) Critical point drying of ethanol-infiltrated, cryofractured biological specimens for scanning electron microscopy. In: Johari O, Corvin I (eds) Scanning electron microscopy, vol I. IIT Research Institute, Chicago, pp 275–282

Inoue S, Richardson JB (1979) A correlated thin section and freeze-fracture study of mouse tracheal epithelium before and after ether anesthesia. Lab Invest 40:583–586

Jones R, Reid L (1978) Secretory cell hyperplasia and modification of intracellular glycoprotein in rat airways induced by short periods of exposure to tobacco smoke, and the effect of the antiinflammatory agent phenylmethyloxadiazol. Lab Invest 39:41–49

Kauffman SL (1980) Cell proliferation in the mammalian lung. Int Rev Exp Pathol 22:131–191

Kennett R, McKearn T, Bechtol K (eds) (1980) Monoclonal antibodies: hybridomas, a new dimension in biological analyses. Plenum, New York

Kleinerman J, Cowdrey CR (1964) The thick-section technique for the study of pulmonary pathology. Am Rev Respir Dis 89:206–213

Kohler G (1981) The technique of hybridoma production. In: Lefkovits I, Pernis B (eds) Immunological methods, vol II. Academic, New York, p 285

Kory RC, Rauterkus LT, Korthy AL, Côté RA (1966) Quantitative estimation of pulmonary emphysema in lung macrosections by photoelectric measurement of transmitted light. Am Rev Respir Dis 93:758–768

Kuhn C, Callaway LA (1975) The formation of granules in the bronchiolar clara cells of the rat: II. enzyme cytochemistry. J Ultrastruc Res 53:66–76

Langston C, Waszkiewicz E, Thurlbeck WM (1979) A simple method for the representative sampling of lungs of diverse size. Thorax 34:527–530

Lauweryns JM, de Bock V, Verhofstad AAJ, Steinbusch HWM (1982) Immunohistochemical localization of serotonin in intrapulmonary neuro-epithelial bodies. Cell Tissue Res 226:215–223

Lechene C (1980) Electron probe microanalysis of biological soft tissues: principle and technique. Fed Proc 39:2871–2880

Lee RMKW, McKenzie R, Kobayashi K, Garfield RE, Forrest JB, Daniel EE (1982) Effects of glutaraldehyde fixative osmolarities on smooth muscle cell volume, and osmotic reactivity of the cells after fixation. J Microsc 125:77–88

Lowrie PM, Tyler WS (1973) Selection and preparation of specific tissue regions for TEM using large epoxy-embedded blocks. In: Arceneaux CT (ed) Proc 31st ann Meet Electron Microsc Soc Am, New Orleans. Claitors, Baton Rouge, pp 324–325

Lum H (1981) Transmission electron microscopic morphometry of pulmonary alveolar macrophages: a comparison of lavaged and in situ macrophages from ozone-exposed and control rats. PhD thesis. University of California, Davis

Luna LG (1968) Manual of histologic staining methods of the Armed Forces Institute of Pathology, third ed. McGraw-Hill, New York

Manabe T (1979) Freeze-fracture study of alveolar lining layer in adult rat lungs. J Ultrastruc Res 69:86–97

Mariassy AT, Plopper CG (1983) Tracheobronchial epithelium of the sheep. I. quantitative light microscopic study of epithelial cell abundance and distribution. Anat Rec 205:263–275

Massaro GD, Massaro D (1972) Granular pneumocytes. Electron microscopic radioautographic evidence of intracellular protein transport. Am Rev Respir Dis 105:927–931

Mathieu O, Claassen H, Weibel ER (1978) Differential effect of glutaraldehyde and buffer osmolarity on cell dimensions: a study on lung tissue. J Ultrastruc Res 63:20–34

Mazzone RW, Kornblau SM (1981) Pinocytotic vesicles in the endothelium of rapidly frozen rabbit lung. Microvasc Res 21:193–211

Mazzone RW, Durand CM, West JB (1979) Electron microscopic appearances of rapidly frozen lung. J Microsc 117:269–284

Mazzone RW, Kornblau SM, Durand CM (1980) Shrinkage of lung after chemical fixation for analysis of pulmonary structure-function relations. J Appl Physiol 48:382–385

McDowell EM, Trump BF (1976) Histological fixatives suitable for diagnostic light and electron microscopy. Arch Pathol Lab Med 100:405–414

McKeever PE, Spicer SS (1979) Demonstration of immune complex receptors on macrophage surfaces and erythrocytic endogenous peroxidase with correlated markers for light microscopy, scanning electron microscopy and transmission electron microscopy. In: Johari O, Becker RP (eds) Scanning electron microscopy, vol III. SEM Inc., Chicago, pp 601–618

McLaughlin RF, Tyler WS, Canada RO (1961) A study of the subgross pulmonary anatomy in various animals. Am J Anat 108:149–165

McLaughlin RF, Tyler WS, Canada RO (1966) Subgross pulmonary anatomy of the rabbit, rat, and guinea pig, with additional notes on the human lung. Am Rev Respir Dis 94:380–387

McNary WF, El-Bermani A-W (1970) Differentiating type I and type II alveolar cells in rat lung by OSO_4 – NaI staining. Stain Technol 45:215–219

Mellick PW, Dungworth DL, Schwartz LM, Tyler WS (1977) Short term morphologic effects of high ambient levels of ozone on lungs of rhesus monkeys. Lab Invest 36:82–90

Meyrick B, Reid L (1975) In vitro incorporation of [³H] threonine and [³H] glucose by the mucous and serous cells of the human bronchial submucosal gland. A quantitative electron microscope study. J Cell Biol 67:320–344

Meyrick B, Reid L (1979) Ultrastructural features of the distended pulmonary arteries of the normal rat. Anat Rec 193:71–98

Meyrick B, Reid L (1982) Pulmonary arterial and alveolar development in normal post natal rat lung. Am Rev Respir Dis 125:468–473

Michel, RP (1982) Arteries and veins of the normal dog lung: qualitative and quantitative structural differences. Am J Anat 164:227–241

Mochizuki I, Setser ME, Martinez JR, Spicer SS (1982) Carbohydrate histochemistry of rat respiratory glands. Anat Rec 202:45–59

Neutra M, Leblond CP (1966) Synthesis of the carbohydrate of mucus in the golgi complex as shown by electron microscope radioautography of globlet cells from rats injected with glucose − ³H. J Cell Biol 30:119–136

Nir I, Pease DC (1976) Polysaccharides in lung alveoli. Am J Anat 147:457–470

Nowell JA, Pawley JB (1980) Preparation of experimental animal tissue for SEM. In: Becker RP, Johari O (eds) Scanning electron microscopy, vol II. SEM Inc., Chicago, pp 1–19

Nowell JA, Tyler WS (1971) Scanning electron microscopy of the surface morphology of mammalian lungs. Am Rev Respir Dis 103:313–328

Nowell JA, Pangborn J, Tyler WS (1972) Stabilization and replication of soft tubular and alveolar systems. A SEM study of the lung. In: Johari O, Corvin I (eds) Scanning electron microscopy, vol II. IIT Research Institute, Chicago, pp 305–312

Ottensmeyer FP (1982) Scattered electrons in microscopy and microanalysis. Science 251:461–466

Pääkkö P (1981) Radiography of excised air-inflated human lungs in autopsy pathology. Diagnostic values and limitations. Acta Univ OULU, series D, number 74 (Anat Pathol Microbiol 12)

Pawley JB, Norton JT (1978) A chamber attached to the SEM for fracturing and coating frozen biological samples. J Microsc 112:169–182

Pawley JB, Nowell JA (1973) Microdissection of biological SEM samples for further study in the TEM. In: Johario O, Corvin I (eds) Scanning electron microscopy. IIT Research Institute, Chicago, pp 333–340

Petrik P (1971) Fine structural identification of peroxisomes in mouse and rat bronchiolar and alveolar epithelium. J Histochem Cytochem 19:339–348

Petrik P, Collet AJ (1974) Quantitative electron microscopic autoradiography of in vivo incorporation of ³H-choline, ³H-leucine, ³H-acetate and ³H-galactose in non-ciliated bronchiolar (Clara) cells of mice. Am J Anat 139:519–534

Phalen RF, Yeh HC, Raabe OG, Velasquez DJ (1973) Casting of the lung in situ. Anat Rec 177:255–264

Phalen RF, Yeh JC, Schum GM, Raabe OG (1978) Application of an idealized model to morphometry of the mammalian tracheobronchial tree. Anat Rec 190:167–176

Pinto da Silva P, Parkison C, Dwyer N (1981) Freeze-fracture cytochemistry: thin sections of cells and tissues after labeling of fracture faces. J Histochem Cytochem 29:917–928

Plopper CG, Dungworth DL, Tyler WS (1973) Pulmonary lesions in rats exposed to ozone. A correlated light and electron microscopic study. Am J Pathol 71:375–394

Plopper CG, Halsebo JE, Berger WJ, Sonstegard KS, Nettesheim P (1983a) Distribution of nonciliated bronchiolar epithelial (Clara) cells in intrapulmonary and extrapulmonary airways of the rabbit. Exp Lung Res 5:79–98

Plopper CG, Mariassy AT, Lollini LO (1983b) Structure as revealed by airway dissection: A comparison of mammalian lungs. Am Rev Respir Dis 128:54–57

Popp JA, Martin JT (1981) Method for the ultrastructural evaluation of rodent nasal mucosa. In: Bailey GW (ed) 39th Ann Proc Electron Miscroscopy Soc Am, Atlanta. Claitors, Baton Rouge, pp 594–595

Pump KK (1973) The pattern of development of emphysema in the human lung. Am Rev Respir Dis 108:610–620

Pump KK (1974) Fenestrae in the alveolar membrane of the human lung. Chest 65:431–436

Raabe OG, Yeh HC, Newton GJ, Phalen RF, Velasquez DJ (1976) Tracheobronchial geometry: human, dog, rat, hamster. Lovelace Foundation for Medical Education and Research LF-53, Albuquerque

Rabinovitch M, Reid LM (1981) Quantitative structural analysis of the pulmonary vascular bed in congenital heart defects. In: Augle A (ed) Pediatric cardiovascular disease. Davis, Philadelphia, p 149

Rana SVS, Agrawal VP, Gautam RK (1979) Histochemical approach to mucin in the trachea and lungs of squirrels, exposed to three chief air pollutants (CO, SO_2 and NO_2). Mikroskopie 35:77–81

Reading CL (1982) Theory and methods for immunization in culture and monoclonal antibody production. J Immunol Methods 53:261–291

Reid A, Heard BE (1962) Preliminary studies of human pulmonary capillaries by india ink injection. Med Thorac 19:215–219

Reznik-Schuller HM, Hague BF (1981) Autoradiographic study of the distribution of bound radioactivity in the respiratory tract of Syrian hamsters given N-[^{3}H] Nitrosodiethylamine. Cancer Res 41:2147–2150

Rick R, Dorge A, Thurau K (1982) Quantitative analysis of electrolytes in frozen dried sections. J Microsc 125:239–247

Roomans GM, Wei X, Seveus L (1982) Cryoultramicrotomy as a preparative method for x-ray microanalysis in pathology. Ultrastruc Pathol 3:65–84

Roth J (1973) Ultrahistochemical demonstration of saccharide components of complex carbohydrate at the alveolar cell surface of the pleura visceralis of mice by means of concanavalin A. Exp Pathol 8:157–167

Roth J, Bendayan M, Orci L (1978) Ultrastructural localization of intracellular antigens by the use of protein A-gold complex. J Histochem Cytochem 26:1074–1081

Rothman AH (1969) Alcian blue as an electron stain. Exp Cell Res 58:177–179

Saffitz JE, Gross RW, Williamson JR, Sobel BE (1981) Autoradiography of phosphatidyl choline. J Histochem Cytochem 29:371–378

Sannes PL, Katsuyama T, Spicer SS (1978) Tannic acid-metal salt sequences for light and electron microscopic localization of complex carbohydrates. J Histochem Cytochem 26:55–61

Sannes PL, Spicer SS, Katsuyama T (1979) Ultrastructural localization of sulfated complex carbohydrates with a modified iron diamine procedure. J Histochem Cytochem 27:1108–1111

Scherle W (1970) A simple method for volumetry of organs in quantitative stereology. Mikroskopie 25:57–60

Schiff RI, Gennaro JF (1979) The role of the buffer in the fixation of biological specimens for transmission and scanning electron microscopy. Scanning 2:135–148

Schneeberger EE (1972) A comparative cytochemical study of microbodies (peroxisomes) in great alveolar cells of rodents, rabbit and monkey. J Histochem Cytochem 20:180–191

Schneeberger EE (1979) Barrier function of intercellular junctions in adult and fetal lungs. In: Fishman AP, Renkin EM (eds) Pulmonary edema. American Physiological Society, Bethesda, p 21

Schneeberger-Keeley EE, Karnovsky MJ (1968) The ultrastructural basis of alveolar-capillary membrane permeability to peroxidase used as a tracer. J Cell Biol 37:781–793

Schreider JP, Raabe OG (1980) Replica casts of the entire respiratory airways of experimental animals. J Exp Pathol Toxicol 4:427–435

Schreider JP, Raabe OG (1981 a) Anatomy of the nasal-pharyngeal airway of experimental animals. Anat Rec 200:195–205

Schreider JP, Raabe OG (1981 b) Structure of the human respiratory acinus. Am J Anat 162:221–232

Schulz WW, McAnalley WH, Reynolds RC (1980) Freeze-fracture study of pulmonary lamellar body membranes in solid crystal phase. J Ultrastruc Res 71:37–48

Schwartz LW, Dungworth DL, Mustafa MG, Tarkington BK, Tyler WS (1976) Pulmonary responses of rats to ambient levels of ozone. Effects of 7-day intermittent of continuous exposure. Lab Invest 34:565–578

Serabjit-Singh CJ, Wolf CR, Philpot RM, Plopper CG (1980) Cytochrome P-450: localization in rabbit lung. Science 207:1469–1470

Sherwin RP, Winnick S, Buckley RD (1967) Response of lactic acid dehydrogenase-positive alveolar cells in the lungs of guinea pigs exposed to nitric oxide. Am Rev Respir Dis 96:319–325

Short DS (1956) Post-mortem pulmonary arteriography with special reference to the study of pulmonary hypertension. J Fac Radiol 8:118–131

Siegesmund KA, Yorde DE, Dragen R (1979) A quantitative immunoperoxidase procedure employing energy dispersive X-ray analysis. J Histochem Cytochem 27:1226–1230

Singer AL, Ariano MA (1981) Localization of cyclic adenosine monophosphate phosphodiesterase in mouse alveolar cells. J Histochem Cytochem 29:1372–1376

Smith FB, Kikkawa Y (1979) The type II epithelial cells of the lung V. Synthesis of phosphatidyl glycerol in isolated type II cells and pulmonary alveolar macrophages. Lab Invest 40:172–177

Smith FB, Kikkawa Y, Diglio CA, Dalen RC (1980) The type II epithelial cells of the lung VI. Incorporation of ^{3}H-choline and ^{3}H-palmitate into lipids of cultured type II cells. Lab Invest 42:296–301

Sorokin SP (1965) On the cytology and cytochemistry of the opossum's bronchial glands. Am J Anat 117:311–338

Sorokin SP (1967) A morphologic and cytochemical study on the great alveolar cell. J Histochem Cytochem 14:884–897

Spicer SS, Schulte BA (1982) Ultrastructural methods for localizing complex carbohydrates. Hum Pathol 13:343–354

Spicer SS, Chakrin LW, Wardell JR (1974) Effect of chronic sulfur dioxide inhalation on the carbohydrate histochemistry and histology of the canine respiratory tract. Am Rev Respir Dis 110:13–14

Spicer SS, Hardin JH, Setser ME (1978) Ultrastructural visualization of sulfated complex carbohydrates in blood and epithelial cells with the high iron diamine procedure. J Histochem Cytochem 10:435–452

Spicer SS, Mochizuki I, Setser ME, Martinez JR (1980) Complex carbohydrates of rat tracheobronchial surface epithelium visualized ultrastructurally. Am J Anat 158:93–109

Spicer SS, Baron DA, Sato A, Schulte BA (1981) Variability of cell surface glycoconjugates – relation to differences in cell function. J Histochem Cytochem 29:994–1002

Springer TA (1981) Monoclonal antibody analysis of complex biological systems. Combination of cell hybridization and immunoadsorbents in a novel cascade procedure and its application to the macrophage cell surface. J Biol Chem 256:3833–3839

Staub NC, Storey WF (1962) Relation between morphological and physiological events in lung studied by rapid freezing. J Appl Physiol 17:381–390

Stephens RJ, Evans MJ (1973) Selection and orientation of lung tissue for scanning and transmission electron microscopy. Environ Res 6:52–59

Sternberger LA (1979) Immunocytochemistry. Prentice-Hall, Englewood Cliffs

Stratton CJ, Wetzstein HY, Hardy T (1980) The ultrastructural histochemistry and stereoscanning electron microscopy of the rodent and amphibian surfactant systems. Anat Rec 197:49–61

Sugai N, Ninomiya Y, Oosaki T (1981) Localization of carbonic anhydrase in the rat lung. Histochemistry 72:415–424

Thiery JP (1967) Mise en evidence des polysaccharides sur coupes fine en microscopie electronique. J Microsc 6:987–1018

Thompson SW (1974) Selected histochemical and histopathological methods. Thomas, Springfield

Thurlbeck WM (1967) The internal surfaces area of nonemphysematous lungs. Am Rev Respir Dis 95:765–773

Tompsett DH (1956) Anatomical techniques. Livingstone, Edinburgh

Turek JJ, Sheares BT, Carlson DM (1982) Substructure of granules from serous cells of porcine tracheal submucosal glands. Anat Rec 203:329–336

Tyler WS, Pearse AGE (1965) Oxidative enzymes of the interalveolar septum of the rat. Thorax 20:149–152

Tyler WS, Pearse AGE, Rhatigan P (1965) Histochemistry of the equine lung: oxidative enzymes of the interalveolar septum. Am J Vet Res 26:960–964

Vaccaro CA, Brody JS (1979) Ultrastructural localization and characterization of proteoglycans in the pulmonary alveolus. Am Rev Respir Dis 120:901–910

Vaccaro CA, Brody JS (1981) Structural features of alveolar wall basement membrane in the adult rat lung. J Cell Biol 91:427–437

Vatter AE, Reiss OK, Newman JK, Lindquist K, Groeneboer E (1968) Enzymes of the lung: I. Detection of esterase with a new cytochemical method. J Cell Biol 38:80–98

Weakley BS (1977) How dangerous is sodium cacodylate? J Microsc 109:249–251

Weibel ER, Limacher W, Bachofen H (1982) Electron microscopy of rapidly frozen lungs: evaluation on the basis of standard criteria. J Appl Physiol 53:516–527

Wetzel MG, Wetzel BK, Spicer SS (1966) Ultrastructural localization of acid mucosubstances in the mouse colon with iron-containing stains. J Cell Biol 30:299–315

Whimster WF (1969) Rapid giant paper sections of lungs. Thorax 24:737–741

Williams MC, Benson BJ (1981) Immunocytochemical localization and identification of the major surfactant protein in adult rat lung. J Histochem Cytochem 29:291–305

Winborn WB, Guerrero DL (1974) The use of a single tissue specimen for both transmission and scanning electron microscopy. Cytobios 10:83–91

Yeh HC, Hulbert AJ, Phalen RF, Velasquez DJ, Harris TD (1975) A stereoradiographic technique and its application to evaluation of lung casts. Invest Radiol 10:351–357

Yoneda K (1978) Ultrastructural localization of phospholipases in the clara cell of rat bronchiole. Am J Pathol 93:745–752

Yoneda K (1982) Regional differences in the intercellular junctions of the alveolar-capillary membrane in the human lung. Am Rev Respir Dis 126:893–897

Yoneda K, Birk MG (1981) The mode of secretion of the clara cell in rat bronchiole: a freeze-fracture study. Exp Lung Res 2:177–185

Young JT (1981) Histopathologic examination of the rat nasal cavity. Fundamental Appl Tox 1:309–312

Zierold K (1982) Cryopreparation of mammalian tissue for x-ray microanalysis in STEM. J Microsc 125:149–156

CHAPTER 10

Morphometry of the Alveolar Region of the Lung

K. E. PINKERTON and J. D. CRAPO

A. What is Morphometry?

Morphometry is the quantitation of shapes or structures as they exist in three dimensions derived from analysis of two-dimensional profiles taken through these structures. Volumes, surface areas, thicknesses, and numerical densities of tissue structures are the most common measurements made using morphometric techniques.

B. Why do Morphometry?

The advantages of using morphometry in the study of lung structure include: (a) quantitation of changes in lung structure in an objective, unbiased manner; (b) greater sensitivity in identifying subtle changes in structure; (c) the capability of rigorously ranking changes in tissue structure caused by different agents or by progressive exposure to the same agent; and (d) the capacity of selectively quantitating changes within specific tissue compartments. The sensitivity of morphometric measurements is particularly beneficial when changes in tissue structure due to the experimental treatment are probable, but not obvious. An important application of morphometry involves those studies in which subjective grading standards suggest changes have taken place, but are inconclusive concerning the relative toxicity of an agent, drug, chemical, or pollutant at that specific exposure and/or dose. Morphometry eliminates the subjective bias found in many grading techniques used to measure structural changes. Morphometry also reduces or eliminates variations in grading between and within observers.

C. Types of Data Obtained by Morphometry

The types of morphometric information that can be obtained in a study of the lung parenchyma are dependent upon the level of resolution used. Light microscopy provides adequate resolution to determine the internal alveolar surface area, proportional volumes of air and tissue, and total number of alveoli present. Measurements by light microscopy are rapid, accurate, and can be done on large numbers of specimens. An additional morphometric measurement commonly used at the light microscopic level of resolution is the mean linear intercept (MLI) which is related to the alveolar surface area and number of alveoli present in the lungs. MLI measurements have been used to study postnatal lung growth (DUNNILL 1962b; DAVIES and REID 1970; BARTLETT 1970), the normal adult human lung (WEIBEL 1963; THURLBECK 1967), and lungs with emphysema (DUNNILL 1962a; SNIDER and KORTHY 1978).

Determination of the volumes, thicknesses, and surface densities of specific alveolar compartments is generally best done using electron microscopy. Volume measurements of air, tissue, and blood can be done using light microscopy on thin (1-μm) plastic sections (HYDE et al. 1978). Electron microscopy is required for adequate resolution of alveolar tissue into epithelium, interstitium, and endothelium (KAPANCI et al. 1969; BURRI et al. 1974; BURRI and WEIBEL 1977), epithelium into type I and type II cells, and interstitium into cellular and noncellular components (CRAPO et al. 1978, 1980; PINKERTON et al. 1982). Subcellular components such as the nucleus, cytoplasm, and cytoplasmic organelles may also be quantitated for specific cell types using morphometric techniques with electron microscopy (VIDIĆ and BURRI 1981; YOUNG et al. 1982).

The thickness of the alveolar septum may be expressed as an arithmetic and/or harmonic mean tissue thickness of the air–blood tissue barrier (WEIBEL and KNIGHT 1964). The arithmetic mean tissue thickness may be further subdivided into the thickness of the epithelial, interstitial, and endothelial compartments (WEIBEL and KNIGHT 1964; CRAPO et al. 1978, 1980; PINKERTON et al. 1982).

The numerical densitiy of particles, cells, or subcellular organelles within the alveolar region of the lungs can also be determined morphometrically. The total number of cells in the lung and the distribution of cells among the various major types of alveolar cells has been determined for both humans and several species of laboratory animals (KAUFFMAN et al. 1974; HAIES et al. 1981; CRAPO et al. 1982, 1983). Estimates of the distribution of cell types within the alveolar interstitium have also been done (CRAPO et al. 1980; PINKERTON et al. 1982; BARRY et al. 1983).

D. Design Strategy for a Morphometric Study of Lung Tissue

I. Light Microscopy or Electron Microscopy

The purpose and types of questions which are to be answered by a morphometric study will determine whether light microscopy alone or light microscopy combined with electron microscopy is needed. The advantages of a light microscopic morphometric study include: (a) rapid, accurate measurements; and (b) the ability to study many specimens and animals without excessive costs. The disadvantages of light microscopy include: (a) the need to determine a correction factor for tissue shrinkage due to paraffin embedding of tissues (WEIBEL 1963); and (b) limitations in the types of alveolar tissue structures which can be easily and reliably quantitated, i. e., airspace, tissue, and capillary blood volumes, alveolar surface area, mean free path lengths, and numbers of alveoli.

Morphometry done with electron microscopy provides the advantages of: (a) quantitative information for specific alveolar tissue compartments and; (b) no need to determine correction factors due to tissue shrinkage since tissues can be embedded in plastics that have negligible shrinkage. The disadvantages of electron microscopy include: (a) higher costs; and (b) substantially greater labor and time required to obtain data.

The quantitation of numbers of lung cells or of volumes of tissue per lung is usually based on a relatively small sample size. It is important, therefore, that the sample be representative of the whole lung. The advantages of optimizing sam-

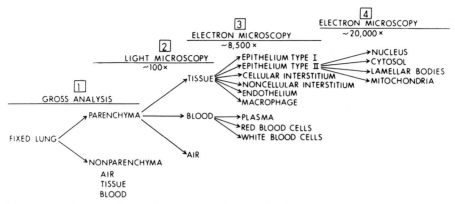

Fig. 1. Flow diagram of a tiered morphometric analysis of lung tissue. The approximate degree of magnification for sampling is given for each level

pling include: (a) reduced cost in carrying out the study since only a small portion of the whole organ is analyzed; (b) greater speed in the determination of values; (c) greater flexibility and scope of variables which can be analyzed; and (d) greater accuracy. If the sample size is adequate and properly taken, the derived values for the whole organ should be a valid estimate of the true values.

Sampling of tissues for morphometric studies is commonly done using a tiered sample approach (Fig. 1). This technique involves the determination of morphometric data at different levels of resolution of structure. An example of the steps required to use tiered sampling to obtain the total volume of lamellar bodies in lung alveolar type II cells in a rat (YOUNG et al. 1982) included: (a) determination of the fraction of the lung that is alveolar region by light microscopy on paraffin step sections (done at approximately × 100); (b) determination of the volume density of alveolar type II cells in the alveolar region by either light microscopy on thin (1-μm) plastic sections (done at approximately × 1,000) or electron microscopy (at a slightly higher magnification); and (c) determination of the volume density of lamellar bodies in type II cells by electron microscopy (done at approximately × 20,000). Tiered sampling in this form can be used to quantitate specific tissue components of the lung with great accuracy while minimizing work load.

Errors in sampling may include incorrect assumptions, the use of convenient estimates which introduce bias, and human error in making measurements. An important assumption of sampling made in most morphometric studies is that the units composing the organ or structures are homogeneously distributed. This means that random sampling of any portion of the structure should be representative of the whole. Preliminary examination of the anatomy of the lung would not appear to satisfy this assumption, since the bronchial tree has a highly ordered pattern of branching. Subpopulation or stratified sampling (COCHRAN 1963) reduces structural inhomogeneities by dividing the lung into distinct structural units or strata. Heterogeneity caused by the tracheobronchial tree is generally handled by dividing the lung into two subpopulations: parenchyma which is defined to include the entire alveolar region including alveolar ducts, and nonparenchyma which is defined as all airways, large blood vessels, and major tissue septa. The fraction of the whole lung that is parenchyma is determined by point counting serial slices or serial step sections through the entire lung (WEIBEL 1963; CRAPO et al. 1978). Once the size of the parenchymal region is known, samples are commonly drawn only from this subpopulation for further morphometric analysis.

Stratified sampling is also used when structural variations exist between different regions of the lung. These variations may include tissue and blood densities which are known to form a gradient from the top to the bottom of large lungs such as human or dog (GLAZIER et al. 1967; GEHR and WEIBEL 1974). Stratified sampling can account for regional differences by subdividing the lung into smaller, more homogeneous strata, and then taking proportionally correct numbers of randomized samples from each stratum. That is, proportionally smaller numbers of samples would be taken from smaller strata. Thus, the mean of all samples would represent a volume-weighted mean of all strata and would correctly represent the whole lung. An alternative approch to stratified sampling is to take the same number of samples from each stratum and then calculate a weighted mean using weight factors based on the size of the strata from which each group of samples is taken. Any sample of lung tissue which comes from only the alveolar (parenchymal) region represents a stratified sample since it is taken from only one of the two major regions (strata) of the lung and must be weighted by the relative volume of this region to give correct data for the total volume of alveolar tissues in a lung. For small animals, it is generally appropriate to assume the alveolar region is homogenous and to sample randomly within it. For larger animals, further stratification of samples from apex to base may be necessary to describe the lung correctly.

II. Animal Selection and Optimal Sample Density

Selection of the appropriate animal model for a morphometric study of lung structure is important and must be based on a number of variables: (a) the number of animals to be used; (b) the duration of the experiment; (c) the cost of animal maintenance; and (d) the need to match human lung structure. Small laboratory animals are easy to maintain and present little difficulty in tissue sampling. Large animals have the advantage of permitting serial biopsies from the same animal with progressive treatment or exposure. However, care is required with large animals to avoid bias in tissue sampling for the reasons discussed previously.

The Fischer 344 rat has been extensively studied over its normal life span (PINKERTON et al. 1982). In this animal, lung growth takes place predominantly during the first 5 months of life and remains relatively stable from 5 to 26 months of age. This characteristic, a stable lung structure, makes the Fischer 344 rat an excellent model for studying the effects of chronic exposure to an inhaled toxin since changes can probably be attributed to the toxin rather than to the effects of aging.

For morphometric studies using electron microscopy, a high work load is required to process and analyze each animal. Therefore, optimization of the number of animals to be studied is important. This is particularly true when changes in tissue structure are subtle following treatment, since larger numbers of animals may be required to determine statistically significant changes. When multiple treatment groups are to be compared with a common control group, the optimum number of control animals to be used should be within the following range

$$1.1 \times n \times \sqrt{t} < \text{number of control animals} < 1.4 \times n \times \sqrt{t},$$

where t is equal to the number of treatment groups and n is equal to the number of animals in each treatment group (WILLIAMS 1972).

The determination of optimum sample size is based upon a number of criteria: (a) the type of information desired from the study; (b) the acceptable limits of error; and (c) the precision with which the techniques used can estimate the values of interest. Therefore, in order to optimize sample density in an electron microscopic morphometric study, the size of each of the following levels of sampling must be considered: (a) the number of animals studied; (b) the number of sites per lung studied; (c) the number of micrographs taken per site; and (d) the number of points or line intercepts counted on each micrograph. For the logic and details of sampling techniques in morphometric studies, the reader should consult any number of stereological texts which deal in depth on this topic (ERÄNKÖ 1955; DeHOFF and RHINES 1968; ELIAS 1967; WEIBEL 1979; UNDERWOOD 1970).

Our experience in carrying out morphometric studies using rats as the animal model (CRAPO et al. 1978; PINKERTON et al. 1982; BARRY et al. 1983) is that variation between animals is relatively small so that experimental groups of 4–8 animals are all that are required to quantify most changes in lung structure. Because rats have substantial homogeneity within the parenchymal region of the lung, we have commonly used only 4 sites per lung to evaluate the entire lung and have taken 15–40 electron micrographs enlarged to $\times 8{,}500$ on 28×36-cm paper from each site. In our experience, the most important variable in determining the accuracy in evaluating any given lung is the total number of micrographs taken; 100–200 points per micrograph is sufficient to evaluate objects having an overall 1% density in the lung. Accuracy is best improved by evaluating more micrographs rather than by counting more than 100–200 points on a single micrograph. Between 40 and 60 micrographs per animal are required to optimize accuracy in evaluating the density of tissues such as alveolar type I epithelium which has a 1%–2% volume density in lung parenchyma.

E. Detailed Methodology

I. Lung Fixation

Intratracheal instillation for lung fixation is most commonly used because it is fast, reproducible, and gives high quality fixation. Disadvantages of intratracheal instillation of fixatives are the loss of the alveolar airspace lining layer and the loss of in vivo septal anatomy since it causes unfolding of the alveolar septum and loss of the effects of surface tension at the air–liquid interface. The effects of intratracheal instillation of fixatives in the volume of blood retained in the pulmonary capillary bed are not clearly known. One study (CRAPO and CRAPO 1983) has suggested that a rapid instillation of glutaraldehyde into an anesthetized animal results in the pulmonary capillary bed being the same volume as that found with flash freezing techniques.

Intravascular perfusion has the distinct advantages of preserving the normal configuration of the alveolar septal wall, preserving portions of the alveolar surface lining layer, and preserving the location of alveolar macrophages within airspaces (no mucus, cells, etc., from airways are washed into the alveolar region). The disadvantages of intravascular perfusion are: (a) it is technically more difficult and time consuming than intratracheal instillation; (b) uniform lung inflation is more difficult to achieve; and (c) high quality fixation of lung cell ultrastructure is more difficult to achieve (because the ratio of fixative volume to tissue volume is much lower). Intravascular perfusion requires opening the chest cavity so that the lungs can be perfused through the right ventricle of the heart initially with saline to remove blood and then with the fixative to fix the lungs. The lungs are held at a physiologically appropriate level of inflation using air at a pressure of 10–20 cm H_2O applied to the trachea. The pressure for vascular perfusion of fixatives is generally 20–30 cm H_2O. The saline wash is for about 30 s and the fixative perfusion must be maintained for prolonged periods to obtain a rigid fixation of the lungs.

The factors that determine the degree of inflation of intratracheally fixed lungs have been extensively evaluated (Hayatdavoudi et al. 1980). To fix lungs in situ the trachea is cannulated and then the abdomen is opened and both hemidiaphragms ruptured to allow the lungs to collapse just prior to the instillation of the fixative (Fig. 2). Many investigators have assumed that the pressure of the fixative is the primary determinant of the degree of inflation achieved. This

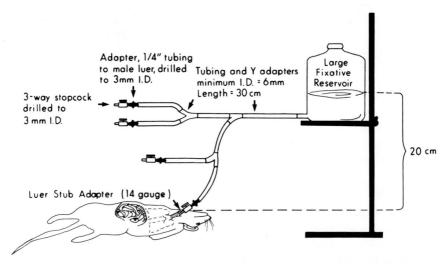

Fig. 2. Rat lung fixation by intratracheal perfusion. 1. The 14-gauge Luer stub adapter is tied into the rat trachea. 2. The abdomen is opened and the hemidiaphragms punctured using blunt forceps. 3. The fixation line is rapidly attached to the tracheal adaptor and the stopcock opened. 4. The fixation pressure is maintained 30 min in situ. The fixative pressure, the length of tubing, and the internal diameter of every component of the tubing and adapters affect the rate of fixative infusion. This system is designed for adult rats. The rate of flow of fixative through the final 14-gauge tubing adaptor is 110–120 ml/min when not attached to a rat. This method of fixation will fix rat lungs at 70%–90% of TLC when 2% buffered glutaraldehyde is used as the fixative

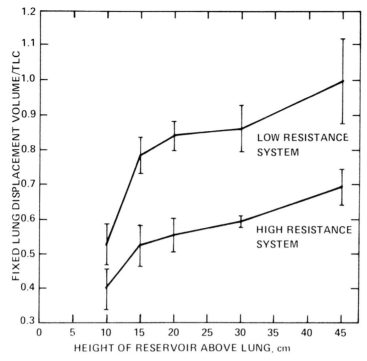

Fig. 3. Degree of inflation achieved in excised glutaraldehyde-fixed lungs at different hydrostatic pressures. *Upper curve* shows the relationship of fixation volume (as a fraction of the physiologic TLC) to fixation pressure when a low resistance (high flow rate) system is used. For the *lower curve* a high resistance (low flow rate) system was used (HAYATDAVOUDI et al. 1980). Note that when low fixative flow rates were used (high resistance), poor inflation of the lung occurred, even in the presence of 20 cm or more pressure on the system. Using high initial fixative flow rates and a pressure of 20–30 cm H_2O, the fixed lungs were reproducibly inflated to 80%–90% of TLC

is true when using slow fixatives such as formalin. Indeed, the fixation is so slow that pressure on the fixative must be maintained for several days in order to produce rigidly fixed lungs. The quality of this type of fixation is not adequate for electron microscopy since much of the ultrastructure is not preserved. When using glutaraldehyde as the fixative, the initial flow rates of the fixative have been found to be much more important than the final pressure applied to the fixative. Using a low resistance system for instilling the fixative (which produces relatively high initial flow rates; Fig. 3) can give a much better and more reproducible degree of lung inflation (HAYATDAVOUDI et al. 1980). The final volume of intratracheal fixed lungs has been found to depend on: (a) the type of fixative used; (b) initial flow rates of the fixative; (c) final pressure of the fixative; (d) whether the lungs were fixed in situ or after excision; and (e) conditions that may affect the volume and/or pressure of blood in the lungs at the initiation of fixation (HAYATDAVOUDI et al. 1980). It appears that glutaraldehyde begins fixation so rapidly that significant fixation occurs during the brief time that fixative flows into the lungs. In working with larger animals we have found that significant regional differences in the degree of inflation will occur if the fixative is instilled over more than 30–60 s. A rule of thumb that works for lungs of all sizes is to adjust the initial flow rate by controlling the resistance in the fixative lines and the initial pressure such that 70%–80% of the estimated lung volume at total lung capacity (TLC) is instilled within the first 10 s. The pressure can then be set at 20–30 cm H_2O and high quality uniform lung fixation at about 80% of TLC will be achieved. For rats (see Fig. 2), this requires a hydrostatic pressure of 20 cm fixative and a total resistance in the tubing to give a fixative flowrate of 110–120 ml/min when the tubing is not attached to the animal (Hayatdavoudi et al. 1980; Pinkerton et al. 1982). The pressure on the fixative is usually maintained for 30 min in situ to insure adequate fixation of the lungs, although this length of time is probably unnecessarily long.

II. Lung Volume Measurement

Following removal of the fixed lungs from the chest cavity, the lungs should be stored in fixative for at least 24 h before further manipulation. This period of time allows the lungs to become further stabilized. We have found that glutaraldehyde-fixed lungs occasionally decrease in volume during this period of time. Determination of the fixed lung volume before stabilization would result in a measurement which will not be an appropriate reflection of the final volume of the lung at the time when samples are taken and morphometric measurements made.

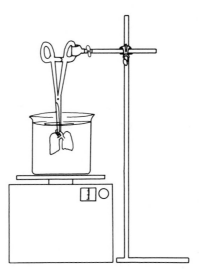

Fig. 4. Determination of fixed lung volume by the weight of displaced fluid. 1. Tare weight is determined with the clamp immersed in the fixative to the same level as used to immerse the lungs. 2. The fixed lungs are clamped at the lower trachea and are then completely suspended in the fixative without touching the sides or bottom of the container. 3. The difference in the tare weight and final weight is equal to the volume of the lungs if the specific gravity of the fluid is 1.0

Two methods most commonly used to determine the volume of the inflation-fixed lung are gravimetric and volumetric measurements of the fluid displaced by the immersed lung. Gravimetric measurement is based upon Archimedes' principle. Since the specific gravity of isotonic saline is approximately 1.0, submersion of the fixed lungs in saline will cause a displacement of saline equal to the volume of the fixed lungs. This displacement of saline is reflected as a change in the weight of the total system. Important considerations which must be met using this procedure are complete immersion of the lungs in the fluid without the lungs touching the sides or the bottom of the vessel containing the fluid (Fig. 4). Gravimetric measurement of volume displacement is highly accurate since a balance can be used to determine the weight of the displaced fluid (and thus the volume) to the nearest 0.1 g (0.1 ml). Volumetric measurement of the fluid displaced by fixed lungs is more appropriate for large lungs where measurement errors are an insignificant proportion of the total lung size.

III. Determination of the Fraction of Lung that is Parenchyma

The first step in many morphometric studies of lung tissue must be to determine the fraction of the total lung volume that is parenchyma (alveolar region). Since nonparenchymal (nonalveolar) tissue is not homogeneously distributed in the lung this analysis must be done on serial sections or uniform step sections taken throughout the entire lobe. Each of these step sections must be sampled with a uniform point density if an unbiased estimate of the fraction of the lobe that is alveolar region is to be obtained. The fraction of the lung composed of the region of interest is simply the number of points falling on the region of interest divided by the total number of points falling on the lung sections.

For small animals where lung slices are small enough to fit on a single light microscopic slide, the alveolar and nonalveolar fractions of the lung can be determined entirely by light microscopy. This is accomplished by step sectioning through an entire lobe of the lungs. The determination of alveolar and nonalveolar tissue fractions by light microscopy is generally based on the criterion that nonalveolar structures consist of all bronchi and bronchioles and all blood vessels with a diameter greater than 25–50 µm. Nonalveolar structures also include interlobular connective tissue. A technique which has been used in our laboratory is to use hematoxylin–eosin-stained step sections as negatives in an enlarger to produce prints of each section on 28 × 36-cm photographic paper. The resulting print is a negative image of the section. The largest section in the series of step sections is enlarged to a magnification in which the image will barely fit on the photographic paper. This magnification is held constant for the printing of all other sections from the same lobe. A test lattice overlay consisting of 112 lines, each 2 cm in length, is used to count points falling on parenchymal and nonparenchymal regions. The ends of each line constitute a point, but only points falling on the section are counted. This technique dramatically speeds up the counting process over that done with an automatic sampling stage light microscope. A light microscope and the original hematoxylin–eosin-stained sections can be used in concert with the prints to improve the evaluation of any area where clarification is required for categorization of points falling on tissues.

For large animals, the methods used to determine the lung parenchymal fraction should include both gross and light microscopic sampling of tissue. Sampling of tissue at the gross level is used in large lungs (such as dog and human) first to determine the fraction of lung occupied by nonalveolar tissues (airways, blood vessels, and major septa) that are large enough to be clearly recognized with the unaided eye (usually those larger than 1 mm in diameter). This requires serial tissue slices through entire lobes of the lung cut at a uniform thickness. One easy approach to analyze these serial gross tissue slices is to photograph them using 35-mm slide film at a constant magnification. Tissue distortion is reduced by photographing each tissue slice while it is immersed in water. These slides can then be projected onto a uniform test lattice on which points falling on the lung sections can be counted. These points are categorized as falling on either parenchyma or nonparenchymal tissue. Since smaller nonparenchymal structures cannot be recognized in the gross specimen, further analysis using light microscopy is necessary to specify the volume of the nonparenchyma. Random light microscopic (paraffin) sections of the lung are point counted to determine the fraction of points falling on small nonparenchymal structures (< 1 mm in size after accounting for shrinkage or compression of the sections) and on parenchyma. Since large nonparenchymal structures would have been counted on the gross tissue slices, any points falling on these structures can be ignored when analyzing for small nonparenchymal structures by light microscopy.

The parenchymal (alveolar) fraction in the lungs of rats has been well studied over the life span of this species. Burri et al. (1974) determined the parenchymal fraction of the lung in neonatal rats and rats up through 5 months of age and obtained values of 0.82. Pinkerton et al. (1982) found the parenchymal fraction in 14- and 26-month-old rats (both male and female) to be 0.81–0.82. In larger animals, the parenchymal fraction has been found to be 82%–90% of the entire lung volume. Weibel (1963) determined the parenchymal fraction in human lung to be 0.90. R. O. Crapo et al. (1982) determined that the parenchymal fraction in mongrel dogs as measured by both gross and light microscopic techniques is 0.82. Recently Knapp and Crapo (1984) found the parenchymal fraction in baboon lung to be 0.85. The human lung may not actually have a parenchymal fraction substantially different from that of other species since Weibel used only gross anatomy to determine the value of 0.90. The addition of light microscopic analysis to detect small nonparenchymal structures would likely reduce the value obtained for humans to near that found for dogs and baboons. In the dog study referred to (R. O. Crapo et al. 1982), the parenchymal fraction determined by gross analysis only was 0.92 which suggests that about 50% of nonparenchymal structures are too small to be easily identified in the gross specimen. The parenchymal fraction of the lung may be significantly affected by differences in the degree of lung inflation since nonparenchymal structures contain less air and are less compliant than the alveolar region. A final consideration is that the parenchymal fraction of the lung has been found to change little after severe lung injury caused by either oxygen (Crapo et al. 1978) or asbestos (Pinkerton et al. 1983). This suggests that in most morphometric studies this fraction can be considered to be a constant if the degree of inflation of the fixed lungs is held constant.

IV. Light Microscopy Analysis

In addition to alveolar – nonalveolar fraction determinations, light microscopy may be used to determine the alveolar airspace, alveolar tissue, and alveolar
capillary blood fractions. Light microscopy may also be used to determine morphometric measurements such as MLI length (mean chord length), alveolar surface area, and alveolar number. Measurements of MLI length (L_m) are commonly
used to evaluate enlargement of airspaces in emphysematous processes. This technique is based upon counting the number of intercepts a random test line of
known length makes with alveolar septa and is expressed as the average length
of the line between intercepts. This method was first proposed by TOMKEIEFF
(1945) and HENNIG (1956) and is based on the following equation

$$L_m = \frac{N \times L}{\sum_{i=1}^{N} m_i}$$

in which L is a line of known length, m is the number of times the line intersects
the alveolar septa, and N is the number of times the line is randomly used on the
tissue sections. This formula assumes the thickness of the alveolar septum to be
negligible and counts one intercept for each septum crossed rather than counting
a separate intercept for each side of a single alveolar septum.

MLI is not a particularly good method to evaluate the presence of emphysema. It can detect airspace enlargement. However, emphysema is not defined only
as airspace enlargement, but rather as destruction of alveolar septa as part of the
mechanism for enlargement of airspaces. MLI is also limited by the fact that as
a linear measurement it changes with the cube root of any change in volume. It
is therefore a relatively insensitive technique for detecting volume changes. Since
the alveolar surface area is represented on both sides of the alveolar septum, the
total alveolar surface area is expressed by the following equation (WEIBEL 1963)

$$S_A = 4 \frac{V_P}{L_m} \, (cm^2/cm^3),$$

where V_P is the volume of the lung parenchyma.

The test line used to count intercepts with the alveolar septa can be placed in
the focal plane of the eyepiece reticle and the relative length of the line calibrated
with a micrometer. All intercept counts must be corrected for errors caused by
section shrinkage and for section compression. Since section compression, caused
by the knife edge, occurs in one dimension only, the orientation of the section can
influence results. This can be partially compensated for by using an arrangement
of perpendicularly crossed lines as the test lattice. An alternative to placing the
test lattice in the eyepiece is to project the microscopic image onto a television
screen and place a test lattice overlay on the screen.

The total number of alveoli N_a within a lung can be estimated by the following
equation (WEIBEL 1963)

$$N_a = n_a^{3/2}/\beta \times q$$

in which n_a is the number of alveolar airspace profiles per unit area found in the
microscopic field, β is a dimensionless shape coefficient which is determined by

the shape of an alveolus, and q is the alveolar fraction of the lungs. The assumptions of this formula include: (a) the objects of interest are randomly distributed within the containing volume; (b) differences in size of the object are randomly distributed; (c) the thickness of the section through the objects of interest is infinitely small compared with the smallest object; and (d) the shape of the object is well defined, that is, it can be mathematically expressed. The limitations of using β are most obvious when objects of interest do not have a uniform shape or one that is well defined in every direction. Values for the shape coefficient β for cylinders and ellipsoids have been derived by WEIBEL and GOMEZ (1962). The value of β for a sphere is 1.38 and for a hemisphere is 1.36. WEIBEL and GOMEZ (1962) determined β for the human alveolus to be 1.55 which assumes the alveolus to be polyhedral in shape. The counting of alveolar profiles or transections per microscopic field is done using a square or rectangle placed in the eyepiece reticle or with an overlay placed on a television screen. The area of the square or rectangle can be measured and only alveolar profiles entirely within the lines are counted, along with alveoli touching the upper and right-hand edges of the square. Alveoli touching the upper left and lower right corners are not counted. This counting rule, described by GUNDERSON (1977), is necessary to eliminate bias and a systematic overestimation of the total number of alveoli.

The random sampling of tissue sections by light microscopy to determine numbers of alveoli and alveolar surface area is best done using an automatic sampling stage microscope. This type of microscope eliminates bias which could be introduced by observer selection of microscopic fields to be analyzed. An automatic stage sampling system can be programmed to make uniform steps in both the x and y directions. The microscopic field can be viewed directly through the eyepiece or on a television screen if a camera is mounted on the microscope as previously described. The test lattice system may consist of several lines of known length placed in the focal plane of the eyepiece reticle or placed on clear acetate over the television screen. Increased speed in movement of the stage and recording of points and intercepts can be accomplished by using a computer interfaced with the automatic sampling stage.

V. Electron Microscopy Analysis

1. Tissue Preparation and Selection

Sampling of tissue at the electron microscopic level of resolution provides the most complete information concerning the alveolar structures of the lung. Sampling of tissue at this level can be directed at the parenchymal portions of the lung since gross and/or light microscopic levels of tissue sampling have been used to determine the nonparenchymal fraction of the lung.

For small animals where the entire lung parenchyma can be assumed to be homogeneous, a number of random blocks, 1–2 mm on a side, are taken with the pleural surfaces excluded and processed for thin sectioning. For larger animals, taking a stratified sample within the lung parenchyma may be necessary if the questions being addressed involve tissue distributions that are not homogeneous. Tissue blocks are processed and embedded using standard techniques for electron microscopy. In the tissue dehydration steps, a graded increase in the concentration of alcohol (50%, 70%, 90%, and 100%) is used to avoid severe osmotic stress on the tissue. Glutaraldehyde-fixed tissue has been shown to be highly resistant to osmotic stress (Mathieu et al. 1978) so that changes in cell sizes and shapes are not significant problems during the embedding steps. Sections 0.5-μm thick are cut from each block and stained to verify the presence of parenchymal tissue. Parenchymal tissue is considered to include alveoli and alveolar ducts. Airways with ciliated epithelium and blood vessels with a diameter greater than 25 μm are usually considered to be nonparenchymal. Sections with large areas containing large blood vessels and/or airways are discarded and another block is taken. The reason for discarding these blocks is to optimize the amount of alveolar tissue which will be sampled on each block by electron microscopy. Small areas of non-parenchymal tissue on a section is not a reason to discard a section since random micrographs of alveolar tissue can be taken around these structures. This should be done to avoid bias that could be introduced by systematically excluding all al-veolar tissue that is adjacent to a nonalveolar structure.

The number of blocks which should be analyzed in a morphometric study of lung tissue is dependent upon the purpose of the study and the relative probability of sampling the tissue structure of interest. Figure 5 provides an easy means of

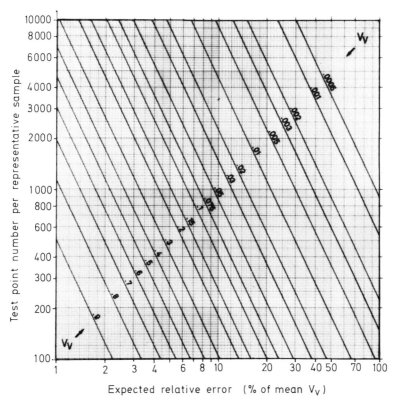

Fig. 5. Nomogram relating test point number to the volume density V_v of the structure being sampled and expected relative standard error (% of mean). The number of test points needed to give a relative standard error in measurement for objects of different volume densities can be read directly from this figure (Weibel 1979)

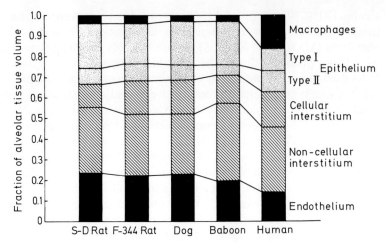

Fig. 6. Composition of the alveolar septum in mammalian lungs. The average volume of each tissue compartment is shown as a fraction of all tissue composing the septum (excluding blood in capillary lumens) (Crapo et al. 1983)

determining the number of points that must be counted to give an expected level of confidence in quantitating structures of different volume densities. The use of this figure plus the fact that 100–200 points is the optimum number to be counted on each micrograph will help determine the total number of micrographs that should be taken from each section or from each animal. Figure 6 gives the relative volume densities of the major tissue compartments in a variety of mammalian lungs. The total tissue as shown in Fig. 6 generally represents less than 6%–10% of the parenchymal volume of the lung because of the presence of large volumes of air and blood.

2. Morphometric Analysis with Electron Microscopy

Electron microscopy offers several levels of resolution at which a morphometric study can be done. The level at which the study is conducted is dependent upon the questions which are to be answered. For studies in which the major alveolar tissue compartments, that is, epithelial, interstitial, and endothelial compartments, are to be determined, a system of random sampling within the entire lung parenchyma is typically used. For studies in which only one or two tissue compartments are to be quantitated, a tiered system of random sampling can be used with selection of the final tier to maximize those tissue compartments of interest. If a specific region of the lungs is to be studied, such as the proximal alveolar regions at the level of the first alveolar duct bifurcation (Barry et al. 1983), strict methods of selective tissue sampling are used. To avoid the introduction of bias, a uniform method in which these regions are isolated and analyzed must be employed. When the volume occupied by a specific region or component of the lung is unknown, tissue values determined morphometrically may be normalized to the length or area of basement membrane included in the sample (Bachofen and

WEIBEL 1977; BARRY et al. 1983). Normalization of tissue values to basement membrane surface area may also be useful when comparing affected and nonaffected regions within the same lung or for simply comparing different regions within the same lung.

3. Volume and Surface Density Measurements

The 0.5-μm-thick sections used to verify the presence of alveolar tissue using light microscopy may also be used for the determination of tissue: air ratios, surface area, and cell number by light microscopy. Silver-gray (60- to 90-nm-thick) sections are cut from the same blocks, placed on grids, and poststained. Mesh grids provide excellent support for the section with a minimum of distortion and the grid bars provide a means of uniformly sampling the section in an unbiased manner.

Only grid squares completely covered by the section are used for analysis. Micrographs are taken from one or more corners of each grid square. If the corner selected contains a nonparenchymal structure such as a large blood vessel or airway, another corner of the grid square is taken. The presence of random debris or similar artifacts could also require another corner to be used. If no corner is satisfactory, no micrograph is taken and the next grid square is considered. Micrographs which would contain only alveolar air are recorded, but not actually photographed. If artifacts or dirt on the specimen are not random then these factors cannot be used as a basis for excluding a specific micrograph since to do so would introduce bias. Morphometry requires large, clean sections to permit an adequate unbiased random sampling of tissue.

Micrographs photographed at $\times 2,000$ on 10×12.5-cm negatives can be printed at a final magnification of $\times 8,500$ on 28×36-cm photographic paper. This magnification will allow excellent resolution and identification of each major alveolar tissue compartment, including separating the thin portions of the alveolar septum into epithelial, basement membrane, and endothelial cell compartments.

An alternative to the printing of micrographs is to use 35-mm direct positive film and project each micrograph. The advantages of slide projection include: (a) the film is cheap; and (b) the process is fast. The major disadvantage is that 35-mm film requires a projection apparatus and the resolution of the projected image (usually on a ground glass screen) is not as good as a print. This problem in resolution may be overcome by enlarging the projected image. Laboratories using this approach commonly work at $\times 10,000$–$11,000$ final magnification of the image on a 30×30-cm ground glass screen (WEIBEL 1979).

The advantages of prints include the following: (a) better resolution; (b) better permanent record in that prints may be written on to record how questions of tissue identifications were resolved; and (c) no projection apparatus is needed. Since only a plastic test lattice overlay is required for counting of point and line intercepts, the entire system is easily portable. The most obvious disadvantages of prints are the time required to produce them, the cost of the photographic paper, and the storage space needed for the prints.

A number of test lattice systems are available for counting. The test lattice most commonly used is an integrated test system described by WEIBEL (1963)

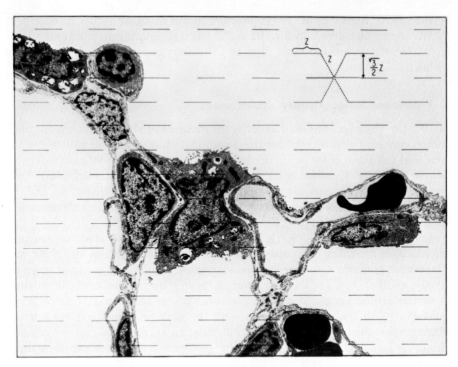

Fig. 7. Multipurpose test lattice overlay consisting of 112 lines of length 2 cm. The end of each line forms a point which is equidistant z from the surrounding six points. Some of the formulae in Table 1 are based on this test lattice

which consists of a series of lines of length Z distributed in a uniform pattern designed to allow uniform sampling over the entire area of the micrograph. The advantages of this overlay are that it allows uniform sampling and is organized so that it simplifies some of the calculations of surface areas, thickness, etc. Figure 7 illustrates this type of counting lattice overlying an electron micrograph of alveolar lung tissue. This illustrated test overlay contains 112 lines of length 2 cm. The volume density of tissue compartments is determined by using the ends of each line as points. The number of points falling upon each individual tissue compartment divided by the total number of test points is the volume density for that particular tissue compartment. The absolute volume per both lungs for each tissue compartment is obtained by multiplying the tissue compartment fraction [Eq. (1), Table 1] by the parenchymal fraction and by the total fixed lung volume.

The surface density of the alveolar epithelium and capillary endothelium is determined by counting the number of times the test line intercepts the airspace–epithelial surface and the plasma–endothelial cell surface respectively. Since the test line is of known length, Eq. (2), Table 1 can be used to determine surface density. In intratracheally fixed lungs, the alveolar epithelial surface is convoluted and ruffled with projections and microvilli. This causes a significant increase in the actual surface area of the alveolar epithelium. The ability to recognize these

Table 1. Formula used in analyzing morphometric data (many of these require the use of the integrated test lattice shown in Fig. 7)

Volume density	$V_V = P_i/P_t$	(1)
Surface density	$S_V = 2I_L$	(2)
Arithmetic mean thickness of:		
Alveolar membrane	$\tau_t = \dfrac{Z \times P_t}{2 \times (I_a + I_c)}$	(3)
Epithelium	$\tau_{ep} = \dfrac{Z \times P_{ep}}{4 \times I_a}$	(4)
Interstitium	$\tau_{in} = \dfrac{Z \times P_{in}}{2(I_a + I_c)}$	(5)
Endothelium	$\tau_{en} = \dfrac{Z \times P_{en}}{4 \times I_c}$	(6)
Harmonic mean thickness	$\dfrac{1}{\pi_h} = \dfrac{3}{2n} \times \displaystyle\sum_{i=1}^{n} \dfrac{1}{I_i}$	(7)
Numerical density	$N_V = N_A/(\bar{D} - 2h + t)$	(8)
	or	
	$N_V = N_A/\bar{D}$ (if $h=0$ and $t=0$)	(9)

P_i = number of points on tissue being studied, P_t = total points
I_L = number of intersections per test line length
Z = length of test line
P_t = number of points falling on tissue
I_a = number of line intersections with the alveolar surface
I_c = number of line intersections with the capillary surface
P_{ep} = test points falling on epithelium
P_{en} = test points falling on endothelium
P_{in} = test points falling on interstitium
π_h = harmonic mean thickness of tissue (air to capillary surface)
I_i = length of random line intercepts crossing the tissue
N_A = number of particle profiles per unit area
$\bar{D}$ = mean caliper diameter of particle
h = correction factor for the height of small cap sections that produce profiles too small to be seen
t = correction factor for the thickness of the section

surface convolutions improves as the magnification is increased. This causes the total epithelial surface area to show an apparent increase as magnification is increased. This is an important consideration in the design of a morphometric study and in the interpretation and comparison of results from different studies.

The basement membrane underlying the epithelium is relatively smooth and its surface area can be used as one relatively reproducible approach to estimate alveolar surface area. Two problems in interpreting basement membrane surface area should be considered. The first is that the basement membrane has many infoldings in the normal lung, in vivo; thus, its surface area represents an estimate of the maximum alveolar surface area rather than the correct surface area of the air–liquid interface in vivo. The second is that around cuboidal epithelial cells the basement membrane follows the cell deep into the alveolar septum and does not provide an estimate of the smoothed air-side surface of the cell as it does for alveolar type I epithelial cells. This problem can be resolved by counting the number of intercepts made by the test line with the basement membrane underlying the type I epithelium and with an imaginary surface of type II epithelial cells which ignores or cuts off all microvilli on the surface of the cell. This gives a slightly modified basement membrane surface area which will estimate the smoothed air-side surface of all epithelial cells while ignoring both extensions of the basement membrane below type II epithelial cells and microvilli at the air-side surface of type II epithelial cells (CRAPO et al. 1982).

4. Arithmetic and Harmonic Mean Tissue Thickness Measurements

The arithmetic mean thickness of tissue in the alveolar septum τ_t is a volume:surface ratio of alveolar tissue [Eq. (3), Table 1]. The arithmetic mean tissue thickness assumes a flat surface with a homogeneous thickness of tissue and can be determined separately for the epithelium, interstitium, and endothelium [Eq. (4–6), Table 1]. There are several problems in interpreting the meaning of "arithmetic mean thicknesses" of tissues by these formulae. First, since it is really a volume:surface ratio it represents the true tissue thickness only when tissue has an identical thickness over all portions of the alveolar septum. This obviously does not hold for lung tissues and the effect of having thick and thin portions of the alveolar septum will be to cause the "arithmetic mean thickness" to underestimate the true thickness. In actual practice the magnitude of this systematic error for normal lung tissue is probably 5%–10% and its importance may be negligible in many experimental designs. The second problem is that this measurement is highly magnification dependent. Increasing the magnification will decrease the calculated septal thickness as the apparent (recognizable) surface area increases. Using a smoothed alveolar surface such as the modified basement membrane surface area described in Sect. E. V. 3 reduces this problem to negligible proportions. Although the arithmetic mean tissue thickness is not a true measurement of septal thickness, its capacity to reflect changes in mean septal thickness owing to fibrosis or edema is excellent.

The harmonic mean tissue thickness [Eq. (7), Table 1] is a value which estimates the effective thickness of tissue with respect to its barrier function to gas exchange. This approach treats the alveolar tissue as a series of resistors in parallel. Efficient gas transfer predominantly occurs across the thin portions of the alveolar system. Thus, changes in tissue structure which lead to thickening of the alveolar septum in areas that are normally thin would be expected to have the greatest impact on gas transfer. The calculation of a harmonic mean thickness weights the thin portions of the septum highest by summing all measurements of septal thickness as their reciprocals, dividing by the number of measurements made, and then taking the reciprocal of this value. Measurements of harmonic mean thickness are independent of surface area or magnification effects and represent the harmonic mean of random linear path lengths across the tissue rather than of path lengths perpendicular to the alveolar surface. In practice, the harmonic mean tissue thickness is determined by using a square lattice test overlay

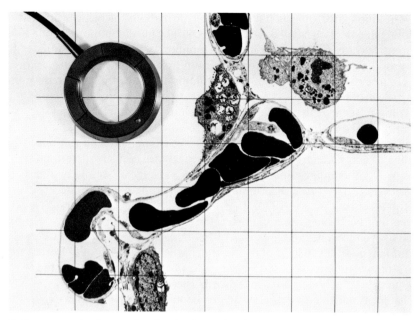

Fig. 8. Square test lattice overlay for the determination of harmonic mean tissue thickness and the tissue component of pulmonary diffusion capacity. A digitizer cursor is shown in the figure

as illustrated in Fig. 8. Using each of the horizontal and vertical lines, which are assumed to be random with respect to alveolar tissue, measurements of line length are made from the airspace surface to the capillary lumen surface using a digitizer table and computer.

5. Numerical Density Measurements

The numerical density of cells or of other particles or structures within the lung can be determined using morphometric techniques. Numerical densities are usually one of the more difficult parameters to determine and in the past this type of data has generally been obtained for cell numbers in the lung (BURRI et al. 1974; HAIES et al. 1981; CRAPO et al. 1980, 1982). Quantitation of subcellular particles has also been done (VIDIĆ and BURRI 1981; YOUNG et al. 1982). A number of approaches to measurements of numerical density have been proposed. Those in most common use employ Eqs. (8) or (9), Table 1. When determining cell numbers, nuclei are usually counted since their borders are distinct and are of more uniform size and shape. Each cell is assumed to have one nucleus. The number of nuclear profiles found per unit area of a random sectioning plane N_A must be divided by the mean caliper diameter of the nuclei $\bar{D}$ to determine the number of nuclei in unit volume of tissue. The mean caliper diameter is defined as the average distance across the particle averaged over all possible orientations of the object. This factor corrects for the fact that the probability of a particle being sectioned by a random plane is proportional to both the size and shape of the object.

Large or enlongated objects have a greater probability of being sectioned by a random plane than do small or round objects. The most common error in a semiquantitative study of lung tissue in which numbers of particles are estimated from their profile frequency on a random section N_A is to assume that this is representative of true particle frequency in a unit volume of tissue. A change in the number of particle profiles seen in a random tissue section may be due to a change in particle volume, a change in particle shape, or a change in particle number.

In Eq. (8), Table 1, the factors $2h$ and t refer to corrections that must be made for missing cap sections $2h$ and section thickness t. Small grazing sections through the edge of a particle are not likely to be recognized, causing determinations of N_A to be slightly underestimated. Counts of N_A assume an infinitely thin section. Thick sections may cause determinations of N_A to be overestimated because of the Holmes effect (WEIBEL 1979). In practice, if the section thickness is less than one-tenth of the mean caliper diameter, the effects of section thickness can be assumed to produce a negligible error ($t = 0$). Similarly, if thin sections are used and resolution is good, the height of cap sections which are likely not to be recognized in the section can be assumed to be negligible ($h = 0$). In this situation the formula for numerical density simplifies to the form listed in Eq. (9), Table 1.

The determination of cell nuclear profile number per unit area N_A has been done on 0.5-μm-thick plastic sections (KAUFFMAN et al. 1974) and by electron microscopy (CRAPO et al. 1983). Electron miscroscopy has the advantage that cell recognition is more accurate, resolution of small sections (cap sections) is enhanced, and section thickness (0.06 μm) is insignificant compared with nuclear size 5–10 μm). The major disadvantage of counting nuclear profiles by electron microscopy is enhanced work load. This can be minimized by using the same electron microscopy sections that are used for volume and surface area measurements and carrying out counts of nuclear profiles directly on the electron microscope rather than on prints. Grid squares completely covered by the tissue section and which contain lung parenchyma are counted, with each nuclear profile being classified according to its cell type. The grid bars form the boundaries for the area counted. Analysis of 20–30 consecutive grid squares (200 mesh grids) per section and evaluating four blocks per animal has been found to provide an adequate sample size to evaluate alveolar cell numbers in rats (CRAPO et al. 1978). For lungs from larger animals, more grid squares must be analyzed since fewer nuclei will be present per grid square owing to the larger airspaces.

In counting numbers of particles in a given section area, the unbiased counting rule described by GUNDERSON (1977) should be used. In counting cells only nuclear profiles located entirely within the grid square or those intersecting the upper and right-hand edges of the grid space are counted. Nuclear profiles which intersect the lower or left-hand grid bar are not counted. In addition, nuclear profiles falling on the lower left corner, the lower right corner, and the upper left corner are not counted, irrespective of whether the profile also contacts the upper or right-hand borders.

To determine the area of the section on which nuclear profiles were counted, the area of one grid square can be determined by photographing the entire grid square at × 500 in the electron microscope and measuring the area by digitization. We have found that the variation in grid square area on 200 mesh grids varies less than 2% on any single grid. However, greater differences do occur between grids. This suggests that at least one grid square needs to be measured from each grid on which nuclei counts are done. The total area counted for nuclear profiles for each section is calculated as the area of the grid square multiplied by the number of measured grid squares counted per section.

Determination of the mean caliper diameter $\bar{D}$ is the most difficult parameter to determine in evaluating numerical densities of particles. Several approaches to this problem are possible, including the following:

1. Assume a uniform shape for the particle being evaluated and calculate $\bar{D}$ from established formulae. This has been done by several investigators (KAUFFMAN et al. 1974; HAIES et al. 1981) who have assumed nuclei of various cell types to be spherical, oblate ellipsoids, or prolate ellipsoids. Formulae are available for calculating $\bar{D}$ from even more complex shapes such as triaxial ellipsoids (GREELEY et al. 1978). Solving for $\bar{D}$ is easiest when the particle in question can be assumed to be a sphere. Even if the particles represent spheres of heterogeneous sizes, the Schwartz-Saltykov technique for diameter analysis can be used to calculate the overall mean caliper diameter for the population of particles. This requires an analysis of about 200 random profiles through the particles (GREELEY and CRAPO 1978). Particles can deviate substantially from spheroidal shape and their mean caliper diameter can be calculated from the Schwartz-Saltykov technique with minimal error. Figure 9 shows that oblate and prolate ellipsoids can reach a ratio

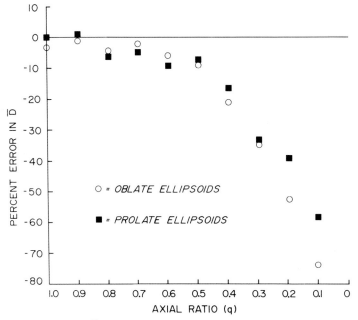

Fig. 9. Percentage error in $\bar{D}$ which results when oblate or prolate ellipsoids or revolution are assumed to be spheres and $\bar{D}$ is determined using the size class analysis method. For each data point, 1,000 random profiles were generated and there are no missed profiles. These elliptical profiles were mathematically converted to a circle of the same area in order to apply a Schwartz-Saltykov "sphere analysis" to the data (GREELEY and CRAPO 1978)

Table 2. Mean caliper diameter of nuclei from major classes of cells found in the alveolar region of mammalian lungs

Type of nucleus	Fischer 344	Sprague–Dawley		
	Rat	Rat	Dog	Human
Alveolar type I cell	$8.29 \pm 1.05_a$	$7.97 \pm 0.66_a$	$7.69 \pm 1.33_a$	$7.85 \pm 0.52_a$
Alveolar type II cell	$7.23 \pm 0.65_a$	$6.92 \pm 0.57_a$	$7.10 \pm 0.53_a$	$7.57 \pm 0.44_a$
Interstitial cells	$7.53 \pm 0.92_a$	$7.64 \pm 1.10_a$	$8.07 \pm 0.93_a$	$7.54 \pm 0.72_a$
Endothelial cells	$7.01 \pm 0.64_a$	8.00 ± 0.76	$7.07 \pm 0.37_a$	8.77 ± 1.09
Alveolar macrophages	$7.53 \pm 0.79_a$	$7.65 \pm 0.54_a$	6.39 ± 0.27	8.33 ± 0.86

All data are given in μm and are mean ± standard deviation. The means are weighted to account for and reduce sampling bias (GREELEY et al. 1978). For each type of cell nucleus, all data connected by the same letter subscript are not statistically different from each other

of short axis to long axis of 0.5 before analysis of random profiles of these particles, using the Schwartz-Saltykov technique to determine $\bar{D}$, creates an error of more than 10%.

2. Three-dimensional reconstruction of particles to determine mean caliper diameter. Serial section reconstruction of lung cell nuclei has been done for a number of animal species (Table 2). Computer algorithms have been used to allow these reconstructions to be done directly in computer memory and $\bar{D}$ to be calculated without shape assumptions (WOODY et al. 1979). This technique requires the preparation of serial 0.5-μm-thick plastic sections. Determination of section thickness is most easily done by measuring the size of a tissue block before and after sectioning with a vernier micrometer. A consecutive ribbon of at least 50 sections should be obtained. These sections are picked up on coverslips 3–5 sections at a time, stained on the coverslips, and mounted on glass slides. Nuclei should be randomly selected by placing a random point on the slide and identifying the nuclear profile whose center is closest to the random point. This technique reduces the potential bias of preferentially selecting large nuclear profiles for analysis. Another form of bias will remain in the analysis because large nuclei also have a larger probability of being intersected by any sectioning plane. It has been shown that their probability of appearing in the sectioning plane is directly proportional to their mean nuclear diameter and that the reciprocal of this factor should be used as a weighting factor to calculate the overall mean caliper diameter of a population of nuclei (GREELEY et al. 1978). Once a nucleus is identified for study from the center section of the serial sections, it is photographed in every section in which it occurs using high resolution light microscopy. For purposes of verification, sections before and after the nucleus begins and ends are also photographed. The particle profiles are digitized into computer memory with careful attention to their orientation with respect to each other so that a vertical stacking distortion is not introduced. This procedure and the computer analysis of the serial sections has been extensively described (GREELEY et al. 1978; WOODY et al. 1979).

3. Determination of particle size by studying sections of varying thickness. This method, which does not directly determine $\bar{D}$, but is a reflection of particle size, was described by LOUD et al. (1978) for myocytes. The procedure uses sections of known varying thickness to count the number of nuclear profiles found per unit area. Thicker sections have a greater probability of intersecting random objects [Eq. (8), Table 1]. Since the size of the nucleus $\bar{D}$ is directly proportional to the probability of being sectioned, N_A will vary linearly with section thickness. Values for N_A obtained from sections of various known thickness can be plotted against section thickness to give a straight line whose slope is a reflection of the numerical density N_V of the object.

4. Determination of particle size by determining the number of particles whose profile remains in sequential sections of known distance apart. The number of particles in a given field is compared with the number of those same particles whose profile remains in a similar field in a section taken a known distance further into the block. The mean caliper diameter of the particles can be easily calculated from these data using the formula

$$\bar{D} = \frac{N_o}{N_r} H,$$

where N_o is the number of particles found in the original section, N_r is the number of those same particles whose profile remains in the subsequent section, and H is the distance between sections. The major limitations in this approach are: (a) it assumes section thickness is small relative to particle size; (b) errors caused by failure to recognize small cap sections of particles are compounded; and (c) the entire technique is critically dependent upon accurate measurement of section thickness in order to calculate the distance between two sections in a series of serial sections.

5. Assume a value for mean caliper diameter. Table 2 gives the $\bar{D}$ values for each major alveolar cell type in normal control rats (Sprague–Dawley and Fischer 344), dogs, baboons, and humans. The values for $\bar{D}$ vary relatively little between cell types and between animals of substantial differences in body size. Exposure to toxicants may or may not alter $\bar{D}$ for specific lung cells. Severe lung injury caused by oxidant exposure (CRAPO et al. 1978) or by asbestos (PINKERTON et al. 1983) have been shown to have little effect on the mean caliper diameter of most lung cell types. After exposure to oxygen, significant effects on $\bar{D}$ were found only for capillary endothelial cells and alveolar type II epithelial cells. However, even these changes represented only a 25% or less variation. One means of determining whether $\bar{D}$ has changed following an exposure is to measure the nuclear profile area of a large series of randomly selected nuclear profiles from both control and treated animals and compare the distributions on these profile areas to determine if any statistical significance exists. This analysis will not completely rule out the possibility that $\bar{D}$ has changed since compensating shape and volume changes could have occurred. If $\bar{D}$ values from the literature are used, it is important that the lung tissue be prepared in the same manner to prevent tissue fixation differences from biasing numerical density estimates (HAIES et al. 1981).

6. Estimation of Lung Function by Morphometric Estimations of Diffusing Capacity

The pulmonary diffusion capacity for carbon monoxide DL_{CO} and its components, membrane diffusing capacity D_m and the pulmonary capillary blood volume V_c are traditionally measured using physiologic techniques and the relationship derived by ROUGHTON and FORSTER (1957)

$$1/DL_{CO} = 1/D_m + 1/\theta V_c$$

where θ is a coefficient which expresses the binding of the test gas (CO) to hemoglobin.

WEIBEL (1970, 1971) has described a technique for estimating the pulmonary diffusion capacity for oxygen (DL_{O2}) using morphometric techniques. The approach follows the ROUGHTON and FORSTER (1957) concepts and permits the calculation of membrane diffusion capacity D_m as the sum of the tissue and plasma barriers to diffusion. All that is required for this calculation are the use of the formulae and constants given in Table 3 and values for tissue densities, surface areas, and harmonic mean thicknesses using techniques already described. Some differences between lung diffusion capacity and the membrane component of diffusion capacity as measured by physiologic and morphometric techniques have been identified (CRAPO and CRAPO 1983), however, the reasons for these differences are not fully explained. Since fixation techniques may affect pulmonary capillary blood volume and thereby the calculation of total lung diffusion capacity, one of the most valuable morphometric parameters to estimate alterations in lung function may be measurement of the membrane component diffusion capacity.

Table 3. Equations used for morphometric estimates of diffusion capacity

Total lung diffusion capacity	$\dfrac{1}{DL} = \dfrac{1}{D_m} + \dfrac{1}{\theta V_c}$	(1)
Membrane diffusion capacity	$\dfrac{1}{D_m} = \dfrac{1}{D_t} + \dfrac{1}{D_p}$	(2)
Tissue barrier	$D_t = K_t \times \dfrac{S_a + S_c}{2 \times \tau_{ht}}$	(3)
Plasma barrier	$D_p = K_p \times \dfrac{S_c + S_e}{2 \times \tau_{hp}}$	(4)
Harmonic mean thickness	$\dfrac{1}{\tau_h} = \dfrac{3}{2n} \times \sum\limits_{i=1}^{n} \dfrac{1}{l_i}$	(5)

$K_t = 3.3 \times 10^{-8}$; $K_p = 4.3 \times 10^{-8}$; $\theta = 0.9-2.5$. V_c = pulmonary capillary blood volume; S_a = surface area of air-tissue interface; S_c = surface area of tissue-blood interface; S_e = surface area of erythrocytes in capillary bed; τ_{ht} = harmonic mean thickness of tissue; τ_{hp} = harmonic mean thickness of plasma; l_i = length of random line intercept

VI. Equipment

A variety of instruments are available for doing morphometric studies. The basic instruments which are most helpful in morphometric studies are a digitizer table and a small computer. The digitizer is useful in measuring areas and lengths with a high degree of accuracy. Most of the formulae used in morphometry are fairly simple; however, a computer is essential in performing the basic calculations because of the large volumes of data that are usually generated. An automated sampling stage for light microscopy is helpful, in particular, for morphometric studies where random sampling is done using light microscopy. The automated sampling stage light microscope can reduce observer bias in selecting areas for study, can increase the uniformity of sampling across single sections, and can increase speed and accuracy (particularly if a computer is used to control movement of the stage and simultaneously record the observed results). However, an automated sampling stage is not imperative since alternative approaches can usually be designed and it has only a minimal role in morphometric studies which utilize electron microscopy.

Automated counting devices have a great appeal for those who are considering morphometry as a research tool, but are in most instances not worth the investment. The quantitation of lung anatomy is simply an application of basic morphometric formulae which can be easily hand calculated or written as a simple computer program to yield the same results as an automated counting device – usually more efficiently and at a much lower cost. The use of a digitizer pad (as is done on many commercially available systems) to record point and line intercept counts automatically is less efficient than recording them by hand because the digitizer requires two operations to record a single point. A simple hand counter or the direct use of a computer to count points is more efficient.

References

Bachofen M, Weibel ER (1977) Alterations of the gas exchange apparatus in adult respiratory insufficiency associated with septicemia. Am Rev Respir Dis 116:589–615

Barry BE, Miller FJ, Crapo JD (1983) Alveolar epithelial injury caused by inhalation of 0.25 ppm of ozone. In: Lee SO, Mustafa MG, Mehlman MA (eds) Adv Mod Envir Tox 5. Princeton Scientific Publishers, Princeton, pp 299–309

Bartlett D (1970) Postnatal growth of the mammalian lung: influence of low and high oxygen tensions. Respir Physiol 9:58–64

Burri PH, Weibel ER (1977) Ultrastructure and morphometry of the developing lung. In: Hodson WA (ed) The development of the lung. Dekker, New York, p 215

Burri PH, Dbaly J, Weibel ER (1974) The postnatal growth of the rat lung. I. Morphometry. Anat Rec 178:711–730

Cochran WG (1963) Sampling techniques, 2nd edition. Wiley, New York

Crapo JD, Crapo RO (1983) Comparison of total lung diffusion capacity and the membrane component of diffusion capacity as determined by physiologic and morphometric techniques. Respir Physiol 51:183–194

Crapo JD, Peters-Golden J, Marsh-Salin J, Shelburne JS (1978) Pathologic changes in the lungs of oxygen-adapted rats. A morphometric analysis. Lab Invest 39:640–653

Crapo JD, Barry BE, Foscue HA, Shelburne J (1980) Structural and biochemical changes in rat lungs occurring during exposures to lethal and adaptive doses of oxygen. Am Rev Respir Dis 122:123–143

Crapo JD, Barry BE, Gehr P, Bachofen M, Weibel ER (1982) Cell numbers and cell characteristics of the normal human lung. Am Rev Respir Dis 126:332–337

Crapo JD, Young SL, Fram EK, Pinkerton KE, Barry BE, Crapo RO (1983) Morphometric characteristics of cells in the alveolar region of mammalian lungs. Am Rev Respir Dis 128:S42–S46

Crapo RO, Crapo JD, Morris AH (1982) Lung tissue and capillary blood volumes by rebreathing and morphometric techniques. Respir Physiol 49:175–186

Davies G, Reid L (1970) Growth of the alveoli and pulmonary arteries in childhood. Thorax 25:669–681

DeHoff RT, Rhines FN (1968) Quantitative Microscopy. McGraw-Hill, New York

Dunnill MS (1962a) Quantitative methods in the study of pulmonary pathology. Thorax 17:320–328

Dunnill MS (1962b) Postnatal growth of the lung. Thorax 17:329–333

Elias H (1967) Stereology. Proceedings of the second international conference for stereology. Springer, Berlin Heidelberg New York

Eränkö O (1955) Quantitative methods in histology and microscopic histochemistry. Little, Brown, Boston

Gehr P, Weibel ER (1974) Morphometric estimation of regional differences in the dog lung. J Appl Physiol 37:648

Glazier JB, Hughes JMB, Maloney JE, West JB (1967) Vertical gradient of alveolar size in lungs of dogs frozen intact. J Appl Physiol 23:694

Greeley D, Crapo JD (1978) Practical approach to the estimation of the overall mean caliper diameter of a population of spheres. J Microsc 114:261–269

Greeley D, Crapo JD, Vollmer R (1978) Estimation of the mean caliper diameter of cell nuclei: I. Serial section reconstruction method and endothelial nuclei from human lung. J Microsc 114:31–39

Gunderson HJG (1977) Notes on the estimation of the numerical density of arbitrary profiles: the edge effect. J Microsc 111:219

Haies DM, Gil J, Weibel ER (1981) Morphometric study of rat lung cells. I. Numerical and dimensional characteristics of parenchymal cell population. Am Rev Respir Dis 123:533–541

Hayatdavoudi G, Crapo JD, Miller FJ, O'Neil JJ (1980) Factors determining degree of inflation in intratracheally fixed rat lungs. J Appl Physiol 48(2):389–393

Hennig A (1956) Bestimmung der Oberfläche beliebig geformter Körper mit besonderer Anwendung auf Körperhaufen im mikroskopischen Bereich. Mikroskopie 11:1–20

Hyde D, Orthoefer J, Dungworth D, Tyler W, Carter R, Lum H (1978) Morphometric and morphologic evaluation of pulmonary lesions in beagle dogs chronically exposed to high ambient levels of air pollutants. Lab Invest 38:455–469

Kapanci Y, Weibel ER, Kaplan HP, Robinson FR (1969) Pathogenesis and reversibility of the pulmonary lesions of oxygen toxicity in monkeys. II. Ultrastructural and morphometric studies. Lab Invest 20:101–118

Kauffman SL, Burri PH, Weibel ER (1974) The postnatal growth of the rat lung. II. Autoradiography. Anat Rec 180:63–76

Knapp MK, Crapo JD (1984) Morphometry of the normal baboon lung. (to be published)

Loud AV, Anversa P, Giacomelli F, Wiener J (1978) Absolute morphometric study of myocardial hypertrophy in experimental hypertension. I. Determination of myocyte size. Lab Invest 38:586–596

Mathieu O, Classen H, Weibel ER (1978) Differential effect of glutaraldehyde and buffer osmolarity on cell dimensions. A study on lung tissue. J Ultrastruct Res 63:20

Pinkerton KE, Barry BE, O'Neil JJ, Raub JA, Pratt PC, Crapo JD (1982) Morphologic changes in the lung during the lifespan of Fischer 344 rats. Am J Anat 164:155–174

Pinkerton KE, Pratt PC, Brody AR, Crapo JD (1984) Fiber localization and its relationship to lung reaction in rats after chronic inhalation of chrysotile asbestos. Amer. J. Path. 117:142–156

Roughton FJW, Forster RE (1957) Relative importance of diffusion and chemical reaction rates in determining rate of exchange of gases in the human lung, with special reference to true diffusing capacity of pulmonary membrane and volume of blood in the lung capillaries. J Appl Physiol 11:290–302

Snider GL, Korthy AL (1978) Internal surface area and number of respiratory air spaces in elastase-induced emphysema in hamsters. Am Rev Respir Dis 117:685–693

Thurlbeck WM (1967) The internal surface area of nonempysematous lungs. Am Rev Respir Dis 95:756–773

Tomkeieff SI (1945) Linear intercepts, areas and volumes. Nature 155:24, 107

Underwood EE (1970) Quantitative stereology. Addision-Wesley, Reading

Vidic B, Burri PH (1981) Quantitative cellular and subcellular changes in the rat type II pneumocyte during early postnatal development. Am Rev Respir Dis 124:174–178

Weibel ER (1963) Morphometry of the human lung. Academic, New York

Weibel ER (1970) An automatic samling stage microscope for stereology. J Microsc 91:1

Weibel ER (1971) Morphometric estimation of pulmonary diffusion capacity. I. Model and method. Respir Physiol 11:54–75

Weibel ER (1979) Stereological methods, vol 1 and 2. Academic, New York

Weibel ER, Gomez DM (1962) A principle for counting tissue structures on random sections. J Appl Physiol 17(2):343–348

Weibel ER, Knight BW (1964) A morphometric study on the thickness of the pulmonary air-blood barrier. J Cell Biol 21:367–384

Williams DA (1972) The comparison of several dose levels with a zero dose control. Biometrics 28:519–531

Woody DM, Woody EZ, Crapo JD (1979) Determination of the mean caliper diameter of lung nuclei by a method which is independent of shape assumptions. J Microsc 118:421–427

Young SL, Crapo JD, Kremers SA, Brumley GW (1982) Pulmonary surfactant lipid production in oxygen-exposed rat lungs. Lab Invest 46:570–576

Biological and Biochemical Analysis

CHAPTER 11

Cellular Kinetics of the Lung

I. Y. R. Adamson

A. Introduction

Cell turnover is a well-recognized normal process whereby dying cells in an organ may be desquamated and replaced by newly divided cells. The dynamics of this process vary with the cell type and, for example, may be rapid for gut epithelium, but very slow for hepatocytes (Leblond et al. 1959). In the adult lung, normal cell turnover ist low with a mitotic rate of about 3 cells per 1,000 at any one time. This is an average value for all the different pulmonary cell types, estimated by Sorokin (1970) to be around 40. However, not all of these are capable of division; some are stem cells that may divide, whereas others are more differentiated and do not usually reenter the mitotic cycle.

In terms of proliferation, the cells of the lung may be grouped into three populations (Baserga 1981). In the first group are cells that continously divide and pass unceasingly through the M, G_1, S, and G_2 phases of the cell cycle. This process may be accelerated in a growing phase such as fetal development and after injury. The second group is comprised of cells that leave the cycle after a number of divisions and then differentiate. These cells are no longer capable of division and will ultimately die. The third group of cells may leave the cycle temporarily and remain dormant in the G_0 phase; a subsequent change in local environment can induce these quiescent cells to reenter the cycle and proliferate. Cell turnover in normal lung will therefore depend on the proportions of cells in these different proliferation groups and most measurements give a composite value vor the whole lung.

Exposure of the lung to a toxin often results in enhanced cell division, usually as a response to cellular injury which is repaired by proliferation of an unharmed stem cell; this process may be followed by differentiation. If these events occur rapidly, normal structure and function is usually restored with minimal sequelae. However, extensive prolonged injury to the various cells of the lung may not be immediately repaired by accelerated cell division alone, and further pathologic changes may develop. Increased mitotic activity in the lung may be accomplished by: (a) accelerated division of continuously dividing cells, and (b) increased entry of G_0 cells into the cycle. Acceleration usually occurs by shortening the G_1 phase which is the most variable for different cell types and is longer in cells with slow growth. Studies to determine the length of specific phases of the cell cycle are difficult because of the cellular heterogeneity and the difficulty of specific cellular identification.

The multicellular nature of the lung also has consequences for many other measurements. Biochemical determinations made on lung extracts give a composite picture for the whole lung and it is often difficult to attribute specific changes to a particular pulmonary cell type. On the other hand, morphological evidence of pulmonary injury and repair in specific cells usually suffers from a lack of functionally related data. Studies that combine structural and functional parameters coupled with kinetic determinations of turnover times and replacement mechanisms for the individual cell types will give more complete information necessary for toxicologic assessment.

B. Use of Cytokinetics in Pulmonary Toxicology

Exposure of the lung to a foreign substance will initially result in an adaptive response. In some cell types, this consists of a metabolic adaptation which is reflected in changes in subcellular components without altering cell turnover (BOYD 1980). In response to particulate material, the number of alveolar macrophages increases as new cells are produced from both blood and interstitial compartments (BOWDEN and ADAMSON 1978; ADAMSON and BOWDEN 1980), thus changing the cellular kinetics of the lung. However, the most common examples of altered cytokinetics occur after necrosis where repair is characterized by enhanced cellular proliferation. It is well established that there is a differential susceptibility of specific lung cells to injury and the patterns of repair, including cell renewal, are also different. In particular, the timing of enhanced cell division is often crucial in determining whether the injury is reversible or whether fibrosis develops. This point is illustrated when considering oxygen toxicity to the lung.

Brief exposure of mice to 90% oxygen produces endothelial injury (KISTLER et al. 1967; BOWDEN et al. 1968a), and on return to air, surviving endothelial cells proliferate rapidly as the lung returns to normal (BOWDEN and ADAMSON 1974). Longer exposure results in a marked decrease in total DNA owing to both endothelial and epithelial cell necrosis (BOWDEN and ADAMSON 1971). On return to air, the DNA level rises sharply owing to sequential increases in endothelial and epithelial proliferation, (ADAMSON and BOWDEN 1974; BOWDEN and ADAMSON 1974), and the lung structure returns to normal in a few days. However, if epithelial necrosis is more severe or prolonged, there is evidence of delayed cell proliferation in the epithelium, associated with fibroblastic proliferation and collagen deposition in the pulmonary interstitium (ADAMSON and BOWDEN 1976; GOULD et al. 1972). In this instance, the postexposure rise in DNA may be attributed to endothelial, epithelial, or fibroblastic cell division, depending upon the time of measurement. There appears to be a link between delayed epithelial repair and fibrosis, suggesting that proliferation and replacement of the surface lining cells is important in controlling the underlying fibroblasts. If so, it becomes vital to determine which cells are capable of proliferation following a toxic insult, as a marker of whether normal or abnormal repair is likely to occur.

Another example of the variable pattern of cellular division following injury is the pulmonary reaction to butylated hydroxytoluene. Initial reports on the toxicity of this compound suggest that primarily it stimulates DNA synthesis in the lung (WITSCHI and SAHEB 1974). More detailed studies indicate that the enhanced DNA synthesis is due to cellular renewal following injury to endothelial and type I epithelial cells (WITSCHI and CÔTÉ 1977; ADAMSON et al. 1977). Values for total DNA and the enzymes associated with DNA synthesis give the overall timing of repair, but are not indicative of the specific cell types involved. Microscopic techniques such as autoradiography have been used to identify cells in DNA synthesis at different times after toxic injury. In this way the biochemical determinations of total DNA can be matched to the percentage of cells in DNA synthesis in lung sections; identification of individual cells gives a breakdown of DNA synthesis by specific lung cell types. After butylated hydroxytoluene, treatment the increase in cell division is due to a rapid epithelial proliferation followed by slower renewal of endothelial cells and a later phase of fibroblast proliferation (ADAMSON et al. 1977).

These examples illustrate briefly the importance of cellular renewal studies in toxicologic investigations. An increase in the rate of cell division is part of the normal reparative pattern in the lung, and if followed by differentiation and restoration of normal structure, the lung may cope adequately with an inhaled cytotoxic substance. However, DNA synthesis does not necessarily occur equally or at the same time in all cell types. Regeneration of a particular cell type may not occur at all, may be delayed, or may be followed by inappropriate differentiation, any of which can lead to further changes in the structure and function of the lung. In these cases, the most common sequel is fibrosis. It is also possible that the switch-on of DNA synthesis may not be controlled and neoplasia might result. These possibilities indicate the need in planning of toxicologic assessment, to correlate the biochemical measurements not only with morphology of the lung, but also with cytodynamic studies to determine changes in the timing and patterns of cell turnover. The principal focus of this chapter is to provide the background information for such studies. This includes the methods of assessing cellular renewal, discussion of the processes of cell division and differentiation to replace the various lung cells, and the kinetics of cell turnover for the specific cell types under normal circumstances.

C. Methods to Determine Cell Turnover

I. Autoradiography

1. General Principles

The process whereby an exposure is made on a photographic emulsion by a radioactive specimen is called autoradiography. A section of tissue containing a radioactive substance is covered by a photographic emulsion for a period of time to allow exposure. Subsequently, it is developed photographically and the precise location of the radioactive molecules is marked by black grains of silver in the exposed emulsion. The grains are formed directly over the cellular site of isotopic incorporation and can be seen in the sections with or without conventional staining.

Although in theory all isotopes will expose a photographic emulsion, only the following low energy β-emitters are useful for autoradiography: ^{3}H, ^{131}I, and ^{35}S. Tritium-labeled compounds are most widely used because of their low energy which will be dissipated in collisions close to source, i.e., they will only expose emulsion closest to the isotope, resulting in good correlation between the location of the silver grains and the site of isotope incorporation.

The composition of the emulsion, which consists of a mixture of small silver halide crystals in gelatin, influences autoradiographic results. For most autoradiographic procedures, the emulsion is melted in darkness and slides with tissue sections are briefly dipped into the gel and allowed to dry. Contact between emitted β-particles from the incorporated isotope and silver halide forms a latent image which produces a metallic silver grain when the slide is subsequently passed through a developing solution. The size of each silver grain will depend on the particular composition of the emulsion. For light microscopy, a grain size of 0.2–0.3 μm is common, but emulsion of much smaller grain size is used in ultrastructural studies where localization of isotope to an organelle or membrane site is required. Detailed information on the theories, experimental procedures, and applications of autoradiography is available (ROGERS 1973; SCHULTZE 1969).

Identification of specific cells and cell types that undergo mitosis and the sequential following of these cells after mitosis is one of the widest applications of autoradiography. It is known that mitosis is preceded by a period of synthesis and, by administering a radioactive precursor of DNA, the nuclei of cells about to divide become radioactivite and can be detected by autoradiography. In addition, after mitosis the two daughter cells will still contain labeled DNA and the fate of these cells may also be followed. The most commonly used substances are tritium-labeled DNA precursors since tritium has a low energy, does not appear to damage cells in the doses used, and can be localized quite precisely.

Tritiated thymidine is the most frequently used compound. It is incorporated into DNA during the S phase which usually lasts 6–8 h (BERTALANFFY (1964a). Although there is some incorporation of thymidine associated with the synthesis of metabolic DNA (PELC 1972), it is generally assumed that almost all the labeling will be in cells of renewing populations. It has been shown that circulating tritiated thymidine is incorporated into nuclei within 1 h of injection (HUGHES et al. 1958; ROGERS 1973), and that once labeled, cells retain the isotope, which may only be diluted by subsequent cell division.

Tissue samples taken after incorporation of tritiated thymidine may be prepared for scintillation counting using standard methods; the level of tritium gives a measure of overall DNA synthesis. Other samples can be sectioned and prepared for autoradiography, usually at the light microscope level. If the identity of the labeled cells is not clear by light microscopy, tissue can be prepared for electron microscopy. Identification of labeled cells can be made in the electron microscope (KOPRIWA 1973; ROGERS 1973).

2. Application to the Lung

The lung as a whole has a low level of cell turnover and, in tissue sections, only 3–4 cells per 1,000 incorporate thymidine under normal conditions; about 30% of these cells are intravascular leukocytes. These values are obtained from autoradiographs and, in most experiments, tissue samples are examined at various times so that changes in DNA synthesis can be plotted serially during an experiment.

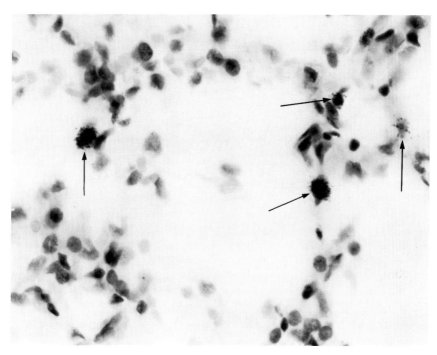

Fig. 1. Lung autoradiograph of 5-μm-thick paraffin section after administration of thymidine ³H. Labeled nuclei can be seen (*arrows*), but precise cellular identification is not possible. Feulgen stain × 1,000

The difference between a labeled cell with many exposed silver grains over the nucleus and an unlabeled cell is readily observed. However, the precise identification of each labeled cell is not so readily determined in the lung and the amount of kinetic data obtained will largely depend on the type of tissue section used.

The early work on cell kinetics relied on paraffin blocks (BERTALANFFY 1964 b) which are large enough for the overall counts of labeled cells to be representative of the whole lung and regional variations among lobes or within a lobe can be determined. However, the section thickness (about 5 μm) makes it difficult to identify the cell types (Fig. 1). In particular, when examining the alveolar walls, it is not easy to differentiate capillary endothelial cells from intravascular cells or from interstitial fibroblasts, and often type II cells cannot be distinguished from alveolar macrophages that are closely adherent to the alveolar wall.

Precise cellular identification can be made on autoradiographs prepared for electron microscopy; the silver grains are electron dense and can be readily recognized (Fig. 2). However, each ultra thin section examined represents a very small sample of the whole lung and very few labeled nuclei are seen in each section. The sampling problems make ultrastructural autoradiography of the lung a very expensive, time-consuming process. It is useful, however, in selective cases to confirm the identity of a labeled population as seen by light microscopy.

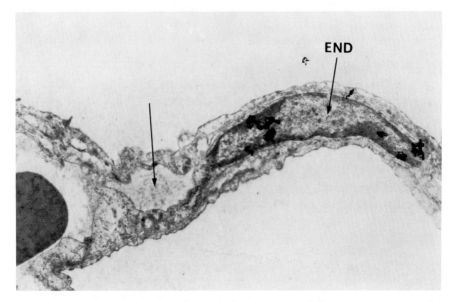

Fig. 2. Electron microscopic autoradiograph showing exposed silver grains over a nucleus, readily identified as an endothelial cell (*END*) lining a capillary. × 6,000

Plastic sections for light microscopy are now being used with increased frequency for autoradiographic studies of the lung. Plastics of the methacrylate group are generally not hard enough for electron microscopy, but can be cut at 0.5–1.0 μm thickness for light microscopy using a glass knife. An autoradiographic of mouse lung after tritiated thymidine injection and embedding in glycol methacrylate is shown in Fig. 3. This technique allows slices through an entire lobe of mouse lung to be embedded in one block. Morphological and autoradiograph differences in different anatomic regions can be examined, and enough cells can be counted for statistical analysis. The chief advantage, however, is the much superior resolution compared with paraffin sections (see Fig. 1). The improved slide quality allows identification of about 95% of cells and so the patterns of DNA labeling in the various pulmonary cells can be followed.

Counts of labeled cells are also more accurate when thinner sections are used. In paraffin sections, all nuclei in the 5-μm section are stained and counted. However, only nuclei containing isotope in the top 2 μm of the section will produce silver grains; below this depth the energy of the tritium will dissipate before reaching the emulsion (ROGERS 1973). Thus, the efficiency of the autoradiographic process is lower so that the percentage of labeled nuclei will be smaller in 5-μm paraffin sections as compared with 1-μm methacrylate sections of the same tissue.

3. Pulse Labeling Experiments

The most common type of study for evaluating changes in lung cell kinetics is the pulse labeling experiment. At intervals after administration of a possible toxin,

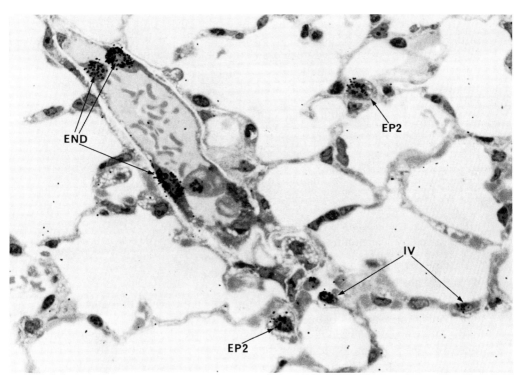

Fig. 3. Autoradiograph of a 0,75-μm-thick methacrylate section from a mouse recovering from exposure to 90% oxygen. Numerous thymidine ^{3}H-labeled nuclei can be seen and cellular identification is possible on this type of section. *EP2* type II cells; *END* endothelium; *IV* intravascular cells. Toluidine blue stain × 1,200 (ADAMSON and BOWDEN 1974)

animals are injected, usually intraperitoneally, with a standard dose of tritiated thymidine (1–2 μCi/g) and killed at a fixed time afterwards, usually 1 h (ADAMSON and BOWDEN 1974; ADAMSON et al. 1977). All the thymidine will be incorporated by cells in the S phase within 30 min, and by killing at 1 h, it is unlikely that any of these labeled cells will have progressed much further in the cycle; some do reach the M phase, but do not divide in the short time available before death.

Several blocks of lung tissue can be prepared from each animal in the experimental group and autoradigraphs prepared. In random microscopic fields, the number of labeled nuclei in a total of about 2,000 cells per section can be determined and a labeling percentage calculated for all lung cells at each time studied. This radiographic index is a measure of overall DNA synthesis in the lung and it has been shown that results of autoradiographic methods correlate well with biochemical markers of DNA synthesis such as thymidine kinase (ADAMSON et al. 1977; WITSCHI and CÔTÉ 1977). One possible error in the determination can occur during an inflammatory response in the lung where there may be a large number of leukocytes in the pulmonary interstitium and alveoli. These are not true lung cells, but cells in transit that add to the overall number of nuclei and, being largely unlabeled, they will lower the observed percentage of labeled cells while increasing the total DNA of the lung.

Once the radiographic index is determined on methacrylate sections, analysis of the labeled cells can be performed in two ways. First, a differential count can be made whereby each labeled nucleus in random fields can be categorized as endothelial, type I or type II epithelial, interstitial, alveolar macrophage, or intravascular. Using a sample of 300 labeled cells per section, differential percentages may be calculated for each cell type (ADAMSON and BOWDEN 1974; ADAMSON et al. 1977). A second possibility is to analyze serially the kinetics of an individual cell population. On autoradiographs, cells of a specific type can be identified and the number labeled and unlabeled recorded. In this way a labeling index can be calculated separately for each cell population in the lung. This approach is particularly useful in analyzing changes that are marked, but limited to one cell type, and so would appear less significant if included with the other normal lung cells in an overall estimation of cell turnover. Changes in cytokinetics of endothelial cells (MEYRICK and REID 1979) and type II epithelial cells (KAUFFMAN 1972) have been studied by determining exclusively the labeling indices of these cell types.

4. Serial Labeling Experiments

Information on the fate of cells after division and on the generation time of a specific population may be obtained by extending the period between the injection of the DNA precursor and killing the animal. Tritiated thymidine is incorporated solely into the DNA molecule during the S phase and, during subsequent division, tritium atoms are distributed approximately equally between the two daughter cells. By examining autoradiographs, this process will be reflected in a halving of the number of silver grains over the nuclei of the daughter cells. The label will halve with each subsequent division until it becomes so dilute it cannot be demonstrated above background grains in the autoradiographs.

Cell turnover in the lung can be determined by injecting a large number of animals with labeled thymidine at day 0 and sacrificing at intervals afterwards. The identity of labeled cells is determined and a count of the grain number made on each type of nucleus. These values are plotted against time to determine the period required for halving of the grain count, which is indicative of the generation time for the particular cell. In normal lung, the overall percentage of cells labeled is low and it is not raised significantly by increasing the dose of thymidine, which will merely give a heavier label per nucleus rather than increase the number of labeled cells. More labeled cells can be obtained by giving three doses of thymidine at 8-h intervals on day 0 to increase the chance of labeling different cells entering the S phase at the time of each injection (BOWDEN and ADAMSON 1980). In a period of cell necrosis, there may be a drop in DNA labeling, but any subsequent phase of repair will result in enhanced synthesis and accelerated mitotic rate of pulmonory cells.

Frequent observations after administration of tritiated thymidine can be used to obtain information on the cell cycle. Cells labeled in the S phase go on to mitosis (M phase) and the numbers of labeled mitotic figures can be counted and compared with unlabeled mitoses from cells in the G_1 phase when the isotope was injected. Although these methods have been used to estimate times of passage through the cell cycle, they are particularly useful for rapidly dividing, single cell

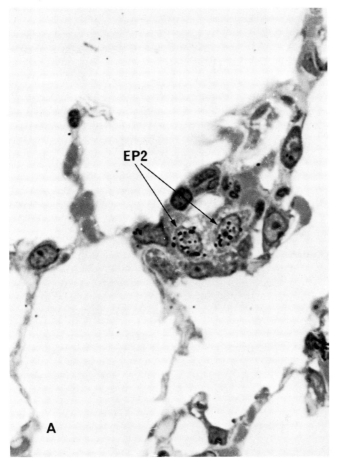

Fig. 4 a, b. Methacrylate sections of mice that received thymidine ^{3}H 2.5 days after removal from 90% O_2. **a** 4 h after injection, epithelial labeling is confined to type II cells (*EP2*); **b** 3 days after isotope injection, grain count in type II cells halves and labeled type I cells (*EP1*) are observed. Toluidine blue stain × 1,500. (ADAMSON and BOWDEN 1974)

populations (QUASTLER and SHERMAN 1959; BERTALANFFY 1964a). Cell cycle determinations in the lung are usually based on the halving of grain counts and the changing pattern of label in a specific cell type, such as the type II cell kinetics in the production of adenomas (DYSON and HEPPLESTON 1975).

Renewal of epithelial cells is an example where the reparative process can be followed by studying the fate of cells labeled during DNA synthesis. In the alveolus, following injury to type I cells, the type II cells proliferate (BOWDEN and ADAMSON 1971; ADAMSON and BOWDEN 1974; EVANS et al. 1975). By injecting tritiated thymidine and killing 1 h later, type II cells incorporate the isotope whereas surviving type I cells remain unlabeled. When the time between thymidine injection and killing is increased, the average number of silver grains in the type II cells drops from 17 to 8 in 3 days, indicating cell division. At that time, labeled type I cells are first observed without injecting more isotope, demonstrat-

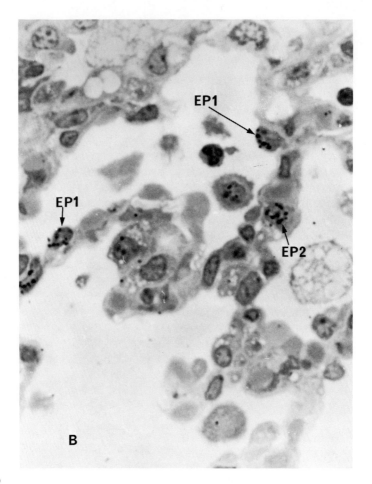

Fig. 4b

ing that the type I cells are derived from dividing type II cells (Fig. 4; ADAMSON and BOWDEN 1974). This process has also been described using these cytokinetic methods for the differentiation of the alveolar epithelium in the fetus (ADAMSON and BOWDEN 1975). Similar experiments have demonstrated that the stem cells of the airway epithelium are basal cells which subsequently differentiate to produce the various cells of the surface lining (BREEZE and WEELDON 1977).

Isotopic labeling may also be used to follow cells in transit; an example is the study of the alveolar macrophage production system. It is known that alveolar macrophages have a dual origin: most arise from blood monocytes that cross through the interstitium to the alveoli while a smaller population arise by division and migration of cells in the pulmonary interstitium (BOWDEN and ADAMSON 1980). These conclusions were made by labeling DNA of mice by tritiated thymidine and serially following the fate of labeled cells. By identifying specific labeled cell types (monocytes in the blood smears, interstitial cells and macrophages in lung sections) and counting the silver grains, temporal relationships can be established to determine whether cells migrate through the lung from blood to al-

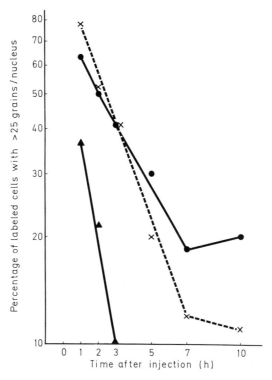

Fig. 5. Semilogarithmic plot showing the serial disappearance of the heaviest labeled cells from normal mice after three injections of thymidine ³H in 8 h. Rapid elimination of la- beled circulating monocytes (*triangles*) correlates with cellular migration from blood through the lung as interstitial cells (*crosses*) and alveolar macrophages (*circles*). The graphs diverge at 1 week, showing a second smaller population of macrophages related to division of heavily labeled interstitial cells. (BOWDEN and ADAMSON 1980)

veolus with or without division. By following the disappearance of the most heavily labeled cells (VAN FURTH and COHN 1968), BOWDEN and ADAMSON (1980) showed that migration from blood to alveolus without division occurs for most cells, whereas a smaller number of macrophages are linked to a slowly dividing population of precursors in the interstitium (Fig. 5).

In many cases, assessment of pulmonary cell kinetics can be made by a com- bination of pulse and serial labeling. From a pulse label study the timing of the maximal thymidine incorporation into a specific cell type is determined. If the ex- periment is repeated and tritiated thymidine given only at the time of the predict- ed peak, the cell type in maximal DNA synthesis will be preferentially labeled. The accelerated turnover of this cell and the fate of its daughters can be deter- mined by serial killing and autoradiography.

II. Mitotic Arrest

Examination of routine tissue sections of lung reveals only an occasional cell in mitosis. In order to increase this number and provide a sufficient dividing population for analysis, the stathmokinetic or mitotic arrest technique has been developed. Although many compounds have the property of arresting cells in metaphase, colchicine or one of its derivatives is the most commonly used. These agents interact with the mitotic spindle, causing a failure to assemble or a disruption, which leads to arrest of mitosis. The number of metaphases seen microscopically will therefore increase with time after drug injection as cells reaching metaphase are arrested and remain in that state. When this time interval is known, the number of cells of a particular type arrested in metaphase over that period can be counted and the time required for the division of the entire population calculated (BERTALANFFY 1964a; ADAMSON and BOWDEN 1974; THORUD et al. 1980).

The mitotic arrest method has one advantage over autoradiography after tritiated thymidine treatment. This latter method will label cells in DNA synthesis, but it is not always certain that all these cells will actually divide since it has been

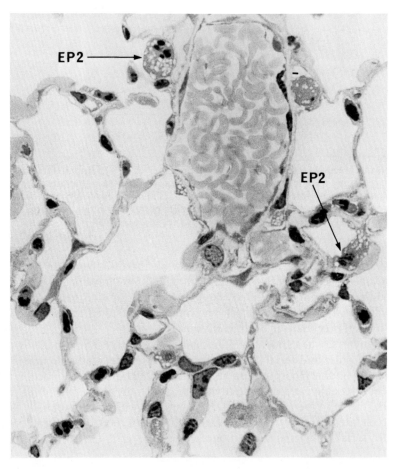

Fig. 6. Type II cells (*EP2*), proliferating in response to type I cell injury by oxygen, are arrested in metaphase by colchicine injection. Methacrylate section, hematoxylin–eosin stain × 1,200

suggested that some DNA synthesis is related to the production of metabolic DNA (PELC 1972). A comparison of the two methods can be made from the results of experiments where animals are injected with colchicine 4 h before killing and the same animals receive tritiated thymidine 1 h before death. From autoradiographs the percentage of labeled nuclei is counted, and on regular histologic sections, the percentage of cells in metaphase is determined.

Colchicine is usually administered in saline at 0.1–0.2 mg per 100 g body weight. The dose most be sufficient to halt all mitoses, but not so high as to produce toxic effects leading to cell necrosis. Animals are usually killed 4–6 h after administration and the tissue prepared for light microscopy. Again for reasons of resolution, plastic sections, about 1 μm thick, are preferred for pulmonary work to allow better identification of cells in mitosis (Fig. 6). As in the case of thymidine injections, the overall percentage of pulmonary cells in mitosis is determined at frequent intervals for test groups of animals and compared with controls. Cells arrested in metaphase can be identified and differential counts made to analyze the mitotic activity of specific pulmonary cell types.

An estimate of cell turnover can be obtained from the percentage of metaphases collected in a 4-h period. In the lung, this value should be obtained for a specific cell type. For example, if 3% of any cell type are arrested in metaphase over a 4-h period, this means that 18% will divide in 24 h and the whole population will turn over in an average of 5.5 days. This value depends on a number of assumptions and on the accurate determination of the daily mitotic rate which may be constant in normal conditions, but may vary widely during a proliferative period in repair (THORUD et al. 1980). The daily rate can be determined more accurately by injecting animals at 4- or 6-h intervals before sacrifice over a 24-h period (BERTALANFFY 1964a). Summation of the mitotic percentages will give the daily mitotic rate of the particular cell population. Detailed discussion of the various parameters of the cell cycle that can be measured by the metaphase arrest technique is the subject of a recent review (WRIGHT and APPLETON 1980).

III. Other Methods

Cell turnover can sometimes be assessed by biochemical methods. The progression of a cell through the cycle to mitosis is accompanied by a doubling of its mass. All cell components must therefore double at some point in the cell cycle and increased synthesis of the various proteins, RNA, and DNA can be measured. Some of the biochemical events are specific to particular phases of the cell cycle and increased enzyme activity can be detected. Enzymes related to DNA synthesis increase specifically in the S phase (BASERGA 1976, 1981; PARDEE et al. 1978).

Changes in cytokinetics that result in alterations in the total cell population of the lung can be measured by morphometric methods. At the ultrastructural level, precise cellular identification can be achieved, but the small sample size is some hindrance to the assessment of overall cell population changes in the lung. Quantitative methods have been established using many tissue blocks and random photography to determine the number of lung cells of a specific type (WEIBEL et al. 1966; CRAPO et al. 1979); changes in cell populations during injury and repair can therefore be monitored by morphometric methods. Morphometry can also be used at the light microscope level, but has limited use in cell turnover studies because of the advantages of the autoradiographic methods.

Techniques such as microfluorometry also have limited application. On an individual cell basis, the content of RNA and DNA can be measured by the intensity of the staining reaction. Cells about to divide double their RNA which can be stained by acridine orange (DARZYNKIEWICZ et al. 1979) and double their DNA, which can be stained by the Feulgen reaction (RUCH 1966). If specific cell types can be identified on histologic slides, the content of RNA or DNA can be measured and sequential changes followed. Since the procedure is carried out on individual cells, it is extremely time consuming to analyze each population of pulmonary cells.

D. Kinetics of Specific Lung Cells

The methods outlined have been widely used to assess cell turnover in the lung. Studies of normal lung have been made to determine the regular renewal system for the specific cell types and this information provides the necessary baseline data for toxicologic studies where alterations in the process or timing of cell turnover may have consequences for the structure and function of the lung. Exposure to inhaled materials may affect all cells from the trachea to the alveolus.

I. Tracheobronchial Cells

Under normal circumstances, mitoses are rarely seen in the tracheobronchial epithelium. Even after thymidine labeling or mitotic arrest techniques, the number of dividing cells observed tends to be small and, coupled with sampling difficulties, these factors partially account for the varied results of published cell turnover studies. Values for cell turnover in the trachea have been reported as 7 days or less (SHORTER et al. 1964, 1966), 48 days (LEBLOND and WALKER 1956), and over 100 days (BLENKINSOPP 1967). It is generally agreed that the renewal time is less in the larger airways; in large bronchi, cell turnover is 18 days compared with 60 days in small bronchi (GOTTESBERGE and KOBERG 1963). From the variability of results obtained in these and other experiments, there is no precise value for the normal turnover rate in this type of epithelium. The reasons for this are partly methodological in the use of isotope conditions and section thickness, sampling of different regions of the airways, and anatomic differences in the various species of animal.

The cells of the tracheobronchial epithelium do not proliferate equally. It has been shwon that the principal proliferative cells are the basal cell and the "intermediate" undifferentiated cell, which can later transform to the ciliated cell type (BLENKINSOP 1967; BINDREITER et al. 1968). The proportion of differentiated cells increases from proximal to distal airway. It is generally accepted that the differentiated cell types do not divide, though there is a low level of tritiated thymidine uptake in some mucous cells (HARRIS et al. 1975). The increase in goblet cells seen after various injuries is believed to be the result of a change in postmitotic differentiation where more mucous than ciliated cells are produced (BREEZE and

WHEELDON 1977). WELLS (1970) has shown that the disease status of the animal affects cell kinetics. Older rats, for example, are prone to chronic respiratory disease and may have focal lesions which produce a local enhanced proliferative activity in the tracheobronchial epithelium.

Regional anatomic differences are most important in selecting sample areas for cytokinetic analysis. Since cell division occurs mainly in basal cells, counts of labeled cells will vary with the proportions of basal to superficial cells in each section. BOLDUC and REID (1976) studied cell turnover at five levels of the bronchial tree and found that the number of dividing cells per 1,000 nuclei decreases progressively to the periphery. In this study they differentiated between extrapulmonary airways, where basal cells are the progenitors, and intrapulmonary airways, where the stem cell appears to be the intermediate cell. The variable cell populations, dividing and nondividing, illustrate the need for standardization in sampling these areas for cytokinetic studies.

II. Bronchiolar Cells

In centrilobular zones of the lung, where the narrow terminal airways meet the gas-exchanging alveoli, the lining cells of the terminal and respiratory bronchioles are particularly vulnerable to injury. They are especially prone to respiratory viruses and to gases such as ozone and nitrogen dioxide. At the level of the bronchiole, basal cells are usually absent and the epithelium consists of approximately two-thirds ciliated and one-third nonciliated cells. The latter appear to be variants of the granulated Clara cells which are regarded as the stem cell population for this region (EVANS et al. 1978). It is generally accepted that the mitotic activity in the distal areas of the lung is lower than that in the higher levels (BOLDUC and REID 1976). Under normal circumstances, the proliferative rate of bronchiolar epithelium is low, ranging from 1.1% of cells in 1-month-old rats (EVANS et al. 1972) to 0.2% in adult rats (SHORTER et al. 1966). A similar low mitotic rate has been observed in monkeys used as controls for an ozone exposure experiment; in the small number examined, 0.2% of cells in the terminal bronchiolar epithelium incorporated tritiated thymidine (CASTLEMAN et al. 1980). In all these studies, the low mitotic rate combined with the relatively small number of cells examined makes it extremely difficult to determine the kinetics of cell renewal, particularly by the labeled mitoses method.

SPENCER and SHORTER (1962) have suggested a brief turnover time of 10 days for bronchiolar cells though variations in the rate may be partly due to cell differences in the epithelium. Studying only Clara cells, KAUFFMAN (1977) followed the decline of silver grains after tritiated thymidine treatment and found that cells in mitosis had a mean cycle time of 30 h. In an earlier study, DIVERTIE et al. (1968) followed the thymidine labeling over a longer period and found some labeled cells in the bronchiolar epithelium up to 8 weeks after injection of isotope, suggesting a prolonged renewal time for the entire population. The long turnover time agrees with the 59-day period found by GOTTESBERGE and KOBURG (1963). This variability in turnover times may again reflect differences in methodology cited earlier, in particular in the identification and counting of specific cell types.

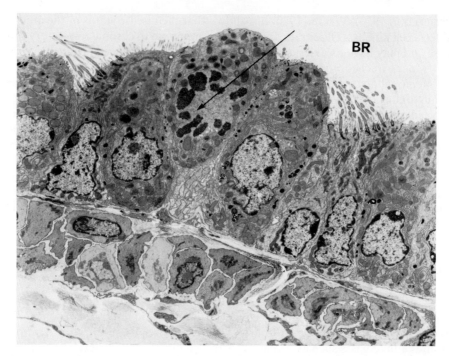

Fig. 7. Mitotic figure (*arrow*) in a nonciliated Clara cell in the terminal bronchiole (*BR*) of a normal mouse. × 5,000

Differential counts of cells synthesizing DNA have seldom been carried out in a large number of normal animals. In a control group of six rats, LUM et al. (1978) found a labeling percentage of approximately 0.25% and, although the number of cells was too low for statistical significance, they showed that almost all the labeling was confined to nonciliated secretory cells. In random sections of normal lung, only occasional mitotic figures are seen in the bronchiolar epithelium and these dividing cells are almost always identified as Clara cells (Fig. 7).

Most of the evidence for the cellular renewal system comes from the reaction of the bronchiole to injury. The low rate of DNA synthesis in the normal epithelium makes a dramatic contrast to the levels of DNA synthesis seen in the reparative phase after ozone or nitrogen dioxide treatment. In a study of young rats, the control labeling index of 1.1% rose dramatically to 23% after 24 h (EVANS et al. 1971); subsequently, the level declined to 5% by 3 days, still considerably above normal values. This indicates a tremendous burst of DNA synthesis over a short period and a rapid turnover rate for the labeled cells.

It is generally agreed that the cellular renewal in repair occurs by the same mechanism as normal turnover, but that the process is accelerated. After exposure to toxic gases, ciliated cells are injured and the stem cell responsible for the enhanced DNA synthesis is the nonciliated cell (EVANS et al. 1971, 1978). When animals are injected with tritiated thymidine and killed up to 15 days later, the fate of the DNA synthesizing nonciliated cells may be followed. By light and electron microscope autoradiography, it was shown that all cells labeled 1 h after thymidine injection are nonciliated. By 4 h, one-third of labeled cells are ciliated and are stable over a 15-day observation period, demonstrating that the nonciliated cell is capable of division and acts as progenitor for the ciliated epithelium. In subsequent experiments, EVANS et al. (1978) have shown that the various nonciliated cell types represent functional phases of the secretory Clara cells. The same cellular renewal system has been described following exposure of various species to different oxidant gases. CASTLEMAN et al. (1980) reported a labeling index of 18% in the bronchiolar epithelium of monkeys after ozone administration. Of these cells, 80% are nonciliated and show mitotic figures.

Changes in cellular renewal seen by autoradiography are often more dramatic than morphological evidence of cell injury, and DNA synthesis can be used as a marker of the site and extent of damage. Whereas injury to the differentiated cell types in the bronchioles may be rapidly repaired, more severe injury to the dividing stem cells is potentially more serious and will be reflected in a lower or delayed increase in cell turnover in the epithelium. This process may be associated with a continuing inflammatory response and later with fibrosis.

III. Alveolar Cells

Kinetic studies of alveolar cells are difficult because of the cellular heterogeneity found in this region of the lung. Basically, the alveolar walls are lined by type II cuboidal and type I squamous epithelium. The blood vessels may be small capillaries or larger venules, veins, and arteries, each lined by thin endothelium. In the septum are various interstitial cells such as fibroblasts, macrophages, and contractile cells while various intravascular leukocytes may also be identified in lung sections. In the alveolar spaces, free macrophages are usually seen. These various cells may be classed as either "itinerant", such as blood cells and macrophage precursors, or "fixed", such as structural cells of the alveolar wall that are replaced by neighboring mitotic activity. In response to inhaled material there may be a response of the macrophagic system to produce more cells and/or there may be direct interaction of the agent on the structural cells; each process can result in alteration to the cytokinetics of the lung.

Early investigations of cell turnover at the alveolar level were hampered by the low mitotic rate and the problems of cellular identification. Using the mitotic arrest technique with paraffin sections, BERTALANFFY (1964b) showed that the mitotic rate is sufficient to balance cell loss and that there are renewing cell populations in the alveolus. Though recognizing the difficulties of cellular identification in a mixed cell population, he classed alveolar cells as vacuolated and nonvacuolated. In the rat, the nonvacuolated cells (now known to be alveolar macrophages) turn over in 8 days whereas vacuolated cells (now identified as type II epithelial cells) are renewed in approximately 28 days (BERTALANFFY and LEBLOND (1953).

Subsequently, SHORTER et al. (1966) used tritiated thymidine labeling to study cytokinetics of normal mice and rats. Although they also had difficulty with cell identification, they found two populations of cells that renew in approximately 7 and 21 days. BOWDEN et al. (1968b) found in mice that labeling of alveolar cells follows a biphasic pattern. The first phase correlates with the disappearance of labeled cells from smears of lavaged cells shown by electron microscopy to be alveolar macrophages; turnover time for these cells was calculated at 7 days. The second phase terminates at 35 days at which time no labeled cells are found. A turnover time of 4–5 weeks was calculated for this different population of alveolar cells, believed to be epithelial.

These and other early studies were limited technically by the inability to make positive cell identification on a large number of dividing cells. EVANS and BILS (1969) used autoradiography at the electron microscope level after tritiated thymidine administration to overcome the problems of cellular identification; however, the number of labeled cells at each time studied was quite low. The percentage of labeled cells in the lung, determined on 1-µm sections, was calculated on two animals per time interval. The overall labeling of about 2% at 1 h after injection declined steadily. In the initial 1- to 4-h period, about 40% of labeled cells in lung sections are leukocytes passing through the capillaries. Endothelial cells make up 30% of the labeled population, 14% are interstitial cells, 6% are type II cells, and 5% are free alveolar macrophages. It should be stressed that these percentages were calculated on totals of about 30 labeled cells in the initial day, down to about 10 labeled cells at 2–4 weeks. These cells represent too small a sample for statistical analysis and, in addition, no grain counts were made to determine cell turnover times.

More recently 0.75 µm plastic sections have been used as a compromise whereby many labeled cells can be counted and sufficiently accurate cellular identification can be made on autoradiographs (ADAMSON and BOWDEN 1974; ADAMSON et al. 1977; BOWDEN and ADAMSON 1974). In these studies, control groups of adult mice have a baseline isotope incorporation 1 h after a pulse of tritiated thymidine of about 0.3%. From differential counts of 300 labeled cells per animal, it has been found that approximately 40% are leukocytes, 11% type II epithelial, 22% endothelial, 25% interstitial, and 2% alveolar macrophages. The changing patterns of cellular labeling can be followed during and after exposure to any potential toxin. Depressed cell division rates of any one cell type will reflect injury; repair will be characterized by a proliferative burst of a particular stem cell. Extended mitotic activity of a stem cell might be indicative of a neoplastic process, whereas predominant interstitial proliferation usually suggests abnormal repair and the development of fibrosis. The processes of normal cell renewal will be considered briefly for each cell type.

1. Alveolar Epithelium

The cuboidal type II cells which contain lamellar bodies (seen as vacuoles by light microscopy) appear to turn over in about 35 days. The effete cells are sloughed off the surface as dead cells, not as macrophages as postulated at one time. The squamous type I epithelium does not incorporate thymidine when given as a pulse, but labeled type I cells are seen if the time between injection and killing is lengthened (EVANS and BILS 1969). Type I cells are susceptible to injury and it is now well established that repair is accomplished by division of type II cells with differentiation of daughter cells to the type I form. This has been shown after treatment with oxygen (ADAMSON and BOWDEN 1974), nitrogen dioxide (EVANS et al. 1975), and various injected drugs (ADAMSON et al. 1977; ADAMSON and BOWDEN 1979). It is likely that this is the normal cell renewal process and a similar mechanism has been described in the developing lung (ADAMSON and BOWDEN 1975). In the fetus, a time for thymidine injection can be chosen when cuboidal epithelial cells exclusively line the air sacs, and are actively dividing. By combined ultrastructural and cytodynamic studies, it was shown that type II cells are the progenitors of type I epithelium.

It is likely that repair and fetal development demonstrate acceleration of the slow cell renewal process taking place in the normal mature lung. In contrast to the normal 4- to 6-week renewal period, type II cell turnover following injury to type I epithelium has been calculated at 2.5–3 days (ADAMSON and BOWDEN 1974).

When type II cells are identified and counted exclusively in normal animals, the percentage labeled is low at about 0.25%–0.5% (KAUFFMAN 1972). For the individual labeled cells, a cell cycle time of about 22 h is reported under normal (KAUFFMAN 1972) and repair conditions (EVANS et al. 1975), though there is some extension after urethane administration (KAUFFMAN 1972). Although there is only a small porportion of cells undergoing mitosis in normal animals, type II cells are resistant to injury and are able to mobilize rapidly a large component of the resting population into mitosis. This is usually a consequence of type I cell injury; sometimes the resulting type II proliferation greatly exceeds the extent of initial damage. On occasion, the proliferated type II cells may not transform to type I epithelium; they may persist as type II cells, particularly in association with fibrotic areas, or they may differentiate to inappropriate metaplastic epithelial cells (ADAMSON 1976; ADAMSON and BOWDEN 1979).

Altered cell kinetics of type II cells can also produce neoplasia. After administration of urethane, an early reduction in epithelial cells is followed by hyperplasia with increased incorporation of tritiated thymidine by type II cells (KAUFFMAN 1976). The labeling index for this cell type rises from 0.2% in controls to 2.3% in the first 6 weeks of exposure. From changes in labeling index, the population doubling time is about 3 weeks and in some areas of the lung, type II cell adenomas are produced. Each cell has the normal cycle time, but there is a greatly increased number in the cell cycle at any one time, though this number decreases with the age of the tumor (DYSON and HEPPLESTON 1975). In these cases, alterations in cell kinetics are exclusive to the type II cell population.

2. Endothelial Cells

Little attention has been paid to the cell turnover of the various types of endothelium in normal lung. BERTALANFFY (1964b) noted that many of the mitoses seen in the lung after colchicine treatment were in endothelial-like cells and estimated the daily percentage at about 0.5%. No estimates were made of turnover, however, owing to the uncertainties of identification. EVANS and BILS (1969) noted by electron microscopy that about 30% of all lung cells labeled by tritiated thymidine were endothelial at 1 h after injection. By 4 weeks, the proportion of labeled endothelial cells was still around 30%, although the total percentage of labeled cells in the alveolar walls dropped from about 2% to 0.3% in the same time. In other words, the absolute number of labeled endothelial cells must also have fallen by a factor of six in the 4-week period, indicating that endothelial cells divide and can be classed as a stem cell population. It can be estimated from the pattern of overall lung labeling and the differential counts that the turnover time of capillary endothelial cells is about 12 days.

There is evidence that endothelial cells are different at various levels of the vasculature. In normal rats, the numbers of Weibel–Palade bodies decrease as the artery moves distally and they are not seen in capillary endothelium. There is little information relating anatomic differences to different renewal rates. MEYRICK and REID (1979) reported variable rates of tritiated thymidine incorporation in different pulmonary vessels in a control group of rats. They found that, 1 h after isotope administration, the percentage of labeled endothelial cells in the hilar pulmonary artery is 0.5%, with a turnover time of 7.5 days, whereas in peripheral arteries, 1.4% of endothelial cells are labeled. At the alveolar walls, they counted the number of labeled cells per unit area of lung periphery; capillary endothelial cells were the most abundant of the cells labeled.

The various types of endothelium appear to have differential susceptibilities to injury and this is reflected in different renewal rates. Following hypoxia, there is a threefold, late increase in endothelial labeling in hilar arteries and a lower, but earlier increase in DNA synthesis in peripheral arteries. No change was found in the endothelium of veins (MEYRICK and REID 1979). In the capillaries, increased labeling of endothelial cells peaked between 3 and 5 days. At high concentration of oxygen, BOWDEN and ADAMSON (1974) also demonstrated a differential reactivity of endothelium. Capillary lining cells are injured and repaired rapidly with an elevated incorporation of tritiated thymidine; cells lining larger vessels remain at control values. From DNA synthesis and mitotic arrest, the capillary endothelium showed accelerated turnover at about 2.5 days.

3. Pulmonary Macrophages

Early studies on the cytodynamics of the alveolar macrophage indicate a turnover time of about 7 days (BERTALANFFY 1964b; BOWDEN et al. 1968b). This value does not represent the life span of the macrophage, but merely the average sojourn of the cell in the alveolus before mucociliary clearance. Although all macrophages are of hematopoietic origin (VAN FURTH and COHN 1968), it appears that some free alveolar cells are derived from dividing precursors in the pulmonary interstitium (VOLKMAN 1976; BOWDEN and ADAMSON 1972). In a study of macrophage kinetics in normal mice, BOWDEN and ADAMSON (1980) showed that there is a dual origin for alveolar macrophages. The major component arises from circulating monocytes while a smaller proportion arise by division and migration of a cell in the interstitium. The usual life span of the macrophage in the alveolus is about 1 week.

The initial response of the alveolar macrophage to an inhaled substance is adaptive in nature with increased lipid and protein synthesis. In overload, the number of free macrophages increases. Although some agents or factors induce

mitotic activity in free alveolar macrophages, the mature cell is usually considered
to be nondividing. Under conditions of particulate loading, the delivery system
is accelerated and continues to supply new cells (BOWDEN and ADAMSON 1979;
ADAMSON and BOWDEN 1980). After exposure to various particulates such as carbon, polystyrene latex, and heat-killed bacteria, the rapid initial efflux of mono-
cyte-derived cells is followed by a mitotic burst in the pulmonary interstitium
(ADAMSON and BOWDEN 1980, 1981). Although the outpouring of alveolar macrophages is accelerated, and circulating monocytes cross the blood–air barrier at
a faster rate than normal, the life span of the macrophage in the alveolus remains
at about 1 week.

Cytokinetic studies of the macrophagic system are complicated by the migration of cells from one anatomic location to another. In serial studies after treatment with tritiated thymidine, initial heavy labeling of marrow is later followed
by increased labeling of blood leukocytes; migrating monocytes subsequently carry the label into the interstitial and alveolar compartments (see Fig. 5). Lung sections examined hours or days after DNA labeling include pulmonary cells labeled
in situ as well as itinerant cells in the vasculature and interstitium. A constant
number of silver grains in such cases is useful for demonstrating migration of a
cell population without division. Mitotic activity can be demonstrated by pulse
labeling or by injecting colchicine and killing the animal soon afterwards; in this
way, dividing interstitial cells have been demonstrated (BOWDEN and ADAMSON
1979, 1980).

A complicating factor in these and other cytokinetic studies is leukocytic labeling. In normal animals pulsed with tritiated thymidine, it is estimated that
30%–40% of labeled cells in the lung are intravascular leukocytes (EVANS and
BILS 1969; BOWDEN and ADAMSON 1979). In serial studies, the labeled leukocytes
gradually disappear and allowances must be made for this in examining overall
percentages of labeled cells in the lung. The problem is more pronounced after
particulate loading or any situation where there is cell injury followed by inflammation which produces a leukocytic chemotactic stimulus in the alveolus or interstitium. The influx of these cells into the lung before and during the macrophagic
response greatly increases the total lung DNA and distorts the percentage of tritiated thymidine-labeled pulmonary nuclei since so many of the cells seen in sections are polymorphonuclear leukocytes.

4. Interstitial Cells

In normal lung, the cells of the interstitium are mainly fibroblasts with some interspersed macrophages. In the alveolar wall, many of these cells appear as fairly
undifferentiated mononuclear cells and it is not easy to distinguish them. There
is cell turnover in the insterstitium and mitotic figures have been seen, particularly
after colchicine injection. After a pulse of tritiated thymidine, EVANS and BILS
(1969) found that 14% of the 30 labeled lung cells seen by electron microscopy
were located in the interstitium. By light microscope autoradiography on methacrylate sections, ADAMSON and BOWDEN (1974) have reported 25% interstitial
cells in 800 labeled pulmonary cells. Whereas some of these cells divide and mi-

grate to produce new alveolar macrophages as already discussed, the bulk of labeled cells are fibroblasts.

No turnover time has been specifically calculated for fibroblasts in the lung. In common with other systems in the body, their proliferation is associated with reparative processes and is usually followed by collagen secretion. Baseline data on lung cell kinetics should include a measure of DNA synthesis in the fibroblast population since changes in this level are a good indication of the onset of fibrosis. Severe injury to either or both endothelial and epithelial surfaces of the lung is associated with fibroblast proliferation, particularly if repair of the surface cells is inhibited (Fig. 8). When endothelial and epithelial injury are rapidly repaired, for example after toxic levels of oxygen (ADAMSON and BOWDEN 1974), there is no kinetic change in the fibroblast population. However, if the epithelial injury is extensive and type II cell proliferation is delayed, fibroblast proliferation occurs (ADAMSON and BOWDEN 1976). A similar result occurs if endothelial regeneration is delayed (ADAMSON et al. 1977). There is also evidence that modified epithelial repair in bleomycin toxicity is associated with fibrosis (ADAMSON and BOWDEN 1979). In this case, increased DNA synthesis is found in the epithelial population, but the postmitotic differentiation is altered and the resultant metaplastic cells overlie areas of fibroblast proliferation and collagen deposition.

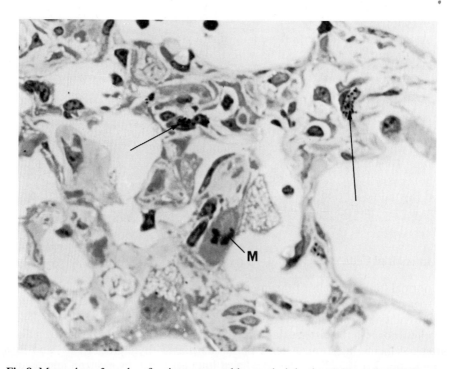

Fig. 8. Mouse lung 3 weeks after intravenous bleomycin injection (120 mg/kg). Following endothelial and epithelial injury, interstitial fibrosis develops. In fibrotic areas, fibroblasts (*arrows*) incorporate a pulse of thymidine ^3H and one cell is seen in mitosis (*M*). Methacrylate section, toluidine blue stain × 1,200

E. Factors Affecting Cell Turnover

The studies outlined provide information on the kinetics of the various cells in the normal lung, including turnover times and processes of cellular renewal which are essential background information for toxicologic investigations. However, a number of factors modify the various measurements of cell kinetics and should be considered when planning a study.

I. Sex, Strain, and Circadian Rhythm

Species differences result in some variations in anatomic structure of the lung and may give some variability in cytokinetics of the various cell types. In addition, the particular strain of mouse and the sex have been shown to be factors that alter rates of cell division (SIMNETT and HEPPLESTON 1966). Using the colchicine arrest technique, these authors found a variable mitotic incidence in three strains of mice and also differences in mitotic rates between male and female animals which could not be accounted for by stages of the estrous cycle. This study illustrates the need, at least for cytodynamic studies, to keep the sex and strain of animal constant to allow more accurate comparisons of cell turnover.

Variations in the mitotic rate of lung cells have been described after tritiated thymidine or colchicine injection at various intervals through a 24-h study period. ROMANOVA (1966) plotted the mitotic index of rat lung cells af 3-h intervals and showed a definite periodicity in mitotic activity in fetal and newborn animals, though it is not clear at which time of day the peaks occur in the rapidly growing lung (SOKOLOVA 1976; DAS et al. 1980). These studies have not identified specific cell types, but rather have analyzed the alveolar wall cells as a whole. The changing proportions of specific cells in the perinatal period may account for the diverse results in the few available studies. In general it is common practice to inject thymidine or colchicine at the same time each day to negate the influence of the circadian rhythm.

II. Age of Animal

Most cytokinetic studies of normal lung cells have been carried out on young adult animals. It is also important to determine the normal cell turnover of pulmonary cells during the growing period. The rate of cell proliferation is highest during the pseudoglandular period of development, about day 16 of gestation in the mouse (KAUFFMAN 1975); subsequently mitotic and thymidine labeling indices fall. ADAMSON and BOWDEN (1975) found that 12% of lung cells are labeled by a pulse of tritiated thymidine at day 17 of gestation in the rat and the value declines sharply to about 2%–3% by day 21. Differential counts of labeled cells reveal that the decline is due to a reduction in epithelial cell division as the process of differentiation progresses and postmitotic type II cells transform to type I epithelium. In mice, KAUFFMAN (1975) showed that the decline in epithelial cell labeling index is associated with an extension of the cell cycle time at the later gestation days.

After birth, the labeling index of alveolar cells averages 2% for at least 2 weeks (ADAMSON and BOWDEN 1975). However, there appears to be a growth spurt around day 4 and there is some diurnal variation to 2 weeks (DAS et al. 1979). In this period of alveolar growth, mitotic activity is prominent in epithelial, endothelial, and fibroblastic cells. In a detailed autoradiographic study, KAUFF-MAN et al. (1974) analyzed the proliferative patterns of each of these cell types up to 3 weeks postnatally. They showed that overall growth is a composite of the three cell populations with peaks in activity occurring at differences times. After 3 weeks, the alveolar walls are thinner, and the lung structure resembles adult lung with the labeling index dropping to the adult value of 0.3%.

An additional factor to consider in studies carried out around the perinatal period is the onset of macrophage production. Very few cells are seen free in the fluid-filled "air sacs" before birth, but the number of alveolar macrophages increases dramatically in the first 10 days after birth (ZELIGS et al. 1977). In addition to the functional significance of these observations there are implications as far as cytokinetics are concerned when this cell type and its precursors become increasingly prominent in the sections of normal lungs. Overall responses, including cytokinetics of the developing macrophagic system to inhaled particulates, have not been determined.

There is also evidence that cell division in the lung slows as animals grow old. This effect was noted in mice studied up to 2 years of age (SIMNETT and HEPPLE-STON 1966), and in rats, BOLDUC and REID (1976) found that the biggest variable in determining mitotic rates in the tracheobronchial tree was the age of the animal. Age differences in cell proliferation have also been described after exposing rats to nitrogen dioxide (EVANS et al. 1977). Young animals respond faster to injury with more rapid proliferation of the repairing type II epithelial cells. A delayed peak in thymidine incorporation is found in 1- to 2-year-old rats; however, a larger percentage of type II cells synthesize DNA. These combined studies indicate the importance of proper age-matched controls for cell kinetic studies in any long-term experiments.

III. Nutrition

It is generally believed that decreased food intake retards DNA synthesis by depressing RNA and protein synthesis. There has been little attention paid to this phenomenon in the lung, though it is clear that some experimentally exposed animals may suffer weight loss or decreased gain as compared with controls. HACK-NEY et al. (1977) studied the thymidine labeling index of 3-month-old mice. Animals starved for 5 days show a dramatic decrease in DNA synthesis in all lung cells and very few labeled cells are seen. The drop in DNA synthesis equals that seen in a properly fed group that is exposed to a high concentration of oxygen. These results suggest that some experimental exposures may affect the appetite and that an observed reduction in cell division may sometimes be due to dietary factors rather than to the direct action of an agent on the lung. In experiments where weight loss or reduced weight gain in growing animals is observed, a pair-feeding experiment may be necessary for the accurate evaluation of any cytokinetic changes in the lung.

F. Cytokinetics of In Vitro Systems

The reaction of lung cells to various potential inhalants may also be assessed using in vitro systems. Among the parameters that should be examined is the mitotic activity of the specific cell types since changes in cytokinetics may indicate interference with the normal cell renewal processes. Autoradiographic methods can be used on cultured cells. A pulse of thymidine (usually about 0.1 µCi per milliliter medium) is added to the cells in culture for 1–2 h, rinsed off, and a smear of cells or cells already attached to glass are prepared, at intervals, for autoradiography. The percentage of cells with silver grains over the nuclei is counted to give the mitotic rate at specific times of culture. Grain counts can also be made and from the halving of grains with each division, the cell turnover time is calculated.

The mitotic arrest technique can also be used by adding colchicine to the culture system. From the percentage of cells arrested in metaphase in a 4-h period, the turnover rate for the whole population is determined. With the great variety of cell culture systems being used, no general statements can be made regarding specific cell turnover in vitro. Each experiment requires its own control to establish baseline data for any toxicologic or other manipulation.

The multicellular nature of the lung suggests that complex cellular interrelationships and control mechanisms operating in vivo may not be appropriately studied in cell cultures and that some in vitro investigations may be better carried out on cultured explants of lung. Again, the cytokinetics of each culture system must be established on normal tissue. SIMNETT and HEPPLESTON (1968) showed that, after 3 days in culture, the rate of DNA synthesis is about three times greater than the rate of mitosis. Later SIMNETT (1972) showed that about 17% of nuclei contained double the normal diploid value, suggesting that a mitotic control mechanism is disturbed by the explantation process.

When normal mouse lung is cultured in medium labeled with tritiated thymidine, the alveolar cells undergoing mitosis are epithelial cells, fibroblasts, and macrophage precursors in the interstitium (BOWDEN and ADAMSON 1972; ADAMSON and BOWDEN 1975). Capillary endothelial cells do not grow well under the conditions used. The percentage of labeled cells and the differential proportion of each cell type can be used as baseline data for the culture of lung at various stages of injury and repair to determine the specific proliferative capacities of each cell type (ADAMSON and BOWDEN 1975). This is of particular importance when assessing cellular repair; preponderance of DNA synthesis in fibroblastic cells, rather than in epithelium or endothelium, is a good indicator of subsequent progression to fibrosis.

G. Conclusions

It is becoming increasingly accepted that the response of the lung to a foreign substance should include data on its effects on the turnover of specific cell types and on the mechanisms of cellular renewal. Metabolic disturbances of a cell may lead to the cycle of cell injury, death, and normal repair with no sequelae, or to abnormal repair with fibrosis, or to abnormal proliferation (hyperplasia or neoplasia), or to altered differentiated function after proliferation. Analysis of the prolifer-

Table 1. Stem cells and their differentiated forms in the various regions of the lung

Location	Progenitor cell	Differentiated cells
Tracheobronchial	Basal	Ciliated, Mucous
Terminal bronchiolar	Clara	Ciliated, Mucous
Alveolar	1. Type II	Type I
		Type II
	2. Endothelial	Endothelial

ative populations and rates of division can give valuable information on which of these processes is under way and the likely functional changes in the lung.

Cytokinetic measurements such as turnover times and analysis of phases of the cell cycle are difficult to carry out in a multicellular organ such as the lung. Some progress has been made, however, by using thin plastic sections for light microscopy; these are large enough to count large numbers of labeled cells at various anatomic locations and are thin enough to allow cellular identification with 95% accuracy. The turnover of a specific cell type may be determined, or the relative proportions of the different labeled cells followed at various experimental periods. In this way, overall biochemical values for DNA synthesis can be broken down to identify changing patterns of mitotic activity in specific cell types.

Various cytokinetic studies demonstrate that not all cell types in the lung are capable of division, but many are the result of postmitotic differentiation. Although most of the evidence comes from studies of reparative mechanisms, there is some confirmatory data from the normal adult lung and from studies of lung development. At all levels of the pulmonary structure, there are certain stem cells that are essential for cellular renewal (Table 1). In a multicellular organ such as lung, however, it is likely that interactions between cells of different type, such as epithelial-mesenchymal interactions, play important roles in control of mitosis and subsequent differentiation. Of particular importance in toxicologic studies are the interrelationships between fibroblasts and the "surface cells", epithelial or endothelial, that regulate proliferation and determine whether or not fibrosis occurs. Division and maturation controls are also disturbed when tumor growth occurs from one of the various pulmonary stem cells. Cytokinetic studies can provide indices of modified cell proliferation and should be included as part of the correlation between structure and function in toxicologic investigations.

References

Adamson IYR (1976) Pulmonary toxicity of bleomycin. Environ Health Perspect 16:116–126

Adamson IYR, Bowden DH (1974) The type 2 cell as progenitor of alveolar epithelial regeneration. A cytodynamic study in mice after exposure to oxygen. Lab Invest 30:35–42

Adamson IYR, Bowden DH (1975) Derivation of type 1 epithelium from type 2 cells in the developing rat lung. Lab Invest 32:736–745

Adamson IYR, Bowden DH (1976) Pulmonary injury and repair. Organ culture studies of murine lung after oxygen. Arch Pathol Lab Med 100:640–643

Adamson IYR, Bowden DH (1979) Bleomycin induced injury and metaplasia of alveolar type 2 cells. Am J Pathol 96:531–544

Adamson IYR, Bowden DH (1980) Role of monocytes and interstitial cells in the generation of alveolar macrophages. II. Kinetic studies after carbon loading. Lab Invest 42:518–524

Adamson IYR, Bowden DH (1981) Dose response of the pulmonary macrophagic system to various particulates and its relationship to transepithelial passage of free particles. Exp Lung Res 2:165–175

Adamson IYR, Bowden DH, Côté MG, Witschi H (1977) Lung injury induced by butylated hydroxytoluene. Cytodynamic and biochemical studies in mice. Lab Invest 36:26–32

Baserga R (1976) Multiplication and division in mammalian cells. Dekker, New York

Baserga R (1981) The cell cycle. N Engl J Med 304:453–459

Bertalanffy FD (1964a) Tritiated thymidine versus colchicine technique in the study of cell population dynamics. Lab Invest 13:871–886

Bertalanffy FD (1964b) Respiratory tissue: structure, histophysiology, cytodynamics. Part II: New approaches and interpretations. Int Rev Cytol 17:213–297

Bertalanffy FD, Leblond CP (1953) The continuous renewal of the two types of alveolar cells in the lung of the rat. Anat Rec 115:515–536

Bindreiter M, Schuppler J, Stockinger L (1968) Zellproliferation und Differenzierung im Tracheal Epithel der Ratte. Exp Cell Res 50:377–382

Blenkinsopp WK (1967) Proliferation of respiratory tract epithelium in the rat. Exp Cell Res 46:144–154

Bolduc P, Reid L (1976) Mitotic index of the bronchial and alveolar lining of the normal rat lung. Am Rev Respir Dis 114:1121–1128

Bowden DH, Adamson IYR (1971) Reparative changes following pulmonary cell injury. Ultrastructural, cytodynamic and surfactant studies in mice after oxygen exposure. Arch Pathol 92:279–283

Bowden DH, Adamson IYR (1972) The pulmonary interstitial cell as immediate precursor of the alveolar macrophage. Am J Pathol 68:521–536

Bowden DH, Adamson IYR (1974) Endothelial regeneration as a marker of the differential vascular responses in oxygen induced pulmonary edema. Lab Invest 30:350–357

Bowden DH, Adamson IYR (1978) Adaptive responses of the pulmonary macrophagic system to carbon. I. Kinetic studies. Lab Invest 38:422–429

Bowden DH, Adamson IYR (1980) Role of monocytes and interstitial cells in the generation of alveolar macrophages. I. Kinetic studies of normal mice. Lab Invest 42:511–517

Bowden DH, Adamson IYR, Wyatt JP (1968a) Reaction of the lung cells to a high concentration of oxygen. Arch Pathol 86:671–675

Bowden DH, Davies E, Wyatt JP (1968b) Cytodynamics of pulmonary alveolar cells in the mouse. Arch Pathol 86:667–670

Boyd MR (1980) Biochemical mechanisms in chemical-induced lung injury: roles of metabolic activation. CRC Crit Rev Toxicol 8:103–176

Breeze RG, Weeldon EB (1977) The cells of the pulmonary airways. Am Rev Respir Dis 116:705–777

Castleman WL, Dungworth DL, Schwartz LW, Tyler WS (1980) Acute respiratory bronchiolitis. An ultrastructural and autoradiographic study of epithelial cell injury and renewal in rhesus monkeys exposed to ozone. Am J Pathol 98:811–840

Crapo JD, Peters-Golden M, Marsh-Salin J, Shelburne JS (1979) Pathologic changes in the lungs of oxygen-adapted rats. Lab Invest 39:640–653

Darzynkiewicz Z, Evenson DP, Staianocoico L, Sharpless TK (1979) Correlation between cell cycle duration and RNA content. J Cell Physiol 100:425–438

Das RM, Jain M, Thurlbeck WM (1979) Diurnal variation of deoxyribonucleic acid synthesis in murine alveolar wall cells and airway epithelial cells. Am Rev Respir Dis 119:81–85

Das RM, Jain M, Thurlbeck WM (1980) Circadian rhythm and proliferation of lung alveolar wall cells during postnatal growth in mice. Am Rev Respir Dis 121:367–371

Divertie M, Shorter R, Titus J (1968) Cell kinetics and tumour formation. Cell turnover in the lungs of mice with hereditary lung tumours. Thorax 23:83–86

Dyson P, Heppleston AG (1975) Cell kinetics of urethane induced murine pulmonary adenomata. I. The growth rate. Br J Cancer 31:405–416

Evans MJ, Bils RF (1969) Identification of cells labeled with tritiated thymidine in the pulmonary alveolar walls of the mouse. Am Rev Respir Dis 100:372–378

Evans MJ, Stephens RJ, Freeman G (1971) Effects of nitrogen dioxide on cell renewal in the rat lung. Arch Intern Med 128:57–60

Evans MJ, Stephens RJ, Cabral LJ, Freeman G (1972) Cell renewal in the lungs of rats exposed to low levels of NO_2. Arch Environ Health 24:180–188

Evans MJ, Cabral LJ, Stephens RJ, Freeman G (1975) Transformation of alveolar type 2 cells to type 1 cells following exposure to NO_2. Exp Mol Pathol 22:142–150

Evans MJ, Cabral-Anderson LJ, Freeman G (1977) Effects of NO_2 on the lungs of aging rats. II. cell proliferation. Exp Mol Pathol 27:366–376

Evans MJ, Cabral-Anderson LJ, Freeman G (1978) Role of the clara cell in renewal of the bronchiolar epithelium. Lab Invest 38:648–655

Gottesberge AM, Koburg E (1963) Autoradiographic investigation of cell formation in the respiratory tract, eustachian tube, middle ear and external auditory canal. Acta Otolaryngol 56:353–361

Gould VE, Tosco R, Wheelis RF (1972) Oxygen pneumonitis in man: Ultrastructural observations on the development of alveolar lesions. Lab Invest 29:499–508

Hackney JD, Evans MJ, Bils RF, Spier CE, Jones MP (1977) Effects of oxygen at high concentrations and food deprivation on cell division in lung alveoli of mice. Exp Mol Pathol 26:350–358

Harris C, Frank A, Barrett L, McDowell E, Trump B, Paradise L, Boren H (1975) Cytokinetics in the respiratory epithelium of the hamster, cow and man. J Cell Biol 67:158 a

Hughes WL, Bond VP, Brecher G, Cronkite EP, Painter RB, Quastler H, Sherman FG (1958) Cellular proliferation in the mouse as revealed by autoradiography with tritiated thymidine. Proc Natl Acad Sci USA 44:476–483

Kauffman SL (1971) Alteration in cell proliferation in mouse lung following urethane exposure. II. Effects of chronic exposure on terminal bronchiolar epithelium. Am J Pathol 64:531–540

Kauffman SL (1972) Alterations in cell proliferation in mouse lung following urethane exposure. III Effects of chronic exposure on type 2 alveolar epithelial cells. Am J Pathol 68:317–323

Kauffman SL (1975) Kinetics of pulmonary epithelial proliferation during prenatal growth of the mouse lung. Anat Rec 183:393–404

Kauffman SL (1976) Autoradiographic study of type II cell hyperplasia in lungs of mice chronically exposed to urethane. Cell Tissue Kinet 9:489–497

Kauffman SL, Burri PH, Weibel ER (1974) The postnatal growth of the rat lung. II Autoradiography. Anat Rec 180:63–76

Kistler GS, Caldwell PRB, Weibel ER (1967) Development of fine structural damage to alveolar and capillary lining cells in oxygen-poisoned rat lungs. J Cell Biol 32:605–628

Kopriwa BM (1973) A reliable, standardized method for ultrastructural electron microscopic radioautography. Histochemistry 37:1–17

Leblond CP, Walker BE (1956) Renewal of cell populations. Physiol Rev 36:255–276

Leblond CP, Messier B, Kopriwa B (1959) Thymidine-H^3 as a tool for the investigation of the renewal of cell populations. Lab Invest 8:296–306

Lum H, Schwartz LW, Dungworth DL, Typer WS (1978) A comparative study of cell renewal after exposure to ozone or oxygen. Response of terminal bronchiolar epithelium in the rat. Am Rev Respir Dis 118:335–345

Meyrick B, Reid L (1979) Hypoxia and incorporation of ^{3}H-thymidine by cells of the rat pulmonary arteries and alveolar wall. Am J Pathol 96:51–70

Pardee AB, Dubrow R, Hamlin JL, Kletzien RF (1978) Animal cell cycle. Ann Rev Biochem 47:715–780

Pelc SR (1972) Metabolic DNA in ciliated protozoa, salivary gland chromosomes and mammalian cells. Int Rev Cytol 32:327–355

Quastler H, Sherman EG (1959) Cell population kinetics in the interstitial epithelium of the mouse. Exp Cell Res 17:420–438

Rogers AW (1973) Techniques of autoradiography, 2nd edn. Elsevier, Amsterdam

Romanova LK (1966) Diurnal periodicity of mitotic cell division in the interalveolar septa of rat lungs. Bull Exp Biol Med 61:689–691

Ruch F (1966) Determination of DNA content by microfluorometry. In: Wied GL (ed) Introduction to quantitative cytochemistry. Academic, New York, p 281

Schultze B (1969) Autoradiography at the cellular level, vol III part B. In: Pollister AW (ed) Physical techniques in biological research. Academic, New York

Shorter RG, Titus JL, Divertie MB (1964) Cell turnover in the respiratory tract. Dis Chest 46:138–142

Shorter RG, Titus JL, Divertie MB (1966) Cytodynamics in the respiratory tract of the rat. Thorax 21:32–37

Simnett JD (1972) Reduplication of DNA content in nuclei from organ cultures of mouse lung. Neoplasma 19:11–18

Simnett JD, Heppleston AG (1966) Cell renewal in the mouse lung. The influence of sex, strain, and age. Lab Invest 15:1793–1801

Simnett JD, Heppleston AG (1968) Rates of DNA synthesis in organ cultures of lung and prostate as measured by tritiated thymidine autoradiography. Lab Invest 19:333–338

Sokolova TN (1976) Diurnal rhythm of mitotic activity in cells of the interalveolar septa of the rat lung and its variation with age. Bull Exp Biol Med 81:251–253

Sorokin SP (1970) The cells of the lungs. In: Nettesheim P, Hanna MG, Deatherage JW (eds) Morphology of experimental respiratory carcinogenesis. US Atomic Energy Commission, Oak Ridge, p 3

Spencer H, Shorter RG (1972) Cell turnover in the respiratory tract. Nature 194–880

Thorud E, Clausen OPF, Bjerknes R, Aarnaes E (1980) The stathmokinetic method in vivo. Time-response with special reference to circadian variations in epidermal cell proliferation in the hairless mouse. Cell Tissue Kinet 13:625–634

Van Furth R, Cohn Z (1968) The origin and kinetics of mononuclear phagocytes. J Exp Med 128:415–436

Volkman A (1976) Disparity in origin of mononuclear phagocyte populations. J Reticuloendothel Soc 19:249–268

Weibel ER, Kistler GS, Scherle WF (1966) Practical stereological methods for morphometric cytology. J Cell Biol 30:23–38

Wells AB (1970) The kinetics of cell proliferation in the tracheobronchial epithelia of rats with and without chronic respiratory disease. Cell Tissue Kinet 3:185–206

Witschi H, Côté MG (1977) Primary pulmonary responses to toxic agents. CRC Crit Rev Toxicol 5:23–66

Witschi H, Saheb W (1974) Stimulation of DNA synthesis in mouse lung following intraperitoneal injections of butylated hydroxytoluene. Proc Soc Exp Biol Med 147:690–693

Wright NA, Appleton DR (1980) The metaphase arrest technique. A critical review. Cell Tissue Kinet 13:643–663

Zeligs BJ, Nerukar LS, Bellanti JA, Zeligs JD (1977) Maturation of the rabbit alveolar macrophage during animal development. 1. Perinatal influx into alveoli and ultrastructural differentiation. Pediat Res 11:197–208

CHAPTER 12

Mucociliary Clearance and Mucus Secretion in the Lung

Jennifer M. Sturgess

A. Introduction

The drainage of the nose, sinuses, and bronchial tree is accomplished by essentially the same biomechanical principles – the mucociliary clearance mechanism. Described originally in the nose (Yates 1924), sinuses (Hilding 1932), and bronchi (Hilding 1957) as "ciliary streaming", the airways are considered to have an overlying, continuous mucous blanket that is dimensionally thin, but has a high viscosity so that it sustains limited traction. Under the motivation of ciliary action, mucus moves as a sheet in the nasal passages and from the bronchial tree to the larynx, passing over the posterior margin to the pharynx. Areas lacking cilia are thought to be cleared by traction of the mucous blanket from surrounding ciliated areas.

In the paranasal sinuses, the velocity of flow varies from the ostium distally. Similar gradients exist also in the bronchial tree. Contrary to many assumptions in models of lung clearance (Barnett and Miller 1966; Blake 1975), the mucociliary escalator is not constant or continuous dynamically from peripheral to central airways. The epithelial cell populations vary progressively, with ciliated and mucus-secreting cells decreasing and nonciliated and Clara cells increasing from central to distal airways. Corresponding changes provide a continuum in the mucous lining, from a glycoprotein-rich biphasic mucous blanket (Kilburn 1968 a) in the major bronchi to a low surface tension, lipid- and protein-rich secretion in the terminal bronchioles (Gil and Weibel 1971).

The bronchial mucosa confers the fundamental properties for mucociliary clearance: propulsive forces are provided by cilia that extend from the epithelial cell surfaces; mucous secretions that originate from specialized secretory cells in the tracheobronchial epithelium and the submucosal glands are discharged into the airway lumen; and fluids and electrolytes are actively transported via the epithelial cells to the periciliary fluid layer. An understanding of the fundamental nature of the clearance mechanism rests with an evaluation of each of these component systems.

The mucociliary transport mechanism and mucus production is a function of the trachea and major bronchi of the airways. The nature of the clearance mechanism in the smaller interpulmonary airways differs considerably from that of the larger airways and many important questions remain to be answered on the mechanisms and controls that exist in different regions of the lung.

B. Bronchial Mucosa:
Normal Structure and Functional Organization

The cellular basis of the clearance mechanism resides in the ciliated epithelium that lines the upper and lower respiratory tract. In the normal trachea and large bronchi, the majority of epithelial cells are ciliated cells, each having 200 or more cilia on its apical surface. Each cilium represents an extension of the cell that is bounded by a specialized plasma membrane and having a structure that is unique and confers motility. The number, length, and distribution of the cilia are not uniform throughout the airways, becoming distally fewer in number, and shorter in length so that the effective clearance function must vary within the bronchial tree, being faster in the larger airways and slower in the more peripheral airways (SERAFINI and MICHAELSON 1977). Although comparative data on clearance from individual airway generations are not yet available, ciliary beat frequency diminishes as one moves from trachea to lobar bronchi (RUTLAND et al. 1982a).

The cell types (Fig. 1) typically observed in the tracheobronchial epithelium (RHODIN 1966) are the basal cells, intermediate cells, ciliated cells, goblet cells, epithelial serous cells, neuroendocrine cells, brush cells, and the specialized cells of the bronchial mucous glands. The number and distribution of these cell types varies in different animal species and are summarized in Table 1. A number of recent reviews describe the detailed ultrastructure of these specific cell types (KUHN

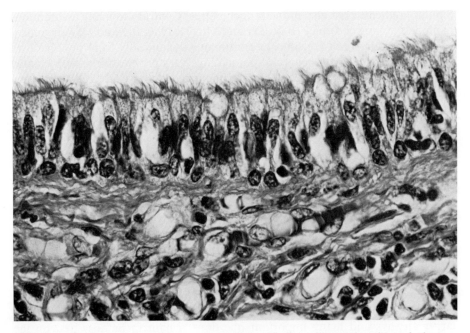

Fig. 1. Longitudinal section of human bronchial epithelium, illustrating the typical pseudostratified epithelium with basal and columnar cell types. Differentiated cells are predominantly ciliated, with approximately 10% of mucus-secreting goblet cells. × 2,100

Table 1. Epithelial cell types in various species identified by electron microscopy (JEFFERY and REID 1977a)

	Human	Monkey	Dog	Cat	Pig	Cow	Rat	Mouse	Hamster	Rabbit	Certain birds
Ciliated	+	+	+	+	+	+	+	+	+	+	+
Goblet (lucent granule)	+	+	+	+	+	−	+	+	+	+	?
Serous (dense granule)	+	−	−	+	−	−	+	−	−	−	−
"Special type" (dog) or nonciliated (mouse)	+	−	+	−	−	−	−	−	−	−	−
Clara	+	+	−	+	+	−	+	+	?	+	−
Intermediate	+	−	−	+	+	−	+	−	−	−	−
Brush	+	−	−	−	+	−	+	−	−	?	−
Basal	+	+	+	+	+	+	+	+	+	+	+
Neuroendocrine	+	−	−	−	−	−	+	+	−	+	+
Globule leukocyte	−	"Migratory"	+	−	−	−	+	−	−	−	−
Lymphocyte	+	"Migratory"	−	−	−	−	+	−	−	−	−
Intraepithelial nerve	+	−	−	+	−	−	+	+	−	+	+

Abbreviations: + identified; − not yet identified; ? unconfirmed

1976; JEFFERY and REID 1977a; BREEZE and WHEELDON 1977; McDOWELL et al. 1978).

In the human proximal airways, the bronchial epithelium is a pseudostratified epithelium. More distally, the epithelium becomes simple in type and progressively thins with a change from columnar cells in the bronchi to cuboidal cell shape in the bronchioles (PACK et al. 1980; MILLER 1932). In contrast to humans, the transition from pseudostratified to simple epithelium may occur more abruptly in smaller mammals such as the rat (RHODIN and DALHAMN 1956) where the transition zone is at the hilus of the lung.

The healthy bronchial epithelium maintains an effective permeability barrier with a continuous lining of cells and competent intercellular junctions. Tight junctions, specialized regions of the plasma membrane of adjoining epithelial cells, are crucial to maintaining the barrier function. By freeze fracture and replication techniques, the tight junction is visualized as a series of parallel arrays of intramembranous particles with random cross arrays. The number and arrangement of the particulate arrays is proportional to the tightness of the intercellular junctions (SCHNEEBERGER and KARNOVSKY 1976; SCHNEEBERGER 1980).

The apical plasma membrane is specialized and has an extracellular coat or glycocalyx. The basolateral membranes are closely apposed in the normal epithelium. In the intact bronchial epithelium, the cells are interconnected to form a continuous sheet that is retained despite regional variation of cellular constituents. The integrity of this sheet is an essential part of the mucociliary defense mechanism.

I. Basal and Intermediate Cells

The basal cells are compact, pyramidal cells that rest on the basement membrane, but do not extend to the airway lumen. Characteristically, the basal cells have a large centrally positioned indented nucleus, sparse endoplasmic reticulum and scattered free ribosomes, small mitochondria and Golgi apparatus. Cytoplasmic fibrils are observed and the cells are interconnected by desmosomes.

The basal cell is presumed to be a progenitor or stem cell for differentiated cell types in airway epithelia. In experimental studies with rats, the cell nuclei near the basement membrane are labeled with tritiated thymidine, suggesting that the basal cell population predominantly proliferates and gives rise to the differentiated epithelial cell types. More recently, goblet cells have been shown to replicate (JEFFERY and REID 1977 b), a potential that is not shared by ciliated epithelial cells (KAUFFMAN 1980). In response to mechanical injury, proliferation of basal cells occurs, producing a multilayered undifferentiated epithelium.

The intermediate or undifferentiated cells closely resemble the basal cells, but are taller and extend towards the lumen, although not necessarily exposed to the

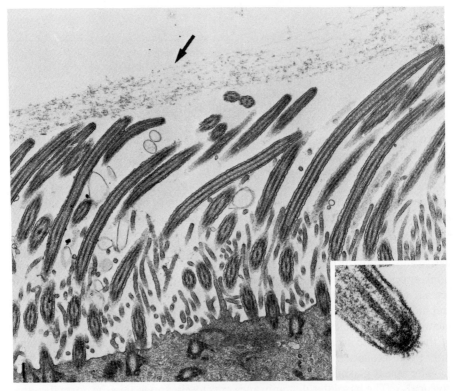

Fig. 2. Electron micrograph of cilia at the apical surfaces of the bronchial epithelium. In section, the cilia exhibit axial filaments or microtubules that originate in a basal body and extend to the tip of the cilium. The cilia are fixed in a waveform and the mucous blanket (*arrow*) is present at the tips. *Inset:* the tip of a cilium, illustrating the "claw-like" structures that have been suggested as having a role in mucus-transport. (STURGESS 1979)

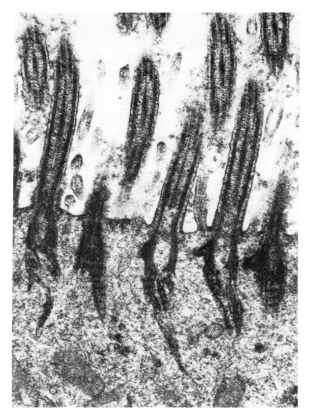

Fig. 3. Electron micrograph of human cilia, showing basal bodies, with lateral spurs, orientated in the direction of movement of the cilia. The striated rootlet has contractile capability and anchors cilia in the cell

airways lumen. The intermediate cell nucleus is large, oval, and surrounded by abundant cytoplasm containing compact mitochondria, profiles of rough endoplasmic reticulum, and sparse Golgi complex. Fewer tonofilaments are present than in the basal cell population. Desmosomes are also less common than in the basal cells. The apical surfaces of the cell are often elaborated into microvilli. The intermediate cell appears to be a precursor for the mucous or ciliated cell type and presumably represents a stage in the differentiation process.

II. Ciliated Cells

The ciliated cell type (Fig. 2) is the predominant cell of the large airways and persists to distal airways and in submucosal gland ducts. The cells are tall, columnar in shape, and approximately 20 μm high. The basolateral cell membranes are attached to basal and intermediate cells through desmosomes. Adjacent ciliated or other specialized cells form junction complexes at the apex with tight junctions at the airway lumen. Each ciliated cell has more than 200 regularly arranged cilia

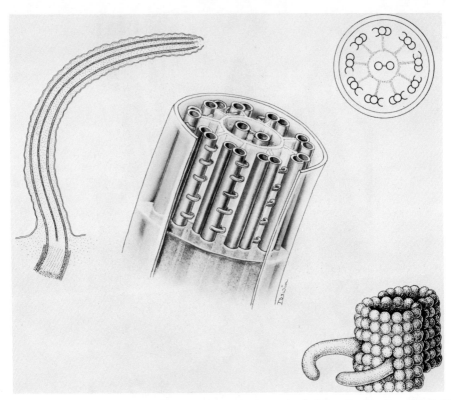

Fig. 4. The ultrastructure of a cilium is illustrated schematically in longitudinal section (*left*) and transverse section (*upper right*), and as a schematic diagram (*center*). The cilium is a cylindrical structure, bounded by a plasma membrane. The ciliary axoneme is composed of a ring of 9 microtubular doublets linked by molecules of a protein, nexin. The individual doublets (*lower right*) are built of tubulin subunits arranged in rows of 13 subunits (complete tubule, A) and 11 subunits (partial tubule, B). The outer doublet tubules have two sets of arms, outer and inner, that contain the enzyme, dynein. Radial spoke linkages connect the outer doublets with a central sheath of protein that surrounds two single microtubules

at its apical surface (RHODIN 1966). The cilia are approximately 6 μm long and 0.2–0.3 μm wide. Fine cell projections and microvilli extend also from the luminal surface between the cilia and may be up to 3 μm long, often with a branching pattern. In the process of ciliogenesis, or in response to irritants or disease, cilia may become sparse, in which case the cells exhibit numerous microvilli (HILDING and HILDING 1966).

The ciliated cell cytoplasm contains scattered rough endoplasmic reticulum towards the cell base with some free ribosomes and tonofilaments. The Golgi complex is well developed and situated on the luminal aspect of the nucleus. Ciliated cells typically have numerous mitochondria, particularly towards the cell apex. This observation has been correlated with the possible role of ciliated epithelial cells in the active transport of ions across the airways epithelia as well as their role in motility. An extensive subjacent cytoskeleton exists at the apical surfaces of the cell with a high density of microtubules and filaments.

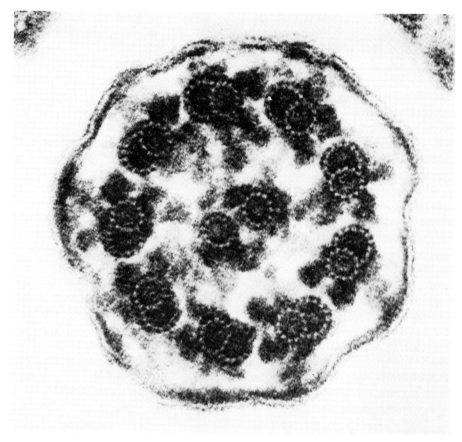

Fig. 5. High resolution transverse section of a cilium, fixed in glutaraldehyde and tannic acid to demonstrate the inner and outer dynein arms, attached to the doublet microtubules. × 400,000

The cilia are specialized motile organelles that are ubiquitous in nature, sharing a common structure and mechanism of action (SLEIGH 1974). Centrioles or basal bodies replicate and migrate to the cell apex and each serves as a microtubule-organizing center for the development of a ciliary axoneme. A lateral spur on the basal body is orientated in the direction of movement of the cilia and a striated rootlet may be present on the basal body and extend deep into the cytoplasm (Fig. 3). Such rootlets are variable in length and may extend to a depth of 10 μm in the human bronchial epithelium. A contractile function has been attributed to these rootlets and their role is considered at this time to provide an anchor for the superficial portion of the cilium (SLEIGH 1979).

1. Cilia

The cilium is a complex organelle capable of motility that has an intrinsic composition ubiquitous throughout the animal kingdom (SATIR 1974). Its unique structural organization (Fig. 4) is based on a series of microtubules that originate from the basal body in the apical portion of the cell and extend almost to the tip of the cilium. The microtubules are comprised of tubulin molecules arranged in a helical pattern to form a hollow cylinder, 25 nm in diameter. The arrangement of microtubules is characteristic for all cilia: an asymmetric ring of nine peripheral doublet microtubules and two single microtubules in the center. Interconnecting linkages between microtubules are provided by nexin, a circumferential link between the outer doublets, radial spoke linkages that connect the outer doublets and the central core, and the central protein sheath. The outer microtubular doublets have accessory hook-like structures, the dynein arms, that function in the sliding of the tubules.

Outer and inner dynein arms (Fig. 5), situated along the length of the doublet tubules are comprised of the enzyme, dynein, that has ATPase activity. The mechanism of ciliary beating has been described in detail (SATIR 1974; SLEIGH 1974, 1977). Essentially, movement is initiated by the sliding of adjacent microtubular doublets. Nexin maintains the axonemal structure and the radial spoke linkages translate the sliding motion of the outer doublets into a bending motion. The bend formation is in a plane perpendicular to the axis of the central tubules and is coordinated between adjacent cilia to generate metachronous waves of ciliary movement. At the tips of the cilia are short projections or "claw-like" structures that have been suggested as having a role in mucus transport (JEFFERY and REID 1977a). Other specialized features of respiratory cilia allow mucus propulsion at an air–fluid interface. Cilia are remarkably stable, motile organelles that may beat independently and, in fact, continue to beat in the airways for up to 173 h postmortem (HILDING 1956) although reduced in motion by accumulation of tenacious strands of mucus.

III. Epithelial Mucus-Secreting Cells

The population of mucus-secreting cells in the airways and the structural arrangement and biochemical nature of the mucous secretions varies distinctly among animal species.

1. Epithelial Mucous Cells

The epithelial mucous or goblet cells (Fig. 6) are tall columnar cells with a slender basal attachment to the basement membrane and a broad apex containing mucous granules giving the classic goblet or chalice shape. Goblet cells may replicate by mitosis or derive from an epithelial cell stem. Goblet cell hypersecretion and hyperplasia occur commonly in response to inhaled irritants (LAMB and REID 1969b; JONES et al. 1973). Junctions between goblet cells and adjoining cells are typically through tight junctions. The cytoplasm towards the base contains extensive rough endoplasmic reticulum and an elaborate Golgi complex. Secretory granules, rich in acid glycoprotein, develop from the Golgi complex and are situated throughout the apical cell cytoplasm in the mature cell. The goblet cell se-

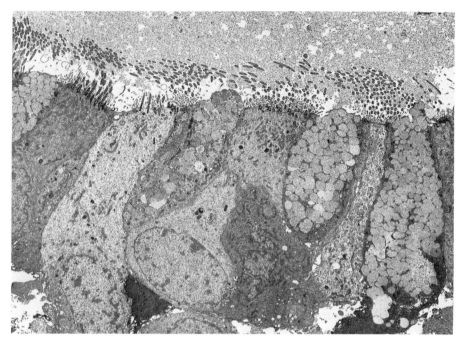

Fig. 6. Electron micrograph of goblet cells from the human bronchial epithelium. These cells have a characteristic shape, determined by the presence of electron-lucent secretory granules that contain mucous glycoproteins. The cells release secretion in response to irritation of the epithelial surface

cretes in response to irritants in the airway lumen and is independent of neurogenic stimuli.

The trachea and major bronchi of human airways contain approximately 10% of goblet cells in the epithelia and the number diminishes in subsequent airway generations so that these cells are rare in the bronchioles (THURLBECK et al. 1975). The numbers of goblet cells are proportionally greater in the cartilaginous walls than in the membranous walls of the human trachea. Such distribution is important to consider in assessing the role of goblet cell populations in the airways. In pathogen-free rats, less than 1% of the total epithelial cell population in the trachea and bronchi are goblet cells.

2. Epithelial Serous Cell

The epithelial serous cell has been described in the trachea and bronchi of the rat and more recently in other species. This cell type is sparse, representing less than 1% of epithelial cells in healthy airways, but may increase significantly in number with respiratory infection or irritation. Typically, apical granules are present that stain for glycoprotein, similar to those of serous cells of the bronchial mucous glands (LAMB and REID 1969a). Similarities exist between the shape of the secretion granules in the epithelial serous cells and those described in the Clara cell of the rat. The cells rest on the basement membrane of the airways and extend to the airway lumen with a microvillous surface. The nucleus is irregular and usually basal in position and the cytoplasm contains abundant rough endoplasmic reticulum and an extensive Golgi complex. The secretion granules that originate in these cells are round, smaller than those of the goblet cells, homogeneous in their electron density, and lacking in osmiophilia. The function of the epithelial serous cell is not clear although it has been considered to contribute lysozyme and other secretory components to the fluid lining of the airways.

IV. Brush Cells

Brush cells are present in the trachea and major bronchi with a distribution and population size that varies considerably among different species. The brush cell is typically pyramidal in shape with a broad base and narrow apex. On the luminal aspect, there is a brush border of broad microvilli up to 200 nm diameter and 0.8 μm long, approximately twice the diameter of the microvilli seen on ciliated cells. Each microvillus has a core of 50- to 70-Å fibrils and bundles of tonofilaments are present throughout the cytoplasm. The role of the brush cell is unknown. Current hypotheses suggest functions as absorptive cells or as chemoreceptors within the airways.

V. Submucosal Glands

The number and distribution of submucosal glands, estimated to be 5,000 in the human lung, are established early in fetal life and are complete by 16 weeks of gestation (THURLBECK et al. 1961). The gland increases in size and complexity with age, up to 13 years in humans. Mucus may be detected cytochemically in the submucosal glands by 24 weeks of gestation, but the nature of the secretions differs from the adult pattern. Mucous and serous cells are present at birth, but the intracellular secretions differentiate fully after the neonatal period.

In the normal airway, the openings of the gland onto the lumen of the airway are narrow and not readily distinguished between surrounding ciliated cells. Following acute mechanical irritation or infection, however, the ducts dilate with concomitant loss of normal ciliated cells so that the ducts leading to submucosal glands are readily observed by the naked eye (NADEL and DAVIS 1977; STURGESS 1977b).

Submucosal glands have a characteristic tubuloacinar structure with a main duct system, the upper portion of which has ciliated and mucus-secreting goblet cells, and the lower portion of which has a specialized region of cells termed the collecting duct (MEYRICK et al. 1969). Secretory cells arise from the duct system and are organized into two types of tubules or acini lined with mucus and serous cells. Myoepithelial cells are located around the secretory tubules and acini and when stimulated may aid in the release of secretory products from the gland into the lumen of the airway. The glands are innervated by both parasympathetic and sympathetic branches of the autonomic nervous system. Hypertrophy and hyperplasia of the mucus-secreting glands are common responses to inhaled irritants and infection (REID 1960). With gland enlargement and hypersecretion, a relative increase occurs in mucous cell types and a shift occurs in cytochemical characteristics of the secretions (LAMB and REID 1969 a, 1972; STURGESS and REID 1973).

VI. Neuroendocrine Cells

Neuroendocrine cells occupy about 1%–2% of bronchial epithelial cells in the adult airways, but are more common in the fetus and newborn. Structurally, the cell has electron-lucent cytoplasm containing dense core vesicles, that may degranulate and release the contents towards the cell base. Groups of neuroendocrine cells may occur also as neuroepithelial bodies. The role of neuroendocrine cells that are characterized as APUD endocrine cells in respiratory function remains controversial. The development of radioimmunoassays has recognized the presence of specific active peptides including vasoactive intestinal peptide (VIP), bombesin, calcitonin, serotonin, and Leu-enkephalin. In parallel with similar cells in the gut, it is possible that these cells may exert a local regulatory mechanism for epithelial function or differentiation. The question yet to be answered is whether this regulation influences cilia, mucus, or ion transport functions in adjacent cells in the epithelial layer.

C. Respiratory Secretions: Source, Composition, and Physicochemical Characteristics

The fluid lining of the respiratory tract involves complex interaction of many different secretions with unique physicochemical properties that are essential for mucociliary clearance. The gel structure of mucus resides in the specific properties of mucous glycoproteins originating from goblet and serous cells of the airways epithelium and from the mucous and serous cells of the submucosal glands. Mucous secretions in the airways form an upper gel layer with a lower layer that bathes the cilia and has a greater fluidity so that the cilia beat freely. The amount of mucus and its unique rheological properties, confer its protective function, the deposition and trapping of inhaled particles and their clearance, and the airways resistance.

I. Extracellular Fluid Lining of Airways

The major airways of the lung (Fig. 7) have an extracellular layer of mucus that extends over large areas of the epithelium and closely follows the contours of the cell surfaces (STURGESS 1977a, b). The continuity of the mucous blanket that exists in the human and rabbit lung may not feature in all mammalian species such as the rat where mucus forms a patchy layer (VAN AS and WEBSTER 1974).

By scanning electron microscopy, the extracellular layer of mucus in the human trachea appears as a smooth cohesive blanket overlying the tips of ciliated cells (Fig. 8). The smooth layer occasionally shows series of overlapping sheets or plaques of mucus. In the main bronchus, the mucous blanket exhibits a more complex three-dimensional arrangement, with series of plaque-like structures that vary in appearance from smooth sheets, to perforated sheets, to open networks

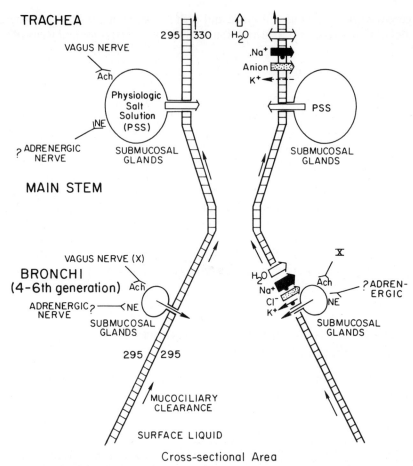

Fig. 7. Schematic representation of airway cross-sectional area. Active ion translocation (*arrow with circle*), passive movement (*arrow*), and relative magnitude of net movements across surface epithelial cells are noted. Osmolality of tracheal surface liquid and projected water flows in various regions are shown. Projections of glandular secretion and regulation are noted. (BOUCHER et al. 1980)

of fibrils. Close to the cell surface, mucus forms more open networks whereas, toward the lumen of the airway, mucus forms more cohesive plaques. The major intrapulmonary airways are characterized by more expanded fibrillar networks with a few smooth sheets of mucus. With successive airway generations, the mucous blanket becomes thinner and less dense.

The fact that the mucous blanket appears smoother and more cohesive in the trachea compared with either main or lobar bronchi, where it becomes a more open expanded structure presumably reflects a change in the macromolecular composition or hydration of secretions in the different airway generations. The thickness of the mucous blanket increases with ascending airway generations, from 0.1 µm in bronchioles to 5 µm in major intrapulmonary airways (LUCHTEL 1976). The thickness and composition of the mucous blanket are important deter-

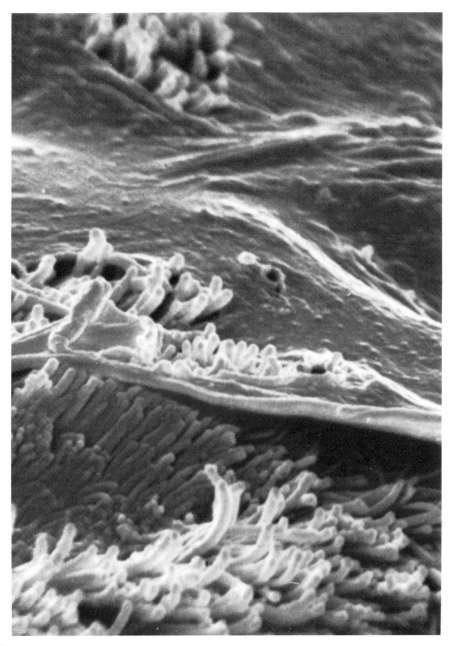

Fig. 8. Scanning electron micrograph of mucous blanket overlying the airway epithelium. The cilia tips are in contact with the mucous layer, but beat in a lower fluid layer of low molecular weight. (STURGESS 1977 a)

minants of the efficiency of the mucociliary clearance mechanism (Silberberg et al. 1977).

The biphasic nature of the mucous blanket in the airways has long been discussed in hypothetical models of mucociliary transport (Lucas and Douglas 1934; Kilburn 1968a; Blake and Winet 1980) and it has been possible to confirm this hypothesis at least in the major bronchi (Sturgess 1977a). The mucous blanket clearly segregates into an upper mucous layer or gel phase, which is separated from the epithelial cells by a serous layer or sol phase. The uppermost layer includes the mucous glycoproteins with characteristic viscoelastic properties. The nature of the lower layer has not been defined clearly, although there is cytochemical evidence that it contains some lysozyme and possibly other serous secretions (Sade et al. 1970; Spicer et al. 1971), and it may be augmented by active transport of ions and water across the tracheobronchial epithelium or from the blood capillaries in the submucosa (Olver et al. 1975). Airway mucus may be separated physically into sol and gel components that vary with physiologic and disease states (Lopez-Vidriero 1973).

Neither the nature nor the source of fluid in the hypophase or sol layer has been defined, although experimental studies with surgical pouches in the dog trachea indicate that it is produced locally in bronchial epithelium (Spicer et al. 1971). Newly secreted mucus from goblet cells and submucosal glands presumably passes through the sol layer, but morphological evidence suggests that it does not diffuse into the sol layer. In the canine and human respiratory tract, goblet cell mucus appears to be discharged through the sol layer as a discrete column that merges with the overlying mucous layer. Similarly, secretions from the submucosal glands pass from the duct to the airway lumen as a continuous layer of mucus that merges directly with the overlying mucous blanket (Sturgess 1977b).

In contrast to the larger airways, the extracellular lining of the bronchioles appears by scanning electron microscopy as a smooth layer (Gil and Weibel 1971; Ebert and Terracio 1975) distinct from the lining in the major bronchi. The appearance reflects the different composition of the secretions in the proximal and distal airways of the lung and, furthermore, implicates the complex network of fibrils in bronchial mucus originating from acidic glycoprotein secretions. In purified form, mucous glycoproteins have been demonstrated to have similar fibrillar networks by scanning electron microscopic studies (Forstner et al. 1976). The complexity of the network and formation of smooth cohesive sheets is proportional to the concentration of macromolecular material in the secretions, the cross-linking and interactions between different glycoproteins, and/or interactions between glycoproteins and electrolytes as well as other proteinaceous material (Forstner et al. 1977). Certainly, the alignment of fibers, and altered structure would be expected to correlate with the rheological or flow properties of the secretions (Litt 1970a, b), and be reflected by variations in rates of mucociliary clearance in the airways (Barton and Lourenco 1973; Puchelle et al. 1976; Chen and Dulfano 1978; Giordano et al. 1978; King and Macklem 1977).

Earlier theories that the lower layer was produced by liquefaction of the upper mucous layer under the shearing force of cilia (Goldfarb and Buchberg 1964) do not appear to be valid since the components of the upper and lower phases can be distinguished using cytochemical techniques. This phase separation resembles a property common to polymer mixtures which segregate effectively in dilute solution and may correlate with different surface tension properties of the sol layer. Such segregation may be a function of the chemical composition of the macromolecules and may provide interfaces for interaction of different macromolecules which may be significant to the protective role of mucous secretions in the respiratory tract.

From a hypothetical consideration, the sol layer has been suggested to originate from alveolar fluid (KILBURN 1968 a) or bronchioli (GIL and WEIBEL 1971), thus providing continuity between alveolar and bronchial clearance. LITT (1970 b) also postulated that alveolar fluid lines the respiratory bronchioles and thus constitutes the sol layer in the terminal bronchioles, while mucus from goblet cells and submucosal glands forms the gel layer. The necessary regulation of the thickness of the sol layer presumably regulates the thickness of the mucous blanket in larger airways. As the mucus is transported towards the trachea, the solid component is increased and mucus becomes more viscoelastic and gel-like. The presence of surfactant, dipalmitoyl lecithin, derived from alveolar epithelial cells, may exert a surface tension effect, facilitating the propulsion of mucus by the differential wettability of cilia (HILLS and BARROW 1979).

II. Chemical Composition of Mucous Secretions

The normal total daily volume of secretions has been variously estimated from 10 ml/day (TOREMALM 1960) to 100 ml/day (REID 1959) in humans, and may increase to 300 ml/day in hypersecretory states.

1. Mucous Glycoproteins

Mucous glycoproteins (REID and CLAMP 1978) are essentially composed of a long protein core to which oligosaccharide side chains are attached (HOLDEN and GRIGGS 1977). The oligosaccharides include an average of 10–16 sugars linked to serine or threonine residues of the protein core (HAVEZ and BISERTE 1968; ROBERTS 1974). The mucous glycoproteins are distinguished from glycoproteins found in sera by the relatively high proportion of carbohydrate, the linkage of the oligosaccharide to serine or threonine through an O-glycosidic bond, and the composition of sugars in the oligosaccharide side chains. These sugars include N-acetylgalactosamine present at the linkage point with the peptide, N-acetylglucosamine, D-galactose, L-fucose, and sialic acids. The last two sugars occupy terminal positions in the side chains and play a major role in the determination of the physiocochemical properties of the mucous glycoproteins. Sulfate is present also in the form of sulfate esters on galactose residues of the glycoproteins. The individual oligosaccharide side chains are heterogeneous with regard to their variable length and branching patterns. Blood group specificity [A, B, H(O), Le^a, and Le^b] exists in mucous glycoproteins and is a function of the carbohydrate sequence in oligosaccharide chains. This leads to a concept that each tissue, individual, and species, has its own specific glycoproteins which are reflected by the composition of these carbohydrate units as well as of the core protein (PIGMAN 1977).

The exact structure of the oligosaccharide side chains remains to be elucidated. In hypersecretory states, variation in the types of acid glycoproteins occurs in both types of secretory cells and appears to involve the pattern of glycosylation of the mucous glycoproteins (Reid 1967; Keal 1971; Lamblin et al. 1977). The assembly of specific sugars in the oligosaccharide chain is regulated by highly specific glycosyltransferase enzymes. The regulation of such enzymes is important in determining the rate of synthesis of mucous glycoproteins and the nature of the mucous macromolecules. The presence of the terminal sugars fucose and sialic acids and of sulfate esters appears to be particularly pertinent to the types of neutral or acid glycoproteins which occur in the respiratory tract.

2. Serum-Type Glycoproteins

Serum-type glycoproteins, the other major component of mucous secretions, are similar to the serum glycoproteins in that they have relatively little carbohydrate in the oligosaccharide side chain, the oligosaccharides are attached to the peptide by an *N*-glycosidic linkage, and the types of sugars are distinct. Although some of the serum-type glycoproteins present in respiratory secretions may be derived by a process of transudation across the bronchial wall (Ryley 1972), most are synthesized in the bronchial wall and are specific to respiratory secretion. Serum-type glycoproteins present in respiratory secretions include serum albumin, orosomucoid, $alpha_1$-acid glycoprotein, haptoglobin, $alpha_2$-macroglobulin, bronchial transferrin, $beta_1$-U-globulin, IgA, IgG, bronchial kallikrein, bronchial lysozyme, and $alpha_1$-antitrypsin (Martinez-Tello et al. 1968; Ryley and Brogan 1973; Masson and Heremans 1973; Bonomo and D'Addabbo 1974).

Apart from the major glycoprotein components, mucous secretions include lipid derived mainly from the surfactant phospholipids formed in more peripheral regions of the lung and their degradation products. In addition, nucleic acid may be present which presumably is derived from exfoliated epithelial cells as well as from inflammatory cells and microorganisms. These constituents increase particularly in respiratory disease. The presence of purulent material in bronchial secretion dramatically influences the viscosity and clearance of mucus.

3. Fluids and Electrolytes

The understanding of fluid and electrolyte transport in bronchial epithelia has provided important new avenues to understand the physiology of the respiratory tract in regard to the transport of fluid and electrolytes into the airways, and the effect on mucociliary clearance in the lung (Olver et al. 1975; Nadel et al. 1979; Marin et al. 1979; Boucher 1980). In vitro, short-circuit techniques have been applied to measure active ion transport across the bronchial wall (Olver et al. 1975). Active ion transport maintains mucus hypertonic, with significantly higher levels of potassium and chloride ions than serum. Before and after birth, the respiratory epithelium secretes Cl^- actively towards the lung lumen, presumably contributing to the alveolar lining fluid and to the periciliary fluid layer of airways. This function persists after birth: pulmonary secretions have persistently high Cl^- and K^+ concentrations relative to plasma. In large airways, Cl^- and Na^+ are actively transported, the active Cl^- flux towards the airway lumen exceeding that of Na^+ towards the submucosa. If the chloride pump is linked to water flow across the epithelium (as in other epithelia) this may be an important de-

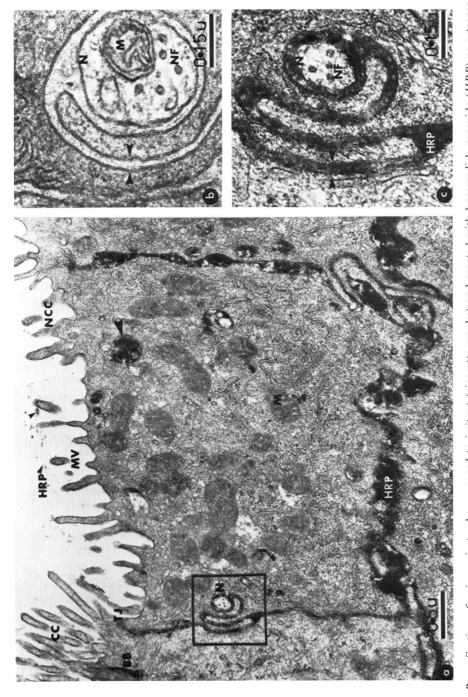

Fig. 9a–c. Section of guinea pig trachea exposed to irritant (cigarette smoke) and reacted with horseradish peroxide (*HRP*) as a tracer for intracellular spaces. Penetration of this dense tracer between the epithelial cells at the basal and lateral margins indicates the disorganization of the intracellular junction complexes. *MV* microvilli, *TJ* tight junction, *CC* ciliated cell, *BB* basal body, *NCC* non-ciliated cell, *M* mitochondria, *N* nerve ending, *NF* nerve fibre (BOUCHER et al. 1980)

terminant of the aqueous phase of airways and alveoli. Control and sites of the resorption of fluid are not known. However, in the dog, studies on sodium and chloride transport in the trachea suggest that net fluid is transported into the lumen, whereas active resorption of fluid appears to be the rule in the normal human and rabbit trachea. In segmental and subsegmental bronchi, sodium and chloride ions are actively absorbed from the airway lumen to the submucosal tissue so that the depth of the fluid layer in the airway surfaces is probably regulated by active ion transport mechanisms. Mucus acts as a polyelectrolyte, having strong anionic surface charge, with terminal COOH residues on the oligosaccharide side chains of the glycoprotein molecules. The presence of cations (Na^+, Ca^{2+}, etc.) has a dramatic effect on mucus, reducing solubility and increasing viscosity (FORSTNER et al. 1977). Thus, the ionic composition and the concentration of mucus are important determinants of the mucous layer also.

The lung liquid and airway lining are not at electrochemical equilibrium with plasma and interstitial fluid. Active transport processes of ions have been identified that allow net transport against an electrochemical gradient. All epithelial cells may have inherent capability to transport Cl^-. Based on the location of ATPase, and the cellular ultrastructure, ciliated cells have been implicated in this process. Defective epithelial transport processes such as paracellular pathways may render airways susceptible to inhaled irritants/infection, etc., by an effect of clearance.

Injury or irritation commonly enhances airway reactivity, for example, by exposure to invironmental pollutants, to cigarette smoke, and to antigen in sensitized airways (BOUCHER et al. 1980). Such toxic insults damage the mucosal barrier, probably at the level of the tight junctions between epithelial cells (Fig. 9). As a result, the epithelium becomes "leaky", increasing access of foreign matter to submucosal tissue and eliminating the normal regulation of electrolytes and water at affected sites in the airways.

III. Rheological Properties of Mucous Secretions

The rheological or flow properties of mucus are critical to normal functioning of the mucociliary clearance mechanism, in pulmonary defense. Mucus is a viscoelastic gel, possessing properties of elasticity and of viscosity that reflects resistance to flow (LITT 1970b). Mucous secretions do not behave as simple newtonian fluids, so that flow cannot be defined only by viscosity (LITT 1973; LUTZ et al. 1973), but show wide variation in viscous and elastic properties, depending on the shearing forces which may be applied. The heterogeneous nature of mucous secretions, their variable hydration, and the variable inclusion of other cellular and macromolecular material in response to injury create difficulties in the interpretation of viscoelastic changes in mucous secretions. The viscosity of normal respiratory secretions has proved difficult to define owing to problems of collection, although the viscosity has been measured for chronic respiratory diseases, including chronic bronchitis, asthma, cystic fibrosis, and bronchiectasis (CHARMAN and REID 1972). In all diseases, the viscosity of purulent, infected secretions may be significantly higher than that of mucoid, clear secretions. The requisite properties for mucociliary transport are not unique to mucus but are shared by other polymeric systems such as guaran, agarose, and gelatin. In these materials, transport rates are dependent on the degree of cross-linking with maximum rates where gel formation occurs (KING et al. 1979; SADE et al. 1975).

With the application of sophisticated approaches to study both the viscous and elastic characteristics of biologic fluids (STURGESS et al. 1970; LITT 1973; DAVIS 1973), the rheological properties of respiratory mucus have received considerable attention during the past decade. A magnetic rheometer has been developed that allows evaluation of microliter quantities (KING and MACKLEM 1977). Mucus has been shown to be viscoelastic (STURGESS et al. 1971; MITCHELL-HEGGS et al. 1974) and theoretically the elastic modulus may be more important than viscosity at the beat frequency estimated for cilia in the respiratory tract (LITT 1970 a). Mucus with high viscosity and with low elasticity will not be cleared effectively (DULFANO et al. 1971; DULFANO and ADLER 1975). While clearance in vitro appears to be independent of mucus viscosity, increased elasticity of mucus decreases mucociliary clearance (DULFANO et al. 1971). On this basis, however, it is difficult to assess the efficacy of mucolytic agents which reduce the "viscosity" of mucus, as their beneficial role in the lung will only exist if one can normalize the physical changes in the secretions to those optimal for clearance (POLU et al. 1978).

At low elasticity (< 10 dyn/cm^2) clearance increases; with increasing elastic modulus (> 10 dyn/cm^3) clearance decreases (SHIH et al. 1977), a paradox that may explain the conflicting results in studies of mucus flow. However, the relationship between clearance and elasticity of mucus is a weak one, with 50% reduction in clearance related to one order of magnitude change in elastic modulus.

Based on theoretical models, in the normal lung, mucus must possess solid properties so that it can flow against forces of gravity and airflow. In disease, increased volumes or composition of secretion occurs with concomitant changes in physicochemical properties of the secretions. Thus, the mucociliary clearance mechanism is exquisitely sensitive to changes in hydration, secretion, epithelial cell function, and ciliary motility. Any imbalance in qualitative or quantitative function will be reflected by impaired clearance, stasis, pooling of secretions, infection, and/or retention of potentially toxic inhaled particles.

D. Fundamental Aspects of Mucociliary Clearance

I. Dynamics of Ciliary Movement

Cilia may beat continually or may beat and then rest in the recovery phase (SLEIGH 1977). The cycle of movement begins with the recovery stroke and ends with the effective stroke, perpendicular to the epithelial surface. At the recovery stroke, a lateral wave excites cilia of adjacent cells, presumably by a direct contact phenomenon, providing for the coordination of epithelial cilia.

Cilia beat at a rate of 10–20 beats/s (Hz) or 600–1,200 beats/min, in the respiratory tract of different mammalian species. The coordinated movement of adjacent cilia generates a metachronous wave of activity that travels in a direction opposite to the flow of mucus (Fig. 10; SLEIGH and AIELLO 1972). The cilia in nor-

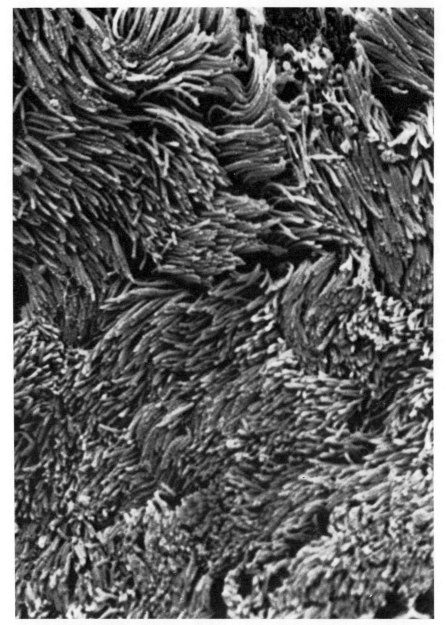

Fig. 10. Scanning electron micrograph of cilia in the trachea, illustrating the metachronous waves of movement

mal airways may carry loads of up to 10 g/cm^2 without dysfunction. The control and coordination of ciliary movement is not fully understood, but appears to be an intrinsic process since ciliary beating may continue in the absence of other vital functions.

However, ciliary beat frequency may be modulated by exogenous factors, such as agonists that accelerate ciliary movement and possibly, serotonin, that excites molluscan gill cilia (GOSSELIN 1966) by premature initiation of the recovery stroke. It may be that ciliary motion is propagated by electrical potential, by the direct contact either between cilia or between cilia and particulate matter, or by a hydrodynamic interaction between adjacent cilia (SLEIGH 1977). In such a system, an impulse will propagate a metachronous wave of ciliary movement.

The effective beat of ciliary motion is normal to the plane of the airway, being twice as effective as a tangential mode (BLAKE 1975). The recovery stroke is tangential; therefore, the velocity of the effective stroke is higher than the recovery stroke. The extension of cilia is thus important to effective movement of the mucous blanket. The ciliary tips are in contact with mucus, a contact that may be enhanced by short "claw-like" projections of the ciliary apex.

The effective force provided by cilia is a direct function of their length and their amplitude of movement. During bending, the force is increased, although effective propulsion of mucus may diminish as the cilium is oblique to the mucus layer. To achieve maximum force with effective propulsion, the optimal length has been calculated theoretically to be 5.5 μm. In the trachea, cilia are typically 6–7 μm in length, approaching this optimal level of function.

II. Relationship of Ciliary Beat and In Vivo Mucociliary Clearance

Ciliary beat frequency may vary considerably from one individual to another. Within the human bronchial tree, early studies revealed no significant differences in the beat frequency of cilia from different airway generations (YAGER et al. 1980). More recently, ciliary beat frequency has been shown to diminish progressively from the trachea to lobar bronchi (RUTLAND et al. 1982a). In addition to beat frequency distally in the bronchial tree, the shorter length of cilia and decreased numbers of ciliated cells will be predicted to contribute significant diminution of propulsive force for the mucociliary clearance mechanism. Variation in ciliary beat has been estimated as 6–7 Hz in the terminal bronchiole to 20–22 Hz in the trachea of the rat. This correlates with movement of mucus from central airways towards the trachea at mucociliary clearance rates that increase significantly in the bullfrog (KILBURN 1967a), rat (VAN As and IRAVANI 1972), dog (ASMUNDSSON and KILBURN 1970), and human (SERAFINI et al. 1976; MORROW et al. 1967; LOURENCO et al. 1971). In addition, physiologic or pathophysiologic changes may occur in peripheral airways that will affect mucociliary clearance; for example, the presence of inflammatory exudate that may lower surface tension of the fluid lining, or the smooth muscle changes that alter airway–fluid interfaces (MACKLEM et al. 1970).

The total cross-sectional area of the human bronchial tree does not increase appreciably from the trachea to the bronchi (1 mm in diameter). In contrast, the circumference of the airways increases cumulatively from 55 mm in the human trachea, to 70–75 mm in the main bronchi, to 300 cm at the tenth generation and then progressively with each bronchial division, to several meters at the level of the respiratory bronchioles (WEIBEL 1963; HORSFIELD and CUMMING 1968).

Conversely, the stream bed available for ciliary flow becomes narrower so that the volume passing any airway must increase progressively as mucus moves upwards in the bronchial tree. In addition, it is assumed that mucus is continually added as the stream advances. This had led to consideration, first, that flow rates vary in different airways, i.e., progressively slower rates of mucociliary transport from trachea to distal airways, and second, that resorption of fluid occurs in the airways to counterbalance secretion (BOUCHER 1980).

In the bronchial tree, bifurcations of major airways are common sites where the normal ciliated epithelia are replaced by nonciliated cells. As mucus passes from a bronchus into the opening of a tributary bronchus, it passes around it, narrowing the surface area of the mucus lining. Ciliary streams do not necessarily rejoin. HILDING (1957) referred to such effects at airway branches as "ciliary narrows". The plane of ciliary beat tends to be oblique, directing the mucous blanket around the bronchial openings.

"Whirlpools" or eddies in the ciliary stream have been described commonly in excised trachea, progressing in the direction of flow and due to the shearing action of the parallel lines of flow moving at unequal rates. These areas may measure up to 0.25 mm in diameter and persist for more than 1 h, in bronchi, on medial walls, and at the carinae. Although these may be artifactual, owing to the nature of the examination, such static whirlpools may act as mechanical or chemical sites of airway damage or irritation.

In the human lung, mucus is secreted mainly by submucosal glands which are confined to the first five generations of bronchi, where cartilage is still existent. Goblet cells contribute mucus in lesser volume and diminish progressively as one descends the bronchial tree so that mucus-secreting potential is minimal at the bronchiolar level in the healthy lung. In distal airways, other secretions such as those of the Clara cells and type II epithelial cells will have a major influence on the nature of the fluid lining.

E. Mucociliary Clearance: Assessment and Flow Rates

Clearance in the nose has been reviewed recently by PROCTOR (1977). In the human nasal mucosa, the mean flow rate is of the order of 4–5 mm/min (PROCTOR et al. 1973; ROSSMAN et al. 1977) and appears to be consistent and accessible for physical measurement. In the lower respiratory tract, one cannot directly extrapolate from nasal clearance rates since embryologically the airways develop separately. It is difficult to extrapolate from tracheal clearance to clearance in successive bronchial generations since differences of several orders of magnitude exist in measured clearance rates, in cell populations, and secretory potentials of each airway. FOSTER et al. (1980) have shown a 2.75:1 ratio of clearance between the trachea and main bronchus in human lungs where average clearance rates are 4.2–6.4 mm/min and 0.9–4.5 mm/min, respectively. Bronchial clearance diminishes further from the central airways to mid and peripheral airways (WILKEY et al. 1980). Lesser, but significant differences exist in the canine bronchi where in vitro clearance rates diminish from an average of 12.6 mm/min in trachea to 8.2, 4.0, and 1.6 mm/min lobar, segmental, and subsegmental bronchi, respectively (ASMUNDSSON and KILBURN 1970).

Many of the factors described contribute to the diminished clearance from central to peripheral airways (THOMSON and PAVIA 1974). Furthermore, bronchial openings delay clearance. Thus, in evaluating mucociliary clearance, it is important to compare mucociliary clearance rates at defined levels in the lung. The efficiency of clearance can be compared only when deposition of particles occurs at the same depth or when clearance rates are defined for airways of similar size.

I. Measurement of Mucociliary Clearance In Vivo

The earliest in vivo techniques to evaluate mucociliary transport rates were based on direct observation of the tracheal mucosa through an incision or "window" (DALHAMN 1955, 1956). Using the cat as an experimental model, transillumination of the exposed trachea has been used to observe transport of carbon and lycopodium particles (LAURENZI et al. 1967). Total lung clearance measurements have been used to define "mucociliary clearance" using noninvasive approaches. The techniques are limited by the geometry of the lung, which hinders visualization of individual airways and may be limited, also, by the variable distribution of markers owing to difficulties inherent in the deposition of uniform aerosol particles in the lung (THOMSON and SHORT 1969). Therefore, most direct measurement of mucociliary clearance is restricted to the trachea and central airways.

1. Radioaerosol Techniques

The most common approach to measure mucociliary clearance in vivo in experimental animal models and in humans is by the inhalation of a radioactively labeled aerosol (ALBERT and ARNETT 1955). γ-Emitting radionuclides with short half-lives have been mostly widely used to label particulates such as albumin microspheres for inhalation. The deposition and clearance may be monitored by external recorders using an approach applied first by BAETJER (1967) to measure total lung clearance. A rapid phase of clearance (up to 6 h) that eliminates approximately 90% of radioactivity, is considered to reflect mucociliary clearance and is followed by a slow phase (24 h or longer) that represents clearance phenomena at the alveobronchiolar level (GREEN 1973). Tracheobronchial clearance is estimated from fast-phase mucociliary clearance time. $^{99}Tc^m$ has been the radionuclide of choice since it has a short half-life (approximately 6 h) and gives a radiation dose of about 2 mrad.

The detection and monitoring of inhaled radioaerosols depends on the dose of radioactivity (CLARKE and PAVIA 1980). At high dose levels, detection has been demonstrated with the gamma camera (SANCHIS et al. 1973), and increasing sensitivity is provided by a single collimated chest counter positioned centrally (TOIGO 1963), by twin detectors (THOMSON et al. 1974), or by a series of detectors positioned around the chest wall (ALBERT et al. 1969a).

The rates of tracheobronchial clearance vary according to the initial deposition pattern that is a function of the mode of inhalation, the physical properties of the aerosol, and the degree of airways obstruction. The size, density, hygroscopicity, and change of aerosol particulates are determinants also of their deposition patterns: larger particles tend to deposit by impaction in central rather than distal airways (LIPPMANN and ALBERT 1969; LIPPMANN 1976). The distribution of deposition depends on the aerodynamic diameter that considers size and density so that particles of greater density behave aerodynamically like larger particles (MORROW 1974; LIPPMANN et al. 1975).

With high flow rate, inhaled particles deposit preferentially in central airways (GOLDBERG and LOURENCO 1973) while large volume inhalation and breath-holding favors peripheral deposition (BOOKER et al. 1967). In obstructive airway disease, aerosols tend to deposit more centrally (THOMSON and SHORT 1969; DOLOVICH et al. 1976), so that clearance patterns must be reviewed carefully to ensure that data do not reflect differences in distribution, rather than clearance. The estimation of mucociliary clearance by inhaled aerosols requires extended observation periods (MORROW et al. 1967) and may be influenced by deposition patterns and physiologic effects as well as by coughing. Using aerosol techniques, biologic half-life may be determined; for normal subjects, the half-life for 1-μm particles varies from 2–3 min in the trachea, 28 min in central airways, to between 3 h and 2 months in distal airways. In contrast, 6-μm particles have a biologic half-life of approximately 1 h (CAMNER et al. 1973a).

2. Cinefiberscopic Techniques

PROCTOR and WAGNER (1966) measured nasal mucociliary clearance by applying a droplet of radioactively labeled albumin on the nasal mucosa and monitored the progression of radioactive labeling with a scintillation camera. Similar techniques have been applied subsequently to measure tracheal and bronchial clearance. Linear velocity may be computed from directional change in the location of radioactivity.

By means of a calibrated fiber optic bronchoscope, the rate of movement of polytetrafluoroethylene (Teflon) disks was measured as an index of tracheobronchial clearance (CAMNER and PHILIPSON 1971; SACKNER et al. 1973). This approach has been applied in experimental models in the dog (WANNER et al. 1975) and sheep (LANDA et al. 1975), and in humans (SANTA CRUZ et al. 1974). Teflon disks, 0.13 mg, are deposited on the tracheal mucosa through a bronchoscope and the movement is recorded on film. The velocity of particles is computed from the recorded images.

With disadvantages in the invasive procedures associated with bronchoscopy and the need for local anesthesia in this procedure, subsequent adaptations of this technique used roentgenographic monitoring (FRIEDMAN et al. 1977) with bismuth trioxide as a marker for the Teflon particles, and using a fluoroscopic image intensifier, recorded on videotape (GOODMAN et al. 1978b). The bismuth-coated particles may be blown into the airway without intubation, thus eliminating the need for bronchoscopy.

3. Bronchoscopic Techniques

Bronchoscopic techniques to deposit ^{99}Tc^m or ^{113}In^m radiolabeled albumin particles (5–7 μm diameter) present an alternate method to determine tracheal clearance. Following deposition of particles at the carina, through a fiber optic bronchoscope, the particle movement is recorded by serial images from a scintillation camera with a wide field of view over a period of about 30–60 min (CHOPRA et al. 1977, 1979). The images are recorded photographically as radioactivity is cleared and the data analyzed to determine rate of clearance.

4. Radioaerosol Bolus Techniques

Based on the deposition of particles in central airways when inhaled at high flow rate, YEATES et al. (1975) developed an alternative procedure, that eliminates bronchoscopy (Fig. 11). Radioactively labeled albumin microspheres (0.5 μm diameter) are inhaled during a series of tidal breaths from a spirometer system so that the microspheres deposit preferentially at bifurcations of the large airways. The distribution and clearance of radioactive boluses are monitored by a scintil-

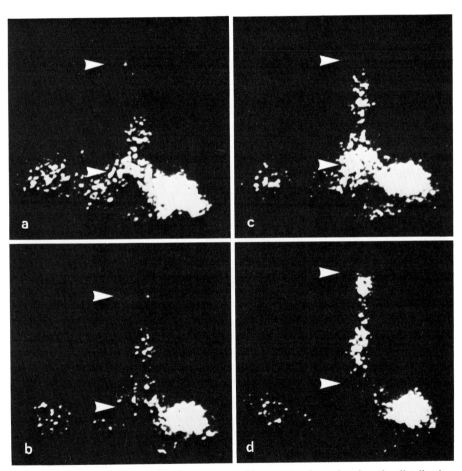

Fig. 11 a–d. Images from scintillation camera of human trachea, showing the distribution of radioactive boluses of technetium-labeled albumin **a** after inspiration at high flow rate, radioactive bolus is concentrated in main carina and central airways. At successive time intervals, the radioactive aerosol is cleared toward the trachea; **b** 10 min; **c** 20 min; **d** 30 min. The linear paths of radioactive boluses in the trachea are recorded as a function of time from the carina (*upper arrow*) to the larynx (*lower arrow*)

lation camera over a period of approximately 30 min. The tracheal mucus velocity or mean tracheal transport rate is derived from the spatial position of individual particles or boluses of labeled particles as a function of time. This procedure is noninvasive and may be conducted without anesthesia.

5. Bronchographic Techniques

In an attempt to improve spatial resolution and measure clearance from airways of different dimensions, tantalum dust labeled with ^{182}Ta has been deposited by catheter at the bifurcation of the trachea and deeper in the lung (EDMUNDS et al. 1970; GAMSU et al. 1973) to measure mucus velocity. The location of the tantalum particles may be monitored by serial chest X-ray examination and the radiographs used to quantify clearance (STITIK et al. 1976). Clearance rates by mucociliary transport are slower than for other insoluble dusts (BIANCO et al. 1974).

Table 2. Techniques for in vivo measurement of mucociliary transport rates

Technique	Species	Marker	Clearance rate (mm/min)	Reference
1. Microscopic observation				
Incised trachea	Rat	Mucus	13.5	DAHLHAMN (1956)
Exposed airways	Rat	Mucus	11	IRAVANI and VAN AS (1972)
Transillumination of airways	Cat	Carbon particles	13–20	LAURENZI et al. (1967)
2. Bronchoscopic techniques				
Bronchoscopy	Dog	India ink	14–15	HILDING (1957)
Cinefiberscopy	Dog	Teflon disks (0.13 mg)	13.5	WANNER et al. (1975)
	Sheep	Teflon disks	17.5	LANDA et al. (1975)
	Human	Teflon disks	20.1	WOOD et al. (1975)
Bronchoscope/gamma camera detection	Human	^{99}Tc^m–albumin (5–7 μm)	15.5	CHOPRA et al. (1979)
Fluoroscopic	Human	BiO$_3$ Teflon disks	10	FRIEDMAN et al. (1977)
	Human	BiO$_3$ Teflon disks	10	GOODMAN et al. (1978 a)
3. Radioaerosol techniques (Scintillation detector)				
Radioaerosol	Dog	^{99}Tc^{m}O$_4$ solution	16	MARIN and MORROW (1969)
	Dog	^{99}Tc^m–labeled resin beads	10.5	PROCTOR et al. (1973)
	Dog	^{99}Tc^m–pertechnetate solution	10	GIORDANO (1978)
	Human	Fe$_2$O$_3$, ^{51}Cr, and polystyrene	14	MORROW et al. (1967)
4. Radioaerosol bolus techniques				
	Human	^{99}Tc^m–albumin microspheres	4.7	YEATES et al (1974, 1976)
	Human	^{99}Tc^m–albumin microspheres		SANCHIS et al. (1973)
5. Bronchographic techniques				
Roentgenographic	Human	Tantalum		GAMSU et al. (1973)

Because of the inherent difficulties and invasive nature of the procedure, the high radiation dose (ALTSHULER et al. 1964) and the requirement for gram quantities of tantalum rather than microgram quantities of radioactively labeled albumin, this procedure has not been applied widely as a tool to monitor mucociliary clearance.

The clearance rates, either nasal or bronchial, may vary widely with different experimental approaches and with different subjects. Typical clearance rates are summarized in Table 2. Variability in mucociliary clearance determined by different procedures has been attributed to many factors, particle mass is probably a critical one as the larger Teflon particles (0.6–1.0 mm diameter, density 3.6) may have considerably different transport rates from albumin microspheres of 6–30 μm dimeter (density 1.0). However, MAN et al. (1980) compared canine tracheal mucous transport and found similar transport with organic particles, (corn and ragweed pollen) and with inorganic particles (chrysotile asbestos, silica, and talc). In beagle dogs, simultaneous clearance measurements were made roentgenographically and by gamma camera, Teflon disks cleared more slowly than ^{99}Tc^m microspheres in the ratio 1 : 1.5 (WOLFF and MUGGENBURG 1979). The effects may be attributable to effects of local radiation (AHMED et al. 1979). This observation differs from studies in humans where up to fivefold faster clearance of Teflon particles has been observed in comparison with radioisotopic techniques by different investigators. In those cases, average clearance were 21.5 mm/min with Teflon particles (SACKNER et al. 1973) and 3.47 mm/min with albumin microspheres (YEATES et al. 1975). The mode of deposition as dry particles or in an aqueous phase, as in aerosolized form, may also influence measured clearance (AHMED et al. 1980).

Regardless of methodological variations, clearance rates vary widely in the human lung; different individuals may exhibit considerable differences in clearance, but the value may be reproducible for that individual (ANDERSEN et al. 1974). The similar values of mucociliary clearance among monozygotic twins suggest that some genetic predisposition may exist among individuals (BOHNING et al. 1975 b).

II. In Vitro Assessment of Mucociliary Function

To assess mucociliary function, attempts have been made to examine beat frequency and waveform using organotypic cultures or explanted mucosal tissue from major airways (BATTISTA and KENSLER 1970 a, b; DI MATTEI and MELCHIORRI 1965). Techniques such as cinephotography in conjunction with oscillographic techniques allow the investigation of waveforms (Table 3). Motion analysis using videotape recording techniques, though providing less resolution, presents alternatives to view ciliary beating. The assessment of ciliary beat frequency in vitro has been limited because of inherent difficulties to a subjective or, at best, semiquantitative evaluation by light microscopy. To measure beat frequency, methods have been applied to provide objective and quantifiable bioassays. These include stroboscopy and laser light scattering spectroscopy (LEE and VERDUGO 1976; VERDUGO et al. 1979). The assay of ciliary movement is limited as the frequency of ciliary beat exceeds the critical flicker fusion frequency. Laser light scattering

Table 3. In vitro techniques for measurement of ciliary beat frequency

Technique	Species	Ciliary beat frequency (Hz)	Reference
Stroboscope	Human	13	Ballenger and Orr (1963)
Photomultiplier with oscilloscope	Human	9.1–16.8	Yager et al. (1978, 1980)
	Human	12.5	Hesse et al. (1981)
	Human	10–14.3	Rutland et al. (1982a)
Videotape with motion analyzer	Human	12.1	Rossman et al. (1980)
	Human		Pedersen and Mygind (1980)
High speed cinematography	Rabbit	18.3	Dalhamn (1955)
	Rabbit	13–29	Sanderson and Sleigh (1981)
	Rat	21.8	Dalhamn (1956)
Laser spectroscopy	Rabbit		Verdugo et al. (1979)

spectroscopy provides a precise measurement of ciliary beat frequency that has been corroborated by comparison with high speed cinematographic techniques (Lee and Verdugo 1976). The principle is based on an analysis of the spectrum of intensity fluctuations of low power laser light reflected from the ciliated epithelial surface. The mean frequency of beating is related to the distribution of frequency of beating in the population of approximately 2,000–4,000 cilia (i.e., 10–20 cells).

Light scattering techniques provide information regarding frequency and frequency distribution of ciliary beat, but do not measure phase coherency. High speed cinematography or video appears to be the only approach to measure the waveform of cilia, but again rests on subjective evaluation, with limitations in resolution. Sample sizes are very small, 35 μm diameter, and, therefore, restricted to only 2–3 cell surfaces. In view of the wide variability that may be seen in ciliary morphology (Sturgess and Turner 1984) in different airway generations, the significance of abnormal ciliary movement must be subject to rigorous criteria and sampling procedures.

F. Factors Affecting Mucociliary Transport

Mucociliary clearance is a sensitive index of mucosal injury in the lung, being dependent on the amount and physiochemical characteristics of the mucus and fluid secretions in the airways and on ciliary activity. It may be affected by various factors.

I. Physiologic Factors

In view of the variation in measured clearance rates, studies on physiologic factors that influence clearance must be interpreted with caution. It is apparent that mucociliary clearance slows with increasing age (Goodman et al. 1978b).

However, the considerable variability among individuals in different age groups suggests that factors other than age are the determinants (PUCHELLE et al. 1979). Posture appears to have little effect on clearance of normal subjects in upright, prone, or supine positions (YEATES et al. 1975; FRIEDMAN et al. 1977; WONG et al. 1977). However, exercise increases clearance (WOLFF et al. 1977). Atmospheric humidity has been reported as having little effect on nasal or tracheal transport rates (CAMNER et al. 1973 b), but mechanical ventilation of dry air through an endotracheal tube (FORBES and GAMSU 1979 a) and inhalation of dry air (FONKALS-RUD et al. 1975) in the dog retards mucociliary clearance, presumably through an effect on airway secretions. Dehydration, furthermore, decreases mucociliary clearance as judged by experimental studies in chick trachea (BAETJER 1973).

The inhalation of aerosols containing water stimulates mucociliary clearance rates in human lung (FOSTER et al. 1976). Aerosols containing hypertonic saline cause twofold increases in clearance and increase in sputum production (PAVIA et al. 1978). The effects of inhaled aerosols, presumably local irritants in the airways, have to be considered in the evaluation of pharmacologic and toxic agents administered by the inhalation route.

Ciliary beat frequency increases as a direct function of temperature in the range 23°–37 °C (YAGER et al. 1978). In the donkey, also, mucociliary clearance increases and has been estimated as 1.7% per °C (LIPPMANN et al. 1975). In vitro, cilia beat at similar rates in the pH range: 4.0–9.5. At lower or higher pH, ciliostasis occurs. Motility alone is not a sensitive index of hydrogen ion effects on mucociliary function, since morphological features of cell damage, including formation of cytoplasmic blebs and expulsion of cells from the epithelium, occur at pH 6.7. Ciliated epithelial cells are less sensitive to alkaline pH, with morphological evidence of damage appearing at pH 9.5 (HOLMA et al. 1977).

X-irradiation causes a transient increase in mucociliary transport by decreased clearance (BALDETORP et al. 1977). Because of differences in transport rates of radioactively labeled particulates in the assessment of mucociliary transport, it has been suggested also that local radiation may act to accelerate mucociliary clearance.

II. Pharmacologic Agents

The mucociliary clearance mechanism is sensitive to many therapeutic agents that variously exhibit pharmacologic activity on mucous and fluid/electrolyte secretions, ciliary activity, and transport (Table 4).

1. Anesthetics

The general anesthetics, halothane and nitrous oxide, have been shown to depress mucociliary clearance in human nasal mucosa (EWERT 1967) and lung (LICHTIGER et al. 1975; GAMSU et al. 1976) and in experimental animals (LIERLE and MOORE 1934; LANDA et al. 1975; FORBES 1976; FORBES and GAMSU 1979 a, b, c). The effects of halothane are reversible after short periods of anesthesia. It is not clear from in vivo observations however, as to the cause or nature of this suppression which may be attributed to premedication and to humidity changes as well as to the di-

Table 4. Summary of neuroleptic, humoral, and exogenous factors reported to influence mucociliary clearance in the respiratory tract

Agent	Total respiratory secretion	Submucosal gland	Goblet cells	Fluid and electrolyte transport	Ciliary activity	Mucociliary clearance
Parasympathomimetic	↑	↑*	−*	↑		↑
Parasympatholytic	↓	↓	−		↓	↓/−
Sympathomimetic						
α-Receptor	↑	↑	−		−	↑
β-Receptor	↑	−*	−*		↑	↑↑
Sympatholytic	−	−		↑	−	
Theophylline	↑	↑			↑	↑
Histamine	↑	−	−	↑	−	
Antihistamine	↓	−	−		↓	
Slow-reacting substance of anaphylaxis	−	−				
Kinins	−	−				
Prostaglandins						
PGF$_2$α	↑	↑	−			↑
PGE$_1$	−	−	−			↓/↑
Serotonin	−	−			↑	
Anesthetics						
Barbiturate						↓
Nitrous oxide						↓
Halothane	↑	↑				↓
Narcotics						
Morphine					↓	↓
Codeine					↓	↓
Methadone					↓	↓
Mucolytics and expectorants						
n-Acetylcysteine	−	−	−		↓	↓
Bromhexine	↑	↑/−				↑/−
Cationic peptides	↑	−	↑			
Polyamines		↑	↑			
Viral or mycoplasma infection	↑	↑*	↑*		↓	↓
Irritants	↑				↓	
(O$_3$, SO$_2$, NO$_2$, CD, Ni)		−*	↑*			↓

Abbreviations: ↑ increase; ↓ decrease; − no effect; * chronic administration may result in hypertrophy or hyperplasia of the mucus-secreting submucosal glands or goblet cells

rect effects of anesthetic gases. In dogs, an induction dose of thiopental without continuing anesthesia does not impair mucociliary clearance (FORBES and GAMSU 1979c), implicating the general anesthetic agents as playing the major ciliodepressant role. Among anesthetics implicated as having a direct suppressant effect on clearance are barbiturates in the rat (IRAVANI et al. 1978), sheep (LANDA et al. 1975), and dog (BRIDGER and PROCTOR 1972; KING et al. 1979). Topical anesthesia with lidocaine at concentrations up to 4% does not significantly influence mucociliary clearance in sheep (LANDA et al. 1975) or in human nasal mucosa (ROSSMAN et al. 1977; FRIEDMAN et al. 1977). At therapeutic dose levels, lignocaine does not influence ciliary function in humans (RUTLAND and COLE 1980).

In vitro, other local anesthetics have variable depressing effects on mucociliary transport that may be a direct ciliotoxic effect that slows or stops ciliary beating and is reversible (CORSSEN and ALLEN 1960). Ciliotoxic concentrations of local anesthetics have been estimated in vivo using explanted human tracheobronchial epithelium, to be 5% lidocaine, 5% procaine, 0.5% chloroprocaine, 10% cocaine, 0.1% tetracaine, and 0.05% dibucaine. Lidocaine, 0.05%, causes ciliostasis in ferret tracheal organ culture (MOSTOW et al. 1979), a model that is also exquisitely sensitive to 0.06 mg/ml methylparaben, causing paralysis of cilia, an effect that is only partially reversible. The experimental studies with explanted bronchial mucosa tend to suggest a greater sensitivity of cilia to anesthetics than that observed in vivo. In the normal physiologic state, mucous secretions may provide some protection against the deleterious ciliotoxic effects of general and local anesthesia.

2. Narcotics

In vivo and in vitro evidence exists that mucociliary transport is depressed by codeine, morphine, and methadone (IRAVANI and MELVILLE 1975; VAN DONGEN and LEVSNICK 1953).

3. Sympathomimetic Agents

The topical, oral, or parenteral administration of β-adrenergic agonists in animals and humans has a dose-dependent stimulation in mucociliary transport. This effect has been demonstrated with isoproterenol (BLAIR and WOODS 1969; KONIETSZKO et al. 1975; FOSTER et al. 1976; SACHNER et al. 1976a, 1979), and norepinephrine in some species (OKESON and DIVERTIE 1970; FOSTER et al. 1976). Selective β_2-adrenoceptor agonists, including carbuterol (SACKNER et al. 1976a), fenoterol (IRAVANI 1972; FELIX et al. 1978), terbutaline (SACKNER et al. 1975; WOOD et al. 1975; CAMNER et al. 1976), clenbuterol (IRAVANI and MELVILLE 1978), reproterol (HESSE et al. 1981), isoetharine (FOSTER et al. 1980), and salbutamol (VAN As 1974), consistently stimulate mucociliary transport.

The adrenergic agonists stimulate ciliary beat frequency directly, presumably through increased levels of cyclic adenosine monophosphate in ciliated cells (VERDUGO et al. 1980). In vivo, additional effects of β-agonists on mucus (STURGESS and REID 1972a, b), fluid, and electrolyte (NADEL et al. 1979; BOUCHER 1981) secretion may exacerbate the direct effects on ciliary function. Effects of sympathomimetic agents on mucociliary transport are not mediated through vascular effects (FOSTER et al. 1976), and β-adrenergic blockers such as propanolol and atenolol do not influence mucociliary clearance in humans (BATAMAN et al. 1980).

4. Parasympathomimetic Agents

Basal mucociliary function is independent of normal vagal tone (BRODY et al. 1972). However, mucociliary transport rates may be modulated by parasympathomimetic agents, indicating that neurogenic stimuli may function to modulate clearance from the baseline levels. Local or systemic administration of acetylcholine and cholinergic agents stimulate ciliary activity (LIPPMAN et al. 1975; CORSSEN and ALLEN 1959; LEE et al. 1980) in vitro as well as promoting the secretion of mucus from the bronchial submucosal glands (STURGESS and REID 1972 a, b) and of fluid/electrolytes from the airway epithelium (BOUCHER 1980). Bethanecol (CAMNER et al. 1974) and methacholine (KING and VIIRES 1979) increase clearance, although methacholine has been reported not to affect ciliary motility directly (OKESON and DIVERTIE 1970).

In contrast, the anticholinergic drugs, atropine and hyoscine given orally cause marked inhibition of ciliary activity (BLAIR and WOODS 1969), mucous secretion (STURGESS and REID 1972 a, b), and mucociliary transport (BLAIR and WOODS 1969; PAVIA and THOMSON 1971; ANNIS et al. 1976; FOSTER et al. 1976; LIPPMANN et al. 1975; SACKNER et al. 1976b) as well as altered deposition of inhaled particles in the lung (BERGER et al. 1978). Blocking mucociliary transport with atropine renders the lung more susceptible to the effects of inhaled dusts (MAZETOV and PANCHENKO 1980). In contrast, to the depressant effect of anticholinergic drugs on mucus transport, methylscopolamine has no significant effect on mucociliary clearance, despite an effect on secretion (CAMNER et al. 1974) and atropine has been reported to promote transport in anesthetized dogs (CHOPRA 1978).

A synthetic anticholinergic bronchodilator, ipratropium bromide, has not been found at human therapeutic levels to inhibit mucous transport in animal models or humans (IRAVANI 1972; SACKNER et al. 1976b; FRANCIS et al. 1977). More recently, RUFFIN et al. (1978) have reported ipratropium to have no effect in patients with chronic bronchitis, but to stimulate clearance in normal individuals.

5. Methylxanthines

Both direct application and systemic administration of theophylline and aminophylline have been reported to increase ciliary movement and mucociliary clearance (SERAFINI et al. 1976; MATTHYS and KOHLER 1980).

6. Histamines and Antihistamines

Histamine has no consistent effect on ciliary motility, mucous secretion, or clearance (GOSSELIN 1966). Antihistamines: diphenhydramine, tripelennamine, and antazoline, have been found to be ciliotoxic, with effects that are often irreversible when applied directly to ciliated epithelia, in vitro (VAN DE DONK et al. 1982b). These agents have little direct effect on the properties of bronchial mucus.

7. Serotonin

Serotonin acts as a pacemaker (DADAIAN et al. 1971) in molluscan gill cilia and, although it occurs naturally, it has an excitatory effect when given exogenously (OKESON and DIVERTHIE 1970). The effect of serotonin is inhibited by antagonists, lysergic acid diethylamide, and dihydroergotamine in this model. Extrapolation of these observations to regulation of ciliary beating in mammalian airways has yet to be established.

8. Mucolytic and Expectorant Drugs

Acetylcysteine decreases the elastic modulus of mucus so that, experimentally, the transport properties of mucus are abnormal (PUCHELLE et al. 1976; MARTIN et al. 1980). However, at human therapeutic concentrations, acetylcysteine causes ciliostasis in organotypic cultures of tracheal epithelium that is only partially reversible (DUDLEY and CHERRY 1978). The changes in mucus properties would appear to be negated therefore by the ciliotoxicity of this agent. In humans, prolonged use of n-acetylcysteine causes depression of mucociliary activity (DREISIN and MOSTOW 1979). This ciliotoxic effect is attributable to the sulfhydryl moiety of the molecule and is found also with L-cysteine, D-cysteine, 2-aminoethanethiol, and n-acetyl-L-homocysteine. In contrast, S-carboxymethylcysteine does not affect the rheological properties of mucus (MARTIN et al. 1980) and has no acute effect on clearance in humans (THOMSON et al. 1975; GOODMAN et al. 1978a). Sodium bicarbonate and L-arginine are mucolytic agents that also inhibit ciliary activity in vitro (DUDLEY and CHERRY 1977).

9. Decongestants

Some minor and reversible effects have been observed when decongestants are applied topically to ciliated epithelia in vivo (SIMON et al. 1977; SAKETHOO et al. 1978). Ephedrine, phenylephrine, xylometazoline, and oxymetazoline have little effect and are less ciliotoxic than phenylpropanolamine, tramazoline, and naphazoline. The hydrophilic compounds are considered to be less ciliotoxic than their lipophilic counterparts (VAN DE DONK et al. 1982a). In an experimental model with chicken trachea in vitro, DUDLEY and CHERRY (1978) found inhibition of ciliary activity with oxymetazoline and phenylephrine.

10. Disodium Cromoglycate

Disodium cromoglycate elicits little effect on ciliary beat frequency in experimental models (BLAIR and WOODS 1969; VAN DE DONK et al. 1982b).

11. Corticosteroid Hormones

The corticosteroids have little effect on respiratory cilia by morphological criteria (LUNDGREN et al. 1977; CLARK 1980). A minor depressant effect that is reversible has been described when they are applied directly in vitro to ciliated epithelia. Beclomethasone diprorionate, administered topically in vivo had no significant effect on tracheal mucous velocity (SACKNER et al. 1977).

12. Antimicrobial Agents

Benzylpenicillin (10,000 U/ml), ampicillin (1%), neomycin (0.35%), polymyxin (0.1%), sulfanilamide (0.4%) have little effect on ciliary movement in vitro. Reversible ciliary arrest has been described however, with topical application of sulfacetamide (10%) and chloramphenicol (0.4%) and irreversible ciliotoxicity with bacitracin (10,000 U/ml) (VAN DE DONK et al. 1982c). The relationship of these findings with topical administration is not predictive for effects of systemic administration of these antimicrobial agents.

13. Cardiac Glycosides

Acetylouabain increases tracheal mucous flow rate in the cat, and is dependent on calcium ions. Digitalis also enhances ciliary activity in a calcium-dependent manner (LAURENZI and YIN 1971).

14. Prostaglandins

Prostaglandins E_1 and $F_2\alpha$ invoke variable responses on mucociliary clearance in patients with asthma (BIERSACK et al. 1978). By inhalation, some patients showed an increase, some a decrease, and some no change in clearance. This effect may have reflected the variation in mucosal injury that occurs in asthma or effects on release of mucus, that may be influenced by prostaglandins.

15. Alcohol

Alcohol causes a significant depressant effect on ciliary beating and on mucociliary transport. Furthermore, dehydration of respiratory secretions occurs with alcohol ingestion, contributing further to decreased mucus transport (BANG et al. 1966).

III. Environmental Factors and Pollutants

The sources of inhaled particulates that influence mucociliary function are diverse in the atmosphere (SCHLESINGER 1973; BALLENGER et al. 1968) and originate from natural processes (e.g., bacteria, pollen, airborne particulates) and artificial particulates such as fly ash, hydrocarbons, nitrogen oxides, metallic and mineral dusts (MASS and LANE 1976), household aerosol products (BORUM et al. 1979), and cigarette smoke (ALBERT and LIPPMANN 1971). Pollutant-induced airways toxicity may be characterized as: (a) oxidant and irritant gases; (b) particulate material including bulk; (c) reactive aldehydes, and (d) heavy metals (BOUCHER 1981). Impaired mucociliary contact and/or sustained exposure of sensitive epithelial or mucosal sites to these inhaled particulates leads to mucosal irritation and thus predisposes to airways hyperreactivity states, with further impairment of mucociliary clearance. Heavy metals (cadmium and nickel) exert such a toxic response (OLSEN and JONSEN 1944; ADALIS et al. 1977, 1978; BOUCHER 1980).

Mucosal injury is caused by inhaled irritants such as ozone (GOLDEN et al. 1978), low levels of nitrogen dioxide (BATTIGELLI et al. 1966; OREHEK et al. 1976), and antigen (BOUCHER et al. 1980) or infection (EMPEY et al. 1976; LAITINEN et al. 1976). It has been postulated that hyperreactivity results from damage to the bronchial mucosa (NADEL 1965). Such changes may result from exfoliation of epithelial cells exposing irritant receptors (HOGG et al. 1968). Increased reactivity to histamine when airway permeability increases (e.g., after 1 h of exposure to cigarette smoke) and the return to normal reactivity (12 h after exposure to cigarette smoke) has lead to a hypothesis that injury causes separation of epithelial tight junctions, particularly as afferent nerve endings exist in close proximity to epithelial tight junctions, and may thus stimulate irritant receptors (BOUCHER et al. 1980).

An alternative mechanism of toxicity induced by noxious particles may be mediated by changes in active ion transport, or in composition or osmolarity of the periciliary fluid layer that interferes with epithelial tight junction complexes by allowing solute diffusion into the junctional compartments, and thus swelling and disruption of the junction. For example, with increased exposure to cigarette smoke, degradation of tight junctions occurs in a progressive and dose-related manner. Questions that remain to be answered are how do mucociliary function, integrity of the bronchial mucosa, mucosal permeability, and hyperreactivity relate. Potential leakines or "airway epithelial hyperpermeability" is one hypothesis (HOGG et al. 1968) which suggests that increased access of agonists to the submucosal and smooth muscle tissues may exist from discontinuity or increased transmembrane potentials in the bronchial epithelium. The airway epithelium and its mucus lining provide a barrier that separates the potential toxic agents in inhaled air from sensitive sites in the submucosal tissue. Any insult that impairs clearance, for example through tight junctions, will increase deposition of toxic substances and their interaction at epithelial cell or basement membrane sites. A resulting increase in the movement to effector sites in the airway wall will therefore potentiate secretion, bronchoconstriction, and other findings typical of hyperactive airways. Toxic agents in vivo, such as ozone, nitrous oxide, heavy metals, sulfur dioxide, and cigarette smoke increase airway epithelial permeability. In vitro, heavy metals such as cadmium, mercury, and zinc also influence the junction complex and perturb mucosal permeability.

Acute irritation of the bronchial mucosa may exert a stimulation of mucociliary transport which may be mediated in part by localized increases in mucus secretion, blood flow, and transudation of fluid into the airways. Longer-term irritation or mechanical injury, however, commonly causes damage to the bronchial epithelium and impairment of clearance (FRASCA et al. 1968). For example, short-term exposure to 5 ppm sulfur dioxide increases mucociliary clearance (NEWHOUSE et al. 1978) while chronic exposure, at 1 ppm, causes impaired mucociliary activity as one of the earliest signs of pulmonary dysfunction (HIRSCH et al. 1975). The effect is probably mediated by loss of ciliated cells in the tracheobronchial tree (ASMUNDSSON et al. 1973) and altered mucus secretion (LAMB and REID 1969 a). Similarly, exposure to ozone (< 0.5 ppm) for short time periods up to 2 h has no effect on mucus transport in vivo in sheep (ABRAHAM et al. 1980 a) and in rats (FRAGER et al. 1979). Higher concentrations (> 1.2 ppm) of ozone, delay mucociliary transport in rats (FRAGER et al. 1979) as does prolonged exposure (PENHA and WERTHAMER 1974). The effect of ozone involves ciliotoxicity and damage to ciliated epithelial cells (CASTLEMAN et al. 1977; CASTERLINE 1980).

Among environmental factors that depress mucociliary function are trichlorethylene that causes ciliostasis in rabbit trachea at 5,000 ppm concentrations (TOMENIUS 1979). Hydrocarbons depress ciliary activity in hamster trachea (OMICHI et al. 1975). Ciliary anomalies and damage are early experimental changes with sufuric acid mist (Schlesinger et al. 1973, 1978, 1979), acrolein (Dahlgren et al. 1972; Izard and Libermann 1978), and benzo[a]pyrene exposure (Reznick-Schueller 1975). Methylmethacrylate vapor at threshold limit values elicits damage and loss of ciliated cells in the trachea, when exposure is prolonged for 6 months (Tansy et al. 1980). In contrast, diesel exhaust (Abraham et al. 1980b), and fluorocarbons such as trichlorofluoromethane and dichlorofluoromethane (Bohning et al. 1975a) have no significant effects on mucociliary transport in vivo.

Dust particles typically influence mucociliary function when augmented by irritants such as nitrogen dioxide and sulfur dioxide. Hydrophilic dusts such as quartz and silica depress mucociliary clearance (Wright 1966) while nonhydrophilic dists, such as carbon, have little apparent effect on mucus secretion or clearance and may be used as inert markers for monitoring function (Camner 1980; Camner and Philipson 1974). Inert plastic dust 1.8–12.5 μm diameter, has no effect on mucociliary function in humans although pulmonary function may be reduced (Andersen et al. 1979). On the other hand, wood workers have marked reductions in mucociliary clearance in the nasal and bronchial mucosa owing to wood dust (Black et al. 1974; Andersen et al. 1976).

Impaired mucociliary function occurs with exposure to 95% oxygen in experimental animals in a concentration- and time-dependent manner in rats (Philpott et al. 1977), mice (Obara et al. 1979), and dogs (Sackner et al. 1976c). Pollutant gases, found in automobile exhaust have an adverse effect on mucociliary transport (Battigelli et al. 1966).

Ciliotoxic substances in cigarette smoke are contained in the gas phase of the smoke and include acrolein, formaldehyde, benzene, hydrogen cyanide, and acetone (Dalhamn 1966). Marijuana smoke also exhibits a ciliotoxic response in human lung (Henderson et al. 1972). There appears to be an inverse relationship between mucociliary clearance rates and number of cigarettes smoked, an effect observed in rabbits (Dalhamn 1970), donkeys (Albert et al. 1969a, 1973, 1974; Aldas et al. 1971), dogs (Isawa et al. 1980). In humans, slowing of mucociliary clearance (Bohning et al. 1975b; Camner et al. 1971; Lippmann et al. 1975) correlates with loss of cilia and changes in the respiratory mucosa (Auerbach et al. 1979).

IV. Infection

Respiratory infection of virus, mycoplasma, or bacterial origin may depress mucociliary clearance. In humans, influenza A virus (Camner et al. 1973b) has a marked effect on mucociliary function. Mycoplasmal pneumonia depresses clearance, and this effect may persist for prolonged periods after infection in human lung (Camner et al. 1978) and hamster trachea (Carson et al. 1979). In chickens, Newcastle disease virus infection depresses mucociliary transport, with the suppression sustained and extended after recovery from infection (Wakabayashi et al. 1977). Hemophilus influenza is ciliotoxic, presumably as a result of local release of toxin and the consequent influence on mucociliary clearance (Denny 1974).

References

Abraham WM, Januszkiewicz AJ, Mingle M et al. (1980a) Sensitivity of bronchoprovocation and tracheal mucous velocity in detecting airway responses to O_3. J Appl Physiol 48(5):789–793

Abraham WM, Kim CS, Januszkiewicz AJ, Welker M, Mingle M, Schreck R (1980b) Effects of a brief low-level exposure to the particulate fraction of diesel exhaust on pulmonary function of conscious sheep. Arch Environ Health 35(2):77–80

Adalis D, Gardner DE, Miller FJ, Coffin DL (1977) Toxic effects of cadmium on ciliary activity using a tracheal ring model system. Environ Res 13(1):111–120

Adalis D, Gardner DE, Miller FJ (1978) Cytotoxic effects of nickel on ciliated epithelium. Am Rev Respir Dis 118(2):347–354

Ahmed T, Januszkiewicz AJ, Landa JF, Brown A, Chapman GA, Kenny PJ, Finn RD, Bondick J, Sackner MA (1979) Effect of local radioactivity on tracheal mucous velocity of sheep. Am Rev Respir Dis 120(3):567–575

Ahmed T, Januszkiewicz AJ, Brown A, Chapman GA, Landa JF (1980) In vitro estimation of tracheal mucous velocity: comparison of a solid and a liquid marker. Clin Respir Physiol 16:533–538

Albert RE, Arnett LC (1955) Clearance of radioactive dust from the human lung. Arch Environ Health 12:99–106

Albert RE, Lippmann M (1971) Bronchial clearance abnormalities in man produced by cigarette smoke and lung disease. Chest 71:59

Albert RE, Lippmann M, Briscoe W (1969a) The characteristics of bronchial clearance in humans and the effects of cigarette smoking. Arch Environ Health 18(5):738–755

Albert RE, Spiegelman RJ, Shatsky S et al. (1969b) The effect of acute exposure to cigarette smoke on bronchial clearance in the miniature donkey. Arch Environ Health 18:30–41

Albert RE, Lippmann M, Peterson HT Jr, Berger J, Sanborn K, Bohning D (1973) Bronchial deposition and clearance of aerosols. Arch Intern Med 131:115–127

Albert RE, Berger J, Sanborn K, Lippmann M (1974) Effects of cigarette smoke components on bronchial clearance in the donkey. Arch Environ Health 29(2):96–101

Aldas JS, Dolovich M, Chalmers R, Newhouse MT (1971) Regional aerosol clearance in smokers and non-smokers. Chest 59:2S

Altshuler B, Nelson N, Kuschner M (1964) Estimation of lung tissue dose from the inhalation of radon and daughters. Health Phys 10:1137–1161

Andersen HC, Solgaard J, Andersen I (1976) Nasal cancer and nasal mucus-transport rates in woodworkers. Acta Otolaryngol (Stokh) 82(3–4):263–265

Andersen I, Camner P, Jensen P, Philipson K, Proctor D (1974) A comparison of nasal and tracheobronchial clearance. Arch Environ Health 29:290–293

Andersen I, Lundqvist GR, Proctor DF, Swift DL (1979) Human response to controlled levels of inert dust. Am Rev Respir Dis 119(4):619–627

Annis P, Landa J, Lichtiger M (1976) Effects of atropine on velocity of tracheal mucus in anesthetised patients. Anesthesiology 44:74–77

Asmundsson T, Kilburn KH (1970) Mucociliary clearance rates at various levels of dog lungs. Am Rev Respir Dis 102:388–397

Asmundsson T, Kilburn KH, McKenzie WN (1973) Injury and metaplasia of airway cells due to SO_2. Lab Invest 29(1):41–53

Auerbach O, Cuyler-Hammond E, Garfinkel L (1979) Changes in bronchial epithelium in relation to cigarette smoking 1955–1960 vs 1970–1977. N Engl J Med 300(8):381–385

Baetjer AM (1967) Effects of ambient temperature and vapour pressure on cilia-mucus clearance rate. J Appl Physiol 23:498–504

Baetjer AM (1973) Dehydration and susceptibility to toxic chemicals. Arch Environ Health 26(2):61–63

Baldetorp L, Hakansson CH, Baldetorp B (1977) Influence of temperature on the activity of ciliated cells during exposure to ionizing radiation. Acta Radiol Ther Phys Biol 16(1):17–26

Ballenger JJ, Orr MF (1963) Quantitative measurement of human ciliary activity. Ann Otol Rhinol Laryngol 72:31–39

Ballenger JJ, McFarland CR, Harding HB, Koll M, Halstead D (1968) The effect of air pollutants on pulmonary clearance. Laryngoscope 78(8):1387–1397

Bang FB, Bang BG, Foard MA (1966) Responses of the upper respiratory mucosa to drugs and viral infections. Am Rev Respir Dis 93:142–149

Barnett B, Miller CE (1966) Flow induced by biological mucociliary systems. Ann NY Acad Sci 130:891–901

Barton AD, Lourenco RV (1973) Bronchial secretions and mucociliary clearance. Arch Intern Med 131:140–144

Bateman JRM, Lennard-Jones AM, Pavia D, Clarke SW (1980) Lung mucociliary clearance in normal subjects during selective and non-selective β-blockade. Clin Sci 58:19P

Battigelli MC, Hengstenberg F, Mannella RJ, Thomas AP (1966) Mucociliary activity. Arch Environ Health 12(4):460–466

Battista SP, Kensler CJ (1970a) Mucus production and ciliary transport activity. In vivo studies using the chicken. Arch Environ Health 20(3):326–338

Battista SP, Kensler CJ (1970b) Use of nonimmersed in vitro chicken tracheal preparation for the study of ciliary transport activity. Cigarette smoke and related components. Arch Environ Health 20(3):318–325

Berger J, Albert RE, Sanborn K, Lippmann M (1978) Effects of atropine and methacholine on deposition and clearance of inhaled particles in the donkey. J Toxicol Environ Health 4(4):587–604

Bianco A, Gibb FR, Kelpper RW et al. (1974) Studies of tantalum dust in the lungs. Radiology 112(3):549–556

Biersack HJ, Hedde JP, Felix R, Winkler C (1978) The effect of prostaglandin E_1-inhalation on ciliary action. Prax Klin Pneumol 32(2):105–107

Black A, Evans JC, Hadfield EH, Macbeth RG, Morgan A, Walsh M (1974) Impairment of nasal mucociliary clearance in woodworkers in the furniture industry. Br J Ind Med 31(1):10–17

Blair AM, Woods A (1969) The effects of isoprenaline, atropine and disodium cromoglycate on ciliary motility and mucous flow measured in vivo in cat. Br J Pharmacol 35(2):379–380

Blake JR (1975) On the movement of mucus in the lung. J Biochem 8:179–190

Blake JR, Winet H (1980) On the mechanics of mucociliary transport. Biorheology 17:125–134

Bohning DE, Albert RE, Lippmann M, Cohen VR (1975a) Effects of fluorocarbons 11 and 12 on tracheobronchial particle deposition and clearance in donkeys. Am Ind Hyg Assoc J 36(12):902–908

Bohning DE, Albert RE, Lippmann M, Foster WM (1975b) Tracheobronchial particle deposition and clearance. A study of the effects of cigarette smoking in monozygotic twins. Arch Environ Health 30(9);457–462

Bonomo L, D'Addabbo A (1974) I-albumin turnover and loss of protein into the sputum in chronic bronchitis. Clin Chim Acta 10:214–222

Booker DV, Chamberlain AC, Rundo J, Muir DCF, Thomson ML (1967) Elimination of 5 micron particles from the human lung. Nature 215:30–33

Borum P, Holten A, Loekkegaard N (1979) Depression of nasal mucociliary transport by an aerosol hair-spray. Scand J Respir Dis 60(5):253–259

Boucher RC (1980) Chemical modulation of airway epithelial permeability. Environ Health Perspect 35:3–12

Boucher RC (1981) Mechanisms of pollutant-induced airway toxicity. In: Brooks SM, Lockey JE, Heuber P (eds) Clin Chest Med 2(3):377–392

Boucher RC, Ranga V, Pare PD, Inoue S, Moroz LA, Hogg JC (1979) Effect of histamine and methacholine on guinea pig tracheal permeability to HRP. J Appl Physiol 45:939–948

Boucher RC, Johnson J, Inoue S, Hulbert W, Hogg JC (1980) The effect of cigarette smoke on the permeability of guinea pig airways. Lab Invest 43:94–100

Breeze RG, Wheeldon EB (1977) The cells of the pulmonary airways. Am Rev Respir Dis 116:705–777

Bridger GP, Proctor DF (1972) Mucociliary function in the dog's larynx and trachea. Laryngoscope 82:218–224

Brody JS, Klempfner G, Staum MM, Vidyassagar D, Kuhl DE, Waldhausen JA (1972) Mucociliary clearance after lung denervation and bronchial transection. J Appl Physiol 32(2):160–164

Camner P (1980) Clearance of particles from the human tracheobronchial tree. Clin Sci 59(2):79–84

Camner P, Philipson K (1971) Tracheobronchial clearance in man studied with monodispersed teflon particles tagged with ^{18}F and ^{99}mTc. Nord Hyg Tidskr 52(1):1–9

Camner P, Philipson K (1974) Mucociliary clearance. Scand J Respir Dis 55(90):45–48

Camner P, Philipson K (1978) Human alveolar deposition of 4 μ teflon particles. Arch Environ Health 36:181–185

Camner P, Philipson K, Arvidsson T (1971) Cigarette smoking in man. Short-term effect on mucociliary transport. Arch Environ Health 23(6):421–426

Camner P, Helstrom PA, Philipson K (1973 a) Carbon dust and mucociliary transport. Arch Environ Health 26(6):294–296

Camner P, Jarstrand C, Philipson K (1973 b) Tracheobronchial clearance in patients with influenza. Am Rev Respir Dis 108:131–135

Camner P, Strandberg K, Philipson K (1974) Increased mucociliary transport by cholinergic stimulation. Arch Environ Health 29(4):220–224

Camner P, Strandberg K, Philipson K (1976) Increased mucociliary transport by adrenergic stimulation. Arch Environ Health 31(2):79–82

Camner P, Jarstrand C, Philipson K (1978) Tracheobronchial clearance 5–15 months after infection with Mycoplasma pneumonia. Scand J Infect Dis 10(1):33–35

Carson JL, Collier AM, Clyde WA Jr (1979) Ciliary membrane alterations occurring in experimental Mycoplasma pneumonia infection. Science 206:349–351

Casterline CL (1980) Irritable airways: early indicator of occupational lung disease. Chest 77:2–4

Castleman WL, Tyler WS, Dungworth DL (1977) Lesions in respiratory bronchioles and conducting airways of monkeys exposed to ambient levels of ozone. Exp Mol Pathol 26(3):384–400

Charman J, Reid L (1972) Sputum viscosity in chronic bronchitis, bronchiectasis, asthma and cystic fibrosis. Biorheology 9:185–199

Chen TM, Dulfano MJ (1978) Mucus viscoelasticity and mucociliary transport rate. J Lab Clin Med 91:423–431

Chopra SK (1978) Effect of atropine on mucociliary transport velocity in anesthetized dogs. Am Rev Respir Dis 118(2):367–371

Chopra SK, Taplin GV, Simmons DH, Elam D (1977) Measurement of mucociliary transport velocity in the intact mucosa. Chest 71:155–158

Chopra SK, Taplin GV, Elam D, Carson SA, Golde D (1979) Measurement of tracheal mucociliary transport velocity in humans – smokers versus nonsmokers (preliminary findings). Am Rev Respir Dis 119:205

Clark TJH (1980) Corticosteroid treatment of asthma. Schweiz Med Wochenschr 110(6):215–218

Clarke SW, Pavia D (1980) Lung mucus production and mucociliary clearance: methods of assessment. Br J Clin Pharmacol 9(6):537–546

Corssen G, Allen CR (1959) Acetylcholine: its significance in controlling ciliary activity of human respiratory epithelium in vitro. J Appl Physiol 14:901–906

Corssen G, Allen CR (1960) Cultured human respiratory epithelium: its use in the comparison of cytotoxic properties of local anesthetics. Anesthesiology 21:237

Dadaian JH, Yin S, Laurenzi GA (1971) Studies of mucus flow in the mammalian respiratory tract. II. The effects of serotonin and related compounds on respiratory tract mucus flow. Am Rev Respir Dis 103(6):808–815

Dahlgren SE, Dalen H, Dalhamn T (1972) Ultrastructural observations on chemically induced inflammation in guinea pig trachea. Virchows Arch [Cell Pathol] 11(3):211–223

Dalhamn T (1955) A method for determination in vitro of the rate of ciliary beat and mucus flow in the trachea. Acta Physiol Scand 33:1–5

Dalhamn T (1956) Mucous flow and ciliary activity in the trachea of healthy rats and rats exposed to respiratory irritant gases. Acta Physiol Scand 36:5–161

Dalhamn T (1966) Effect of cigarette smoke on ciliary activity. Am Rev Respir Dis 93:108–114

Dalhamn T (1970) In vivo and in vitro ciliotoxic effects of tobacco smoke. Arch Environ Health 21(5):633–634

Davis SS (1973) Techniques for the measurement of the rheological properties of sputum. Bull Eur Physiopathol Respir 9:47

Denny FW (1974) Effect of a toxin produced by Haemophilus influenzae on ciliated respiratory epithelium. J Infect Dis 129(2):93–100

Di Mattei P, Melchiorri P (1965) Effects of organophosphorus esters on the ciliary movement and their use for the detection of organophosphorus compounds. Arch Int Pharmacodyn Ther 153:339–345

Dolovich MB, Sanchis J, Rossman C, Newhouse MT (1976) Aerosol penetrance: a sensitive index of peripheral airways obstruction. J Appl Physiol 30:468–471

Dreisin RB, Mostow SR (1979) Sulfhydryl-mediated depression of ciliary activity: an adverse effect of acetylcysteine. J Lab Clin Med 93(4):674–678

Dudley JP, Cherry JD (1977) The effect of mucolytic agents and topical decongestants on the ciliary activity of chicken tracheal organ cultures. Pediatr Res 11(8):904–906

Dudley JP, Cherry JD (1978) Effects of topical nasal decongestants on the cilia of a chicken embryo tracheal organ culture system. Laryngoscope 88(1):110–116

Dulfano MJ, Adler KB (1975) Physical properties of sputum. VII. Rheological properties and mucociliary transport. Am Rev Respir Dis 112:341–347

Dulfano MJ, Adler K, Phillippoff W (1971) Sputum visco-elasticity in chronic bronchitis. Am Rev Respir Dis 104:88–98

Ebert RV, Terracio MJ (1975) Observations on the secretions of the bronchioles with the scanning electron microscope. Am Rev Respir Dis 112:491–496

Edmunds LH, Graf PD, Sagel SS, Greenspan SH (1970) Radiographic observations of clearance of tantalum and barium sulfate particles from airways. Invest Radiol 5:131–141

Empey DW, Laitmen LA, Jacobs L, Gold WM, Nadel J (1976) Mechanisms of bronchial hyper-reactivity in normal subjects after upper respiratory infection. Am Rev Respir Dis 113:131–139

Ewert G (1967) The effect of two topical anaesthetic drugs on the mucus flow in the respiratory tract. Ann Otol 76:359–367

Felix R, Hedde JP, Zwicker HJ, Winkler C (1978) Mucociliary clearance during beta-adrenergic stimulation with fenoterol. Prax Klin Pneumol 32(12):777–782

Fonkalsrud EW, Sanchez M, Higashijima I, Arima E (1975) A comparative study of the effects of dry vs humidified ventilation on canine lungs. Surgery 78(3):373–380

Forbes AR (1976) Halothane depresses mucociliary flow in the trachea. Anesthesiology 45:59–63

Forbes AR, Gamsu G (1979a) Lung mucociliary clearance after anesthesia with spontaneous and controlled ventilation. Am Rev Respir Dis 120(4):857–862

Forbes AR, Gamsu G (1979b) Mucociliary clearance in the canine lung during and after general anesthesia. Anesthesiology 50(1):26–29

Forbes AR, Gamsu G (1979c) Depression of lung mucociliary clearance by thiopental and halothane. Anesth Analg 58(5):387–389

Forstner JF, Forstner GG, Sturgess JM (1976) Physical changes induced in mucin by calcium: implications for the obstructive complications in cystic fibrosis. In: Proceedings of the 7th intern. cystic fibrosis conference, Paris. L'Association Française de Lutte contre la Mucoviscidose, Paris, p 31

Forstner G, Sturgess JM, Forstner J (1977) Malfunction of intestinal mucus and mucus production. In: Elstein M, Parke DV (eds) Mucus in health and disease. Plenum, New York

Foster WM, Bergofsky EH, Bohning DE, Lippmann M, Albert RE (1976) Effect of adrenergic agents and their mode of action on mucociliary clearance in man. J Appl Physiol 41(2):146–152

Foster WM, Langenback E, Bohning D, Bergofsky EH (1978) Quantitation of mucus clearance in peripheral lung and comparison with tracheal and bronchial mucus transport velocities in man: adrenergics return depressed clearance and transport velocities in asthmatics to normal. Am Rev Respir Dis 117:327–341

Foster WM, Langenback E, Bergofsky EH (1980) Measurement of tracheal and bronchial mucus velocities in man: relation to lung clearance. J Appl Physiol 48(6):965–971

Frager NB, Phalen RF, Kenoyer JL (1979) Adaptations to ozone in reference to mucociliary clearance. Arch Environ Health 34(1):51–57

Francis RA, Thompson ML, Pavia D, Douglas RB (1977) Ipratropium bromide: mucociliary clearance rate and airway resistance in normal subjects. Br J Dis Chest 71(3):173–178

Frasca JM, Averbach O, Parks VR et al. (1968) Electron microscopic observations of the bronchial epithelium of dogs. II. Smoking dogs. Exp Mol Pathol 9:380–399

Friedman M, Dougherty R, Nelson SR, White RP, Sackner MA, Wanner A (1977) Acute effects of an aerosol hair spray on tracheal mucociliary transport. Am Rev Respir Dis 116(2):281–286

Friedman M, Stott FD, Poole DO, Dougherty R, Chapman RP, Watson H, Sackner MA (1977) A new roentgenographic method for estimating mucous velocity in airways. Am Rev Respir Dis 115:67–72

Gamsu G, Weintraub RM, Nadel JA (1973) Clearance of tantalum from airways of different caliber in man evaluated by a roentgenographic method. Am Rev Respir Dis 107:214–224

Gamsu G, Singer MM, Vincent HH, Berry S, Nadel JA (1976) Post-operative impairment of mucus transport in the lung. Am Rev Respir Dis 114:673–679

Gil J, Weibel ER (1971) Extracellular lining of bronchioles after perfusion fixation of rat lungs for electron microscopy. Anat Rec 169:185–199

Giordano AM, Holsclaw D, Litt M (1978) Mucus rheology and mucociliary clearance: normal physiologic state. Am Rev Respir Dis 118:245–250

Goldberg IS, Lourenco RV (1973) Deposition of aerosols in pulmonary disease. Arch Intern Med 131:88–91

Golden JA, Nadel J, Boushey HA (1978) Bronchial hyper-irritability in healthy subjects after exposure to ozone. Am Rev Respir Dis 118:287–294

Goldfarb H, Buchberg AS (1964) The rheology of human respiratory tract mucus and its relationship to ciliary activity. Clin Res 12:291

Goodman RM, Yergin BM, Sackner MA (1978 a) Effects of S-carboxymethylcysteine on tracheal mucus velocity. Chest 74:615–618

Goodman RM, Yergin BM, Landa JF, Golinvaux MH, Sackner MA (1978 b) Relationship of smoking history and pulmonary function tests to tracheal mucus velocity in nonsmokers, young smokers, ex-smokers, and patients with chronic bronchitis. Am Rev Respir Dis 117:205–214

Gosselin RE (1966) Physiologic regulators of ciliary motion. Am Rev Respir Dis 93:41–59

Green GM (1973) Alveobronchiolar transport mechanisms. Arch Intern Med 131:109–114

Havez R, Biserte G (1968) Etude biochimique des secretions bronchiques. In: Hypersecretion bronchique. Colloque international de pathologie thoracique, Lille, p 43

Henderson RL, Tennant FS, Guerry R (1972) Respiratory manifestations of hashish smoking. Arch Otolaryngol 95:248–251

Hesse H, Kasparek R, Mizera W, Unterhulzner C, Konietzko N (1981) Influence of reproterol on ciliary beat frequency of human bronchial epithelium in vitro. Arzneimittelforsch 31:716–718

Hilding AC (1932) Physiology of drainage of nasal mucus: experimental work on accessory sinuses. Am J Physiol 100:664–670

Hilding AC (1956) On cigarette smoking, bronchial carcinoma and ciliary action. Ann Otol Rhinol Laryngol 65:736–746

Hilding AC (1957) Ciliary streaming in the lower respiratory tract. Am J Physiol 191:404–410

Hilding DA, Hilding AC (1966) Ultrastructure of tracheal cilia and cells during regeneration. Ann Otol Rhinol Laryngol 75:281–295

Hills BA, Barrow RE (1979) The contact angle induced by DPL at pulmonary epithelial surfaces. Respir Physiol 38:173–183

Hirsch JA, Swenson EW, Wanner A (1975) Tracheal mucous transport in Beagle dogs after long term exposure to 1 ppm sulfur dioxide. Arch Environ Health 75:249–253

Hogg JC, Macklem PT, Thurlbeck WM (1968) Site and nature of airway obstruction in chronic obstructive lung disease. N Engl J Med 278:1355–1360

Holden KG, Griggs LJ (1977) Respiratory tract. In: Horowitz MI, Pigman W (eds) The glycoconjugates, vol 1. Mammalian glycoproteins and glycolipids. Academic, New York

Holma B, Lindegren M, Andersen JM (1977) pH Effects on ciliomotility and morphology of respiratory mucosa. Arch Environ Health 32:216–226

Horsfield K, Cumming G (1968) Morphology of the bronchial tree in man. J Appl Physiol 24:373–383

Iravani J (1972) Flimmeraktivitor unter besonderer Berücksichtigung von Berotec. Int J Clin Pharmacol 4:20

Iravani J, Melville GN (1975) Wirkung von Pharmaka und Milicuänderungen auf die Flimmertätigkeit der Atemwege. Respiration 32:157

Iravani J, Melville GN (1978) Beta sympathomimetic effects and mucociliary function of the respiratory passages. Kolloq Bad Reichenhaller Forschungsanst Kr Atmungsorgane 1:90–97

Iravani J, Van As A (1972) Mucus transport in the tracheobronchial tree of normal and bronchitic rats. J Pathol 106:81–93

Iravani J, Melville GN, Horstmann G (1978) Tracheobronchial clearance in health and disease: with special reference of interciliary fluid. Ciba Found Symp 54:235–252

Isawa T, Hirano T, Teshima T, Konno K (1980) Effect of non-filtered and filtered cigarette smoke on mucociliary clearance mechanism. Tokoho J Exp Med 130:189–197

Izard C, Libermann C (1978) Acrolein. Mutat Res 47:115–138

Jeffery PK, Reid L (1977a) The respiratory mucous membrane. In: Brain JD, Proctor DF, Reid L (eds) Respiratory defense mechanisms. Marcel-Dekker, New York (Lung biology in health and disease, vol 5)

Jeffery PK, Reid L (1977b) Ultrastructural features of the airway lining epithelium in the developing rat and human lung. J Anat 120:295–320

Jones R, Bolduc P, Reid L (1973) Goblet cell glycoprotein and tracheal gland hypertrophy in rat airways: the effect of tobacco smoke with or without the anti-inflammatory agent phenylmethyloxadiazole. Br J Exp Pathol 54:229–239

Kauffman SL (1980) Cell proliferation in the mammalian lung. Int Rev Exp Pathol 22:131–191

Keal EE (1971) Biochemistry and rheology of sputum in asthma. Postgrad Med J 47:171–177

Kilburn KH (1967a) Mucociliary clearance from bullfrog (Rana catesbiana) lung. J Appl Physiol 23:804–810

Kilburn KH (1967b) Cilia and mucus transport as determinants of the response of lung to air pollutants. Arch Environ Health 14:77–91

Kilburn KH (1968a) A hypothesis for pulmonary clearance and its implications. Am Rev Respir Dis 98:449–463

Kilburn KH (1968b) Theory and models for cellular injury and clearance failure in the lung. Yale J Biol Med 40:339–351

King M, Macklem PT (1977) Rheological properties of microliter quantities of normal mucus. J Appl Physiol 42:797–802

King M, Viires N (1979) Effect of methacholine chloride on rheology and transport of canine tracheal mucus. J Appl Physiol 47:26–31

King M, Engel LA, Macklem PT (1979) Effect of pentobarbital anesthesia on rheology and transport of canine tracheal mucus. J Appl Physiol 46:504–509

Konietzko N, Klopfer M, Adam WE, Matthys H (1975) Die mukociliare Klarfunktion der Lunge unter β-adrenerger Stimulation. Pneumonologie 152:203–208

Kuhn C (1976) The cells of the lung and their organelles. In: Crystal RC (ed) The biochemical bases of pulmonary function. Marcel-Dekker, New York, pp 3–48

Laitinen LA, Elkin RB, Empey DW, Jacobs L, Mills J, Gold WM, Nadel JA (1976) Changes in bronchial reactivity after administration of live attenuated virus. Am Rev Respir Dis [Suppl 4] 113:194

Lamb D, Reid L (1969 a) Histochemical types of acidic glycoproteins produced by mucous cells of the tracheobronchial glands in man. J Pathol 98:213–229

Lamb D, Reid L (1969 b) Goblet cell increase in rat bronchial epithelium after exposure to cigarette smoke. Br Med J 1:33–35

Lamb D, Reid L (1972) The tracheobronchial submucosal glands in cystic fibrosis: a qualitative and quantitative histochemical study. Br J Dis Chest 66:239–247

Lamblin G, Lafitte JJ, Lhermitte M et al. (1977) Mucins from cystic fibrosis sputum. Mod Probl Pediatr 19:153–164

Landa JF, Hirsch JA, Lebeaux MI (1975) Effects of topical and general anesthetic agents on tracheal mucous velocity of sheep. J Appl Physiol 38:946–948

Laurenzi GA, Yin S (1971) Mucus flow in the mammalian respiratory tract. I. Beneficial effects of acetyl ouabain on respiratory tract mucus flow. Am Rev Respir Dis 103:800–807

Laurenzi GA, Yin S, Collins B, Guarneri JJ (1967) Mucus flow in the mammalian trachea. N Engl J Med 279:333–336

Lee TK, Man SF, Connolly TP, Noujaim AA (1980) Simultaneous comparison of canine tracheal transport of anion exchange resin particles to albumin microaggregates and sulfur colloid. Effects of subcutaneous methacholine chloride and intravenous hypertonic saline. Am Rev Respir Dis 121:487–494

Lee WI, Verdugo P (1976) Laser light-scattering spectroscopy: a new application in the study of ciliary activity. Biophys J 16:1115–1119

Lichtiger M, Landa JF, Hirsch JA (1975) Velocity of tracheal mucus in anesthetized women undergoing gynecological surgery. Anesthesiology 42:753–756

Lierle DM, Moore PM (1934) Effects of drugs on ciliary activity of mucosa of upper respiratory tract. Arch Otolaryngol 19:55–65

Lippmann M (1976) Mucociliary clearance of insoluble particles deposited on the bronchial tree. In: Aharonson EF (ed) Air pollution and the lung. Wiley, New York, pp 79–82

Lippmann M, Albert R (1969) The effect of particle size on the regional deposition of inhaled aerosols in the human respiratory tract. Am Ind Hyg Assoc J 30:257–275

Lippmann M, Albert RE, Yeates DB, Berger JM, Foster WM, Bohning DE (1975) Factors affecting mucociliary transport. Inhaled Part. 4(1):305–319

Litt M (1970 a) Flow behaviour of mucus. Ann Otol 80:330–335

Litt M (1970 b) Mucus rheology: Relevance to mucociliary clearance. Arch Intern Med 126:417–423

Litt M (1973) Basic concepts of mucus rheology. Bull Eur Physiopathol Respir 9:33–46

Lopez-Vidriero MT (1973) Individual and group correlations of sputum viscosity and airway obstruction. Bull Eur Physiopathol Resp 9:339–347

Lourenco RV, Klimek MF, Borowski CJ (1971) Deposition and clearance of 2 micron particles in the tracheobronchial tree of normal subjects – smokers and non-smokers. J Clin Invest 50:1411–1420

Lucas A, Douglas LC (1934) Principles underlying ciliary activity in the respiratory tract. II. A comparison of nasal clearance in man, monkey and other mammals. Otolaryngology 20:518–541

Luchtel D (1976) Ultrastructural observations on the mucous layer in pulmonary airways. J Cell Biol 70:350 a

Lundgren R (1977) Scanning electron microscopic studies of bronchial mucosa before and during treatment with beclomethasone diproprionate inhalations. Scand J Respir Dis 101:179–187

Lutz R, Litt M, Chakrin LW (1973) Physiocochemical factors in mucus rheology. In: Gabelnick HL, Litt M (eds) Rheology of biological systems. Thomas, Springfield, p 119

Macklem PT, Proctor DF, Hogg JC (1970) The stability of peripheral airways. Respir Physiol 8:191–203

Man SF, Noujaim AA, Lee TK, Gibney RT, Logus JW (1980) Canine tracheal mucus transport of particulate pollutants: comparison of radiolabelled corn pollen, ragweed pollen, asbestos, silica and talc to Dowex anion exchange particles. Arch Environ Health 35:283–286

Marin MG, Morrow PE (1969) Effect of changing inspired O_2 and CO_2 levels on tracheal mucociliary transport rate. J Appl Physiol 27:385–388

Marin MG, Davis B, Nadel JA (1979) Effect of histamine on electrical and ion transport properties of tracheal epithelium. J Appl Physiol 46:205–210

Martin R, Litt M, Marriott C (1980) The effect of mucolytic agents on the rheologic and transport properties of canine tracheal mucus. Am Rev Respir Dis 121:495–500

Martinez-Tello FJ, Braun DG, Blanc WA (1968) Immunoglobulin production in bronchial mucosa and bronchial lymph nodes, particularly in cystic fibrosis of the pancreas. J Immunol 101:989–1003

Mass MJ, Lane BP (1976) Effect of chromates on ciliated cells of rat tracheal epithelium. Arch Environ Health 31:96–100

Masson PL, Heremans JF (1973) Sputum proteins. In: Dulfano M (ed) Sputum, fundamentals and clinical pathology. Thomas, Springfield, pp 412–475

Matthys H, Kohler D (1980) Effect of theophylline on mucociliary clearance in man. Eur J Respir Dis 109:98–102

Mazetov GS, Panchenko KI (1980) Implication of motility disturbances of the mucosal ciliated epithelium of airways in the pathogenesis of duct-induced diseases of the respiratory organs (experimental study). Vestn Otorinolaringol 42:39

McDowell EM, Barnett LA, Glavin F, Trump BF (1978) The respiratory epithelium. I. Human bronchus. J Natl Cancer Inst 61:539–549

Meyrick B, Sturgess JM, Reid L (1969) A reconstruction of the duct system and secretory tubules of the human bronchial submucosal gland. Thorax 24:729–736

Miller WS (1932) The epithelium of the lower respiratory tract. In: Cowdry EV (ed) Special cytology. Oxford University Press, London, p 133

Mitchell-Heggs P, Palfrey AJ, Reid L (1974) The elasticity of sputum at low shear rates. Biorheology 11:417–426

Morrow PE (1974) Aerosol characterization and deposition. Am Rev Respir Dis 110:88–99

Morrow PE, Gibb FR, Gazioglu KM (1967) A study of particle clearance from the human lungs. Am Rev Respir Dis 96:1209–1221

Mostow SR, Dreisin RB, Manawadu BR, Laforce FM (1979) Adverse effects of lidocaine on methylparaben on tracheal ciliary activity. Laryngoscope 89:1697–1701

Nadel JA (1965) Structure-function relationships in the airways. Bronchoconstriction mediated via vagus nerve or bronchial arteries, peripheral lung constriction mediated via pulmonary arteries. Med Thorac 22:231–243

Nadel JA, Davis B (1977) Autonomic regulation of mucus secretion and ion transport in airways. In: Lichtenstein LM, Austen KF (eds) Asthma: physiology, pharmacology and treatment. Academic, New York, p 197

Nadel JA, Davis B, Phipps RJ (1979) Control of mucus secretion and ion transport in airways. Annu Rev Physiol 41:369–381

Newhouse MT, Wolff RK, Dolovich M, Obminski G (1978) Effect of TLV levels of SO_2 and H_2SO_4 on bronchial clearance in exercising man. Arch Environ Health 33:24–32

Obara H, Sekimoto M, Iwai S (1979) Alterations to the bronchial and bronchiolar surfaces of adult mice after exposure to high concentrations of oxygen. Thorax 34:479–485

Okeson GC, Divertie MB (1970) Cilia and bronchial clearance: the effects of pharmacologic agents and disease. Mayo Clin Proc 45:361–373

Olsen I, Jonsen J (1944) Effect of cadmium acetate, copper sulphate and nickel chloride on organ cultures of mouse trachea. Acta Pharmacol Toxicol (Copenh) 44:120–127

Olver RE, Davis B, Marin MG, Nadel JA (1975) Active ion transport across canine tracheal epithelium. A possible control system for mucociliary transport. Chest 67:57S

Omichi S, Kita H, Kubora T (1975) Effects of hydrocarbons on ciliary activity of the respiratory tract. Jpn J Hyg 30:139

Orehek J, Massari JP, Gayrard P, Grimoud G, Charpin J (1976) Effect of short term, low level nitrogen dioxide exposure on bronchial sensitivity in asthmatic patients. J Clin Invest 57:301–307

Pack RJ, Al-Ugaily LH, Morris G, Widdicombe JG (1980) The distribution and structure of cells in the tracheal epithelium of the mouse. Cell Tissue Res 208:65–84

Pavia D, Thomson ML (1971) Inhibition of mucociliary clearance from the human lung by hyoscine. Lancet 1:449–450

Pavia D, Thomson ML, Clarke SW (1978) Enhanced clearance of secretions from the human lung after the administration of hypertonic saline aerosol. Am Rev Respir Dis 117:199–203

Pavia D, Bateman JRM, Sheahan NF, Clarke SW (1979) Effect of ipratropium bromide on mucociliary clearance and pulmonary function in reversible airways obstruction. Thorax 34:501–507

Pedersen M, Mygind N (1980) Ciliary motility in the "immotile cilia syndrome". First results of microphoto-oscillographic studies. Br J Dis Chest 74:239–244

Penha PD, Werthamer S (1974) Pulmonary lesions induced by long term exposure to ozone. Arch Environ Health 29:282–289

Philpott DE, Harrison GA, Turnbill C, Black S (1977) Ultrastructural changes in tracheal epithelial cells exposed to oxygen. Aviat Space Environ Med 48:812–818

Pigman W (1977) Mucus glycoproteins. In: Horowitz MI, Pigman W (eds) The glycoconjugates, vol 1. Mammalian glycoproteins and glycolipids. Academic, New York, p 137

Polu JM, Puchelle E, Sadoul P (1978) Current concepts of bronchial fluidifiers. Nouv Presse Med 7:557–563

Proctor DF (1977) The upper airways. I. Nasal physiology and defense of the lungs. Am Rev Respir Dis 115:97–129

Proctor DF, Wagner H Jr (1966) Mucociliary particle clearance in the human nose. In: Davis CN (ed) Inhaled particles and vapours II. Pergamon, New York, pp 25–35

Proctor DF, Andersen I, Lundquist G (1973) Clearance of inhaled particles from the human nose. Arch Intern Med 131:132–139

Puchelle E, Girard F, Zahm JM (1976) Rheology of bronchial secretions and mucociliary transport. Bull Eur Physiopathol Respir 76:771–779

Puchelle E, Zahm JM, Bertrand A (1979) Influence of age on bronchial mucociliary transport. Scand J Respir Dis 60:307–313

Reid L (1959) Chronic bronchitis and hypersecretion of mucus. Lect Sci Basis Med 8:235–254

Reid L (1960) Measurement of bronchial mucous glands: a diagnostic yardstick in chronic bronchitis. Thorax 15:132–141

Reid L (1967) Bronchial mucus production in health and disease. Williams and Wilkins, Baltimore, p 87

Reid L, Clamp JR (1978) Biochemical and histochemical nomenclature of mucus. Br Med Bull 34:5–8

Reznik-Schueller H (1975) Ciliary alterations in hamster respiratory tract epithelium after exposure to carcinogens and cigarette smoke. Cancer Lett 1:7–13

Rhodin JAG (1966) Ultrastructure and function of human tracheal mucosa. Am Rev Respir Dis 93:1–15

Rhodin J, Dalhamn T (1956) Electron microscopy of the tracheal ciliated mucosa in rat. Z Zellforsch 44:345–412

Roberts GP (1974) Isolation and characterization of glycoprotein from sputum. Eur J Biochem 50:265

Rossman CM, Dolovich J, Dolovich M, Wilson W, Newhouse MT (1977) Cystic fibrosis-related inhibition of mucociliary clearance in vivo in man. J Pediatr 90:579–584

Rossman CM, Forrest JB, Lee RM, Newhouse MT (1980) The dyskinetic cilia syndrome. Ciliary motility in immotile cilia syndrome. Chest 78:580–582

Ruffin RE, Wolff RK, Dolovich MB, Rossman CM, Fitzgerald JD, Newhouse MT (1978) Aerosol therapy with SCH 1000. Short term mucociliary clearance in normal and bronchitic subjects and toxicology in normal subjects. Chest 73:501–506

Rutland J, Cole PJ (1980) Non-invasive sampling of nasal cilia for measurement of beat frequency and study of ultrastructure. Lancet 2:564–565

Rutland J, Griffin W, Cole PJ (1982a) Human ciliary beat frequency in epithelium from intrathoracic and extrathoracic airways 1–3. Am Rev Respir Dis 125:100–105

Rutland J, Griffin W, Cole PJ (1982b) An in vitro model for studying the effects of pharmacological agents on human ciliary beat frequency. Effect of lignocaine. Br J Clin Pharmacol 13:679–683

Ryley HC (1972) An immunoelectrophoretic study of the soluble secretory proteins of sputum. Biochim Biophys Acta 271:300

Ryley HC, Brogan TD (1973) Quantitative immunoelectrophoretic analysis of plasma proteins in the sol phase of sputum from patients with chronic bronchitis. J Clin Pathol 26:852–856

Sackner MA, Rosen MJ, Wanner A (1973) Estimation of tracheal mucus velocity by bronchofiberscopy. J Appl Physiol 34:495–499

Sackner MA, Landa LF, Hirsch JA, Zapata A (1975) Pulmonary effects of oxygen breathing. Ann Intern Med 82:40–43

Sackner MA, Epstein S, Wanner A (1976a) Effect of beta adrenergic agonist aerosolized by freon propellant on tracheal mucous velocity and cardiac output. Chest 69:593–598

Sackner MA, Chapman GA, Dougherty RD (1976b) Effects of nebulised SCH 1000 and atropine sulphate on tracheal mucous velocity and lung mechanics in anaesthetised dogs. Am Rev Respir Dis 113:131

Sackner MA, Hirsch JA, Epstein S, Rywlin AM (1976c) Effect of oxygen in graded concentrations upon tracheal mucous velocity. A study in anesthetised dogs. Chest 69:164–167

Sackner MA, Reinhart M, Arkin B (1977) Effects of beclomethasone diproprionate on tracheal mucous velocity. Am Rev Respir Dis 115:1069–1070

Sackner MA, Yergin BA, Brito M, Januszkiewicz A (1979) Effect of adrenergic agonists on tracheal mucous velocity. Bull Eur Physiopathol Respir 15:505–511

Sade J, Elezier N, Silberberg A, Nevo AC (1970) The role of mucus in transport by cilia. Am Rev Respir Dis 102:48–52

Sade J, Meyer FA, King M, Silberberg A (1975) Clearance of middle ear effusions by the mucociliary system. Acta Otolaryngol (Stockh) 79:277–282

Saketkhoo K, Yergin BM, Januszkiewicz A, Kovitz K, Sackner MA (1978) The effect of nasal decongestant on nasal mucous velocity. Am Rev Respir Dis 118:251–254

Sanderson MJ, Sleigh MA (1981) Ciliary activity of cultured rabbit tracheal epithelium; beat pattern and metachrony. J Cell Sci 47:331–347

Sanchis J, Dolovich M, Rossman C, Wilson W, Newhouse M (1973) Pulmonary mucociliary clearance in cystic fibrosis. New Engl J Med 288:651–654

Santa Cruz R, Landa J, Hirsch J, Sackner MA (1974) Tracheal mucus velocity in normal man and patients with obstructive lung disease: effects of terbutaline. Am Rev Respir Dis 109:458–463

Satir P (1974) The present status of the sliding microtubule model of ciliary motion. In: Sleigh MA (ed) Cilia and flagella. Academic, London, pp 131–142

Schlesinger RB (1973) Mucociliary interaction in the tracheobronchial tree and environmental pollution. Bioscience 23:567–572

Schlesinger RB, Lippmann M, Albert RE (1978) Effects of short term exposures to sulfuric acid and ammonium sulphate aerosols upon bronchial airway function in the donkey. Am Ind Hyg Assoc J 39:275–286

Schlesinger RB, Halpern M, Albert RE, Lippmann M (1979) Effect of chronic inhalation of sulfuric acid mist upon mucociliary clearance from the lungs of donkeys. J Environ Pathol Toxicol 2:1351–1367

Schneeberger EE (1980) Heterogeneity of tight junction morphology in extrapulmonary and intrapulmonary airways of the rat. Anat Rec 198:193–208

Schneeberger EE, Karnovsky MJ (1976) Substructure of intercellular junctions in freeze fractured alveolar-capillary membranes of mouse lung. Cir Res 38:404–411

Serafini SM, Michaelson ED (1977) Length and distribution of cilia in human and canine airways. Bull Eur Physiopathol Respir 13:551–559

Serafini SM, Wanner A, Michaelson ED (1976) Mucociliary transport in central and intermediate size airways. Effects of aminophylline. Bull Eur Physiopathol Respir 12:415–422

Shih CK, Litt M, Khan MA, Wolfe DP (1977) Effect of non-dialysable solids concentration and visceolasticity on ciliary transport of tracheal mucus. Am Rev Respir Dis 115:989–995

Silberberg A, Meyer FA, Gilboa A, Gelman RA (1977) Function and properties of epithelial mucus. In: Elstein M, Parke DV (eds) Mucus in health and disease. Plenum, London, pp 91–102

Simon H, Drettner B, Jung B (1977) Measurement of transport of mucous membrane in the human nose with Cr^{51}-labelled resin beads. Acta Otolaryngol (Stockh) 83:378–390

Sleigh MA (1974) Cilia and flagella. Academic, London, p 500

Sleigh MA (1977) The nature and action of respiratory tract cilia. In: Brain JD, Proctor DF, Reid LM (eds) Respiratory defense mechanisms. Marcel-Dekker, New York, pp 192–288

Sleigh MA (1979) Contractility of the roots of flagella and cilia. Nature 277:263–264

Sleigh MA, Aiello E (1972) The movement of water by cilia. Acta Protozool 11:265–277

Spicer SS, Charkrin LW, Wardell JR, Kendrick W (1971) Histochemistry of mucosubstances in the canine and human respiratory tracts. Lab Invest 25:483–490

Stitik FP, Smith JC, Swift DL, Proctor DF (1976) Tantalum inhalation bronchography. Am Rev Respir Dis 113:411

Sturgess JM (1977a) The mucous lining of major bronchi in the rabbit lung. Am Rev Respir Dis 115:819–827

Sturgess JM (1977b) Bronchial mucous secretion in cystic fibrosis. Mod Probl Pediatr 19:129

Sturgess JM (1977c) Structural organization of mucus in the lung. In: Sanders CL, Schneider RP, Dagle GE, Ragan HA (eds) Pulmonary macrophages and epithelial cells. Energy Research and Development Administration, Oakridge, p 149

Sturgess JM (1979) Mucous secretions in the respiratory tract. In: Levison H (ed) Symposium on the chest. Pediatr Clin North Am 26:481–502

Sturgess JM, Reid L (1972a) An organ culture study of the effects of drugs on the secretory activity of the human bronchial submucosal gland. Clin Sci 43:533

Sturgess JM, Reid L (1972b) The secretory activity of human bronchial submucosal glands in vitro. Exp Mol Pathol 16:362

Sturgess JM, Reid L (1973) The effect of isoprenaline and pilocarpine on (a) bronchial mucus-secreting tissue and (b) pancreas, salivary glands, heart, thymus, liver and spleen. Br J Exp Pathol 54:388

Sturgess JM, Palfrey AJ, Reid L (1970) The viscosity of bronchial secretion. Clin Sci 38:145–156

Sturgess JM, Palfrey AJ, Reid L (1971) Rheological properties of sputum. Rheol Acta 10:36

Sturgess JM, Chao J, Wong J et al. (1979) Cilia with defective radial spokes. A cause of human respiratory disease. N Engl J Med 300:53–56

Sturgess JM, Turner JAP (1984) Ultrastructural pathology of cilia in the immotile cilia syndrome. Persp Ped Path 8:133–161

Tansy MF, Hohenleitner FJ, White DK, Oberly R, Landin WE, Kendall FM (1980) Chronic biological effects of methylmethacrylate vapour. Environ Res 21:117–125

Thomson ML, Pavia D (1973) Long term tobacco smoking and mucociliary clearance from the human lung in health and disease. Arch Environ Health 26:86–89

Thomson ML, Pavia D (1974) Particle penetration and clearance in the human lung. Arch Environ Health 24:214–219

Thomson ML, Short MD (1969) Mucociliary function in health, chronic obstructive airways disease and asbestosis. J Appl Physiol 26:535–539

Thomson ML, Pavia D, McNicol MW (1973) A preliminary study of the effect of guia-phenesin on mucociliary clearance from human lung. Thorax 28:742–747

Thomson ML, Pavia D, Gregg J, Stark JE (1974) Bromhexine and mucociliary clearance in chronic bronchitis. Br J Dis Chest 68:21–27

Thomson ML, Pavia D, Jones CJ, McQuiston TAC (1975) No demonstrable long-term effect of 5-carboxymethylcysteine on clearance of secretions from the human lung. Thorax 30:669–673

Thurlbeck WM, Benjamin B, Reid L (1961) Development and distribution of mucous glands in the fetal human trachea. Br J Dis Chest 55:54–64

Thurlbeck WM, Malaka D, Murphy K (1975) Goblet cells in the peripheral airways in chronic bronchitis. Am Rev Respir Dis 112:65

Toigo A (1963) Clearance of large carbon particles from the human tracheal tree. Am Rev Repir Dis 87:487–492

Tomenius L, Holma B, Ehrner-Samuel H, Kylin B, Tebrock O, Thomasen M (1979) Effect of trichlorethylene on cilia activity in rabbit trachea. Acta Pharmacol Toxicol 44:65–70

Toremalm NG (1960) The daily amount of tracheobronchial secretions in man. Acta Oto-laryngol 52:43–53

Van As A (1974) The role of selective Beta$_2$-adrenoceptor stimulants in the control of ciliary activity. Respiration 31:146

Van As A, Iravani J (1972) Mucous transport in the tracheobronchial tree of normal and bronchitis rats. J Pathol 106:81–93

Van As A, Webster I (1974) The morphology of mucus in mammalian airways. Environ Res 7:1–12

Van de Donk HJM, Jadoenath S, Zuidema J, Merkus FWHM (1982a) The effects of drugs on ciliary motility. I. Decongestants. Int J Pharmacol 12:57–65

Van de Donk HJM, Van Egmond ALM, Van den Heuvel AGM, Zuidema J, Merkus FWHM (1982b) The effect of drugs on ciliary motility. III. Local anaesthetics and anti-allergic drugs. Int J Pharmacol 12:77–85

Van de Donk HJM, Van Egmond ALM, Zuidema J, Merkus FWHM (1982c) The effects of drugs on ciliary motility. II. Antimicrobial agents. Int J Pharmacol 12:67–76

Van Dongen K, Levsnick H (1953) The action of opium alkaloids and expectorants on the ciliary movements in the air passages. Arch Int Pharmacodyn Ther 93:261–277

Verdugo P, Hinds TR, Vincenzi FF (1979) Laser light-scattering spectroscopy: preliminary results on bioassay of cystic fibrosis factor(s). Pediatr Res 13:131–135

Verdugo P, Johnson NT, Tam PY (1980) Beta-adrenergic stimulation of respiratory ciliary activity. J Appl Physiol 48:863–871

Wakabayashi M, Bang BG, Bang FB (1977) Mucociliary transport in chickens infected with Newcastle disease virus and exposed to sulfur dioxide. Arch Environ Health 32:101–103

Wanner A (1977) Clinical aspects of mucociliary transport. Am Rev Respir Dis 116:73–125

Wanner A, Zarzecki S, Hirsch J, Epstein S (1975) Tracheal mucous transport in experimental canine asthma. J Appl Physiol 39:950

Weibel ER (1963) Morphometry of the human lung. Academic, New York

Wilkey DD, Lee PS, Hass FJ, Gerrity TR, Yeates DB, Lourenco RV (1980) Mucociliary clearance of deposited particles from the human lung: intra- and inter-subject reproductivity, total and regional lung clearance, and model comparisons. Arch Environ Health 35:294–303

Wolff RK, Muggenburg BA (1979) Comparison of two methods of measuring tracheal mucous velocity in anaesthetized Beagle dogs. Am Rev Respir Dis 120:137–142

Wolff RK, Dolovich MB, Obmirski G, Newhouse MT (1977) Effects of exercise and eucapnic hyperventilation on bronchial clearance in man. J Appl Physiol 43:46–50

Wong JW, Keens TG, Wannamaker EM, Douglas PT, Crozier N, Levison H, Aspin N (1977) Effects of gravity on tracheal mucus transport rates in normal subjects and in patients with cystic fibrosis. Pediatrics 60:146–152

Wood RE, Wanner A, Hirsch J, Farrell PM (1975) Tracheal mucociliary transport in patients with cystic fibrosis and its stimulation by terbutaline. Am Rev Respir Dis 111:733–738

Wright AW (1966) Effects of industrial dust on ciliated epithelium. Am Rev Respir Dis 93:103–107

Yager JA, Chen TM, Dulfano MJ (1978) Measurements of the frequency of ciliary beats of human respiratory epithelium. Chest 73:627–633

Yager JA, Ellman H, Dulfano MJ (1980) Human ciliary beat frequency at three levels of the tracheobronchial tree. Am Rev Respir Dis 121:661–665

Yates AL (1924) Methods of estimating activity of ciliary epithelium within the sinuses. J Laryngol Otol 39:554–560

Yeates DB, Aspin N, Levinson H, Bryan AC (1974) Measurements of mucociliary transport rates in man. Fed Proc 33:365

Yeates DB, Aspin N, Levison H, Jones M, Bryan AC (1975) J Appl Physiol 39:481–495

Yeates DB, Sturgess JM, Kahn SR, Levison H, Aspin N (1976) Mucociliary transport in trachea of patients with cystic fibrosis. Arch Dis Child 51:28–33

CHAPTER 13

General Enzymology of the Lung

M. G. MUSTAFA

A. Introduction

It is now well documented that biochemical and enzymatic changes occur in lung tissue in response to injury. The reaction of inhaled toxic agents with lung tissue is often regional. Depending upon the solubility, reactivity, and other physical and chemical properties, the toxic agents may react variably with the airway epithelium, terminal bronchioles, and/or alveolar parenchyma as they travel through the conducting airways to the gas exchange area. The regional or focal nature of injury tends to lower the sensitivity of quantitative biochemical and enzymatic changes. Lung tissue preparations generally include both injured and uninjured portions of lung tissue, thus diluting the effects. Quantitative determinations are convenient with high level exposures, which cause massive lung injury, producing large changes in enzymatic and other biochemical parameters. When focal or subtle changes occur with low level exposures, quantitative expressions become difficult, but are still possible if a set of sensitive parameters can be examined, or a battery of tests can be carried out. Measurements of a variety of parameters will have the virtue that all biochemical and enzymatic parameters do not change to the same extent, and some may not change at all. It is from a plot of all the parameters examined that a definitive answer can be derived whether or not a given toxic agent has produced lung injury.

Biochemical and enzymatic changes in the lung are attributed to cell injury and/or death caused by toxic agents, and then to multiplication of metabolically active cells occurring as a part of the repair process. Consequently, two types of changes have been observed: an injury phase in which enzymatic and metabolic activities are either depressed or adversely affected, and a reparative phase in which these activities are elevated. The sequence of these events parallels that of morphological changes that occur in response to toxic lung injury.

There are several unique problems with lung tissue that must be considered when making data presentation. Any tissue, organelle, or enzyme preparation from the whole lung is likely to have contributions from a great variety of cells (SOROKIN 1970). Thus, biochemical and metabolic parameters or their changes as measured in these preparations will provide values averaging the relative contributions of various cell types. Caution should be exercised when interpreting the data, particularly to indicate whether the changes are due to one or more structural lung cells or recruited inflammatory cells, viz., macrophages, leukocytes, etc. A separate assessment of the relative contributions of recruited cells may be made by isolating then from the alveolar spaces.

Quantitative expressions of data, such as are conventionally made for other tissues, in terms of units per gram wet tissue, per milligram dry tissue, or per milligram protein or DNA, are not always suitable for lung tissue. Wet weight of the lung is often unstable owing to injury from toxic exposures and accumulation of edema fluid and/or blood in the alveolar or interstitial spaces. Even with the normal lung, perfusion through the vascular bed to remove the blood, or lavage through the airways to harvest or remove the free cells may alter wet weight of the lung owing to buffer solution trapped in capillary or extravascular spaces. Likewise, data presentation per milligram dry weight is not valid because of variable amounts of solutes derived from edema fluid or added buffer solution. Lung injury from toxic exposures, accumulation of edema fluid and/or inflammatory cells, and proliferation of metabolically active cells result in alterations of protein and DNA content of the lung, making data presentation per miligram protein or DNA unsuitable.

Expression of data on a per lung basis (WITSCHI 1975) seems to overcome many of these difficulties, and has become a common practice, although periodically units per milligram protein or DNA are also used whenever appropriate. The variations in lung weights of a group of normal animals of the same age, sex, and body weight are negligible. Units of enzyme activities per lung of these animals are strikingly similar. Once we have resorted to data expression per lung, the vascular perfusion and/or endobronchial lavage can be carried out routinely so as to eliminate the influence of the blood cells and/or inflammatory cells on lung tissue enzyme activities.

B. Tissue Preparation

Although inhalation exposures are generally conducted in vivo, the biochemical and enzymatic parameters applied to assess the toxic effects are studied with lung tissue in vitro. Occasionally, however, in vivo biochemical studies are carried out. For in vivo studies, the substrates or precursors are delivered to the lung by an intravenous or intraperitoneal injection, or by an intratracheal instillation. The effects of inhaled toxic agents are then examined on the utilization of substrates or incorporation of precursors (see Sects. C.V.–VII). The in vitro studies involve a variety of tissue preparations including the whole lung, tissue slices, isolated cells, tissue homogenate, and subcellular fractions, viz., nuclei, mitochondria, lysosomes, microsomes, lamellar bodies, and cytosol. Since the whole lung (isolated lung perfusion) studies have been covered in Chap. 6, only limited information as it becomes pertinent will be discussed in this chapter.

I. Isolation of Lung

To remove the lung from the chest cavity, animals are anesthetized by an intraperitoneal injection of sodium pentobarbital (50–60 mg/kg) or are anesthetized in a bell jar with 4% halothane. After the animal becomes unconscious, the lung and heart are exposed by a midline thoracotomy. If intended, the endobronchial lavage and vascular perfusion are carried out at this point. For lung lavage, the trachea is cannulated; for perfusion, the pulmonary artery is cannulated and the left atrium is then excised. Cold (4 °C) physiologic saline (0.9% or 0.154 M NaCl) is commonly used for lavage or perfusion. The lung is then removed from the chest cavity; the individual lobes are separated, rinsed in cold saline, blotted on a filter paper, and weighed. The lung weight after lavage and/or perfusion is not accurate; it is taken to facilitate allocation of tissue for different purposes.

II. Isolation of Cells

Many cell types that make up the lung tissue do not apparently respond equally or uniformly to inhaled toxic agents. Because metabolic studies are generally carried out in tissue slices or subcellular fractions of the whole lung, the specific question as to which cells respond to the toxic agent remains unanswered or only partly answered. Separation of lung cells into defined populations would considerably lessen the information gap in this regard. For example, after toxic lung injury there is a proliferation of metabolically active cells, such as the alveolar type II cells (KAUFFMAN 1972; EVANS et al. 1973; ADAMSON and BOWDEN 1974; WITSCHI 1976; MASON and WILLIAMS 1977). Isolation into pure forms would provide a tremendous opportunity to study type II cell metabolic behavior and related phenomena in response to inhaled toxicants.

Separation of structural lung cells and their isolation into pure forms are rather tedious. Attempts have been made to isolate epithelial cells from the trachea and major bronchi, and type II alveolar epithelial cells from the parenchyma. The method of cell dispersion and the subsequent separation into defined populations are the two major steps in lung cell isolation. Several investigators have used various combinations of mechanical, chemical, and enzymatic methods to disperse lung tissue into individual cells. GOULD (1976) and MASON et al. (1976) have reviewed the various techniques for lung tissue dispersion. An inherent problem with these techniques is that during the dispersion process the individual cells undoubtedly receive various degrees of injury, resulting in alternations of metabolic activities. Nonetheless, research in this direction remains promising.

1. Alveolar Macrophages

Isolation of alveolar free cells by tracheobronchial lavage, particularly the alveolar macrophages, and their use in metabolic studies are relatively common.

2. Tracheobronchial Epithelial Cells

The most numerous cells in the tracheobronchial epithelium are the ciliated cells and the mucus-secreting cells. Other cells with specialized functions occur, but much less in numbers. Isolated cell preparations from the tracheobronchial surface will contain mostly the ciliated and mucous cells. In an earlier attempt, SPENCER (1958) devised a procedure for the preparation of epithelial cells from human trachea in which a sucrose solution containing ethylenediaminetetraacetate (EDTA) was used as the cell dispersing agent. The sucrose-EDTA solution was layered over the tracheal epithelium, and the epithelial cells were gently brushed with a narrow pipette mouth. By this procedure, the author was able to obtain enough cells from 1 cm^2 tracheal or bronchial surface to carry out biochemical studies. The procedure was later adopted by Nasr et al. (1971) for isolation of epithelial cells from rat trachea. An average of 1.5×10^6 cells were obtained from a rat trachea.

3. Dispersed Parenchymal Cells

Dispersion of lung parenchyma into individual cells has been attempted in several laboratories. A typical preparation generally contains a mixture of structural cells and free cells of the lung. The usefulness of such preparations is rather limited, but the techniques represent an initial success in isolating metabolically active lung parenchymal cells.

In an attempt by Wolfe et al. (1968), minced rabbit lung tissue was first incubated with collagenase and then with DNAase, resulting in a dispersion of individual pneumocytes. The cells thus obtained were a mixture of alveolar epithelial cells, alveolar macrophages, other monocytes, and polymorphonuclear leukocytes. It was not possible to separate them into specific cell types. The isolated cells were able to carry out metabolic activities, viz., oxidation of glucose and succinate, and incorporation of palmitate into lipids at rates similar to lung slices.

Gould et al. (1972) applied a similar method in which they intratracheally filled the isolated rabbit lung with a buffer containing fetal calf serum, DNAase, and several proteolytic enzymes, viz., collagenase, pronase, chymotrypsin, and elastase. The tissue was then cut into small cubes, and incubated in the same medium. The dispersed cells were isolated, and the yield of viable cells (in terms of weight) was greater than 50% of the original lung weight. The cells thus isolated were of several types. They were able to incorporate palmitate into lipids.

Ayuso et al. (1973) adapted a similar technique for rat lung. They were able to prepare a cell suspension representing 25% of the original lung weight. The cell types were a mixture, and they were metabolically active. They metabolized glucose, including incorporation of ^{14}C from glucose into lipids and proteins. Endogenous O_2 consumption was somewhat low in the cell preparation compared with tissue slices.

4. Alveolar Type II Epithelial Cells

Two major cell types that form the alveolar epithelium are the membranous type I cells and the granular type II cells. The type I cells form a thin layer over most of the alveolar wall, and their metabolic function is considered to be limited based on their content of few mitochondria and other organelles. The type II cells are metabolically active, and contain numerous mitochondria, endoplasmic reticula, lamellar inclusions, and other organelles. A great deal of effort has been made to seperate alveolar type II cells and to isolate them into pure forms.

The methods thus far applied to dissociate parenchymal cells have resulted in inclusion of blood-borne cells and alveolar macrophages in the preparation. Kikkawa and Yoneda (1974) described a method for rat lung in which they tried to eliminate the problem by perfusing the pulmonary vascular bed and lavaging the alveoli through trachea prior to mincing. The minced lung was subjected to a mechanical shaking to remove additional macrophages and blood-borne cells. The minced lung upon incubation with trypsin yielded up to 10^7 cells per rat lung.

Based on electron microscopy, 30% of the cells were alveolar type II cells, and they were all morphologically intact. The residual alveolar macrophages from the cell suspension were removed by allowing them to ingest barium sulfate and thus increase their weight. When the cell suspension was layered on a discontinuous Ficoll gradient (Sigma Chemical Company, St. Louis, Missouri), the pure fraction of type II cells remained above the density of 1.047, and the "heavy" macrophages appeared at the bottom under centrifugal force. The type II cell fraction, with purity of 90%, represented 6% of the original cells. By centrifuging further, a purity of 95% was achieved. The cells were morphologically intact, and were 93% viable based on trypan blue exclusion.

Subsequently, KIKKAWA et al. (1975) adapted the method for rabbit lung, and successfully isolated type II epithelial cells. By this method up to 3×10^7 cells per rabbit lung were obtained. They have characterized the type II cells with respect to protein and lipid content, and synthesis of phospholipids. The isolated type II cells actively incorporated choline and palmitate into disaturated lecithin.

MASON et al. (1976) used a somewhat different method to isolate type II cells. Using warm saline (37 °C), they perfused the rat lungs to remove the blood-borne cells, and lavaged the lungs to remove the macrophages. A heavy emulsion of fluorocarbon was then instilled through the airways to allow the remaining macrophages to ingest the heavy material. The subsequent procedure was to carry out a trypsin digestion, mincing of the lung, agitation of the minced tissue in a flask, filtration of the cells through gauze and nylon mesh, and layering of the cells on an albumin discontinuous density gradient. The preparation of type II cells thus obtained was 76% pure (range 56%–86%), and the cells were viable based on trypan blue exclusion.

III. Preparation of Tissue Slices

Although the isolated perfused lung provides an intact organ system, tissue slices offer a multicellular system in which at least several layers of cells remain intact. Some of the metabolic studies carried out in the two systems seem to compare well, suggesting the functional usefulness of tissue slices (O'NEIL and TIERNEY 1974; FISHER 1976). Studies with lung tissue slices have shown that the system can be routinely used for various metabolic activities with reproducible results.

Depending upon the experimental design, the lung may be perfused and/or lavaged, and for the purpose of measuring O_2 consumption the organ should be degassed to remove trapped air. To prepare lung tissue slices, the individual lobes are sliced with a tissue slicer (McIlwain, Brinkmann Instruments, Westbury, New York, or Stadie-Riggs, A.H. Thomas Company, Philadelphia, Pennsylvania, type) unidirectionally, producing 1-mm-thick sheets. A bidirectional cutting will produce rectangular slices, but these are metabolically less efficient than the sheet slices, possibly because of too many bruised or cut cells per unit tissue mass (O'NEIL and TIERNEY 1974; O'NEIL et al. 1977; WOODS et al. 1980). Slices thicker than 1 mm are also not efficient, possibly because of limited substrate diffusion through the multiple cell layer (CALDWELL and WITTENBERG 1974; LEVY and HARVEY 1974; O'NEIL and TIERNEY 1974; O'NEIL et al. 1977). The sliced tissue is weighed and transferred to individual flasks for incubation. Most commonly,

Krebs-Ringer buffer at physiologic pH is used as the medium (Umbreit et al. 1972), but the exact ingredients may vary, depending upon the experimental design and objective.

IV. Preparation of Subcellular Fractions

The procedure for tissue fractionation and isolation of subcellular organelles is an adaptation of methodology generally applied to other tissues and organs. Typical preparations include homogenate, nuclei, mitochondria, lysosomes, microsomes, and cytosol. These subcellular fractions from the liver or other tissues are well characterized with respect to the isolation procedure and purity. The reader is referred to reviews of the isolation techniques by De Duve (1971 a, b). Working with lung tissue is a little tedious compared with other tissues, such as liver or heart. The following presentation will point out some of the difficulties and the precautionary measures.

1. Homogenate

Lung tissue homogenization is carried out in the following ways. The lungs from small animals, e.g., mice, rats, and young guinea pigs and rabbits, are relatively easy to homogenize with a glass–Teflon (polytetrafluoroethylene) homogenizer. This method of homogenization is preferred when preparing mitochondria or other subcellular organelles. Hook et al. (1972) used glass–Teflon, glass–glass, and two-blade-type homogenizers while preparing lung microsomes, and upon comparing marker enzyme activities concluded that the glass–Teflon homogenizer was superior to all others. For lung tissue from larger animals, e.g., adult guinea pigs and rabbits, sheep and dogs, the glass–Teflon homogenizer may not be suitable because of the fibrous and spongy nature of the tissue. A Polytron homogenizer (Brinkmann Instruments, Westbury, New York) is generally used. However, owing to excessive tissue grinding in a Polytron homogenizer, the mitochondria and other subcellular organelles are damaged. For preparation of soluble enzymes such a homogenization procedure may be useful. Another method of homogenization may be a low speed tissue chopping in a Waring blender followed by homogenization of the chopped tissue in a glass–Teflon homogenizer. Although the yield of a subcellular fraction is not great by this method, the structure of the subcellular organelles is better preserved.

The medium for tissue homogenization usually consists of 0.15 M sucrose, 0.15 M mannitol, 1 mM Tris-chloride, and 1 mM Tris-EDTA at pH 7.5 (henceforth called sucrose–mannitol medium) (Mustafa and Cross 1974a; Mustafa et al. 1977). Approximately an 8% w/v homogenate is prepared, which is then filtered through a two-layer cheesecloth or gauze, and adjusted to a final volume of 2 ml per mouse lung, 10 ml per rat lung, or 10 ml per gram lung tissue of other animals. The overall operation starting from thoracotomy through homogenization should not take longer than 5–10 min, and the tissue should be kept ice-cold at all times.

It should be noted that variations exist in the media used for tissue homogenization and the subsequent isolation of subcellular organelles. An all-sucrose medium, even though routinely used for heart or liver tissue, is not considered suitable for lung tissue because of some degree of agglutination of subcellular organelles. An all-mannitol medium (0.3 M, isotonic) may be preferred, but is not feasible because of possible precipitation of mannitol in an ice-cold solution. Another combination of sucrose and mannitol (70 mM and 210 mM, respectively) has been used by some workers (FISHER et al. 1973; VALDIVIA 1973). A completely ionic medium, e.g., 0.15 M NaCl or KCl, is not recommended because mitochondria become uncoupled in this medium. However, MATSUBARRA and TOCHINO (1971) used 0.15 M KCl as the medium of choice while preparing lung microsomes, since this permitted considerable elimination of hemoglobin from the preparation. A vascular perfusion of the lung before homogenization, however, should eliminate much of the hemoglobin source. The selection of a homogenizing medium may become important, depending upon the purpose. In addition, the presence of a buffer (1 mM Tris-chloride) and a chelator of divalent cations (1 mM Tris-EDTA) in the medium is considered desirable. The homogenate should be filtered through cheesecloth or gauze in order to remove large particles and unbroken cells.

After preparing the homogenate, it can be used directly for various biochemical and enzymatic determinations. Otherwise, the homogenate is fractionated by differential centrifugation to prepare, as desired, nuclei, mitochondria, microsomes, lysosomes, and cytosol, according to the scheme shown in Fig. 1. The scheme is basically derived from procedures used for liver tissue, but modified by various authors for lung tissue (HOOK et al. 1972; DE LUMEN et al. 1972; MUSTAFA and CROSS 1974a; MUSTAFA et al. 1977). Whereas this scheme is a guideline

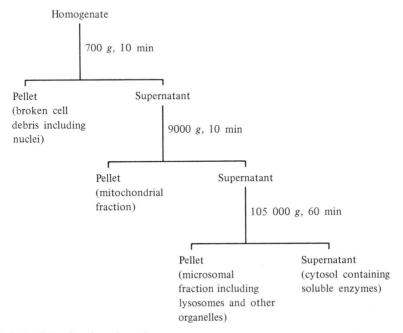

Fig. 1. Subcellular fractionation scheme

for fractionation of lung homogenate on a routine basis, the individual fractions collected as such are by no means "pure", but are merely "rich" in the given organelles.

2. Nuclei

Lung tissue nuclei are not usually prepared routinely, and only limited studies have been carried out to date. Yazdi et al. (1971), and Yazdi and Gyorkey (1971, 1973) isolated nuclei from human lung tissue and also from lung tumors. The isolated nuclei were morphologically intact, and suitable for biochemical studies. Smith et al. (1971) prepared morphologically intact nuclei from tracheal epithelium of hamster. All these methods were conventional, and included separation of nuclear fraction from tissue homogenate and then purification by centrifugation through a high density sucrose medium. The specific methods for preparation of nuclei from a variety of tissues have been reviewed by Roodyn (1969). The reader is referred to those methods outlined in the review for selection and/or adaptation of one for lung tissue. For a routine preparation of nuclei, the pellet obtained after centrifugation of homogenate at 700 g (Fig. 1) should serve as the starting material. The nuclei isolated from lung tissue are heterogeneous when one considers the various cell types in the lung.

3. Mitochondria

Lung mitochondria have been isolated from several animal species, including rat (Reiss 1966; Fisher et al. 1973; Mustafa 1974; Mustafa and Cross 1974a; Mustafa et al. 1973, 1977; Singh et al. 1976), rabbit (Reiss 1965, 1966), sheep (Mustafa et al. 1971), and monkey (Mustafa and Cross 1974a). In addition, mitochondria have been prepared from sheep lung macrophages (Mustafa and Cross 1971). The methods used for these preparations have certain variations with respect to tissue homogenization and isolation medium (see Sect. B.IV.1).

a) Preparation of Coupled Mitochondria

In order to prepare relatively tightly coupled mitochondria, no undue time lapse should occur between killing the animal and the assay of mitochondria. For small animals (mice or rats) a single or a few lungs, and for larger animals a single lung or a portion of it should be used at one time. Lung mitochondria rapidly lose their coupling ability in isolation, unlike liver, heart, or kidney mitochondria.

The animals are anesthetized by an intraperitoneal injection of sodium pentobarbital (50–60 mg/kg), or better yet they are decapitated (without anesthesia). The lungs are quickly removed, rinsed with an ice-cold sucrose–mannitol medium, minced, washed once, and homogenized in a glass–Teflon homogenizer (0.15 mm clearance) allowing only one or two strokes of the pestle. The homogenate (approximately 5% w/v), after filtering through two layers of cheesecloth, is centrifuged first at 700 g for 10 min to remove the nuclei and broken cell debris, and then at 9,000 g for 10 min to sediment the mitochondrial fraction. The mitochondrial fraction thus obtained (as a pellet) may be washed once by resuspending in sucrose–mannitol medium and then centrifuging between the low and the high speeds as already indicated. However, the washing step may be omitted, and the pellet of mitochondria-rich fraction, after resuspension in a minimal volume (0.2 ml per mouse lung or 1 ml per rat lung), should be used for assay of coupled phosphorylation immediately.

b) Preparation of Mitochondria for General Enzymatic Assays

The animals are anesthetized, a thoracotomy performed, a vascular perfusion and an endobronchial lavage carried out, and the lung prepared as described in Sect. B.I. The lung lobes are minced, and homogenized in the sucrose–mannitol medium using a glass–Teflon homogenizer (0.15 mm clearance) allowing three strokes of the pestle. The subsequent procedure, including the sedimentation of the mitochondrial fraction, is the same as described for coupled mitochondria, except the fraction is washed 2–3 times before the final pellet is resuspended in a minimal volume.

c) Characteristics of Isolated Mitochondria

Mitochondria are intracellular organelles characterized by certain well-defined structural and biochemical properties. They carry out specific reactions, including oxidation via the electron transport chain and coupled phosphorylation. Most work in the laboratory is carried out in a "crude" preparation of mitochondria; to prepare a "pure" preparation is not practicable on a routine basis primarily because the speeds set for the differential centrifugation are to harness as much of the mitochondrial population as possible in a given fraction. Thus, there is the possibility of contamination by nuclei or nuclear debris, fragments of membranes, including endoplasmic reticulum, lysosomes, and other subcellular organelles.

Lung mitochondria are rather inhomogeneous, both in terms of their cellular sources and structural appearances. Many cell types contribute to a given preparation. A relatively large contribution probably results from the alveolar type II cells which are rich in mitochondria. Two important characteristics of lung mitochondria are relatively high adenosine triphosphatase (ATPase) activity and membrane permeability. In isolated lung mitochondria, the ATPase activity shows some degree of latency, but it becomes almost fully stimulated in the presence of Mg^{2+} (REISS 1966). Isolated lung mitochondria show some degree of permeability to added NADH or cytochrome c (MUSTAFA and CROSS 1974 a). Mitochondria prepared from animal lungs exposed to toxic substances, or those prepared under harsh conditions, may show much greater permeability. Addition of cytochrome c (5–10 μM) to a suspension of homogenate or mitochondria actually stimulates oxygen consumption with oxidation of a substrate (REISS 1966; MUSTAFA and CROSS 1974 a).

4. Lysosomes

Lysosomes are a heterogeneous group of cytoplasmic, membrane-bound organelles which contain a large number of hydrolytic enzymes. The hydrolysis of a variety of compounds occurs as they are taken into lysosomes by endocytosis.

The classes of compounds include proteins, nucleic acids, polysaccharides, glyco-proteins, and others.

The characteristic function of lysosomes is to carry out intracellular digestion, including participation in such processes as metamorphosis, tissue regression, differentiation, and inflammation. Lysosomes have been identified in most animal cells. The highest activities of lysosomal enzymes are located in some specific tissues and cells, e.g., liver, kidney, spleen, intestine, leukocytes, and macrophages. In the lung, the lysosomal enzyme activities are of particular interest because of the alveolar macrophage and other inflammatory cells. Alveolar macrophages carry out phagocytosis, the process of ingesting foreign materials into the cell in membrane-bound vacuoles, or phagosomes. Breakdown of the ingested materials occurs as the lysosomal enzymes are introduced into the phagosomes. The fusion of the two structures, lysosomes and phagosomes, results in a single vacuole where the digestion is carried out. The role of alveolar macrophages, including the involvement of lysosomal enzymes, in defense of the lung have been reviewed by Allison (1971) and Bowden (1973). Some of the lysosomal enzymes of alveolar macrophages studied include hydrolases, hyaluronidase, elastase-like protease, and phospholipases A_1 and A_2 (Fanson and Waite 1973).

The separation of lysosomes from other organelles has remained a difficult task. In the fractionation of liver homogenate, lysosomes sediment with the light mitochondria and heavy microsomes. In most routine studies these lysosome-rich fractions are used. There are several procedures for preparation of lysosomes in sufficient purity. Sawant et al. (1964) have described a procedure for rat liver, and Shibko and Tappel (1965) for rat kidney by which lysosomes are prepared by subfractionation of the light mitochondrial fraction. A single density gradient centrifugation of the mitochondrial or light mitochondrial fraction does not allow a sufficient separation of lysosomes from mitochondria. The important marker enzyme activities in liver and kidney lysosomes are: acid phosphatase, acid deoxyribonuclease, β-glucuronidase, β-galactosidase, aryl sulfatases A and B, acid ribonuclease, and the cathepsins (Tappel 1968).

Only limited studies have been carried out with lung lysosomes. Manning et al. (1966) have shown that rat lung homogenate is moderately rich in acid phosphatase. De Lumen et al. (1972) have studied the subcellular distribution of twelve acid hydrolases in rat lung. In general, the distribution profile is similar to liver lysosomal enzymes in rats and guinea pigs. A fraction rich in lysosomes has been obtained from the light mitochondrial fraction. In this fraction, the specific activities of various enzymes have been shown to increase 3.6–15.7 times that in the original homgenate. A partially purified preparation of lung lysosomes from rabbit has been obtained by Hoffman (1972). Hydrolase activities have also been observed in the lamellar body of alveolar type II cells (Goldfischer et al. 1968; Diaugustine 1974). Other studies include distribution of alkaline phosphatase in lung tissue (Fredricsson 1956), hydrolytic enzymes in bronchial epithelium (Spencer 1959), and increase in hydrolytic enzyme activities in the lung with ozone exposure (Dillard et al. 1972). In all these preparations, an important question that has not been answered is the relative contribution of alveolar macrophages and other inflammatory cells.

5. Microsomes

Unlike the nuclei, mitochondria, and lysosomes, which are discrete cytoplasmic organelles, "microsome" is an operational term, referring to the cell fraction sedimenting at centrifugal speeds exceeding 10,000 g (DE DUVE 1971 a, b; REID 1967). In a conventional fractionation of liver homogenate, the larger and/or denser bodies (nuclei, mitochondria, and much of the lysosomes) are spun down at a speed of 10,000 g within a short time (usually 10 min), and the resulting supernatant is referred to as "postmitochondrial" fraction. To date, most isolation procedures of microsomes involve a prolonged centrifugation of postmitochondrial fraction at high speeds (also referred to as ultracentrifugation, usually 105,000 g for 60–90 min). The pellet thus obtained represents vesicles of membrane fragments usually derived from the endoplasmic reticulum, but the cytoplasmic membrane and membranes of other organelles are also present. The endoplasmic reticulum may be smooth (agranular) or rough (granular), and the microsomal preparation is a mixture of the two, including ribosomes or clusters of ribosomes (polysomes).

A wide variety of enzymatic activities are associated with the microsomal vesicles. Two of the classical functions are protein synthesis, and detoxification of foreign substances (xenobiotics), including drug. Typical markers for the liver microsomes include the activities of glucose-6-phosphatase, Na^+-,K^+- and Mg^{2+}-ATPase, and NADPH-cytochrome c reductase, and the presence of hemoprotein, cytochrome P-450 and the ribonucleoprotein particles, ribosomes (TATA 1969).

Various procedures developed for isolation of microsomes are for studying either the enzymes of the endoplasmic reticulum or the protein-synthesizing activities of the ribosomes. TATA (1969) reviewed the procedures and recommended the conditions that should satisfy the two purposes. Attempts have been made to separate microsomes into smooth and rough membranes, such as by using a discontinuous gradient of 0.25 and 1.3 M sucrose (DALLNER et al. 1966). However, based on the distribution of marker enzyme activities or protein-synthesizing activities, the isolation procedures for microsomes are found to be arbitrary. This is evident from the report of LEWIS and TATA (1973), who found the microsomal markers (glucose-6-phosphatase and ribosomal RNA content) associated with all fractions of a liver homogenate. By a quantitative examination of these markers they demonstrated that as much as 40%–60% could be associated with the low speed fractions, and the remainder with the conventional microsomal fraction. The microsomal vesicles (or fragments of endoplasmic reticulum) could be separated from the 600 g pellet containing broken cell debris, red blood cells, and nuclei by buoyant density gradient centrifugation.

Lung microsomes have been prepared and studied, often in comparison with liver microsomes, by a number of workers (GARFINKEL 1963; OPPELT et al. 1970; BREYER 1971; MATSUBARA and TOCHINO 1971; BEND et al. 1972; FOUTS and DEVEREUX 1972; HOOK et al. 1972). Certain discrepancies apparently exist between lung and liver microsomes, e.g., glucose-6-phosphatase activity is poor in lung microsomes (HOOK et al. 1972). From the point of preparation, hemoglobin contamination remains a problem if 0.25 M sucrose is used as the lung homogenization medium (Bend et al. 1972). The hemoglobin contamination is greatly eliminated if 0.15 M KCl is used as the homogenization medium (Matsubara and Tochino 1971). Based on the enzymatic criteria, the procedure by Bend et al. (1972) provides a microsomal preparation with sufficient yield and purity. However, none of the media is suitable for mitochondria, and therefore cannot be used for lung homogenization inasmuch as both mitochondria and microsomes are to be prepared from the same homogenate. The sucrose–mannitol medium (see Sect. B.IV.3) may yet be considered the most suitable medium, and hemoglobin can be greatly eliminated if the lung is perfused prior to homogenization.

6. Lamellar Bodies and Other Organelles

Lamellar bodies are membranous organelles located in alveolar type II cells. Based on autoradiographic and ultrastructural studies, and analysis of chemical composition, it appears certain that the lamellar bodies are the site of saturated phospholipid synthesis in the lung (Kikkawa and Spitzer 1969; Williams et al. 1971; Williams 1974; Hoffman 1972; Page-Roberts 1972; Adamson and Bowden 1973; Gil and Reiss 1973; Morgan and Morgan 1973; Valdivia 1973; Diaugustine 1974). Isolation of these organelles in pure form should permit detailed studies of surfactant lipid synthesis. To date, several laboratories have reported preparations of lamellar bodies. The methods for bovine lung by Williams et al. (1971) and for guinea pig lung by Valdivia (1973) involve a digestion of lung tissue with a proteolytic enzyme and then a differential centrifugation. Other workers have prepared lamellar bodies from lung homogenates of rats (Page-Roberts 1972; Gil and Reiss 1973) and rabbits (Hoffman 1972) without the digestion procedure, and the lamellar bodies are removed by flotation rather than sedimentation. This latter method permits isolation of the organelles with an intact outer membrane. More recently, Williams (1974) has reviewed the isolation procedures.

It is now well documented that the capillary endothelium of the lung is involved in the metabolism of a variety of vasoactive substances. Studies of Bakhle (1968) and Sander and Higgins (1971) have augmented the concept that the enzyme converting angiotensin I to angiotensin II, is associated with a microsomal or mebrane-rich fraction of endothelial cell origin. Further studies by Ryan and Smith (1971) and Ryan et al. (1972) have demonstrated that the enzymes for conversion of angiotensin I and dephosphorylation of AMP are localized in the plasma membrane, more specifically the pinocytic vesicles, of endothelial cells. Ryan and Smith (1971) have developed a procedure for isolation of the pinocytic vesicles, which involves an incubation of homogenate with lead nitrate and AMP. The incubation results in deposition of lead phosphate on walls of the pinocytic vesicles, thus facilitating their separation by a low speed centrifugation. The vesicles thus prepared are sufficiently pure and capable of carrying out the conversion of angiotensin I, as well as other enzymatic functions, e.g., bradykinin hydrolysis and 5′-nucleotidase activity.

The presence of peroxisomes (microbodies) has been demonstrated in the bronchiolar epithelial (Clara) cells and alveolar type II cells by histochemical techniques and electron microscopy (Petrik 1971). Peroxisomes are a separate class of organelles with defined morphological properties and enzyme content, and they can be isolated by a density gradient centrifugation (DE DUVE and BAUDHUIN 1966, BAUDHUIN 1974). They contain such enzymes as urate oxidase, D-amino acid oxidase, α-hydroxy acid oxidase, and catalase. Their isolation from lung tissue has not yet been reported, but they remain potentially useful for studies of toxic lung damage.

7. Cytosol

Cytosol, the supernatant fraction obtained after a high speed centrifugation of homogenate, generally contains a large number of cytoplasmic (soluble) enzymes. The lung cytosol may not be as rich in the varieties or concentrations of soluble enzymes as the liver cytosol; the overall profile of lung enzyme activities has not yet been determined. A comparative study of enzyme activities in the cytosol of lung and liver tissue has been carried out by WITSCHI (1973a). On a per milligram protein basis, some of the enzyme activities are fairly comparable between lung and liver tissues. On a per cell or per organ basis, however, many of the enzyme activities are much lower in lung than liver tissue. This is because the lung contains much less soluble protein per cell than the liver. Furthermore, certain specific enzyme activities may be high in certain types of cells in the lung, but the cytosol fraction prepared from the whole lung may mask the critical differences in the enzyme activities and substrate utilization of specific cells.

It should be pointed out once again that many investigators express enzyme activities on a per milligram protein basis. Whereas in normal circumstances this may be reasonable, in lung injury the values may be grossly affected by extrapulmonary fluids and proteins. The problem can be overcome by expressing enzyme activities per lung. It is therefore necessary to keep the procedures quantitative, beginning with lung homogenization through cytosol preparation.

C. Biochemical and Enzymatic Determinations

This section will describe the various biochemical and enzymatic parameters used in assessing toxic lung damage. Other objectives are to discuss the relative merits and usefulness of various biochemical methods, including recommendation of the need for more techniques for sensitive and accurate determination of toxic effects.

I. Body Weight and Lung Weight

The body weight of animals provides an index of overall growth. Growth of experimental animals may be affected by exposure, and less weight relative to control animals may signify the toxic nature of an exposure. Most commonly, a lack of food and water consumption may cause a decrease in weight gain during an exposure over a period of days or weeks. With a severe or high level exposure, the weight difference between the exposed and control animals may become large. A drastic diminution of body weight or failure to gain weight may affect enzymatic activities in the lung (SCHOLZ and RHOADES 1971; MASSARO 1973a; KIMBALL et al. 1976) and perhaps also in other tissues or organs. In that situation,

Table 1. Lung weight, and lung protein and DNA content of small rodents [a]

Parameter	Rodent species and strains			
	Swiss/Webster mouse	Long–Evans rat	Webster rat	Sprague–Dawley rat
Lung weight (g)	0.19	1.17	1.40	1.34
Protein (mg/lung)	15.76	85.93	144.97	143.60
DNA (mg/lung)	0.82	8.06	11.46	10.19

[a] MUSTAFA et al. (1982)

a separate control for the weight loss should be used (MUSTAFA and TIERNEY 1978).

The lung weight of animals is essentially the same when they are of the same species, age, and sex (Table 1). This parameter serves as an important index for toxic lung damage. Both low and high level exposures are found to cause significant, often overwhelming, changes in lung weight. Pulmonary edema (e.g., perivascular, interstitial, or alveolar edema), hemorrhage, and/or accumulation of inflammatory cells are the major causes of increase in lung weight during acute, high level exposures, and sometimes in the early phase of low level exposures. A large increase in lung weight that may result under such conditions reflects a gross injury of the lung. An increase in lung weight may also be observed after low level exposures. Such a gain, which occurs over a few days or longer period of time, generally reflects an increase in cellular mass of the lung, including an accumulation of inflammatory cells. After an initial injury, the subsequent reparative and/or proliferative processes (EVANS et al. 1973; MUSTAFA 1974; STEPHENS et al. 1974; DUNGWORTH et al. 1975; WITSCHI and COTE 1976) are thought to be responsible for the increase in lung weight.

Conventionally, an alteration of lung weight is expressed as the ratio or percentage change in the ratio of dry weight to wet weight. The dry weight of the lung is taken after placing it in an oven at 105 °C for 24 h or until the weight is constant. Under normal conditions, the dry weight: wet weight ratio of the lung is 0.22: 1. Alternatively, the percentage lung weight: body weight ratio is expressed as an index of alterations in lung weight (ELSAYED et al. 1982a; ELSAYED and MUSTAFA 1982). Alterations in lung weight or lung weight: body weight ratio have been observed with exposure to ozone (FUKASE et al. 1978; ELSAYED et al. 1982 a, b; MUSTAFA et al. 1982), nitrogen dioxide (ELSAYED and MUSTAFA 1982), and cadmium particles (BOULEY et al. 1977), and administration of butylated hydroxytoluene or hydroxyanisole (OMAYE et al. 1977).

II. Lung Protein and DNA Content

The protein and DNA contents of the lung are altered by lung damage. These two parameters serve as important indices of pollutant toxicity in the lung, as has been shown for ozone (EVANS et al. 1971; WERTHAMER et al. 1974; ELSAYED et al. 1982 a; MUSTAFA et al. 1982), nitrogen dioxide (OSPITAL ET AL. 1981; ELSAYED and MUSTAFA 1982), quartz dusts (ENGELBRECHT and BESTER 1968), butylated hydroxytoluene (WITSCHI and SAHEB 1974; SAHEB and WITSCHI 1975; WITSCHI et al. 1976; ADAMSON et al. 1977; OMAYE et al. 1977), hydrazine compounds (D'SOUZA and BHIDE 1975), and nickel carbonyl (HACKETT and SUNDERMAN 1968).

In acute high level exposures, pulmonary edema, hemorrhage, and inflammatory cells cause an increase in protein content. In low level exposures, the increase in protein content is primarily due to increased synthesis in the lung (see Sect. C.VI), although inflammatory cells are thought to contribute in part. Protein in lung homogenate (or in other subcellular fractions) is determined by the method of LOWRY et al. (1951). Other methods may be used, but this method is considered most suitable. Table 1 provides some typical data for protein content in the lungs of mice and rats.

In acute, high level exposures, when the lung weight increases owing to edema, the DNA content per lung often remains constant, but declines per milligram protein. After low level exposures, the DNA content is found to increase, reflecting cellular proliferation (see Sect. C.VII). However, a part of the increase in DNA content may result from the accumulation of inflammatory cells. Typical values for DNA content in the lungs of mice and rats are shown in Table 1.

III. Oxygen Consumption and Energy Metabolism

Oxygen consumption and energy metabolism, i.e., production and utilization of energy such as in the form of ATP, are among the fundamental processes of cellular metabolism. The major sites for these cellular processes are mitochondria. Alterations of mitochondrial functions provide sensitive indicators of cell damage. Such alterations can be conveniently measured in isolated mitochondria and in homogenate, cells, and tissue slices. Oxygen consumption in lung homogenate requires the presence of an added substrate, but in isolated cells, tissue slices, or isolated intact lung, it can occur without added substrates. Endogenous substrates of the cell support oxygen uptake. The following procedures are described for routine studies.

Assay of O_2 consumption in lung tissue slices, cells, homogenate or mitochondria can be carried out by two methods: using a respirometer (manometric or volumetric type) in which O_2 uptake is measured in volume, or using an oxygraph with an O_2 electrode (polarographic technique) in which O_2 uptake is measured in concentration (or activity). The general principles of the two methods have been discussed by various authors (UMBREIT et al. 1972; SLATER 1967; ESTABROOK 1967; PACKER 1967).

For use in manometric or volumetric respirometers, the assay medium (usually, a phosphate-buffered system) is saturated with O_2. This is particularly useful when tissue slices or intact cells are employed for O_2 consumption. The O_2 saturation generates a large gradient of O_2 between the medium and the center of tissue slices or cells, and facilitates the O_2 diffusion process. In the O_2 polarographic method, an air-saturated medium is used. Typically, a buffered medium (with an osmolarity of 0.3) contains 260 and 230 μM O_2 at 25 °C and 30 °C, respectively.

Both the respirometric and polarographic methods have certain advantages and disadvantages unique to each. Oxygen consumption can be determined in all types of tissue preparation using a respirometer, but the technique is time consuming and laborious. The polarographic technique is much more rapid, but large particulate tissues (e.g., slices) may pose a problem. After the initial uptake, as the O_2 concentration drops in the reaction vessel, O_2 diffusion into tissue becomes rate-limited, causing a decline in the rate of O_2 uptake. With proper caution, e.g., using a limited amount of sliced tissue which will allow a linear initial rate, the difficulty may be overcome.

1. Tissue Slices

Oxygen consumption has been measured in lung tissue slices from a number of animal species, including humans (Table 2). The overall procedure is the same for tissue slices from other organs, except that it is necessary to degas the lung before slicing in order to remove trapped oxygen. The O_2 consumption of lung tissue slices is most commonly determined by using manometric or volumetric respirometers. In another approach, the polarographic method (i.e., an O_2 elec-

Table 2. Oxygen consumption in lung tissue slices

Species	O_2 uptake [a]	Reference
Rat	129	EDSON AND LELOIR (1936)
	107	STADIE et al. (1945)
	129	BARRON et al. (1947)
	73	SIMON et al. (1947)
	144	KREBS (1950)
	48 [b]	CALDWELL and WITTENBERG (1974)
	148	LEVY and HARVEY (1974)
	90 [b, c]	MUSTAFA et al. (1977)
	125 [b, c, d]	MUSTAFA et al. (1977)
	21 [e]	ROSENTHAL and DRABKIN (1944)
	114 [e]	HERAN et al. (1961)
Rabbit	111	BARRON et al. (1947)
	134	KREBS (1950)
	31 [e]	ROSENTHAL and DRABKIN (1944)
Dog	48	STADIE et al. (1945)
	82	KREBS (1950)
	29 [b]	AVIADO (1959)
Human	34	STRAUSS (1964)
	29 [e]	ROSENTHAL and DRABKIN (1944)
	23 [e]	HERAN et al. (1961)

[a] Expressed as μl/min per gram dry tissue at 37 °C
[b] Calculated on the basis of dry weight = 22% of wet weight
[c] Measured at 30 °C
[d] In the presence of 2,4-dinitrophenol (an uncoupler)
[e] Measured in tissue mince

trode) has been used (CALDWELL and WITTENBERG 1974; MUSTAFA et al. 1977). The incubation medium for most studies has been a phosphate-buffered system (UMBREIT et al. 1972) without bicarbonate or CO_2. For the respirometric method (manometric or volumetric) the buffer is generally saturated with 100% O_2 in order to ensure a large driving gradient for O_2 diffusion into the central cell layers of tissue slices. According to CALDWELL and WITTENBERG (1974), the oxygen consumption is maximal when O_2 tension in the medium is 100–200 mm Hg. For the polarographic method the buffer should be saturated with air.

There is a variation in the O_2 uptake values for lung tissue slices from various animal species (Table 2). Even though the lung tissue samples from various species were studied using similar techniques, the O_2 consumption for smaller animals (mouse, rat, guinea pig, and rabbit) was appreciably higher than that for larger animals (cat, dog, sheep, cow, and horse) (BARRON et al. 1947; KREBS 1950). The difference may be attributed to increased proportions of connective tissue (which is metabolically poor) and/or relatively slow tissue metabolism in the lungs of larger animals. Measurement of O_2 uptake in lung tissue slices provides a sensitive parameter for assessing toxic lung damage. Studies of oxygen toxicity (STADIE et al. 1945), ozone exposure (MUSTAFA et al. 1977), phosgene poisoning (SIMON et al. 1947), and other forms of lung injury (AVIADO 1959; STRAUSS 1964) have shown that this parameter changes appreciably in injured tissue relative to control.

2. Isolated Cells

Isolated lung cells consume oxygen. The reported O_2 uptake values (μl/min per gram dry weight) are 26 for rat lung cells (AYUSO et al. 1973) and 101 for rabbit lung cells (GOULD et al. 1972). PEREZ-DIAZ et al. (1977a) have reported a value of 126 natom/h per 10^6 cells isolated from rat lung. Despite its great promise, the O_2 consumption in isolated lung cells cannot be used as a sensitive parameter for assessing lung damage. This is because the cells may have already received an injury during isolation, and the baseline for the metabolic behavior of structural cells in isolation remains uncertain. The O_2 consumption in isolated alveolar macrophages has been studied (MUSTAFA and CROSS 1971; MUSTAFA et al. 1971). Because these cells become exposed to inhaled toxic agents, and they can be conveniently isolated, their O_2 consumption can be used as a suitable parameter.

3. Homogenate

In earlier studies with lung homogenate, BARRON et al. (1947) and SIMON et al. (1947) found the rate of O_2 consumption to be slower than in lung tissue slices. They attributed the slow rate to the loss of nicotinamide adenine dinucleotide (NAD) caused by a high NADase activity present in lung homogenate. These findings apparently had a discouraging effect on further studies of oxidative metabolism using lung homogenate. In a tissue or cell homogenate, the compartmentation of cell constituents is destroyed. The control of substrate availability and O_2 utilization, which exists between the mitochondria and cytoplasm, is lost. The O_2 consumption in a homogenate is therefore slow and limited unless external substrates are added to the system.

Table 3. Relative rates of oxygen uptake for oxidation of various substrates in rat lung homogenate and mitochondria [a]

Substrate	O_2 uptake [b]	
	Homogenate	Mitochondria
2-Oxoglutarate	6	30
Succinate	8	41
Glycerol-1-phosphate	6	28
Ascorbate–Wurster's blue	7	34

[a] Mustafa (1974)
[b] Expressed as nmol/min per milligram for oxidation of substrates in state 3, i.e., in the presence of ATP plus glucose and hexokinase; reaction at 30 °C

Table 4. Relative rates of oxygen uptake for oxidation of substrates in lung homogenates from mouse and rat [a]

Species	Substrate	O_2 uptake [b]
Swiss/Webster mouse	Succinate	240
	Ascorbate + cytochrome c	720
Long–Evans rat	Succinate	868
	Ascorbate + cytochrome c	3355
Webster rat	Succinate	1297
	Ascorbate + cytochrome c	5639
Sprague–Dawley rat	Succinate	1037
	Ascorbate + cytochrome c	3903

[a] Mustafa et al. (1982)
[b] Expressed as nmol/min per lung for oxidation of substrates in state 3, i.e., in the presence of ATP plus glucose and hexokinase; reaction at 30 °C

Oxygen uptake in lung homogenate has been measured in the presence of various substrates, including some of the intermediates of the tricarboxylic acid cycle. The list has been discussed for mitochondria, and the rates of O_2 consumption for oxidation of some substrates in homogenate are shown in Tables 3 and 4. Because of convenience and rapidity, the polarographic method is most commonly used for assay of O_2 uptake in homogenate and mitochondria.

4. Mitochondria

Isolated lung mitochondria are able to oxidize a wide variety of substrates, including the intermediates of the tricarboxylic acid cycle. However, the list presented is not exhaustive since there are many other compounds which are oxidizable in mitochondria. Typical substrates are: isocitrate, 2-oxoglutarate (α-ketoglutarate), malate, and succinate among the tricarboxylic acid cycle intermediates; pyruvate and glycerol-1-phosphate (α-glycerophosphate) which are products of glycolysis; fatty acids, e.g., palmitate; amino acids, e.g., glutamate; monoamines, e.g., tyramine, and 3-hydroxytyramine; artificial substrates, e.g., ascorbate plus tetra-methyl-*p*-phenylenediamine (TMPD), ascorbate plus cytochrome *c* (LEHNINGER 1965; WAINIO 1970). Ketone bodies, e.g., 3-hydroxybutyrate (β-hydroxy-butyrate), which are good substrates for mitochondria from heart and other or-gans, are poorly oxidized in lung mitochondria (FISHER et al. 1973; MUSTAFA and CROSS 1974b). For a rapid assay or characterization of lung mitochondrial O_2 up-take, the recommended substrates covering all three segments of the respiratory chain (LEHNINGER 1965; WAINIO 1970) are: 2-oxoglutarate (an NAD-linked sub-strate), succinate (an FAD-linked substrate), and ascorbate plus TMPD (a sub-strate for the terminal region of the respiratory chain (Tables 3 and 4).

The rate of mitochondrial O_2 uptake may vary markedly, depending upon the respiratory states (LEHNINGER 1965; WAINIO 1970). When measured polaro-graphically, "coupled" mitochondria suspended in an isotonic buffer may exhibit a slow rate of O_2 uptake, referred to as "endogenous respiration". Upon addition of an oxidizable substrate, the O_2 uptake increases, showing a steady rate (state 4 or resting respiration). A marked further increase occurs immediately after addi-tion of adenosine diphosphate (ADP) (state 3 or active respiration). Since ADP is added in finite quantity (inorganic phosphate being already present in excess), the O_2 uptake returns to the previous resting rate (state 4) as soon as ADP is used up. The rapid O_2 uptake for this brief period is also referred to as "phosphory-lating respiration", and the ADP:O ratio is calculated by dividing µmoles ADP added by µatoms oxygen consumed during this period. Another index, called the respiratory control ratio (RCR), is calculated by dividing the state 3 (phosphory-lating) rate by the state 4 rate (obtained after ADP is used up). The reader is re-ferred to ESTABROOK (1967) for further details. Both the ADP:O ratio and RCR are sensitive parameters of mitochondria, and are a measure of functional integ-rity. As the mitochondria become fully uncoupled, the O_2 uptake rate attains maximal (state 3). It is in this state that O_2 uptake should be compared in mitochondria from different sources (Table 5), e.g., control and exposed animals. Most commonly, the state 3 conditions are achieved by adding ATP plus glucose and hexokinase.

When measured manometrically or volumetrically, the oxidative phosphory-lation is assayed in terms of P:O ratio. A "phosphorylation trap" is established by adding ATP plus glucose and hexokinase, which constantly supplies ADP for phosphorylation to ATP. Subsequently, inorganic phosphate (Pi) is determined in the control and experimental flasks, and the difference in the amount of Pi be-comes numerically equal to the number of moles of ATP formed. The reader is referred to UMBREIT et al. (1972) for specific details.

Some of the properties of lung mitochondria are shown in Table 6. Based on these values, it appears that the lung mitochondria thus far isolated in various lab-oratories are not as tightly coupled as the liver and heart mitochondria. The cause of this difference is not known. Preparational artifacts and/or the presence of sur-factant with a "detergent-like behavior" may be responsible.

Alterations of oxidative and energy metabolism in the lung occur under a variety of conditions. These include alterations of oxygen consumption with lung distension (FARIDAY and NAIMARK 1971), hemorrhagic shock (SAYEED and BAUE 1971), lung pathology (HERAN et al. 1961; FRITTS et al. 1963; STRAUSS 1964), ad-

Table 5. Oxygen uptake in lung mitochondria from several animal species

Species	O_2 uptake[a]	Reference
Rat	50	Sayeed and Baue (1971)
	53	Fisher et al. (1973)
	45	Mustafa and Cross (1974a)
Guinea pig	25	Kyle and Riesen (1970)
Rabbit	67[b]	Reiss (1966)
	57[c]	Chen (1967)
	60	Mustafa and Cross (1974b)
	25	Fisher et al. (1973)
Sheep	52	Mustafa and Cross (1974b)
	24	Fisher et al. (1973)
Monkey	42	Mustafa and Cross (1974a)

[a] Expressed as nmol/min per milligram protein for oxidation of succinate in state 3, i.e., in the presence of ADP plus inorganic phosphate, or ATP plus glucose and hexokinase at 30 °C unless otherwise indicated
[b] At 37 °C
[c] At 34 °C

Table 6. Oxidative phosphorylation and respiratory control in lung mitochondria

Species	Substrate	ADP:O	P:O	Respiratory control ratio
Rat[a]	2-Oxoglutarate	2.70		3.2
	Succinate	1.75		3.3
	Glycerol-1-phosphate	1.55		2.2
	Ascorbate–Wurster's blue	0.96		2.0
Rabbit[b]	Succinate		1.70	
Monkey[a]	2-Oxoglutarate	2.60		3.0
	Succinate	1.60		3.3
	Glycerol-1-phosphate	0.48		2.4

[a] Mustafa and Cross (1974a)
[b] Reiss (1966)

ministration of amino acid analogs (Baudach et al. 1971), phosgene poisoning (Simon et al. 1947), hyperoxia (Stadie et al. 1945; Currie et al. 1974; Sanders et al. 1974), and exposure to ozone (Mustafa et al. 1973, 1977, 1982; Mustafa 1974; Mustafa and Cross 1974a; Mustafa and Lee 1976; Elsayed et al. 1982a), nitrogen dioxide (Mustafa et al. 1979, 1980; Elsayed and Mustafa 1982), and silica dusts (Kilroe-Smith and Breyer 1963; Breyer et al. 1964). Alterations of marker enzyme activities in lung mitochondria have been observed with tubercle bacilli infection of the lung (Segal 1966), silicosis (Singh et al. 1976), exposure to silica dusts (Jamieson and Van den Brenk 1962; Bardell and Fowler 1971), and exposure to nitrogen dioxide (RAMAZZOTTO et al. 1971). Other functions of lung mitochondria that are altered include oxidative phosporylation with cigarette smoke (KYLE and RIESEN 1970) and ozone exposure (MUSTAFA and CROSS 1974 a), and membrane permeability (MUSTAFA and CROSS 1974 a).

IV. Glucose Metabolism

Glucose is an important substrate for lung metabolism. Glucose metabolism by the glycolytic pathway, and the hexose monophosphate (HMP) shunt pathway is important for the normal and injured lung, since a variety of intermediates, including energy (ATP) and reducing compounds (NADH and NADPH), are derived from this substrate. It is somewhat unusual that the metabolic functions of the lung occur in more aerobic conditions than those of other organs, but lung tissue converts a large quantity of glucose to lactate, a process that generally occurs in anaerobic conditions. With adequate O_2 supply, glucose utilization in most tissues leads to pyruvate formation, which is then commonly oxidized through the mitochondrial tricarboxylic acid cycle. The conversion of pyruvate to lactate occurs when O_2 supply is rate-limiting. In the normal lung, as much as half the glucose consumed is converted to lactate (Table 7), and this may be increased when the lung is injured (TIERNEY 1971, 1974a, b; YOUNG and TIERNEY 1977; TIERNEY et al. 1977).

1. Glycolytic Pathway

Glucose metabolism in the lung is generally studied using tissue slices and isolated perfused lung. In the rat, both systems are comparable, showing a glucose consumption of 11–15 µmol/h per gram wet tissue (O'NEIL and TIERNEY 1974). Most commonly, tissue slices are incubated in a medium containing Krebs–Ringer bicarbonate buffer (UMBREIT et al. 1972) and in an atmosphere of 95% O_2/5% CO_2 (O'NEIL and TIERNEY 1974). The common parameters of glucose metabolism are the consumption of glucose, production of pyruvate, lactate, and carbon dioxide, and incorporation of glucose carbons into lipid and protein fractions of lung tissue. Studies by SCHOLZ et al. (1972), YEAGER and HICKS (1972), YEAGER and MASSARO (1972), LEVY and HARVEY (1974), O'Neil and TIERNEY (1974), LONGMORE and MOUNING (1976), HAMOSH et al. (1978), and WARSHAW et al. (1980) have shown the relative rates of these parameters using lung tissue slices (Table 8). Some of these parameters have also been studied in isolated perfused lungs

Table 7. Glucose consumption and lactate production in rat lung tissue slices

Glucose consumption[a]	Lactate production[a]	Reference
15.0	14.2	YEAGER and HICKS (1972)
12.9	14.1	O'NEIL and TIERNEY (1974)
13.2	13.2	POSTLETHWAIT and MUSTAFA (1981)

[a] Expressed in µmol/h per lung

Table 8. Utilization of glucose carbon for other metabolic intermediates in
lung slices

Parameter	Distribution of radioactivity from uniformly labeled glucose ^{14}C (%)[a]	
	Rat[b]	Rabbit[c]
Carbon dioxide	23	19
Lactate	40	29.7
Glycogen	1	
Lipid	5	4.4
Amino acid	9	
Protein	2	1.4
Nucleic acid		0.4
Total	80	54.9
Isotope recovery (%)	89	84
Hexose monophosphate shunt activity (% of glucose uptake)	4.2	3.8

[a] Glucose uptake (μmol/h per gram wet tissue) was 19.8 for rat and 10.2 for
rabbit
[b] LEVY (1971)
[c] YEAGER and MASSARO (1974)

(O'NEIL and TIERNEY 1974; RHOADES 1974) and lung cells (AYUSO et al. 1973). Of
the glucose consumed, 20%–25% is apparently oxidized to CO_2, and this may
correspond to a sizable fraction of the overall O_2 consumption observed in lung
tissue slices. Incorporation into proteins and lipids accounts for another significant fraction of glucose consumed. Of particular note, the glucose carbon incorporated into lipids is found mostly in the phospholipid, lecithin (phosphatidylcholine) (SALISBURY-MURPHY et al. 1966), and the incorporation apparently occurs via the formation of glycerol-1-phosphate (FELTS 1964).

Alterations in lung glucose uptake and lactate production have been observed
with exposure to pulmonary carcinogens (SYDOW and WILDNER 1971), lung edema (YOUNG et al. 1980), lung distension (FARIDAY and NAIMARK 1971), sympathetic stimulation (GLAVIANO et al. 1967), lack of ventilation (STUBBS et al. 1977),
and exposure to carbon monoxide (BASSETT and FISHER 1976), hyperoxia (CHVA-
PIL and PENG 1975; TIERNEY et al. 1977; ROBINSON et al. 1978; BASSETT and FISHER
1979), ozone (MUSTAFA et al. 1977), and nitrogen dioxide (OSPITAL et al. 1976).
These studies have shown that alterations in glucose metabolism may offer both
sensitive and early indicators of lung tissue injury.

In addition to measurements of glucose uptake and production of metabolites, the activities of marker enzymes: hexokinase (HK), phosphofructokinase
(PFK), pyruvate kinase (PK), lactate dehydrogenase (LDH), and aldolase, and
the LDH isozymes pattern have been studied. RADY et al. (1980) observed an increase of HK, PFK, PK, and LDH activities in mouse lung after administration
of carcinogenic chemicals, and BUCKLEY and BALCHUM (1967a) observed an increase of LDH and aldolase activities in guinea pig lungs following nitrogen di-

oxide exposure. The lung LDH isozymes pattern showed a shift with beryllium carcinogenesis (REEVES 1967), administration of carcinogenic chemicals (RADY et al. 1980), and exposure to nitrogen dioxide (BUCKLEY and BALCHUM (1967b) and ozone (CHOW et al. 1977). An alteration of lung aldolase activity was shown by RAMAZOTTO and RAPPAPORT (1971) using in vitro nitrogen dioxide exposure.

2. Hexose Monophosphate Shunt

The alternate pathway for glucose oxidation, known as the hexose monophosphate (HMP) shunt or pentose phosphate pathway, seems to have a significant metabolic role in lung tissue injury and repair. Glucose oxidation by this pathway produces ribose which may be incorporated into nucleic acids. However, the major interest remains with the formation of NADPH from NADP by the two initial steps of this pathway, catalyzed by glucose-6-phosphate dehydrogenase (G6PD) and 6-phosphogluconate dehydrogenase (6PGD). By furnishing the reducing equivalent, NADPH participates in numerous reductive and biosynthetic reactions. Some of these reactions that are considered important for the lung include synthesis of fatty acids and surfactant, and reduction of oxidized glutathione (GSSG) to its reduced form (GSH), which in turn participates in the prevention of oxidative and peroxidative damage to cells and tissues. (A further discussion appears in Sect. C.VII.)

The HMP shunt pathway is often studied by following the activities of G6PD and 6PGD, i.e., the formation of NADPH from NADP. These two enzyme activities are determined spectrophotometrically by the method adapted by OSPITAL et al. (1981). An alternate method, as adapted by O'NEIL and TIERNEY (1974), involves determination of the ratio of $^{14}CO_2$ produced from glucose-1 ^{14}C and glucose-6 ^{14}C in a system of lung tissue slices or isolated perfused lung. As the ratio becomes greater than 1, the HMP shunt is thought to become the major pathway for glucose oxidation.

In addition to the glycolytic pathway, the HMP shunt pathway is also altered in lung injury. Exposure to a toxic agent generally causes an increased activity of this pathway as observed for hyperoxia (TIERNEY et al. 1973; KIMBALL et al. 1976), ozone (DE LUCIA et al. 1972; CHOW and TAPPEL 1972, 1973; CHOW et al. 1976; MUSTAFA and LEE 1976; MUSTAFA et al. 1977), nitrogen dioxide (LUNAN et al. 1977; MUSTAFA et al. 1979, 1980; OSPITAL et al. 1981), and paraquat (ROSE et al. 1976). Paraquat and diquat administration also causes a decrease of the NADPH : NADP ratio in the lung at the initial phase (WITSCHI et al. 1977). The HMP shunt, therefore, provides important parameters for assessing toxic lung damage.

V. Lipid Metabolism

Lipid metabolism in the lung has been studied with much interest ever since specific lipids were found to be the major components of lung surfactant. Particularly, dipalmitoylphosphatidylcholine, which is a unique phospholipid and key surfactant component, became the target of study from the points of biosynthesis, metabolism, and its role in surfactant function. Lung lipid metabolism has been elegantly reviewed by several authors (FELTS 1964; DARRAH and HEDLEY-WHYTE

1969; Harlan and Said 1969; Heinemann and Fishman 1969; Masoro 1973; Naimark 1973; Tierney 1974 a, b; Mason 1976). The studies of lung lipid metabolism generally involve characterization of lipids present in lung tissue, cells, or subcellular organelles (e.g., analysis of various lipid species) and biosynthesis using labeled substrates or precursors.

Lung tissue can incorporate acetate and glycerol into lipids, and can also esterify free fatty acids. Popjak and Beeckmans (1950) injected acetate ^{14}C intravenously into rabbits, and after 20 h found that the specific activity of fatty acids in phospholipids was 30 times greater in the lung than in the liver, and it was generally higher in the lung than in other organs. The specific activity of fatty acids in triglycerides was also much greater in the lung than in the liver. Likewise, injected acetate ^{14}C and glycerol ^{14}C were incorporated into phosphatidylcholines (lecithin) and triglycerides in the lung (Lands 1958). However, the ratios of labeled acetate to glycerol incorporated into two classes of lipids were different, suggesting that the diglyceride used for their synthesis was not the same. Wang and Meng (1972) examined a series of substrates, viz., glucose, acetate, pyruvate, and several fatty acids, for their contribution to in vitro lipogenesis in rat lung slices. Both glucose and acetate were rated satisfactory substrates. Fatty acids were readily taken up, and incorporated into lipids. Other studies on substrate utilization include those of Chida and Adams (1967), Naimark and Klass (1967), Gassenheimer et al. (1972), Scholz et al. (1972), Rhoades (1974), and Hamosh et al. (1978).

From the studies of Salisbury-Murphy et al. (1966) and Gilder and McSherry (1972), it is certain that the rate of utilization of free fatty acids by lung tissue depends upon their concentration in the medium. The presence of exogenous glucose in the incubation medium is essential for maximal incorporation of fatty acids. Inhibition of oxidative and energy metabolism, e.g., by cyanide, hypoxia, or low temperature, decreases the esterification of palmitate (Naimark and Klass 1967). Other conditions that affect the uptake of fatty acids or other substrates include altered gas tensions (Newman and Naimark 1968), starvation (Scholz and Rhoades 1971; Scholz 1972), and anoxia (Bassett et al. 1973). Young and Tierney (1972) injected labeled palmitate bound to albumin intravenously into rats, and found that approximately 2% of the palmitate appeared in the lung, and that esterification was complete within 30 min. Of this, up to 90% of labeled palmitate appeared in phospholipids, 30% being in the form of dipalmitoylphosphatidylcholine. In a study comparing the effectiveness of several substrates, Abe and Tierney (1977a) found that labeled glycerol, palmitate, and lysophoshatidylcholine, upon incubation with rat lung slices, incorporated radioactivity into phosphatidylcholine. The incorporation of radioactivity from lysophosphatidylcholine was about ten times greater than that from glycerol or palmitate. The results suggest lysophosphatidylcholine is an important precursor for phosphatidylcholine synthesis.

Studies of lipid synthesis in the lung can be carried out in intact animals, isolated perfused lungs, tissue slices, isolated cells, or subcellular fractions. Some of these studies include those of Tombropoulos (1971, 1973), Naimark (1966), Spitzer et al. (1969), Akino et al. (1971), Scholz and Rhoades (1971), Abe et al. (1972), Abe and Akino (1972), Mason et al. (1972), Wang and Meng (1972,

1974), DARRAH and HADLEY-WHYTE (1973), GOLDNER and BRUMLEY (1974), HALLMAN and GLUCK (1974), and MORIYA and KANOH (1974).

In the biosynthetic process, the routes of substrate entry seem to make a difference to the pathways of synthesis and utilization of substrates. Certain intermediates or precursors cannot enter the cells, and therefore are not appropriate for study in isolated lungs, tissue slices, or cells. For example, selective and enzymatic regulation of synthesis observed under in vivo conditions may be lost when tissue homogenate or a subcellular fraction is used (HILL et al. 1968). Pathways of synthesis can be studied by using labeled substrates and a system approximating the physiologic conditions. ABE and TIERNEY (1977 b) have studied lipid synthesis using two different routes of substrate delivery: through vascular perfusion (i.e., via the capillary endothelial surface) using isolated lungs, and through the cut edges of cells or tissues using lung slices. They observed that the isolated perfused lungs consumed about one-third as much lysophosphatidylcholine as did tissue slices. Such a difference may be due to the pulmonary endothelial surface in the perfused lungs, which may regulate the uptake of circulating precursors, or it may be due to a direct and greater access of substrates to alveolar cells in tissue slices. In addition, the slicing of tissues may cause a release of enzymes into the medium, which would then act upon the substrates and alter their ability to penetrate cellular membranes.

In addition to biosynthesis, formation, and elongation of fatty acids in lung tissue have been studied by HEINEMANN (1961), SCHILLER and BENSCH (1971), SCHILLER and DONABEDIAN (1973), and GROSS and WARSHAW (1974). Much of the synthetic activities apparently occur in the alveolar type II and bronchiolar nonciliated (Clara) cells (BUCKINGHAM et al. 1966; NIDEN 1967; CHEVALIER and COLLET 1972; Petrik and COLLET 1974).

A series of marker enzyme activities related to lipid biosynthesis and lipolysis have been studied in lung tissue. These include the activities of choline kinase and choline phosphotransferase (FARRELL et al. 1974), acyl transferase (FROSOLONO et al. 1971), lipid N-methyltransferase (MORGAN 1969), choline phosphokinase, phosphorylcholine cytidyl transferase, CDP-choline:1,2-diglyceride choline phosphotransferase (CHIDA et al. 1973), phosphorylcholine glyceride transferase and other lecithin biosynthetic enzymes (ZACHMAN 1973 a, b), phosphatidic acid phosphohydrolase (MEBAN 1972; JOHNSTON et al. 1975), phospholipase A (OHTA and HASEGAWA 1972; OHTA et al. 1972), and esterases (O'HARE et al. 1971).

Various toxic inhalants may affect lung lipid metabolism, including substrate utilization, rate of synthesis, and composition of lipids. FLETCHER and WYATT (1970, 1972) observed alterations in lipid synthesis and composition after paraquat poisoning. ABE and TIERNEY (1976) observed that the dipalmitoylphosphatidylcholine content in rat lung was not altered after 3 days of exposure to 100% oxygen, but it doubled within 2 days during recovery from the hyperoxic lung injury. Exposure to nitrogen dioxide also causes alterations of lipid metabolism (BLANK et al. 1978). In addition, peroxidation of unsaturated lipids is considered to be an important mechanism by which a number of toxic agents can cause lung injury. Two oxidant pollutants, e.g., ozone and nitrogen dioxide, are implicated as the inducers of lipid peroxidation in the lung (MENZEL 1970, 1976; MUDD and FREEMAN 1977). A further discussion appears in Sect. C.IX.

VI. Protein Metabolism

Protein metabolism in the lung has been studied to a limited extent, mostly from the point of view of synthesis. The basic knowledge and methodology applied to the lung are essentially derived from studies carried out in the liver and other selected systems. However, such a methodology is not always directly applicable to the lung because of its heterogeneity of cell types. The rates and extent of protein synthesis or metabolism apparently differ for different cell types. Despite these difficulties, protein synthesis and certain aspects of metabolism in the lung have been carried out both in normal conditions and in injury or adverse conditions. Often new techniques have been devised to overcome the problems inherent in the study of lung tissue.

To date, protein synthesis in the lung has been studied using intact animals (MASSARO et al. 1970a, 1971a, b; WITSCHI 1974), isolated perfused lungs (ASKOSAS and HUMPHREY 1958; TRENTALANCE and MANGIATINI 1968a, b), tissue slices (MASSARO et al. 1967; LOW 1974; HAMOSH et al. 1978), organ and tissue culture (MATSUYA and YAMANE 1970; SMITH et al. 1974; STONER 1974; HUSSAIN et al. 1978; HUSSAIN and BHATNAGAR 1979a, b; BHATNAGAR et al. 1979), and cell-free systems (FITSCHEN 1967a, b; MASSARO et al. 1970a; COLLINS and CRYSTAL 1975).

In the in vivo studies, a radiolabeled amino acid is injected intravenously or intraperitoneally, and the incorporation into lung protein is determined after an appropriate interval of time. The in vivo technique is useful in determining the time course and nature of protein synthesis. MASARO et al. (1970a) have demonstrated that labeled amino acids in the blood enter the amino acid pool of the lung, and then are incorporated into lung proteins. Protein synthesis is particularly active in the alveolar type II epithelial cells, as demonstrated by in vivo labeling and autoradiographic studies (CHEVALIER and COLLET 1972; MASSARO and MASSARO 1972).

In vitro studies, particularly with isolated perfused lungs, tissue slices, and cell-free systems, are attractive because systemic effects on lung protein synthesis can be avoided, and quantitative information on the rate and extent of synthesis can be obtained. COLLINS and CRYSTAL (1976) and CRYSTAL (1976) have reviewed the studies on biosynthesis of lung proteins, including collagen, and provided a comparison of various in vivo and in vitro approaches utilized to date. In addition to synthesis, several aspects of analytic and metabolic studies have been carried out. These include lung protein secretion (MASSARO et al. 1970a) and transport (DICKIE and MASSARO 1974), turnover of surfactant protein (SPITZER and NORMAN 1971), lung collagen heterogeneity (BRADLEY et al. 1974a), and alterations with age (BRADLEY et al. 1974b).

Protein synthesis and metabolism in the lung have been studied to determine the effects of a variety of environmental agents. These include effects of carinogens, e.g., uracil mustard (ABELL et al. 1967) and diethylnitrosamine (WITSCHI 1973b), and other chemicals and gases, e.g., paraquat (WITSCHI 1973c), ethionine (WITSCHI 1974), carbon tetrachloride (OGAWA 1972; OKUDA 1973; WITSCHI 1974), thiourea (HOLLINGER et al. 1974), ozone (OKUDA 1973; WERTHAMER et al. 1974; HUSSAIN et al. 1974, 1976, CHOW et al. 1976; MUSTAFA et al. 1977), and hyperoxia (GACAD and MASSARO 1973; MASSARO 1973b; MASSARO and MASSARO

1974; Bhatnagar et al. 1978). Other conditions that affect lung protein synthesis are hypoxia (Chvapil et al. 1970), starvation (Gacad et al. 1972; Massaro 1973a), pulmonary artery ligation (Massaro et al. 1971a, b), and various metabolic factors (Massaro et al. 1971c). Some of the specific proteins studied in the lung include collagen (Davis and Reeves 1971; Bradley et al. 1974a, b; Chvapil and Peng 1975; Hussain et al. 1976; Hussain and Bhatnagar 1979a, b), glycoproteins (De Luca et al. 1971; Bonanni et al. 1973; Levart and Louisot 1973), mucins (Ellis et al. 1972), and proteins associated with surfactant (Spitzer and Norman 1971; Dickie et al. 1973). Protein synthesis has also been studied in alveolar macrophages under certain conditions, e.g., to examine the effects of tobacco smoke (Yeager 1969; Holt and Keast 1973; Low 1974) and phagocytosis (Massaro et al. 1970b).

VII. Nucleic Acid Metabolism

Biochemical and metabolic studies with ribonucleic acid (RNA) and deoxyribonucleic acid (DNA) in the lung are essentially based on methodology developed for other organs or tissues. Typical studies involve biosynthesis of RNA and DNA in terms of incorporation of precursors in order to examine the effects of toxicants on the lung. The DNA content of normal lung increases after birth until the animal matures. Lung growth and DNA content then stabilize, except when the lung is injured or a portion is removed surgically. With lung injury, DNA and RNA biosynthesis increases, which is apparent from increased incorporation of labeled precursors into these macromolecules. Romanova et al. (1967) have examined nucleic acid synthesis and mitotic activity during compensatory lung growth.

For studies of DNA biosynthesis in vivo, usually radioactivity thymidine is injected intravenously, and its incorporation into DNA is measured at appropriate time intervals. Several studies have been reported that used this method to examine the toxic effects on lung tissue (Northway et al. 1972; Witschi 1973a, b, 1974; Witschi and Saheb 1974; Witschi et al. 1976; Aronson et al. 1976). Autoradiographic studies of thymidine incorporation have shown the sites and kinetics of cell renewal in the lung, particularly after an injury (Kleinerman 1970; Evan et al. 1971, 1975, 1976, 1977, 1978).

Kaufman et al. (1972a, b) and Kaufman (1976) have studied RNA metabolism in tracheal epithelium. For studies of RNA biosynthesis, the radiolabeled precursor used for lung tissue is uridine (Bieber et al. 1971; Witschi 1972, 1973 a, b). In a subsequent review, Witschi (1975) has pointed out that whereas orotic acid is useful for the liver, uridine proves to be a much better precursor for RNA in the lung.

VIII. Sulfhydryl Metabolism

Sulfhydryl (SH) groups are constituents of tissue proteins, serum proteins, enzymes, coenzymes, amino acids, and other compounds. The presence of SH groups is essential for the functions of many enzymes and proteins, including those of membranes. These functions may be lost if the SH groups at the active sites are oxidized or altered by an agent. For the purpose of assay, the sulfhydryl compounds are divided into soluble and insoluble forms. The soluble form consists of low molecular weight substances, including reduced glutathione (GSH), which are grouped as nonprotein sulfhydryls (NPSH). The insoluble form, grouped as protein sulfhydryls (PSH), comprises the SH group of enzymes, proteins, and membranes.

The NPSH compounds, particularly GSH, constitute a major pool of cellular reducing compounds, and may be important in determining the cellular redox state. Glutathione is a tripeptide (γ-glutamylcysteinylglycine), which is widely distributed among living cells. Its concentration in the cells may be appreciable, ranging from 0.1 to 5 mM, but only a minor fraction of it may be in the oxidized (GSSG) form (JOCELYN 1972). GSH and NPSH contribute to important biologic processes, including normal structure and function of cells. They participate in numerous biochemical reactions either as a substrate, cosubstrate, or cofactor for enzymes (BOYLAND and CHASSEAUD 1969; JOCELYN 1972, FLOHE et al. 1974; KOSOWER and KOSOWER 1976). GSH is thought to play specific roles in mitotic cells, and may therefore be essential for regenerating, repairing, or proliferating systems (KOSOWER and KOSOWER 1976). GSH is also thought to play protective roles against free radical-mediated or peroxidative damage (LITTLE and O'BRIEN 1968 a; O'BRIEN and LITTLE 1969; DE LUCIA et al. 1972, 1975; CHOW and TAPPEL 1972, 1973; COFFIN and STOKINGER 1977). Other NPSH compound, e.g., coenzyme A and lipoic acid (thioctic acid), are involved in acetylation and oxidative decarboxylation reactions, respectively.

In interactions with the biologic system, many environmental agents behave as metabolic inhibitors. A target of these agents is the SH groups with which they bind, causing an inactivation of the related biochemical system. Binding of toxicants with SH groups may occur in three different ways, oxidation to disulfide, mercaptide formation, and alkylation. Of these reactions, alkylation is usually irreversible, and oxidation and mercaptide formation are reversible under favorable conditions.

Another role of GSH or NPSH is cellular detoxification. Several workers have reported specific reactions of GSH with foreign compounds, including toxic metals (BOYLAND and CHASSEAUD 1969; JOLLOW et al. 1974). Participation in a variety of reactions is possible because GSH contains five potential ligands for complex formation with metal ions: an SH group, an NH_2 group, two COOH groups, and two peptide linkages (KOSOWER and KOSOWER 1976). GSH and other NPSH are capable of undergoing one-electron or two-electron oxidations. Reactions of SH groups with free radicals and metal ions are usually one-electron oxidations, and biologically common. Two-electron oxidations are relatively more complex, and may be of biologic significance, e.g., in thiol–disulfide interchange reactions (KOSOWER and KOSOWER 1976). Cellular reserves of GSH or NPSH can be depleted either reversibly or irreversibly. Various enzymatic reactions utilizing GSH, e.g., in glutathione peroxidase activity, lead to oxidation of GSH to GSSG, and GSH can be regenerated enzymatically using reducing equivalents of NADPH. Irreversible losses of GSH or NPSH occur when SH groups form complexes with heavy metals, e.g., mercury, or other environmental agents (JOLLOW et al. 1974).

Sulfhydryl metabolism in the lung has been widely studied in relation to oxidant effects. Several authors have demonstrated that acute ozone exposure results in an oxidation of GSH or NPSH in lung tissue, and an inhibition of enzymes that are dependent on SH groups for their activities (MOUNTAIN 1963; MUDD et al. 1971; DE LUCIA et al. 1972, 1975). Other reports suggest that oxidants may cause lung cellular injury by oxidizing SH groups either directly or via free radical reactions (FAIRCHILD et al. 1959; NASR 1967; MENZEL 1970; COFFIN and STOKINGER 1977).

1. Measurement of Sulfhydryls

The whole lung homogenate is used for assay of sulfhydryls. The method of SEDLAK and LINDSAY (1968) is adapted to determine nonprotein sulfhydryls (NPSH), and total sulfhydryls (TSH), i.e., SH groups of both protein and nonprotein molecules. The level of protein sulfhydryls (PSH) is then obtained as the difference between TSH and NPSH (DE LUCIA et al. 1972). The procedure specifically adapted for NPSH has been described by DE LUCIA et al. (1975). A normal rat lung (weighing approximately 1 g) contains an average of 1.6 µmol NPSH, of which up to 90% may be GSH. Glutathione (GSH and GSSG) is directly determined by a procedure adapted by DE LUCIA et al. (1975). Two other methods, as described by SRIVASTAVA and BEUTLER (1968) and TIETZE (1969), may be consulted. Although in vitro oxidation of GSH produces mainly GSSG, e.g., by ozone exposure (MUDD et al. 1969; MENZEL 1971) and by lipid peroxides (LITTLE and O'BRIAN 1968 b), measurements of GSH oxidized in vivo show that only 1%–3% of total glutathione occurs in the GSSG form (SRIVASTAVA and BEUTLER 1968; TIETZE 1969). Other disulfide forms, namely mixed disulfides (PSSG) consisting of PSH and GSH, appear to be common, and have been shown to occur in lung tissue (DE LUCIA et al. 1975), mammalian erythrocytes (ALLEN and JANDL 1961), ascites tumor cells (MODIG 1968), human eye lens (HARDING 1969), and several rat tissues (HARRAP et al. 1973) as a significant fraction of the total sulfhydryls present. The method for determination of PSSG in lung homogenate has been described by DE LUCIA et al. (1975). Chemical reduction of PSSG in lung homogenate yields GSH. Under in vivo conditions, the formation of PSSG in the lung seems to be a transient phenomenon, i.e., PSH and GSH eventually return to normal levels (DE LUCIA et al. 1975). Sulfhydryl groups (PSH and NPSH), including GSH, can also be assayed by histochemical techniques (ASGHAR et al. 1975), particularly if their occurrence in cells or cellular sites is to be determined.

2. Assay of Enzyme Activities Related to Sulfhydryl Metabolism

A series of enzyme activities related to glutathione and other NPSH metabolism can be routinely assayed using lung cytosol. Glutathione is thought to be an effective free radical scavenger. In particular, the lipid hydroperoxides formed are reduced to alcohols in the presence of GSH, and the reaction is catalyzed by glutathione peroxidase (LITTLE and O'BRIAN 1968 a, b; CHOW and TAPPEL 1972, 1973). In this reaction, GSH (or other NPSH, if involved) is oxidized to the disulfide, S–S, form. The disulfides, including GSSG, are then reduced to the corresponding sulfhydryls in the presence of NADPH and the appropriate enzymes.

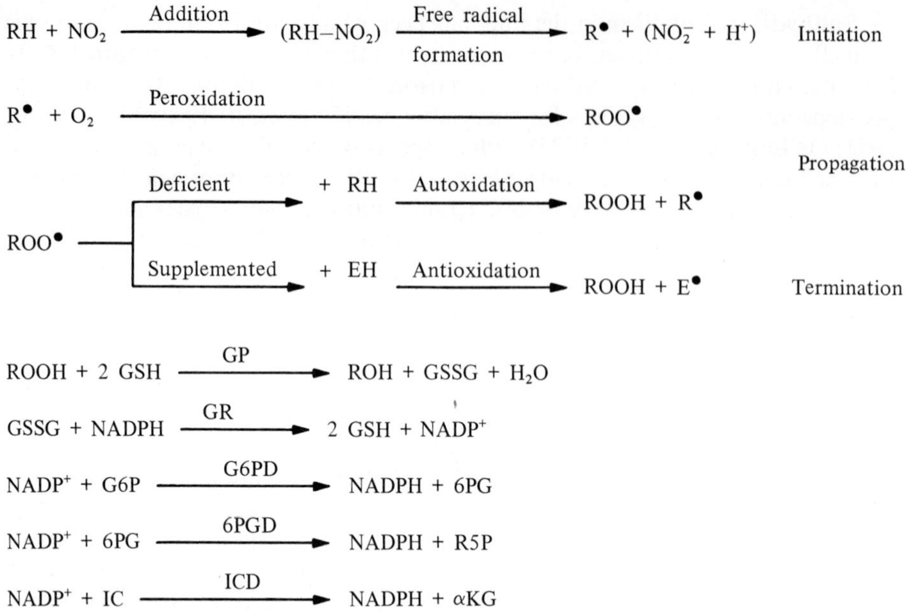

$$RH + NO_2 \xrightarrow{\text{Addition}} (RH{-}NO_2) \xrightarrow[\text{formation}]{\text{Free radical}} R^\bullet + (NO_2^- + H^+) \qquad \text{Initiation}$$

$$R^\bullet + O_2 \xrightarrow{\text{Peroxidation}} ROO^\bullet$$

Propagation

$$ROO^\bullet \begin{cases} \xrightarrow{\text{Deficient} \quad + \text{ RH} \quad \text{Autoxidation}} ROOH + R^\bullet \\ \xrightarrow{\text{Supplemented} \quad + \text{ EH} \quad \text{Antioxidation}} ROOH + E^\bullet \qquad \text{Termination} \end{cases}$$

$$ROOH + 2\,GSH \xrightarrow{GP} ROH + GSSG + H_2O$$

$$GSSG + NADPH \xrightarrow{GR} 2\,GSH + NADP^+$$

$$NADP^+ + G6P \xrightarrow{G6PD} NADPH + 6PG$$

$$NADP^+ + 6PG \xrightarrow{6PGD} NADPH + R5P$$

$$NADP^+ + IC \xrightarrow{ICD} NADPH + \alpha KG$$

Fig. 2. Scheme of a possible mode of action for NO_2 and vitamin E in rat lung. Abbreviations: *RH* lipid; *R*$^\bullet$ lipid radical; *ROO*$^\bullet$ lipid peroxide radical; *EH* vitamin E; *E*$^\bullet$ vitamin E radical; *ROOH* lipid hydroxyperoxide; *ROH* lipid alcohol; *GSH* reduced glutathione; *GSSG* oxidized glutathione; *NADPH* reduced nicotinamide adenine dinucleotide phosphate; *NADP*$^+$ oxidized nicotinamide adenine dinucleotide phosphate; *G6P* glucose-6-phosphate; *G6PD* glucose-6-phosphate dehydrogenase; *6PG* 6-phosphogluconate; *6PGD* 6-phosphogluconate dehydrogenase; *R5P* ribulose-5-phosphate; *IC* isocitrate; *ICD* isocitrate dehydrogenase; and αKG α-ketoglutarate

A scheme has been postulated by Elsayed and Mustafa (1982) as shown in Fig. 2.

Glutathione peroxidase (GP) activity is assayed spectrophotometrically by coupling the reduction of a hydroperoxide (cumene hydroperoxide) to oxidation of NADPH through the glutathione reductase reaction (Ospital et al. 1981, adapted from Little and O'Brien 1968a). Glutathione reductase (GR) catalyzes the reduction of GSSG to GSH using the reducing equivalent of NADPH. The assay involves spectrophotometric determination of NADPH oxidation (at 340 nm) in the presence of GSSG and cytosol (Ospital et al. 1981, adapted from Horn 1965). Oxidation of GSH may also form mixed disulfides, e.g., PSSG or others. Disulfide reductase (DR) catalyzes the reduction of a broad spectrum of disulfides. The assay involves spectrophotometric determination of a disulfide reduction, 5-5'-dithiobis(2-nitrobenzoic acid) (DTNB) (at 412 nm), in the presence of NADP and cytosol (Ospital et al. 1981, adapted from Tietze 1970). Glutathione disulfide transhydrogenase (GDT) catalyzes the reduction of disulfides by transferring the reducing equivalent of GSH, which in turn is oxidized to GSSG. The assay, as described by Ospital et al. (1981), is an adaptation of method used by Tietze (1970).

IX. Lipid Peroxidation

It is now well recognized that lipid peroxidation (autoxidation of unsaturated lipids) is an important molecular mechanism for the deleterious effects of a variety of harmful agents (MEAD 1976; BUS et al. 1976; PLAA and WITSCHI 1976). Generally, free radicals initiate an autoxidation of unsaturated lipids in the membrane which then propagates randomly. The subsequent accumulation of fatty acid epoxides and peroxides in tissues leads to injury and death of cells. Exposure to ozone, nitrogen dioxide, or high concentrations of oxygen are thought to initiate this type of peroxidative damage in the lung (THOMAS et al. 1968; GOLDSTEIN et al. 1969; ROEHM et al. 1971; CHOW and TAPPEL 1972, 1973; CROSS et al. 1976; MENZEL 1976; MUDD and FREEMAN 1977; WITSCHI and COTE 1977; MUSTAFA and TIERNEY 1978).

Despite the importance of this mechanism in tissue damage, a quantitative determination of lipid peroxidation remains difficult, and its in vivo occurrence or assessment is controversial. Several procedures are currently applied for measuring lipid peroxidation. Any one of these products can ascertain the occurrence of lipid peroxidation, but cannot provide a quantitative measure of the overall process.

1. Conjugated Dienes

Lipids contain nonconjugated dienes or polyenes. Upon attack by a free radical or an agent capable of abstracting a hydrogen atom, the dienes or polyenes show a shift of double bond positions leading to conjugation. The conjugated dienes are measured in tissue extracts by ultraviolet spectrophotometry (absorption maximum at 233 nm with a shoulder due to ketone dienes between 260 and 280 nm). The conjugated trienes show an absorption maximum at 288 nm. The method has been described by several workers (RECKNAGEL and GHOSAL 1966; HAASE and DUNKLEY 1969; SELL and REYNOLDS 1969). A limitation of the method is that it is nonspecific, and the extinction coefficients used for biologic systems are only approximate. Since the conjugated dienes are formed of fatty acids containing at least two sets of double bonds, the peroxidation of monoenoic fatty acids will remain undetected by this method.

2. Fatty Acid Epoxides

Unsaturated lipids can be converted to epoxides in tissues by processes similar to those occurring with polycyclic aromatic hydrocarbons (SIMS and GROVER 1974; KADIS 1978). The epoxide-containing lipids have been demonstrated in rat lung, and lipid peroxidation is apparently a major cause of epoxide formation, since oxidant exposures increase lipid epoxides in rat lung (SEVANIAN et al. 1979, 1980 a). The measurement of lipid epoxides (epoxides of fatty acids and cholesterol) offers another sensitive index of lipid peroxidation. The assay procedure involves extraction of epoxides and analysis by gas chromatography–mass spectroscopy (SEVANIAN et al. 1979, 1980 a, b).

3. Malonaldehyde

The measurement of lipid peroxidation by the thiobarbituric acid (TBA) test has been widely used. Malonaldehyde, a dialdehyde, is a breakdown product of fatty acids containing two or more sets of double bonds. A color reaction that occurs between malonaldehyde and TBA (TBA–malonaldehyde chromatophore with an absorption maximum at 532 nm) serves as an index for lipid peroxidation in tissues. The test system has been reviewed by several authors (Barber and Bernhein 1967; Slater 1972; Logani and Davies 1980). More recently, Asakawa and Matsushita (1980) have shown that metal ions, such as ferrous iron, are important in the assay because they seem to accelerate the release of TBA-reacting materials from lipid hydroperoxides. Accordingly, the TBA test can accurately represent the amount of fatty acid hydroperoxides, either as malonaldehyde or other TBA-reacting materials originating from hydroperoxides (Terao and Matsushita 1981). Although the method offers a reliable index of lipid peroxidation, there may still be some problems. An absence of malonaldehyde or TBA-reacting material may not be an indication of the absence of lipid peroxidation. This is because malonaldehyde may be metabolized in tissue, as reported by several workers (Recknagel and Ghoshal 1966a; Horton and Packer 1970). Lipid peroxides are also reported to be metabolized in tissues (Little and O'Brien 1968a; O'Brien and Little 1969; Chow and Tappel 1972). In addition, malonaldehyde will not be formed from lipids with fatty acids containing only one set of double bonds.

4. Fluorescent Products

The peroxidation of polyunsaturated fatty acids forms not only hydroperoxides, but also a great many carbonyl compounds, including malonaldehyde. The carbonyl compounds, being highly reactive, undergo reactions with a variety of tissue components, giving rise to fluorescent products. Specifically, the carbonyl compounds react with the amino groups of proteins, amino acids, and phospholipids (phosphatidylethanolamine) to form fluorescent compounds (Chio and Tappel 1969). Malonaldehyde undergoes decomposition, and the decomposition products react with proteins (Shin et al. 1972). Malonaldehyde also reacts with DNA, yielding fluorescent products (Reiss et al. 1972). Dillard and Tappel (1973) have shown that the fluorescent chromophores derived from phosphatidylethanolamine (lipid soluble) and phenylalanine (water soluble), and those associated with age pigment (lipofuscin) have similar spectral characteristics. The major fluorescent species arising from lipid peroxidation appear to be conjugated Schiff base fluorophores, which are formed as the products of cross-linking of two primary amines with malonaldehyde (Chio and Tappel 1969). The assay method involves extraction, and analysis by fluorospectrophotometry (Trombly and Tappel 1975). The measurement of fluorescent compounds may provide sensitive and selective markers of lipid peroxidation in vitro and in vivo (Tappel 1980; Logani and Davies 1980). However, the extraction procedure may yield components that are fluorescent, but not necessarily lipid peroxidation products.

5. Hydrocarbon Gases

The release of low molecular weight hydrocarbon gases in exhaled air was first observed by RILEY et al. (1974), who treated mice with carbon tetrachloride, a known inducer of lipid peroxidation. Since then, several laboratories have measured hydrocarbon gases as an index of lipid peroxidation in vivo (HAFEMAN and HOEKSTRA 1977; DILLARD et al. 1977; DOWNEY et al. 1978; ICHINOSE and SAGAI 1982). The hydroperoxides resulting from lipid peroxidation undergo decomposition to alkoxy radicals, which then ultimately give rise to hydrocarbon gases. Theoretically, various hydrocarbons can be generated, but ethane and pentane have been detected. Because of multiplicity of products and lack of their quantitation, it is difficult to develop a quantitative relationship between lipid peroxidation and release of hydrocarbon gases. The source of hydrocarbons is also debatable (GELMONT et al. 1981).

There is another technique, developed by MAY and MCCAY (1968), which exploits the loss of polyunsaturated fatty acids as an index for the detection and assessment of lipid peroxidation. In this method, the total fatty acid profile of the tissue lipids is determined by gas–liquid chromatography before and after lipid peroxidation. The amount of polyunsaturated fatty acids lost in the peroxidized lipids is determined by comparison with the control profile. The method has the virtue that it directly assesses the fatty acids destroyed, and hence can provide a quantitative measure of lipid peroxidation in biologic systems.

X. Other Enzyme Activities and Metabolic Pathways

In addition to those already discussed, a series of enzyme activities, either serving as markers or carrying out key reactions of certain metabolic pathways in the lung, have been studied in a variety of contexts.

1. Histochemical Localization of Enzyme Activities

Histochemical studies are excellent in localizing enzyme activities in cells or subcellular organelles. This is particularly important for the lung, which is composed of heterogeneous cell types, not all of which are metabolically very active. The oxidative enzyme pattern in the lung has been studied by TYLER and PEARSE (1965), and AZZOPARDI and THURLBECK (1967, 1968, 1969). Some of the cells and tissue sites that have received attention are the interalveolar septum (alveolar type II cells), bronchial mucous glands, and bronchiolar nonciliated (Clara) cells. A variety of enzyme activities, including those of mitochondrial oxidative, cytoplasmic glycolytic, and hexose monophosphate shunt pathways have been identified. Other histochemical studies include localization of lactate dehydrogenase activity in alveolar type II cells after nitric oxide or nitrogen dioxide exposure (SHERWIN et al. 1968, 1972; YUEN and SHERWIN 1971).

2. Enzyme Activities Related to Detoxification

There are mechanisms (other than the airway mucociliary transport and the alveolar macrophage clearance) by which the lung can defend itself to a degree against toxic damage. In one type of mechanism, considered extrinsic, the protection is afforded when certain nutrients or chemicals are present (Mustafa and Tierney 1978). An example of this mechanism is the antioxidant protection of the lung against ozone, nitrogen dioxide, and hyperoxia provided by vitamin E (Kann et al. 1964; Chow and Tappel 1972, 1973; Fletcher and Tappel 1973; Mustafa 1975; Sato et al. 1976; Elsayed and Mustafa 1982), ascorbate (Willis and Kratzing 1974; Fukase et al. 1975), sulfhydryl compounds (Fairchild et al. 1959; Jamison and Van den Brenk 1964), selenium (Elsayed et al. 1982b; Cross et al. 1977), and other chemicals and drugs (Giri et al. 1975; Sahebjami et al. 1974).

The other type of mechanism is referred to as intrinsic or metabolic defense. In this category, several metabolic pathways are thought to be involved in either prevention of toxic damage or repair of tissue after injury (Mustafa and Tierney 1978). Examples are the HMP shunt producing NADPH, sulfhydryl metabolism utilizing GSH, and others. The toxicity caused by hyperoxia, ozone, nitrogen dioxide, and many other chemical agents often involves free radical reactions, as well as reactions of toxic products that are generated. Normal cells may contain enzymatic mechanisms that serve to eliminate free radicals and peroxides or toxic metabolites. Examples of such enzymatic mechanisms are superoxides dismutase, glutathione peroxidase, catalyse, and others.

Oxygen toxicity is related, at least in part, to the production of superoxide anion, which is a free radical. The enzyme superoxide dismutase (SOD), which acts upon this free radical, is ubiquitous in oxygen-metabolizing cells (Fridovich 1974). The enzyme is expected to offer protection against oxygen-mediated free radical damage at the cellular and organ levels. A stimulation of SOD activity has been observed with hyperoxia in lung tissue (Crapo and Tierney 1974; Autor et al. 1976; Kimball et al. 1976; Liu et al. 1977; Frank et al. 1977, 1978a; Nirurkar et al. 1978), and in alveolar macrophage (Fisher et al. 1974a; Rister and Baehner 1976, 1977). The stimulation is considered to be specific for hyperoxia (Douglas et al. 1977; Liu et al. 1977; Crapo et al. 1978a; Stevens and Autor 1980), although Robinson et al. (1978) failed to observe it in this condition. Others reported a stimulation of SOD with ozone (Mustafa et al. 1975), nitrogen dioxide (Crapo et al. 1978a), butylated hydroxytoluene (Omaye et al. 1977), and paraquat (Montgomery 1977) injury of the lung. The assay of SOD requires some attention. There are two types of SOD in lung tissue, and their assay conditions are different (Crapo et al. 1978a). The assay methods have been reviewed by McCord et al. (1977). A method for preparation of lung SOD (Crapo et al. 1978b) and an immunologic assay (Crapo and McCord 1976) have also been reported.

Glutathione peroxidase activity (already discussed in Sect. C.VIII) is reported to be associated with destruction of lipid peroxides, but Cross and Last (1977) did not observe any correlation between this enzyme activity and pulmonary oxygen toxicity.

3. Other Enzyme Activities

Some of the other enzyme activities in the lung that can be used as markers for toxic lung injury include microsomal mixed-funtion oxidase, a variety of cytosolic enzymes, and selected enzymes of certain cell types. Mixed-function oxidation and xenobiotic metabolism in the lung are among the important nonrespiratory functions. Hook and Bend (1976) have reviewed the subject, and it will be discussed in Chap. 14.

Some of the enzymes studied in lung cytosol include those that mediate biosynthesis, degradation, and phosphorylation of pyrimidines (Witschi 1972, 1973 a), carry out glycolysis, viz., hexokinase, phosphofructokinase, aldolase, and pyruvate kinase (Sydow and Wildner 1971), metabolize prostaglandin F_2 (Granstrom 1971), act as esterases (Vatter et al. 1968; Brebner and Kalow 1970), and hydrolyse lysolecithin (lysolecithin acyl hydrolase) (Gershon and Gatt 1976). The lung participates in the metabolism of circulating prostaglandins (Piper et al. 1970). Two enzymes that participate in this metabolism are prostaglandin dehydrogenase and prostaglandin Δ^{13}-reductase. In addition, lung tissue also synthesizes and releases prostaglandins into the circulation. Exposure to hyperoxia or toxic gases results in alterations of both synthesis and metabolism in the lung (Chaudhari et al. 1979). In addition, Wilson (1972) has reported the lung enzyme patterns in young and old mice.

D. Conclusion

The nonrespiratory functions of the lung, particularly the metabolic parameters, have received increased attention because of their usefulness in assessing lung damage due to toxicity or disease. The methodology applied to the lung is generally an adaptation of that used for other organs and tissues, although the tissue structure and cellular composition of the lung often make it difficult to work with this organ. This chapter provides a summary of information on lung enzymology and related biochemistry applicable to the assessment of toxic lung damage.

References

Abe M, Akino T (1972) Comparison of metabolic heterogeneity of glycerolipids in rat lung and liver. Tokoho J Exp Med 106:343–355

Abe M, Tierney DF (1976) Lipid metabolism of rat lung during recovery from lung injury. Fed Proc 35:479

Abe M, Tierney DF (1977 a) Lung lipid metabolism after 7 days of hydrocortisone administration to adult rats. J Appl Physiol 42:202–205

Abe M, Tierney DF (1977 b) Lysophosphatidylcholine (LPC) incorporation into phosphatidylcholine (PC) of rat lung tissue slices (TS) and isolated perfused lungs (IPL). Fed Proc 36:480

Abe M, Akino T, Ohno K (1972) The formation of lecithin from lysolecithin in rat lung supernatant. Biochim Biophys Acta 280:275–280

Abell CW, Rosini LA, DiPao O (1967) Effects of uracil mustard on DNA, RNA, and protein biosynthesis in tissues of A-J mice. Cancer Res 27:1101–1108

Adamson IYR, Bowden DH (1973) The intracellular site of surfactant synthesis. Autoradiographic studies on murine and avian lung explants. Exp Mol Pathol 18:112–124

Adamson IYR, Bowden DH (1974) The type 2 cell as progenitor of alveolar epithelial regeneration. Lab Invest 30:35–42

Adamson IYR, Bowden DH, Cote MF, Witschi HP (1977) Lung injury induced by butylated hydroxytoluene. Cytodynamic and biochemical studies in mice. Lab Invest 36:26–32

Akino T, Abe M, Arai T (1971) Studies on the biosynthetic pathways of molecular species of lecithin by rat lung slices. Biochim Biophys Acta 248:274–281

Allen DW, Jandl JH (1961) Oxidative hemolysis and precipitation of hemoglobin. II. Role of thiols in oxidant drug action. J Clin Invest 40:454–475

Allison AC (1971) Lysosomes and the toxicity of particulate pollutants. Arch Intern Med 128:131–138

Aronson JF, Johns LW, Pietra GG (1976) Initiation of lung cell proliferation by trypsin. Lab Invest 34:529–536

Asakawa T, Matsushita S (1980) Coloring conditions of thiobarbituric acid test for detecting lipid hydroperoxides. Lipids 15:137–140

Asghar K, Reddy BG, Krishna G (1975) Histochemical localization of glutathione in tissues. J Histochem Cytochem 23:774–779

Askosas BA, Humphrey JH (1958) Formation of antibody by isolated perfused lungs of immunized rabbits. Biochem J 70:212–222

Autor AP, Frank L, Roberts RJ (1976) Developmental characteristics of pulmonary superoxide dismutase: relationship to idiopathic respiratory distress syndrome. Pediatr Res 10:154–158

Aviado DM (1959) Therapy of experimental pulmonary edema in the dog with special reference to burns of the respiratory tract. Circ Res 7:1018–1030

Ayuso MS, Fisher AB, Perilla R, Willamson JR (1973) Glucose metabolism by isolated rat lung cells. Am J Pathol 225:1153–1160

Azzopardi A, Thurlbeck WM (1967) The oxidative enzyme pattern in developing and adult mice and adult rabbits. Lab Invest 16:706–716

Azzopardi A, Thurlbeck WM (1968) Oxidative enzyme pattern of the bronchial mucous glands. Am Rev Respir Dis 97:1038–1045

Azzopardi A, Thurlbeck WM (1969) The histochemistry of the nonciliated bronchiolar epithelial cell. Am Rev Respir Dis 99:516–525

Bakhle YS (1968) Conversion of angiotensin I to angiotensin II by cell-free extracts of dog lung. Nature 220:919–921

Barber AA, Bernheim F (1967) Lipid peroxidation: its measurement, occurrence and significance in animal tissues. Adv Gerontol Res 2:355–403

Bardell D, Fowler AK (1971) Inhibition of dehydrogenase activity in lung tissue due to breathing oxygen at atmospheric pressure. Aerosp Med 42:432–435

Barron ESG, Miller ZB, Bartlett GR (1947) Studies of biological oxidations. XXI. The metabolism of lung as determined by study of slices and ground tissue. J Biol Chem 171:791–800

Bassett DJ, Fisher AB, Rabinowitz JL (1973) Effect of anoxia on lipid synthesis by the lung. Fed Proc 32:364

Bassett DJP, Fisher AB (1976) Metabolic response to carbon monoxide by isolated rat lungs. Am J Physiol 230:658–663

Bassett DJP, Fisher AB (1979) Glucose metabolism in rat lung during exposure to hyperbaric O_2. J Appl Physiol 45:943–949

Baudach H, Widow W, Peck U, Behrendt G (1971) Über die Beeinflussung der Sauerstoffaufnahme von Lungengewebeschnitten durch THAM und Antibiotika. Z Exp Chir 4:236–240

Baudhuin P (1974) Isolation of rat liver peroxisomes. In: Fleischer S, Packer L (eds) Biomembrane, part A. Academic, New York, pp 356–368 (Methods in enzymology, vol 31)

Bend JR, Hook GER, Easterling RE, Gram TE, Fouts JE (1972) A comparative study of the hepatic and pulmonary microsomal mixed-function oxidase systems in the rabbit. J Pharmacol Exp Ther 182:206–217

Bhatnagar RS, Hussain MZ, Streifel J, Tolentino M, Enriquez B (1978) Alterations of collagen synthesis in lung organ culture by hypertoxic environment. Biochem Biophys Res Commun 83:392–397

Bhatnagar RS, Hussain MZ, Belton JC (1979) Applications of lung organ culture in environmental investigations. In: Lee SD, Mudd JB (eds) Assessing Toxic effects of environmental pollutants. Ann Arbor Science Publishers, Ann Arbor, pp 121–149

Bieber MM, Cogan MG, Durbridge TC, Rosan RC (1971) Oxygen toxicity in the newborn guinea-pig lung. The incorporation of tritiated uridine into monoribosomes. Biol Neonatorum 17:35–43

Blank ML, Dalbey W, Nettesheim P, Price J, Creasia D, Snyder F (1978) Sequential changes in phospholipid composition and synthesis in lungs exposed to nitrogen dioxide. Am Rev Respir Dis 117:273–280

Bonanni F, Levinson SS, Wolf G, De Luca L (1973) Glycoproteins from the hamster respiratory tract and their response to vitamin A. Biochim Biophys Acta 297:441–451

Bouley G, Dubreuil A, Despaux N, Boudene C (1977) Toxic effects of cadmium microparticles on the respiratory system: an experimental study on rats and mice. Scand J Work Environ Health 3:116–121

Bowden DH (1973) The alveolar macrophage and its role in toxicology. CRC Crit Rev Toxicol 2:95–124

Boyd MR (1977) Evidence for the Clara cell as a site of cytochrome P-450 dependent mixed function oxidase activity in lung. Nature 269:713–715

Boyland E, Chasseaud LG (1969) The role of glutathione and glutathione-S-transferases in mercapturic acid biosynthesis. Adv Enzymol 32:173–219

Bradley K, McConnell-Breul S, Crystal RG (1974a) Lung collagen heterogeneity. Proc Natl Acad Sci USA 71:2828–2832

Bradley KH, McConnell-Breul SD, Crystal RG (1974b) Lung collagen composition and synthesis: Characterization and changes with age. J Biol Chem 249:2674–2683

Brebner J, Kalow W (1970) Soluble esterases of human lung. Can J Biochem 48:970–978

Breyer MG, Kilroe-Smith TA, Prinsloo H (1964) Changes in activities of respiratory enzymes in lungs of guinea-pigs exposed to silica dust. II. Comparison of the effects of quartz dust and lampblack on the succinate oxidase system. Br J Ind Med 21:32–34

Breyer U (1971) Metabolism of the phenothiazine drug perazine by liver and lung microsomes from various species. Biochem Pharmacol 20:3341–3351

Buckingham S, Heinemann HO, Sommers SC, McNary WF (1966) Phospholipid synthesis in the large pulmonary alveolar cell. Am J Pathol 48:1027–1041

Buckley RD, Balchum OJ (1967a) Enzyme alterations following nitrogen dioxide exposure. Arch Environ Health 14:687–692

Buckley RD, Balchum OJ (1967b) Effects of nitrogen dioxide on lactic dehydrogenase isozymes. Arch Environ Health 14:424–428

Bus JS, Aust SD, Gibson JE (1976) Paraquat toxicity: proposed mechanism of action involving lipid peroxidation. Environ Health Perspect 16:139–146

Caldwell PRB, Wittenberg BA (1974) The oxygen dependency of mammalian tissue. Am J Med 57:447–452

Chaudhari A, Sivarajah K, Warnock R, Eling TE, Anderson MW (1979) Inhibition of pulmonary prostaglandin metabolism by exposure of animals to oxygen or nitrogen dioxide. Biochem J 184:51–57

Chen RF (1967) Removal of fatty acids from serum albumin by charcoal treatment. J Biol Chem 242:173–181

Chevalier G, Collet AJ (1972) In vivo incorporation of choline-^{3}H, Leucine-^{3}H and galactose-^{3}H in alveolar type II pneumocytes in relation to surfactant synthesis. A quantitative radioautographic study in mouse by electron microscopy. Anat Rec 174:289–310

Chida N, Adams FH (1967) Incorporation of acetate into fatty acids and lecithin by lung slices from fetal and newborn lambs. J Lipid Res 8:335–341

Chida N, Hirono H, Nishimura Y, Arakawa T (1973) Choline phosphokinase, phosphorylcholine cytidyltransferase and CDP-choline; 1,2-diglyceride cholinephosphotransferase activity in developing rat lung. Tokoho J Exp Med 110:273–282

Chio KS, Tappel AL (1969) Synthesis and characterization of the fluorescent products derived from malonaldehyde and amino acids. Biochemistry 8:2821–2827

Chow CK, Tappel AL (1972) an enzymatic protective mechanism against lipid peroxidation damage to lungs of ozone-exposed rats. Lipids 7:518–524

Chow CK, Tappel AL (1973) Activities of pentose shunt and glycolytic enzymes in lungs of ozone-exposed rats. Arch Environ Health 26:205–208

Chow CK, Hussain MZ, Cross CE, Dungworth DL, Mustafa MG (1976) Effects of low levels of ozone on rat lungs. I. Biochemical responses during recovery and reexposure. Exp Mol Pathol 25:182–188

Chow CK, Cross CE, Kaneko JJ (1977) Lactate dehydrogenase activity and isoenzyme pattern in lungs, erythrocytes, and plasma of ozone-exposed rats and monkeys. J Toxicol Environ Health 3:877–884

Chvapil M, Peng YM (1975) Oxygen and lung fibrosis. Arch Environ Health 30:528–532

Chvapil M, Hurych J, Mirejovska E (1970) Effect of long-term hypoxia on protein synthesis in granuloma and in some organs of rats. Proc Soc Exp Biol Med 135:613–617

Coffin DL, Stokinger HE (1977) Biological effects of air pollutants. In: Stern AC (ed) Airpollution, vol 2. Academic, New York, pp 231–361

Collins JF, Crystal RG (1975) Characterization of cell-free synthesis of collagen by lung polysomes in a heterologous system. J Biol Chem 250:7332–7342

Collins JF, Crystal RG (1976) Protein synthesis. In: Crystal RG (ed) The biochemical basis of pulmonary function, vol 2. Marcel Dekker, New York, pp 171–212

Crapo JD, McCord JM (1976) Oxygen induced changes in pulmonary superoxide dismutase assayed by antibody titrations. Am J Physiol 231:1196–1203

Crapo JD, Tierney DF (1974) Superoxide dismutase and pulmonary oxygen toxicity. Am J Physiol 226:1404–1407

Crapo JD, Sjostrom K, Drew RT (1978a) Tolerance and cross-tolerance using NO_2 and O_2. I. Toxicology and biochemistry. J Appl Physiol 44:364–369

Crapo JD, McCord JM, Fridovich I (1978b) Preparation and assay of superoxide dismutases. In: Fleischer S, Packer L (eds) Biomembranes, part D: biological oxidations – mitochondrial and microbial systems. Academic, New York, pp 382–393 (Methods in enzymology, vol 53)

Cross CE, Last JA (1977) Lack of correlation between glutathione peroxidase activities and susceptibility to O_2 toxicity in rat lungs. Res Commun Chem Pathol Pharmacol 17:433–446

Cross CE, De Lucia AJ, Reddy AK, Hussain MZ, Chow CK, Mustafa MG (1976) Ozone interaction with lung tissue: biochemical approaches. Am J Med 60:929–935

Cross CE, Hasegawa G, Reddy KA, Omaye ST (1977) Enhanced lung toxicity of O_2 in selenium-deficient rats. Res Commun Chem Pathol Pharmacol 16:695–706

Crystal RG (1976) Biochemical processes in the normal lung. In: Bouhuys A (ed) lung cells in disease. North-Holland, Amsterdam, pp 17–38

Currie WD, Pratt PC, Sanders AP (1974) Hyperoxia and lung metabolism. Chest (Suppl) 66:19S–21S

Dallner G, Siekevitz P, Palade GE (1966) Biogenesis of endoplasmic reticulum membrane. II. Synthesis of constitutive microsomal enzymes in developing rat hepatocyte. J Cell Biol 30:97–117

Darrah HK, Hedley-Whyte J (1969) Abnormalities in lung chemistry. Anesth Analg (Cleve) 48:148–165

Darrah HK, Hedley-Whyte J (1973) Rapid incorporation of palmitate into lung: site and metabolic fate. J Appl Physiol 34:205–213

Davis HV, Reeves AL (1971) Collagen biosynthesis in rat lungs during exposure to asbestos. Am Ind Hyg Assoc J 32:599–602

De Duve C (1971a) Tissue fractionation: past and present. J Cell Biol 50:20D–55D

De Duve C (1971b) General principles. In: Roodyn DB (ed) Enzyme cytology. Academic, New York, pp 1–26

De Duve C, Baudhuin P (1966) Peroxisomes (microbodies and related particles). Physiol Rev 46:323–357

De Luca L, Anderson H, Wolf G (1971) The in vivo and in vitro biosynthesis of lung tissue glycopeptides. Arch Intern Med 127:853–857

De Lucia AJ, Hoque PM, Mustafa MG, Cross CE (1972) Ozone interaction with rodent lung. Effect on sulfhydryls and sulfhydryl-containing enzyme activities. J Lab Clin Med 80:559–566

De Lucia AJ, Mustafa MG, Hussain MZ, Cross CE (1975) Ozone interaction with rodent. III. Oxidation of reduced glutathione and formation of mixed disulfides between protein and nonprotein sulfhydryls. J Clin Invest 55:794–802

De Lumen BO, Taylor S, Urribarri N, Tappel AL (1972) Subcellular localization of acid hydrolases in rat lungs. Biochim Biophys Acta 268:597–600

DiAugustine RP (1974) Lung concentric lamellar organelle. Hydrolase activity and compositional analysis. J Biol Chem 249:584–593

Dickie K, Massaro D (1974) Protein transport by lung. Proc Soc Exp Biol Med 145:154–156

Dickie KJ, Massaro GD, Marshall V, Massaro D (1973) Amino acid incorporation into protein of surface-active lung fraction. J Appl Physiol 34:606–614

Dillard CJ, Tappel AL (1973) Fluorescent products from reactions of peroxidizing polyunsaturated fatty acids with phosphatidyl ethanolamine and phenylalanine. Lipids 8:183–189

Dillard CJ, Urribarri N, Reddy K, Fletcher B, Taylor S, De Lumen B, Langberg S, Tappel AL (1972) Increased lysosomal enzyme activities in lungs of ozone-exposed rats. Arch Environ Health 25:426–431

Dillard CJ, Dumelin EE, Tappel AL (1977) Effect of dietary vitamin E on expiration of pentane and ethane by the rats. Lipids 12:109–114

Douglas JS, Curry G, Geffkin SA (1977) Superoxide dismutase and pulmonary ozone toxicity. Life Sci 20:1187–1192

Downey JE, Irving DH, Tappel AL (1978) Effects of dietary antioxidants on in vivo lipid peroxidation in the rat as measured by pentane production. Lipids 13:403–407

D'Souza RA, Bhide SB (1975) Profiles of protein biosynthesis in isoniazid (INH) and hydrazine sulfate (HS) treated mice. Indian J Cancer 21:439–445

Dungworth DL, Castleman WL, Chow CK, Mellick PW, Mustafa MG, Tarkington BK, Tyler WS (1975) Effect of ambient levels of ozone on monkeys. Fed Proc 34:1670–1674

Edson NL, Leloir LF (1936) Ketogenesis-antiketogenesis. V. Metabolism of ketone bodies. Biochem J 30:2319–2332

Ellis DB, Munro JR, Stahl GH (1972) Biosynthesis of respiratory tract mucins. III. Metabolism of aminosugars by tracheal mucosal extracts. Biochim Biophys Acta 289:108–116

Elsayed NM, Mustafa MG (1982) Dietary antioxidant and the biochemical response to oxidant inhalation. I. Influence of dietary vitamin E on the biochemical effects of nitrogen dioxide exposure in rat lung. Toxicol Appl Pharmacol 66:319–328

Elsayed NM, Mustafa MG, Postlethwait EM (1982a) Age-dependent pulmonary response of rats to ozone exposure. J Toxicol Environ Health 9:835–848

Elsayed NM, Hacker AD, Mustafa MG, Kuehn K, Schrauzer G (1982b) Effects of decreased gluthathione peroxidase activity on the pentose phosphate cycle in mouse lung. Biochem Biophys Res Commun 104:564–569

Engelbrecht FM, Bester JCP (1968) The in vivo effects of quartz and carbon dusts on the activity of cytochrome c oxidase and the DNA and RNA content of lung tissue. S Afr Med J 42:1142–1145

Estabrook RW (1967) Mitochondrial respiratory control and the polarographic measurement of ADP:O ratios. In: Estabrook RW, Pullman ME (eds) Methods in enzymology, vol 10. Academic, New York, pp 41–47

Evans MJ, Mayr W, Bils RF, Loosli CG (1971) Effects of ozone on cell renewal in pulmonary alveoli of aging mice. Arch Environ Health 22:450–453

Evans MJ, Cabral LJ, Stephens RJ, Freeman G (1973) Renewal of alveolar epithelium in the rat following exposure to NO_2. Am J Pathol 70:171–194

Evans MJ, Cabral LJ, Stephens RJ, Freeman G (1975) Transformation of alveolar type 2 cells to type 1 cells following exposure to nitrogen dioxide. Exp Mol Pathol 22:142–150

Evans MJ, Johnson LV, Stephens RJ, Freeman G (1976) Renewal of the terminal bronchiolar epithelium in the rat following exposure to NO_2 or O_3. Lab Invest 35:246–257

Evans MJ, Cabral-Anderson LJ, Freeman G (1977) Effects of NO_2 on the lungs of aging rats. II. Cell proliferation. Exp Mol Pathol 27:366–376

Evans MJ, Cabral-Anderson LJ, Freeman G (1978) Role of the Clara cell in renewal of the bronchiolar epithelium. Lab Invest 38:648–655

Fairchild EJ, Murphy SD, Stokinger HE (1959) Protection by sulfur compounds against the air pollutants ozone and nitrogen dioxide. Science 130:861–862

Fanson RC, Waite M (1973) Lysosomal phospholipases A_1 and A_2 of normal and bacillus Calmette Guerin-induced alveolar macrophages. J Cell Biol 56:621–627

Fariday EE, Naimark A (1971) Effect of distension on lung metabolism of excised dog lung. J Appl Physiol 31:31–37

Farrell PM, Lundgren DW, Adams AJ (1974) Choline kinase and choline phosphotransferase in developing fetal rat lung. Biochem Biophys Res Commun 57:696–701

Felts JM (1964) Biochemistry of the lung. Health Phys 10:973–979

Fisher AB (1976) Oxygen utilization and energy production. In: Crystal RG (ed) The biochemical basis of pulmonary function. Marcel Dekker, New York, pp 75–104

Fisher AB, Scarpa A, LaNoue KF, Bassett D, Williamson JR (1973) Respiration of rat lung mitochondria and the influence of Ca^{++} on substrate utilization. Biochemistry 12:1438–1445

Fisher AB, Diamond S, Mellen S (1974) Effect of oxygen exposure on metabolism of the rabbit alveolar macrophage. J Appl Physiol 37:341–345

Fisher HK, Clements JA, Wright RR (1973) Enhancement of oxygen toxicity by the herbicide paraquat. Am Rev Respir Dis 107:246–252

Fitschen W (1967a) Studies on monkey lung ribosomes. Chemical and physical properties. S Afr J Med Sci 32:112–118

Fitschen W (1967b) Studies on monkey lung ribosomes. Cell-free protein synthesis: comparison of free and membrane-bound ribosomes. S Afr J Med Sci 32:119–131

Fletcher BL, Tappel AL (1973) Protective effects of dietary alpha-tocopherol in rats exposed to toxic levels of ozone and nitrogen dioxide. Environ Res 6:165–175

Fletcher K, Wyatt I (1970) The composition of lung lipids after poisoning with paraquat. Br J Exp Pathol 51:604–610

Fletcher K, Wyatt I (1972) The action of paraquat on the incorporation of palmitic acid into dipalmitoyl lecithin in mouse lungs. Br J Exp Pathol 53:225–230

Flohe L, Benohr HC, Siess H, Waller HD, Wendel A (eds) (1974) Symposium on glutathione. Thieme, Stuttgart

Fouts JR, Devereux TR (1972) Developmental aspects of hepatic and extrahepatic drug-metabolizing enzyme systems: microsomal enzymes and components in rabbit liver and lung during the first month of life. J Pharmacol Exp Ther 183:458–468

Frank L, Autor AP, Roberts RJ (1977) Oxygen toxicity and hyaline membrane disease: the effect of hyperoxia on pulmonary superoxide dismutase activity and the mediating role of plasma or serum. J Pediatr 90:105–110

Frank L, Wood D, Roberts RJ (1978a) The effect of diethyldithiocarbamate (DDC) on oxygen toxicity and lung enzyme activity in immature and adult rats. Biochem Pharmacol 27:251–254

Frank L, Yam J, Roberts RJ (1978b) The role of endotoxin in protection of adult rats from oxygen-induced lung toxicity. J Clin Invest 61:269–275

Fredricsson B (1956) The distribution of alkaline phosphatase in the rat lung. Acta Anat 26:246–256

Fridovich I (1974) Superoxide dismutase. Adv Enzymol 41:35–97

Fritts HW Jr, Strauss B, Wichern W Jr, Courand A (1963) Utilization of oxygen in lung of patients with diffuse, nonobstructive pulmonary disease. Trans Assoc Am Phys 76:302–311

Frosolono MF, Slivka S, Charms BL (1971) Acyl transferase activities in dog lung microsomes. J Lipid Res 12:96–103

Fukase O, Isomura K, Watanabe H (1975) Effect of ozone on vitamin C in vivo. Taiki-osen Kenkyu 10:13–16

Fukase O, Isomura K, Watanabe H (1978) Effects of exercise on mice exposed to ozone. Arch Environ Health 32:198–201

Gacad G, Massaro D (1973) Hyperoxia: influence on lung mechanics and protein synthesis. J Clin Invest 52:559–565

Gacad G, Dickie K, Massaro D (1972) Protein synthesis in lung: influence of starvation on amino acid incorporation into protein. J Appl Physiol 33:381–384

Garfinkel D (1963) A comparative study of electron transport in microsomes. Comp Biochem Physiol 8:367–379

Gassenheimer L, Rhoades RA, Scholz RW (1972) In vivo incorporation of ^{14}C-1-palmitate and ^{3}H-U-glucose into lung lecithin. Respir Physiol 15:268–275

Gelmont D, Stein RA, Mead JF (1981) The bacterial origin of rat breath pentane. Biochem Biophys Res Commun 102:932–936

Gershon ZLB, Gatt S (1976) Lysolecithinase activity in subcellular fractions of rat organs. Biochem Biophys Res Commun 69:592–598

Gil J, Reiss OK (1973) Isolation and characterization of lamellar bodies and tubular myelin from rat lung homogenates. J Cell Biol 58:152–171

Gilder H, McSherry CK (1972) An improved method for measuring the incorporation of palmitic acid into lung lecithin. Am Rev Respir Dis 106:556–562

Giri SN, Benson J, Siegel DM, Rice SA, Schiedt M (1975) Effects of pretreatment with anti-inflammatory drugs on ozone-induced lung damage in rats. Proc Soc Exp Biol Med 150:810–814

Glaviano VV, Yo S, Masters T (1967) Levels of lactate in lung tissue during sympathetic stimulation. Am J Physiol 213:437–440

Goldfischer S, Kikkawa Y, Hoffman L (1968) The demonstration of acid hydrolase activities in the inclusion bodies of type II alveolar cells and other lysosomes in the rabbit lung. J Histochem Cytochem 16:102–109

Goldner RD, Brumley GW (1974) Comparative incorporation of P^{32} into lung phosphatidyl choline in mammals with different metabolic and pulmonary morphologic characteristics. Proc Soc Exp Biol Med 145:1343–1347

Goldstein BD, Buckley RD, Cardenas R, Balchum OJ (1970) Ozone and vitamin E. Science 169:605–606

Gould KG (1976) Dispersal of lung into individual viable cells. In: Crystal RG (ed) The biochemical basis of pulmonary function. Marcel Dekker, New York, pp 49–71

Gould KG, Clements JA, Jones AL, Felts JM (1972) Dispersal of rabbit lung into individual viable cells: a new method for the study of lung metabolism. Science 178:1209–1210

Granstrom E (1971) Metabolism of prostaglandin R_2 in guinea-pig lung. Eur J Biochem 20:451–458

Gross I, Warshaw JB (1974) Enzyme activities related to fatty acid synthesis in developing mammalian lung. Pediatr Res 8:193–199

Haase G, Dunkley WL (1969) Ascorbic acid and copper in linoleate oxidation. I. Measurement of oxidation by ultraviolet spectrophotometry and the thiobarbituric acid test. J Lipid Res 10:555–560

Hackett RL, Sunderman FW Jr (1968) Pulmonary alveolar reaction to nickel carbonyl. Arch Environ Health 16:349–362

Hafeman DG, Hoekstra WG (1977) Lipid peroxidation in vivo during vitamin E and selenium deficiency in the rat as monitored by ethane evolution. J Nutr 107:666–672

Hallman M, Gluck L (1974) Phosphatidyl glycerol in lung surfactant. I. Synthesis in rat lung microsomes. Biochem Biophys Res Commun 60:1–7

Hamosh M, Shechter Y, Hamosh P (1978) Metabolic activity of developing rabbit lung. Pediatr Res 12:95–100

Harding JJ (1969) Glutathione-protein mixed disulfides in human lens. Biochem J 114:88P–89P

Harlan WR Jr, Said SI (1969) Selected aspects of lung metabolism. In: Bittar EE, Bittar N (eds) The biological basis of medicine, vol 6. Academic, New York, pp 357–384

Harrap KR, Jackson RC, Smith CA, Hill BT (1973) The occurrence of protein-bound mixed disulfides in rat tissues. Biochim Biophys Acta 310:104–110

Heinemann HO (1961) Free fatty acid production by rabbit lung tissue in vitro. Am J Physiol 201:607–610

Heinemann HO, Fishman AP (1969) Nonrespiratory functions of mammalian lung. Physiol Rev 49:1–47

Heran J, Mandell P, Weill G, Florange W (1961) Metabolic studies of surgical specimens of the human lung. I. Tissue consumption of oxygen. Rev Agressol 2:411–415

Hill EE, Husbands DR, Lands WEM (1968) The selective incorporation of ^{14}C-glycerol into different species of phosphatic acid, phosphatidylethanolamine, and phosphatidylcholine. J Biol Chem 243:4440–4451

Hoffman L (1972) Isolation of inclusion bodies from rabbit lung parenchyma. J Cell Physiol 79:65–72

Hollinger MA, Giri SN, Hwang F, Budd E (1974) Effect of thiourea on rat lung protein synthesis. Res Commun Chem Pathol Pharmacol 8:319–326

Holt PG, Keast D (1973) The effect of tobacco smoke on protein synthesis in macrophages. Proc Soc Exp Biol Med 142:1243–1247

Hook GER, Bend JR (1976) Minireview: pulmonary metabolism of xenobiotics. Life Sci 18:279–290

Hook GER, Bend JR, Hoel D, Fouts JE, Gram TE (1972) Preparation of lung microsomes and a comparison of the distribution of enzymes between subcellular fractions of rabbit lung and liver. J Pharmacol Exp Ther 182:474–490

Horn HD (1965) Glutathione reductase. In: Bergmeyer HU (ed) Methods of enzymatic analysis (revised). Academic, New York, pp 875–879

Horton AA, Packer L (1970) Mitochondrial metabolism of aldehydes. Biochem J 116:19P–20P

Hussain MZ, Bhatnagar RS (1979a) Enhanced collagen synthesis in lung organ culture in the presence of mercury. Environ Intl 2:33–35

Hussain MZ, Bhatnagar RS (1979b) Involvement of superoxide in the paraquat-induced enhancement of lung collagen synthesis in organ culture. Biochem Biophys Res Commun 89:71–76

Hussain MZ, Mustafa MG, Cross CE, Tyler WS (1974) Increased protein synthesis in lung after sub-acute exposure of rats and monkeys to ozone. Fed Proc 33:1468

Hussain MZ, Cross CE, Mustafa MG, Bhatnagar RS (1976) Hydroxyproline contents and prolyl hydroxylase activities in lungs of rats exposed to low levels of ozone. Life Sci 18:897–904

Hussain MZ, Belton JC, Bhatnagar RS (1978) Macromolecular synthesis in organ cultures of neonatal rat lungs. In Vitro 14:740–745

Ichinose T, Sagai M (1982) Studies on biochemical effects of nitrogen dioxide. III. Changes of the antioxidative protective systems in rat lungs and of lipid peroxidation by chronic exposure. Toxicol Appl Pharmacol 66:1–8

Jamieson D, Van Den Brenk HAS (1962) Pulmonary damage due to high pressure oxygen breathing in rats. 2. Changes in dehydrogenase activity of rat lung. Aust J Exp Biol Med Sci 40:51–56

Jamieson D, Van Den Brenk HAS (1964) The effect of antioxidants on high pressure oxygen toxicity. Biochem Pharmacol 13:159–164

Jocelyn PC (ed) (1972) Biochemistry of the SH groups. Academic, New York

Johnston JM, Schultz FM, Jiminez JM, MacDonald PC (1975) Phospholipid biosynthesis: the activity of phosphatidic acid phosphohydrolase in the developing lung and amnionic fluid. Chest (Suppl) 67:19S–21S

Jollow DJ, Mitchell JR, Zampaglione N, Gillette JR (1974) Bromobenzene-induced liver necrosis: protective role of glutathione and evidence for 3,4-bromobenzene oxide as the hepatotoxic metabolite. Pharmacology 11:151–169

Kadis B (1978) Steroid epoxides in biologic system: a review. J Steroid Biochem 9:75–81

Kann HE, Mengel CE, Smith W, Horton B (1964) Oxygen toxicity and vitamin E. Aerosp Med 35:840–844

Kauffman SL (1972) Alterations in cell proliferation in mouse lung following urethane exposure. III. Effects of chronic exposure on type 2 alveolar epithelial cell. Am J Pathol 68:317–323

Kaufman DG (1976) Biochemical studies of isolated hamster tracheal epithelium. Environ Health Perspect 16:99–110

Kaufman DG, Baker MS, Harris CC, Smith JM, Boren H, Sporn MB, Saffiotti U (1972a) Coordinated biochemical and morphological examination of hamster tracheal epithelium. J Natl Cancer Inst 49:783–792

Kaufman DG, Baker MS, Smith JM, Henderson WR, Harris CC, Sporn MB, Saffiotti U (1972b) RNA metabolism in tracheal epithelium: alteration in hamsters deficient in vitamin A. Science 177:1105–1108

Kikkawa Y, Spitzer R (1969) Inclusion bodies of type II alveolar cells: species differences and morphogenesis. Anat Rec 163:525–541

Kikkawa Y, Yoneda K (1974) The type II epithelial cell of the lung. I. Method of isolation. Lab Invest 30:76–84

Kikkawa Y, Yoneda K, Smith F, Packard B, Suzuki K (1975) The type II epithelial cells of the lung. II. Chemical composition and phospholipid synthesis. Lab Invest 32:296–302

Kilroe-Smith TA, Breyer MG (1963) Changes in activities of respiratory enzymes in lungs of guinea-pigs exposed to silica dust. Br J Ind Med 20:243–247

Kimball RE, Reddy K, Peirce TH, Schwartz LW, Mustafa MG, Cross CE (1976) Oxygen toxicity: augmentation of antioxidant defense mechanisms in rat lung. Am J Physiol 230:1425–1431

Kleinerman J (1970) Effects of nitrogen dioxide in hamsters: autoradiographic and electron microscopic aspects. AEC Symp Ser 18:271–279

Kosower NS, Kosower EM (1976) The glutathione-glutathione disulfide system. In: Pryor WA (ed) Free radicals in biology, vol II. Academic, New York, p 55

Krebs HA (1950) Body size and tissue respiration. Biochim Biophys Acta 4:249–269

Kyle JL, Riesen WH (1970) Stress and cigarette smoke effects on lung mitochondrial phosphorylation. Arch Environ Health 21:492–497

Lands WEM (1958) Metabolism of glycerolipids. A comparison of lecithin and triglyceride synthesis. J Biol Chem 231:883–888

Lehninger AL (1965) The mitochondrion. Benjamin, New York

Levart C, Louisot P (1973) Biosynthese des glycoproteines dans le parechyme pulmonaire. I. Activite mannosyltransferase dans les fractions subcellulaires des pneumocytes. Can J Biochem 51:931–938

Levy SE (1971) The role of glucose in lung metabolism. The role of glucose as an energy substitute for the lung. Clin Res 19:515

Levy SE, Harvey E (1974) Effect of tissue slicing on rat lung metabolism. J Appl Physiol 37:239–240

Lewis JA, Tata JR (1973) Protein-synthesis activity of rat liver microsomal fraction that sediments at 600 g. Biochem Soc Trans 1:585–586

Little C, O'Brien PJ (1968a) An intracellular GSH peroxidase with a lipid peroxide substrate. Biochem Biophys Res Commun 31:145–150

Little C, O'Brien PJ (1968b) The effectiveness of a lipid peroxide in oxidizing protein and nonprotein thiols. Biochem J 106:419–423

Liu J, Simon LM, Phillips JR, Robin ED (1977) Superoxide dismutase (SOD) activity in hypoxic mammalian systems. J Appl Physiol 42:107–110

Logani MK, Davies RE (1980) Lipid oxidation: biological effects and antioxidants – a review. Lipids 15:485–495

Longmore WJ, Mourning JT (1976) Lactate production in isolated perfused rat lung. Am J Physiol 231:351–354

Low RB (1974) Protein biosynthesis by the pulmonary alveolar macrophage: conditions of assay and the effects of cigarett smoke extract. Am Rev Respir Dis 110:446–477

Lowry OH, Rosebrough NJ, Farr AL, Randall RJ (1951) Protein measurement with the Folin phenol reagent. J Biol Chem 193:263–275

Lunan KD, Short P, Negi D, Stephens RJ (1977) Glucose-6-phosphate dehydrogenase response of postnatal lungs to NO_2 and O_3. In: Sanders CL, Schneider RP, Dagle GE, Raga HA (eds) Pulmonary macrophage and epithelial cells. US Atomic Energy Commission, Oak Ridge, pp 236–247

Manning JP, Babson AL, Buttler MC, Priester SF (1966) Determination of acid phosphatase activity in tissue homogenates. Can J Biochem 44:755–761

Mason RJ (1976) Lipid metabolism. In: Crystal RG (ed) The biochemical basis of pulmonary function. Marcel Dekker, New York, pp 127–169

Mason RJ, Williams MC (1977) Type II alveolar cell. Defender of the alveolus. Am Rev Respir Dis 115 (Suppl):81–91

Mason RJ, Huber G, Vaughan M (1972) Synthesis of dipalmitoyl lecithin by alveolar macrophages. J Clin Invest 51:68–73

Mason RJ, Williams MC, Greenleaf ED (1976) Isolation of lung cells. In: Bouhuys A (ed) Lung cells in disease. North-Holland, Amsterdam, pp 39–52

Masoro EJ (1973) Development of the enzymes of lipid biosynthesis in the human fetus. In: Villee Ca, Villee DB, Zuckerman J (eds) Respiratory distress syndrome. Academic, New York, pp 7–27

Massaro D (1973a) Hyperoxia: influence of food deprivation on protein synthesis by lung. Proc Soc Exp Biol Med 143:602–603

Massaro D (1973b) Protein synthesis in rat lung: recovery from exposure to hyperoxia. J Appl Physiol 35:32–34

Massaro D, Handler A, Bottoms L (1967) Alveolar cells: protein biosynthesis. Am Rev Respir Dis 96:957–961

Massaro D, Weiss H, Simon MR (1970a) Protein synthesis and secretion by lung. Am Rev Respir Dis 101:198–206

Massaro D, Kelleher K, Massaro G, Yeager H Jr (1970b) Alveolar macrophages: depression of protein synthesis during phagocytosis. Am J Physiol 218:1533–1539

Massaro D, Weiss H, White G (1971a) Pulmonary artery ligation. Effect on in vitro protein synthesis. Arch Intern Med 126:861–862

Massaro D, Weiss H, White G (1971b) Protein synthesis by lung following pulmonary artery ligation. J Appl Physiol 31:8–14

Massaro D, Simon MR, Steinkamp H (1971c) Metabolic factors affecting protein synthesis by lung in vitro. J Appl Physiol 30:1–6

Massaro GD, Massaro D (1972) Granular pneumocytes: electron microscopic radioautographic evidence of intracellular protein transport. Am Rev Respir Dis 105:927–931

Massaro GD, Massaro D (1974) Adaptation to hyperoxia. Influence on protein synthesis by lung, and on granular pneumocyte ultrastructure. J Clin Invest 53:705–709

Matsubara T, Tochino Y (1971) Electron transport systems of lung microsomes and their physiological functions. J Biochem (Tokyo) 70:981–991

Matsuya Y, Yamane I (1970) Changes in cellular properties during the long-term serial culture of lung cells of newborn hamster and the transformation in A cells. Tokoho J Exp Med 1–2:37–49

May HE, McCay PB (1968) Reduced triphosphopyridine nucleotide oxidase-catalyzed alterations of membrane phospholipids. J Biol Chem 243:2288–2295

McCord JM, Crapo JD, Fridovich I (1977) Superoxide dismutase assays: a review of methodology. In: Michelson AM, McCord JM, Fridovich I (eds) Superoxide and the superoxide dismutases. Academic, New York, pp 11–17

Mead JF (1976) Free radical mechanisms of lipid damage and consequences for cellular membranes. In: Pryor WA (ed) Free radicals in biology, vol 1. Academic, New York, p 51

Meban C (1972) Localization of phosphatidic acid phosphatase activity in granular pneumonocytes. J Cell Biol 53:249–252

Menzel DB (1970) Toxicity of zone, oxygen and radiation. Annu Rev Pharmacol Toxicol 10:379–394

Menzel DB (1971) Oxidation of biologically active reducing substances by ozone. Arch Environ Health 23:149–153

Menzel DB (1976) The role of free radicals in the toxicity of air pollutants (nitrogen oxides and ozone). In: Pryor WA (ed) Free radicals in biology, vol 2. Academic, New York, pp 181–201

Modig H (1968) Cellular mixed disulfides between thiols and proteins, and their possible implication for radiation protection. Biochem Pharmacol 17:177–186

Montgomery MR (1977) Paraquat toxicity and pulmonary superoxide dismutase. An enzymic deficiency of lung microsomes. Res Commun Chem Pathol Pharmacol 16:155–158

Morgan TE (1969) Isolation and characterization of lipid N-methyl transferase from dog lung. Biochim Biophys Acta 178:21–34

Morgan TE, Morgan BK (1973) Surfactant synthesis, storage, and release by alveolar cells. In: Villee CA, Villee DB, Zuckerman J (eds) Respiratory distress syndrome. Academic, New York, pp 117–125

Moriya T, Kanoh H (1974) In vivo studies on the de novo synthesis of molecular species of rat lung lecithins. Tokoho J Exp Med 112:241–256

Mountain JT (1963) Detecting hypersensitivity to toxic substances. Arch Environ Health 6:357–365

Mudd JB, Freeman BA (1977) Reaction of ozone with biological membranes. In: Lee SD (ed) Biochemical effects of environmental pollutants. Ann Arbor Science, Ann Arbor, pp 97–133

Mudd JB, Leavitt R, Ongun A, McManus TT (1969) Reaction of ozone with amino acids and proteins. Atmos Environ 3:669–681

Mudd JB, McManus TT, Ongun A, McCullough TT (1971) Inhibition of glycolipid biosynthesis in chloroplasts by ozone and sulfhydryl reagents. Plant Physiol 48:335–339

Mustafa MG (1974) Augmentation of mitochondrial oxidative metabolism in lung tissue during recovery of animals from acute ozone exposure. Arch Biochem Biophys 165:531–538

Mustafa MG (1975) Influence of dietary vitamin E on lung cellular sensitivity to ozone in rats. Nutr Rep Int 11:473–476

Mustafa MG, Cross CE (1971) Pulmonary alveolar macrophage. Oxidative metabolism of isolated cells and mitochondria and effect of cadmium ion on electron and energy transfer reactions. Biochem 10:4176–4185

Mustafa MG, Cross CE (1974a) Effects of short-term ozone exposure on lung mitochondrial oxidative and energy metabolism. Arch Biochem Biophys 162:585–594

Mustafa MG, Cross CE (1974b) Lung cell mitochondria: rapid oxidation of glycerol-1-phosphate but slow oxidation of 3-hydroxybutyrate. Am Rev Respir Dis 109:301–303

Mustafa MG, Lee SD (1976) Pulmonary biochemical alterations resulting from ozone exposure. Ann Occup Hyg 19:17–26

Mustafa MG, Tierney DF (1978) State of the art – biochemical and metabolic changes in the lung with oxygen, ozone, and nitrogen dioxide toxicity. Am Rev Respir Dis 118:1061–1090

Mustafa MG, Peterson PA, Munn RJ, Cross CE (1971) Effects of cadmium on metabolism of lung cells. In: Englund HM, Berry WT (eds) Proceedings of the 2nd international clean air congress. Academic, New York, pp 143–151

Mustafa MG, DeLucia AJ, York GE, Arth C, Cross CE (1973) Ozone interaction with rodent lung. II. Effects on oxygen consumption of mitochondria. J Lab Clin Med 82:357–365

Mustafa MG, Macres SM, Tarkington BK, Chow CK, Hussain MZ (1975) Lung superoxide dismutase (SOD). Clin Res 23:138A

Mustafa MG, Hacker AD, Ospital JJ, Hussain MZ, Lee SD (1977) Biochemical effects of environmental oxidant pollutants in animal lungs. In: Lee SD (ed) Biochemical effects of environmental pollutants. Ann Arbor Science, Ann Arbor, pp 59–96

Mustafa MG, Elsayed N, Lim JST, Postlethwait E (1979) Effects of nitrogen dioxide on lung metabolism. In: Grosjean D (ed) Nitrogenous air pollutants: chemical and biological implications. Ann Arbor Science, Ann Arbor, pp 165–178

Mustafa MG, Faeder EJ, Lee SD (1980) Biochemical effects of nitrogen dioxide on animal lungs. In: Lee SD (ed) Nitrogen oxides and their effects on health. Ann Arbor Science, Ann Arbor, pp 161–179

Mustafa MG, Elsayed NM, Quinn CL, Postlethwait EM, Gardner DE, Graham JA (1982) Comparison of pulmonary biochemical effects of low-level ozone exposure on mice and rats. J Toxicol Environ Health 9:857–865

Naimark A (1966) Pulmonary blood flow and the incorporation of palmitate-1-^{14}C by dog lung in vivo. J Appl Physiol 21:1292–1298

Naimark A (1973) Cellular dynamics and lipid metabolism in the lung. Fed Proc 32:1967–1971

Naimark A, Klass D (1967) The incorporation of palmitate-1-^{14}C by rat lung in vitro. Can J Physiol Pharmacol 45:597–607

Nasr ANM (1967) Biochemical aspects of ozone intoxication. J Occup Med 9:589–597

Nasr ANM, Dinman BD, Bernstein IA (1971) An experimental approach to study the toxicity of nonparticulate air pollutants. Arch Environ Health 22:538–544

Newman D, Naimark A (1968) Palmitate-^{14}C uptake by rat lung: effect of altered gas tensions. Am J Physiol 214:305–312

Niden AH (1967) Bronchiolar and large alveolar cell in pulmonary phospholipid metabolism. Science 158:1323–1324

Nirurkar LS, Zeligs BJ, Bellanti JA (1978) Changes in superoxide dismutase, catalase and glucose-6-phosphate dehydrogenase activities of rabbit alveolar macrophages: induced by postnatal maturation and/or in vitro hyperoxia. Photochem Photobiol 28:781–786

Northway WH, Petriceks R, Shahinian L (1972) Quantitative aspects of oxygen toxicity in the newborn: inhibition of lung DNA synthesis in the mouse. Pediatrics 50:67–72

O'Brien PJ, Little C (1969) Intracellular mechanisms for the decomposition of a lipid peroxide. II. Decomposition of a lipid peroxide by subcellular fractions. Can J Biochem 47:493–499

Ogawa K (1972) A study on non-respiratory function of the lung with special reference to protein synthesis system of pulmonary tissue. I Jpn Soc Intern Med 61:251–261

O'Hare KH, Newman JK, Vatter AE, Reiss OK (1971) Esterases in developing and adult rat lung. II. An electrophoretic analysis. J Histochem Cytochem 19:116–123

Ohta M, Hasegawa H (1972) Phospholipase A activity in rat lung. Tokoho J Exp Med 108:85–94

Ohta M, Hasegawa H, Ohno K (1972) Calcium dependent phospholipase A_2 activity in rat lung supernatant. Biochim Biophys Acta 280:552–558

Okuda E (1973) A study on non-respiratory function of the lung with reference to the nucleic acid and protein synthesis of pulmonary tissue. Jpn J Thoracic Dis 11:261–269

Omaye ST, Reddy AK, Cross CE (1977) Effect of butylated hydroxytoluene and other antioxidants on mouse lung metabolism. J Toxicol Environ Health 3:829–836

O'Neill JJ, Tierney DF (1974) Rat lung metabolism: glucose utilization by isolated perfused lungs and tissue slices. Am J Physiol 226:867–873

O'Neil JJ, Sanford RL, Wasserman S, Tierney DF (1977) Metabolism in rat lung tissue slices: technical factors. J Appl Physiol 43:902–906

Oppelt WW, Zange M, Ross WE, Remmer H (1970) Comparison of microsomal drug hydroxylation in lung and liver of various species. Res Commun Chem Pathol Pharmacol 1:43–56

Ospital JJ, Elsayed N, Hacker AD, Mustafa MG, Tierney DF (1976) Altered glucose metabolism in lungs of rats exposed to nitrogen dioxide. Am Rev Respir Dis 113:108

Ospital JJ, Hacker AD, Mustafa MG (1981) Biochemical changes in rat lungs after exposure to nitrogen dioxide. J Toxicol Environ Health 8:47–58

Packer L (1967) Experiments in cell physiology. Academic, New York

Page-Roberts BA (1972) Preparation and partial characterization of lamellar body fraction from rat lung. Biochim Biophys Acta 260:334–338

Perez-Diaz J, Carballo B, Ayuso-Parrilla MS, Parrilla R (1977a) Preparation and metabolic characterization of isolated rat lung cells. Biochimie 59:411–416

Perez-Diaz J, Martin A, Ayuso-Parrilla MS, Parrilla R (1977b) Metabolic features of isolated rat lung cells. I. Factors controlling glucose utilization. Am J Physiol 232:E394–E401

Petrik P (1971) Fine structural identification of peroxisomes in mouse and rat bronchiolar and alveolar epithelium. J Histochem Cytochem 19:339–348

Petrik P, Collet AJ (1974) Quantitative electron microscopic autoradiograph of in vivo incorporation of ^{3}H-choline, ^{3}H-leucine, ^{3}H-acetate and ^{3}H-galactose in non-eiliated bronchiolar (Clara) cells of mice. Am J Anat 139:519–534

Piper PJ, Vane JR, Wyllie JH (1970) Inactivation of prostaglandins by the lungs. Nature 225:600–604

Plaa GL, Witschi HP (1976) Chemicals, drugs, and lipid peroxidation. Annu Rev Pharmacol Toxicol 16:125–141

Popjak G, Beeckmans M (1950) Extrahepatic lipid synthesis. Biochem J 47:233–238

Postlethwait EM, Mustafa MG (1981) Fate of inhaled nitrogen dioxide in isolated perfused rat lung. J Toxicol Environ Health 7:861–872

Rady P, Arany I, Bojan F, Kertal P (1980) Effect of carcinogenic and non-carcinogenic chemicals on the activities of four glycolytic enzymes in mouse lung. Chem Biol Interact 31:209–213

Ramazzotto LJ, Rappaport LJ (1971) The effect of nitrogen dioxide on aldolase enzyme. Arch Environ Health 22:379–380

Ramazzotto L, Jones CR, Cornell F (1971) Effect of nitrogen dioxide on the activities of cytochrome oxidase and succinic dehydrogenase on homogenates of some organs of the rat. Life Sci 10(2):601–604

Recknagel RO, Ghoshal AK (1966) Lipoperoxidation as a vector in carbon tetrachloride hepatetoxicity. Lab Invest 15:132–148

Reeves AL (1967) Isozymes of lactate dehydrogenase during beryllium carcinogenesis in the rat. Cancer Res 27:1895–1899

Reid E (1967) Membrane systems. In: Roodyn DB (ed) Enzyme cytology. Academic, New York, pp 321–406

Reiss OK (1965) Properties of mitochondrial preparations from rabbit lung. Med Thoracalis 22:100–103

Reiss OK (1966) Studies of lung metabolism. I. Isolation and properties of subcellular fractions from rabbit lung. J Cell Biol 30:45–57

Reiss U, Tappel AL, Chio KS (1972) DNA-malonaldehyde reactions: formation of fluorescent products. Biochem Biophys Res Commun 48:921–926

Rhoades RA (1974) Net uptake of glucose, glycerol, and fatty acids by the isolated perfused rat lung. Am J Physiol 226:144–149

Riley CA, Cohen G, Lieberman M (1974) Ethane evolution: a new index of lipid peroxidation. Science 183:208–210

Rister M, Baehner RL (1976) The alteration of superoxide dismustase, catalase, glutathione peroxidase, and NAD(P)H cytochrom c reductase in guinea pig polymorphonuclear leukocytes and alveolar macrophages during hyperoxia. J Clin Invest 58:1174–1184

Rister M, Baehner RL (1977) Effect of hyperoxia on superoxide anion and hydrogen peroxide production of polymorphonuclear leucocytes and alveolar macrophages. Br J Haematol 36:241–248

Robinson LA, Wolfe WG, Salin ML (1978) Alterations in cellular enzymes and tissue metabolism in the oxygen toxic primate lung. J Surg Res 24:359–365

Roehm JN, Hadley JC, Menzel DB (1971) Oxidation of unsaturated fatty acids by ozone and nitrogen dioxide. Arch Environ Health 23:142–148

Romanova LK, Leikina EM, Antipova KK (1967) Nucleic acid synthesis and mitotic activity during development of compensatory hypertrophy of the lung in rats. Bull Exp Biol Med (USSR) 63:303–306

Roodyn DB (1969) Some methods for the isolation of nuclei from mammalian cells. In: Birnie GD, Fox SM (eds) Subcellular components: preparation and fractionation. Plenum, New York, pp 15–42

Rose MS, Smith LL, Wyatt I (1976) The relevance of pentose phosphate pathway stimulation in rat lung to the mechanism of paraquat toxicity. Biochem Pharmacol 25:1763–1767

Rosenthal O, Drabkin DL (1944) The oxidative response of normal and neoplastic tissues to succinate and to phenylenediamine. Cancer Res 4:487–494

Ryan JW, Smith U (1971) A rapid, simple method for isolating pinocytic vesicles and plasma membrane of lung. Biochim Biophys Acta 249:177–180

Ryan JW, Smith U, Niemeyer RS (1972) Angiotensin I: metabolism by plasma membrane of lung. Science 176:64–66

Saheb W, Witschi HP (1975) Lung growth in mice after a single dose of butylated hydroxytoluene. Toxicol Appl Pharmacol 33:309–319

Sahebjami H, Gacad G, Massaro D (1974) Influence of corticosteroid on recovery from oxygen toxicity. Am Rev Respir Dis 110:566–571

Salisbury-Murphy S, Rubinstein D, Beck JC (1966) Lipid metabolism in lung slices. Am J Physiol 211:988–992

Sander GE, Higgins CG (1971) Subcellular localization of angiotensin I converting enzyme in rabbit lung. Nature (New Biol) 230:27–29

Sanders AP, Pratt PC, Currie WD (1974) Pulmonary oxygen toxicity and gas mixtures: B. Biochemistry. In: Trapp WG, Banister EW, Davison AJ, Trapp PA (eds) Proceedings of the fifth international congress of hyperbaric medicine. Simon Fraser University, Burnaby, British Columbia, pp 93–101

Sato S, Kawakami M, Maeda S, Takishima T (1976) Scanning electron microscopy of the lungs of vitamin E-deficient rats exposed to a low concentration of ozone. Am Rev Respir Dis 113:809–821

Sawant PL, Shibko S, Kumta US, Tappel AL (1964) Isolation of rat-liver lysosomes and their general properties. Biochim Biophys Acta 85:82–92

Sayeed MM, Baue AE (1971) Mitochondrial metabolism of succinate, B-hydroxybutyrate, and -ketoglutarate in hemorrhagic shock. Am J Physiol 220:1275–1281

Schiller H, Bensch K (1971) De novo fatty acid synthesis and elongation of fatty acids by subcellular fractions of lung. J Lipid Res 12:248–255

Schiller H, Donabedian RK (1973) Elongation and esterification of fatty acids in lung by a microsomal fraction. Am J Physiol 224:1006–1010

Scholz RW (1972) Lipid metabolism by rat lung in vitro. Utilization of citrate by normal and starved rats. Biochem J 126:1219–1224

Scholz RW, Rhoades RA (1971) Lipid metabolism by rat lung in vitro: effect of starvation and re-feeding on utilization of (U-^{14}C)-glucose by lung slices. Biochem J 124:257–264

Scholz RW, Woodard BM, Rhoads RA (1972) Utilization in vitro and in vivo of glucose and glycerol by rat lung. Am J Physiol 223:991–996

Sedlak J, Lindsay BH (1968) Estimation of total, protein-bound, and nonprotein sulfhydryl groups in tissue with Ellman's reagent. Anal Biochem 25:192–205

Segal W (1966) Enhancement of succinate oxidation in lung and liver mitochondria of tuberculous mice. Arch Biochem Biophys 113:750–757

Sell DA, Reynolds ES (1969) Liver parenchymal cell injury. VIII. Lesions of membranous cellular components following iodoform. J Cell Biol 41:736–752

Sevanian A, Mead JF, Stein RA (1979) Epoxides as products of lipid autoxidation in rat lungs. Lipids 14:634–643

Sevanian A, Mead JF, Stein RA (1980a) Lipid epoxidation in the lung: major isolable products of lipid autoxidation in vivo. In: Bhatnagar RS (ed) Molecular basis of environmental toxicity. Ann Arbor Science, Ann Arbor, pp 213–228

Sevanian A, Stein RA, Mead JF (1980b) Epoxide hydrolase in rat lung preparations. Biochim Biophys Acta 614:489–500

Sherwin RP, Winnick S, Buckley RD (1967) Response of lactic acid dehydrogenase-positive alveolar cells in the lungs of guinea-pigs exposed to nitric oxide. Am Rev Respir Dis 96:319–323

Sherwin RP, Dibble J, Weiner J (1972) Alveolar wall cells of the guinea-pigs: increase in response to 2 ppm nitrogen dioxide. Arch Environ Health 24:43–47

Shibko S, Tappel AL (1965) Rat-kidney lysosomes: isolation and properties. Biochem J 95:731–741

Shin BC, Huggins JW, Carraway KL (1972) Effects of pH, concentration and aging on the malonaldehyde reaction with proteins. Lipids 7:229–233

Simon FP, Potts AM, Gerrard RW (1947) Metabolism of isolated lung tissue: normal and in phosgene poisoning. J Biol Chem 167:303–311

Sims P, Grover PL (1974) Epoxides in polycyclic aromatic hydrocarbon metabolism and carcinogenesis. Adv Cancer Res 20:165–274

Singh J, Viswanathan PN, Pandey SD, Zaidi SH (1976) Changes in mitochondrial enzyme activity of rat lung during the development of silicosis. Life Sci 20:367–374

Slater EC (1967) Manometric methods and phosphate determination. In: Estabrook RW, Pullman ME (eds) Methods of enzymology, vol 10. Academic, New York, pp 19–29

Slater TF (1972) Free radical mechanisms in tissue injury. Pion, London, pp 1–283

Smith BT, Torday JS, Giroud CJP (1974) Evidence for different gestational-dependent effects of cortisol on cultured fetal lung cells. J Clin Invest 53:1518–1526

Smith SM, Sporn MB, Berkowitz DM, Kakefuda T, Callan E, Saffiotti U (1971) Isolation of enzymatically active nuclei from epithelial cells of the trachea. Cancer Res 31:199–202

Sorokin SP (1970) The cells of the lungs. AEC Symp Ser 21:3–41

Spencer B (1958) A cytological basis for the biochemical study of bronchial epithelium. J Histochem Cytochem 6:105–111

Spencer B (1959) The biochemistry of epithelia. Hydrolytic enzymes of human bronchial epithelim. Biochem J 71:500–507

Spitzer HL, Norman JR (1971) The biosynthesis and turnover of surfactant lecithin and protein. Arch Intern Med 127:425–435

Spitzer HL, Norman JR, Morrison K (1969) In vivo studies of (Me-^{3}H)choline and (1,2-^{14}C$_2$)choline incorporation into lung and liver lecithins. Biochim Biophys Acta 176:584–590

Srivastava SK, Beutler E (1968) Accurate measurement of glutathione content of human, rabbit, and rat blood cells and tissues. Anal Biochem 25:70–76

Stadie WC, Riggs BC, Haugaard N (1945) Oxygen poisoning. IV. The effect of high oxygen pressure upon the metabolism of liver, kidney, lung and muscle tissue. J Biol Chem 160:209–216

Stephens RJ, Solan MF, Evans MJ, Freeman G (1974) Early response of lung to low levels of ozone. Am J Pathol 74:31–42

Stevens JB, Autor AP (1980) Proposed mechanism for neonatal rat tolerance to normobaric hyperoxia. Fed Proc 39:3138–3143

Stoner GD (1974) Hormone-mediated differentiation of mouse lung adenoma cells. In Vitro 9:381

Strauss B (1964) In vitro respiration of normal and pathologic human lung. J Appl Physiol 19:503–509

Stubbs WA, Kelly DM, Walters FJ, Alberti KGMM (1977) The metabolic characteristics of the ventilated and non-ventilated perfused rat lung. Biochem Soc Trans 5:1312–1314

Sydow G, Wildner GP (1971) Glykolytische Enzyme und Glykolyse in Lunge und primaren Lungenkarzinomen des Menschen. Acta Biol Med Ger 27:651–654

Tappel AL (1968) Lysosomes. In: Florkin M, Stotz EH (eds) Cytochemistry. Elsevier, Amsterdam, pp 77–98 (Comprehensive biochemistry, vol 23)

Tappel AL (1975) Vitamin E. Nutr Today 6:4

Tappel AL (1980) Measurement of an protection from in vivo lipid peroxidation. In: Pryor WA (ed) Free radicals in biology, vol III. Academic, New York, pp 1–47

Tata JR (1969) Preparation and properties of microsomal and submicrosomal fractions from animal cells. In: Birnie GD, Fox SM (eds) Subcellular components: preparation and fractionation. Plenum, New York, pp 83–107

Terao J, Matsushita S (1981) Thiobarbituric acid reaction of methyl arachidonate monohydroperoxide isomers. Lipids 16:98–101

Thomas HV, Meuller PK, Lyman RL (1968) Lipoperoxidation of lung lipids in rats exposed to nitrogen dioxide. Science 159:532–534

Tierney DF (1971) Lactate metabolism in rat lung tissue. Arch Intern Med 127:858–860

Tierney DF (1974a) Intermediary metabolism of the lung. Fed Proc 33:2232–2237

Tierney DF (1974b) Lung metabolism and biochemistry. Annu Rev Physiol 36:209–231

Tierney DF, Levy SE (1976) Glucose metabolism. In: Crystal RG (ed) The biochemical basis of pulmonary function. Marcel Dekker, New York, pp 105–125

Tierney DF, Ayers L, Herzog S, Yang J (1973) Pentose pathway and production of reduced nicotinamide adenine dinucleotide phosphate. Am Rev Respir Dis 108:1348–1351

Tierney DF, Ayers L, Kasuyama RS (1977) Altered sensitivity to oxygen toxicity. Am Rev Respir Dis 115 (Suppl):59–65

Tietze F (1969) Enzymic method for quantitative determination of nanogram amounts of total and oxidized glutathione. Applications to mammalian blood and other tissues. Anal Biochem 27:502–522

Tietze F (1970) Disulfide reduction in rat liver. Arch Biochem Biophys 138:177–188

Tombropoulos EG (1971) Lipid synthesis by lung subcellular particles. Arch Intern Med 127:408–412

Tombropoulos EG (1973) Palmitate incorporation into lipids by lung subcellular fractions. Arch Biochem Biophys 158:911–918

Trentalance A, Mangiatini MT (1968a) Ricerche sulla sintesi proteica in organi isolati e perfusi. I. Sintesi de proteine plasmatiche e tissutali de parte del fegato e del polmone di ratto. Boll Soc Ital Biol Sper 44:1219–1222

Trentalance A, Mangiatini MT (1968b) Ricerche sulla sintest proteica in organi isolati e perfusi. II. Sintesi de proteine plasmatiche e tissutali da parte del polmone di coniglio. Boll Soc Ital Biol Sper 44:1222–1226

Trombly R, Tappel AL (1975) Fractionation and analysis of fluorescent products of lipid peroxidation. Lipids 10:441–447

Tyler WS, Pearse AGE (1965) Oxidative enzymes of the interalveolar septum of the rat. Thorax 20:149–152

Umbreit WM, Burris RH, Stauffer JF (1972) Manometric and biochemical techniques, 5th edn. Burgess, Minneapolis, pp 64–99, pp 144–147

Valdivia E (1973) Isolation and identification of pulmonary lamellar bodies from guinea-pigs. Prep Biochem 3:19–30

Vatter AE, Reiss OK, Newman JK, Lindquist K, Groeneboer E (1968) Enzymes of the lung. I. Detection of esterase with a new cytochemical method. J Cell Biol 38:80–98

Wainio WW (1970) The mammalian mitochondrial respiratory chain. Academic, New York, pp 77–151

Wang MC, Meng HC (1972) Lipid synthesis by rat lung in vitro. Lipids 7:207–211

Wang MC, Meng HC (1974) Synthesis of phospholipids and phospholipid fatty acids by isolated perfused rat lung. Lipids 9:63–67

Warshaw JB, Terry ML, Ranis MB (1980) Metabolic adaptation in developing lung. Pediatr Res 14:296–299

Weber KC, Visscher MB (1969) Metabolism of the isolated canine lung. Am J Physiol 217:1044–1052

Werthamer S, Penha PD, Amral L (1974) Pulmonary lesions induced by chronic exposure to ozone. I. Biochemical alterations. Arch Environ Health 29:164–166

Williams CH (1974) The isolation of lung lamellar bodies. In: Fleischer S, Packer L (eds) Biomembrane, part A. Academic, New York, pp 419–425 (Methods in enzymology, vol 31)

Williams CH, Vail WJ, Harris RA, Green DE, Valdivia E (1971) The isolation and characterization of the lamellar body of bovine lung. Prep Biochem 1:37–45

Willis RJ, Kratzing CC (1974) Ascorbic acid in rat lung. Biochem Biophys Res Commun 59:1250–1253

Wilson PD (1972) Enzyme patterns in young and old mouse livers and lungs. Gerontologia 18:36–54

Witschi H-P (1972) A comparative study of in vivo RNA and protein synthesis in rat liver and lung. Cancer Res 32:1686–1694

Witschi H-P (1973a) Qualitative and quantitative aspects of the biosynthesis of ribonucleic acid and of protein in the liver and the lung of the Syrian golden hamster. Biochem J 136:781–788

Witschi H-P (1973b) The effects of diethylnitrosamine on ribonucleic acid and protein synthesis in the liver and lung of the Syrian golden hamster. Biochem J 136:789–794

Witschi H-P (1973c) The biochemical pathology of rat lung after acute paraquat poisoning. Toxicol Appl Pharmacol 25:485–486

Witschi H-P (1974) A comparative study of in vivo RNA and protein synthesis in rat liver and lung. Cancer Res 32:1686–1694

Witschi H-P (1975) Exploitable biochemical approaches for the evaluation of toxic lung damage. In: Hayes WJ (ed) Essays in toxicology, vol 6. Academic, New York, pp 125–191

Witschi H-P (1976) Proliferation of type II alveolar cells: a review of common response in toxic lung injury. Toxicology 5:267–277

Witschi H-P, Cote MG (1976) Biochemical pathology of lung damage produced by chemicals. Fed Proc 35:89–94

Witschi H-P, Cote MG (1977) Primary pulmonary responses to toxic agents. CRC Crit Rev Toxicol 5:23–66

Witschi H-P, Saheb W (1974) Stimulation of DNA synthesis in mouse lung following intraperitoneal injection of butylated hydroxytoluene. Proc Soc Exp Biol Med 147:690–693

Witschi H-P, Kacew S, Tsang BK, Williamson D (1976) Biochemical parameters of BHT-induced cell growth in mouse lung. Chem Biol Interact 12:29–40

Witschi H-P, Kacew S, Hirai KI, Cote MG (1977) In vivo oxidation of reduced nicotinamide-adenine dinucleotide phosphate by paraquat and diquat in rat lung. Chem Biol Interaction 19:143–160

Wolfe BMJ, Rubinstein D, Beck JC (1968) The metabolism isolated pneumocytes from rabbit lung. Can J Biochem 46:151–154

Woods HF, Meredith A, Tucker GT, Shortland JR (1980) Ciba Found Symp 78 (new series):61–83

Yazdi E, Gyorkey F (1971) Biochemical study of nuclei isolated from normal lung and lung tumors. II. Nuclear RNAs of low molecular weight. J Natl Cancer Inst 47:765–770

Yazdi E, Gyorkey F (1973) RNA synthesis in isolated nuclei of human lungs. Am J Pathol 70:30a

Yazdi E, Gyorkey F, Busch H, Gyorkey P (1971) Biochemical study of nuclei isolated from normal lung and lung tumors. I. Isolation of nuclei and characterization of nuclear RNA. J Natl Cancer Inst 47:212–219

Yeager H Jr (1969) Alveolar cells: depression effect of cigarette smoke on protein synthesis. Proc Soc Exp Biol Med 131:247–250

Yeager H Jr, Hicks PS (1972) Glucose metabolism in lung slices of late fetal, newborn, and adult rats. Proc Exp Biol Med 141:1–3

Yeager H Jr, Massaro D (1972) Glucose metabolism and glycoprotein synthesis by lung slices. J Appl Physiol 32:477–482

Young SL, Tierney DF (1972) Dipalmitoyl lecithin secretion and metabolism by the rat lung. Am J Physiol 222:1539–1544

Young SL, Tierney DF (1977) Metabolic activity of the lung. Int Anesthesiol Clin 15:1–17

Young SL, O'Neill JJ, Kasuyama RS, Tierney DF (1980) Glucose utilization by edematous rat lungs. Lung 157:165–177

Yuen TGH, Sherwin RP (1971) Hyperplasia of type 2 pneumocytes and nitrogen dioxide (10 ppm) exposure. Arch Environ Health 22:178–188

Zachman RD (1973a) The enzymes of lecithin biosynthesis in human newborn lungs. III. Phosphorylcholine glyceride transferase. Pediatr Res 7:632–637

Zachman RD (1973b) Enzymes of lecithin biosynthesis in human neonatal lung. In: Villee CA, Villee DB, Zuckerman J (eds) Respiratory distress syndrome. Academic, New York, pp 295–309

CHAPTER 14

The Pulmonary Mixed-Function Oxidase System

T. E. GRAM

A. Introduction

In 1974 TIERNEY wrote: "In terms of phylogeny, the lung is a relatively new organ, but it has been in existence longer than have biochemists and physiologists. Why, then, have its metabolism and biochemistry been ignored until recently?" Since then, considerable progress has been made in our knowledge of basic lung biochemistry, including the pulmonary mixed-function oxidase or monooxygenase system. Much of this recent research has been spurred by the need to identify and quantify the pulmonary effects of a variety of inhaled toxic pollutants and synthetic pneumotoxins.

Lung, gastrointestinal tract, and skin are the three "primary portals" through which animals and humans are exposed to hazardous potentially toxic substances in the environment. Having entered the lung, a substance may produce toxicity by virtue of a local effect on the cells of the lung itself (O_3, NO_2) or a systemic effect following transalveolar absorption into the circulating blood (HCN). Each minute, between 4 and 6 l of air, which may contain potentially toxic substances, are passed over a surface whose area is about 70 m^2. Foreign compounds may also damage the lung itself through their presence in the systemic blood, persuing the lung.

B. Cell Types of Lung

The vast majority of studies of mixed-function oxidation have been conducted with liver, an organ in which two cell types comprise more than 90% of the cells (GRAM 1980) and one of those (Kupffer cells) is essentially devoid of monooxygenase activity. Thus, studies in liver are performed on a virtually pure population of cells. By contrast, mammalian lung is comprised of "well over 40 distinctive cell types" (SOROKIN 1970) which raises the question whether monooxygenase activity is concentrated in only a few cell types or is generally distributed throughout all cells.

SOROKIN (1970) has proposed that four cell types, all of epithelial origin, are unique to the lung. They are: (a) the nonciliated bronchiolar or Clara cells; (b) the membranous pneumocytes or type I cells; (c) the granular pneumocytes or type II cells; and (d) the pulmonary alveolar macrophages (PAM). The nonciliated bronchiolar epithelial or Clara cells are cuboidal cells which form domes protruding into the bronchiolar lumen. They are interspersed with ciliated cells. The characteristic feature of Clara cells is the presence of numerous cytoplasmic electron-dense bodies which migrate from the base to the apex of the cell and are apparently extruded onto the bronchiolar surface by exocytosis. Another noteworthy characteristic of Clara cells is the presence, particularly at the apex of the cell, of an extremely highly developed smooth endoplasmic reticulum (Kuhn 1976, 1978; Plopper et al. 1980).

The type I cell is somewhat unremarkable in ultrastructural terms. The cell and its flat cytoplasm are poor in organelles; however, limited numbers of mitochondria, free ribosomes, and short cisternae of rough endoplasmic reticulum are evident (Kuhn 1976). Histochemical findings suggest that type I cells are metabolically relatively inactive.

Type II cells, by contrast, are metabolically active and widely believed to be the site of pulmonary surfactant biosynthesis (Morgan 1971). Type II cells have a large, centrally located nucleus and an abundance of cytoplasmic structures: lamellar bodies, mitochondria, free ribosomes, rough endoplasmic reticulum, Golgi apparatus, and multivesicular bodies. A variety of metabolically active enzymes have been demonstrated histochemically.

PAM can be distinguished by their relatively large size, rounded shape, the presence of pseudopodia, and their usual location in the alveolar space or alveolar surface. The predominant cytoplasmic structure of PAM is lysosomes which can be readily demonstrated histochemically or in purified cell fractions following cellular disruption. Mitochondria, Golgi apparatus, and free ribosomes are also present.

C. Drug Oxidation by Lung

The mixed-function oxidase system, whether of lung, liver, or placenta is remarkable in its lack of substrate specificity. A compound needs only to be lipophilic and relatively nonionized at physiologic pH to be a substrate. Accordingly, the monooxygenase system catalyzes the oxidation of a variety of drugs and other foreign chemical compounds (food additives, pesticides, chemical carcinogens, etc.) For this reason, the term xenobiotic (foreign to life) was coined (Mason 1965) to describe collectively the substrates for this enzyme system. However, the monooxygenase system also catalyzes the hydroxylation of certain endogenous substrates such as steroids, bile acids, and fatty acids. The terms monooxygenase or mixed-function oxidase have been largely retained because they describe the mechanism and reactants–products of the reaction

$$R-H + O_2 \rightarrow R-OH + HOH.$$

Thus, both atoms of oxygen enter into the reaction, one being inserted into the substrate while the other is reduced to water.

Drug biotransformation or metabolism was once equated with "detoxication" or biological inactivation; indeed, this is generally the case. But more recent work has shown that certain xenobiotics can be metabolically activated to highly reactive chemical intermediates which may interact with vital tissue macromolecules and cause a variety of toxic sequelae (e. g., acetaminophen, furosemide, chloramphenicol, and carbon tetrachloride).

I. Pulmonary Cell Fractionation and the Preparation of Microsomes

Prior to 1970, no studies had been published dealing with the systematic subfractionation of lung homogenates (nuclei, lysosomes, mitochondria, microsomes, cytosol) accompanied by verification of the fractions by electron microscopy or marker enzymes, or both; all information available pertained to whether lung contained monooxygenase activity or not. MATSUBARA and TOCHINO (1971) and HOOK et al. (1972) fractionated rabbit lung homogenate according to standard differential centrifugation techniques. Cell fractions were characterized by marker enzyme distribution or electron microscopy, or both, and were compared with simultaneously prepared liver fractions.

In general, the subcellular distribution of marker enzymes and biochemical constituents was very similar in lung and liver and a number of clear trends emerged (Table 1). Enzymes employed as "markers" in liver distributed themselves in a similar pattern in lung fractions; DNA predominated in the crude nuclear fraction while monoamine oxidase and succinate cytochrome c reductase were found primarily in the mitochondrial fraction. The lysosomal markers were also found in this fraction, but is should be remembered that under simple differential centrifugation, mitochondria and lysosomes cosediment (REISS 1966).

Table 1. Distribution of marker enzymes in subcellular fractions of rabbit lung (values are percentages of the total activity in the four cell fractions found in each fraction)

Enzyme or constituent		Cell fractions			
		Nuclear	Mitochondrial	Microsomal	Cytosol
Nuclear marker	DNA	77	8	3	3
Mitochondrial marker	Monoamine oxidase	8	77	13	2
	Succinate cytochrome c reductase	15	81	4	0
Lysosomal marker	Aryl sulfatase	7	85	5	3
	Acid phosphatase	5	63	22	10
Microsomal marker	RNA	10	22	62	7
	Glucose-6-phosphatase	51	36	10	3
Monooxygenase components	Aniline-4-hydroxylase	19	24	55	2
	Benzphetamine-N-demethylase	20	21	56	3
	Biphenyl-4-hydroxylase	18	23	60	0
	NADPH-cytochrome c reductase	5	22	72	1
	Cytochrome P-450	2	44	53	0
Cytosol marker	Glucose-6-phosphate dehydrogenase	11	16	8	65

Data assembled from MATSUBARA and TOCHINO (1971) and HOOK et al. (1972)

Table 2. Mixed-function oxidase activities in subcellular fractions of liver and lung (data are expressed as nmol product formed per milligram protein per minute)

Parameter	Nuclear	Mitochondrial	Microsomal	Cytosol	Microsomal lung/liver
Benzphetamine-N-demethylase					
Lung	3.2	1.7	9.0	0.5	1.11
Liver	5.4	1.7	8.1	0.3	
Biphenyl-4-hydroxylase					
Lung	1.1	0.7	3.7	0	1.12
Liver	0.6	0.7	3.3	0.1	
NADPH-cytochrome c reductase					
Lung	4.2	10.3	42.7	0.9	0.90
Liver	7.2	7.8	47.7	2.0	
Cytochrome P-450					
Lung	0.01	0.01	0.24	0	0.13
Liver	0.30	0.37	1.82	0	
Aniline-4-hydroxylase					
Lung	0.12	0.08	0.23	0.01	0.43
Liver	0.17	0.10	0.53	0.01	

Data from Hook et al. (1972)

Glucose-6-phosphatase, a classical marker for microsomes (endoplasmic reticulum) in liver was smeared across more rapidly sedimenting pulmonary cell fractions; in addition, the total activity of glucose-6-phosphatase in lung was less that 5% that of liver. The mixed-function oxidase components were concentrated in the microsomal fraction of the lung. Electron micrographs revealed that the monooxygenase activities in the nuclear and mitochondrial fractions were largely the result of microsomal contamination.

For quantitative purposes, the absolute mixed-function oxidase activities in rabbit liver and lung are presented in Table 2. Expressed per milligram microsomal protein, the activities of benzphetamine-N-demethylase, biphenyl-4-hydroxylase, and NADPH-cytochrome c reductase activities were very similar in microsomes of rabbit liver and lung. Aniline hydroxylase activity of lung was less that 50% that of liver (actually closer to 35% in subsequent experiments). To place these specific activities (activity per milligram protein) in proper perspective, it should be pointed out that the yield of microsomal protein per gram liver is about 2–3 times that from lung and that in the adult rabbit, the total liver mass is about 8 times that of lung. These factors would appear to minimize the role of lung in whole body clearance of drugs, but this topic will be discussed in Sect. F.

The kinetic behavior of monooxygenases in lung and liver are very similar: both require NADPH or an NADPH-generating system for maximal activity and activity was not enhanced by the addition of NADH (Bend et al. 1972; Gram 1973). Both systems require oxygen or air and are inhibited by nitrogen (anaerobiosis) and by carbon monoxide; similarly, both are inhibited by ferricytochrome c and by SKF 525-A (2-diethylaminoethyl-2,2-diphenylvalerate) in vitro. They had similar K_m values for a variety of substrates and similar temperature and pH optima (BEND et al. 1972).

II. Pragmatic Considerations in the Preparation of Pulmonary Microsomes

Lungs, dissected free of large blood vessels and airways, are finely divided by passage through a tissue press or carefully diced with scissors. Phosphate buffers (0.1 M), 0.25 M sucrose, Tris-HCl, and 0.15 M KCl–50 mM Tris-HCl have been used successfully as homogenizing media (GRAM 1980). We routinely use a polytetrafluoroethylene (Teflon)–glass homogenizer immersed in ice (A.H. Thomas Company, Philadelphia, Pennsylvania, size C with 0.15–0.22 mm clearance, attached to an electric drill ($\sim$2,500 rpm) for this purpose. The tissue is homogenized in 2 volumes w/v of buffer by 10–15 up and down excursions of the pestle and diluted to 1:4 w/v with buffer. The diluted homogenate is then centrifuged (0°–4 °C) at about 10,000 g (20 min) and the resulting postmitochondrial supernatant is centrifuged at 105,000 g for 60–75 min to sediment microsomes. The supernatant (cytosol) phase is removed, the microsomes resuspended by homogenization in buffer, and resedimented to remove traces of hemoglobin. The usual yield of microsomal protein from rodent lung is 5–10 mg per gram tissue. Attempts to increase microsomal protein yield have utilized brief sonication of the whole lung homogenate (FOUTS and DEVEREUX 1973) or rehomogenization of the 10,000 g pellet (GRAM 1980) which have increased microsomal protein yield up to twofold without reducing enzymic specific activity. Lung microsomes have also been successfully prepared using the calcium aggregation method (LITTERST et al. 1975 b).

III. The Microsomal Monooxygenase System of Mammalian Lung

1. Kinetic Aspects and Substrate Spectrum

Summarizing what we know about this system in rabbit lung:

1. The enzyme system is localized in the microsomal fraction of lung and requires NADPH and oxygen for optimal activity. NADH substitutes poorly for NADPH in supporting monooxygenase activity ($\sim$20%) and the two nucleotides do not act synergistically (HOOK et al. 1972; BEND et al. 1972; GRAM 1973).
2. The enzyme is inhibited by oxidized cytochrome c and by carbon monoxide, probably implicating the mediation of the flavoprotein enzyme NADPH-cytochrome c reductase and the hemoprotein cytochrome P-450. It is also inhibited by the traditional hepatic microsomal enzyme inhibitor SKF 525-A (GRAM 1973).
3. In rabbit lung, levels of cytochrome P-450 are less that 20% those of liver whereas activities of NADPH-cytochrome c reductase in the two organs are very similar (HOOK et al. 1972).
4. Apparent K_m values for several substrates did not differ in lung and liver while V_{max} differed in all cases, being higher in lung or liver depending upon the sub-

strate. Other kinetic properties in the two organs such as temperature (35°–45 °C) and pH optima (pH 7–8) did not differ (Bend et al. 1972).
5. Substrate difference spectra with type I substrates (ΔA_{max}) were always lower in magnitute in lung (30%–60%) and with aniline, a type II substrate, the spectrum was anomalous.
6. Lung microsomes (Matsubara et al. 1974; Capdevila et al. 1975) had a high affinity for hemoglobin and aggregated around a microfibrillar matrix when isolated (Hook et al. 1972; Johannessen et al. 1977).

Some of the numerous metabolic pathways recorded in the lung are presented in Table 3. In addition, the pulmonary monooxygenase system catalyzes the oxidation of fatty acids, steroid hormones, and other endogenous compounds.

Table 3. Oxidation reactions [a] catalyzed by lung microsomes

Reaction	Reference
1. Hydroxylation	
A. Aromatic	
1. Benzene → phenol	Harper et al. (1973)
2. Cyclohexane → cyclohexanol	Guengerich (1977)
3. Benzo[a]pyrene → 3-hydroxybenzo[a]pyrene	Grover et al. (1974)
4. Aniline → 4-hydroxyaniline	Matsubara and Tochino (1971), Hook et al. (1972)
5. Biphenyl-4-Hydroxylase	Hook et al. (1972)
Biphenyl-2-Hydroxylase	Burke and Prough (1976)
B. Aliphatic	
1. p-Xylene → p-methylbenzylalcohol	Carlone and Fouts (1974)
2. Decane → 1-decanol	Ichihara et al. (1969)
2. Epoxidation	
A. Benz[a]anthracene → 5,6-epoxide	Grover et al. (1973)
B. Benzo[a]pyrene → 4,5-epoxide	Grover et al. (1974)
Epoxide hydrolase	Smith et al. (1978)
3. Dealkylation	
A. N-Dealkylation	
1. N-Methylaniline	Devereux and Fouts (1974)
2. Aminopyrine	Bend et al. (1972)
Ethylmorphine	
Benzphetamine	
N-Methyl-p-chloroaniline	
3. 3-Methyl-4-monomethylaminoazobenzene	Gilman and Conney (1963)
B. O-Dealkylation	
1. p-Nitroanisole	Ichikawa et al. (1969)
2. 7-Ethoxycoumarin	Devereux et al. (1979)
3. Ethoxyresorufin	Burke et al. (1977), Sipal et al. (1979)
4. Acetophenetidin	Welch et al. (1972)
4. N-Oxidation	
A. N,N-Dimethylaniline	Devereux and Fouts (1974)
B. Perazine	Breyer (1971)

[a] Relative to liver microsomes, sulfoxidation and deamination have not yet been reported

Moreover, the lung appears to be equipped with a full complement of conjugative enzymes (glucuronyl transferases, N-acetyltransferases, etc.) found in other organs.

2. Species Differences in Pulmonary Monooxygenase Activity

Much of the work performed has utilized rabbits, primarily because of the relatively high levels of enzyme activity found in this species. A survey of five common laboratory species (LITTERST et al. 1975 a) has confirmed this generalization (Table 4). Most of the other species examined including humans (Table 5) had low or insignificant lung enzyme levels.

Table 4. Enzyme activities in several animal species expressed as liver/lung (specific enzyme activities)

Enzyme	Rabbit	Rat	Mouse	Hamster	Guinea pig
Benzphetamine Demethylase	1.23	0.16			
Biphenyl-4-hydroxylase	1.10				
Cytochrome P-450	0.13	0.07	0.15	0.07	0.10
NADPH-cytochrome c reductase	0.90	0.29	1.22	0.35	0.41
Aniline-4-hydroxylase	0.33	0.05	0.22	0.19	0.25
Aminopyrine demethylase	0.40	0.30	0.05	0.20	0.07
Glutathione S-aryltransferase	0.24	<0.05	0.29	0.08	0.08
N-Acetyltransferase (p-aminobenzoic acid)	1.11	0.33	0.25	0.15	0.34
Uridine diphosphate glucuronyltransferase (p-nitrophenol)	0.06	0.18	0.68	0.18	<0.05

Abstracted in part from LITTERST et al. (1975 a)

Table 5. Monooxygenase activities in human lung and liver microsomes (values are means from 3–9 individual cases)

	Lung	Liver	Lung/liver
Benzo[a]pyrene hydroxylase (pmol per milligram protein per minute)	0.23	34.5	0.007
Ethoxycoumarin O-deethylase (pmol per milligram protein per minute)	13.3	585	0.023
Phenacetin O-deethylase (pmol per milligram protein per minute)	4.2	1441	0.003
Cytochrome P-450 (nmol per milligram protein)	Undetectable	0.58	
Cytochrome b_5 (nmol per milligram protein)	0.009	0.400	0.022
NADPH-cytochrome c reductase (nmol per milligram protein per minute)	33	177	0.19

Abstracted from McMANUS et al. (1980)

3. Differential Control of Monooxygenase Activities in Lung and Other Organs

It is now clear that the biologic mechanisms that control monooxygenase activity in lung and other organs are quite different. This is true of intestine, adrenal, placenta, gonads, skin, liver, and other organs. For example, there is a three- to fourfold difference in the levels of monooxygenase activity in the livers of male and female rats. No such sex difference exists in the lungs of these animals (LITTERST et al. 1977). Similarly, pretreatment of animals with an enzyme inducer such as phenobarbital increases hepatic monooxygenase activity two- to fourfold, but is without effect on pulmonary enzymes (LITTERST et al. 1977). Marked differences have been noted in the patterns of postnatal development of monooxygenase systems in liver and lung (FOUTS and DEVEREUX 1972). Finally, monooxygenase enzymes in liver are known to be markedly depressed during deficiency of vitamin C (SIKIC et al. 1977; KUENZIG et al. 1977) or vitamin A (MIRANDA et al. 1979), but lung enzymes in these deficiency states remain unaffected.

4. Purification and Reconstitution of the Rabbit Pulmonary Monooxygenase System

In 1968 LU and COON first described resolution, purification, and reconstitution of the microsomal monooxygenase from rabbit liver microsomes. Some 8 years later, using similar techniques ARINC and PHILPOT (1976) reported partial (32-fold) purification of cytochrome P-450 from rabbit lung microsomes. The authors solubilized the phospholipid microsomal membranes with Na-cholate, employed ammonium sulfate precipitation and chromatography on DEAE-cellulose and hydroxyapatite. They found that use of 20% glycerol, which was a key to stabilizing hepatic cytochrome P-450 during purification, failed to stabilize pulmonary P-450. Their best preparation contained 7.4 nmol cytochrome P-450 per milligram protein with yields of 10%–15% and was free of NADPH-cytochrome c reductase activity and cytochrome P-420, a partially denatured form of cytochrome P-450. It copurified with epoxide hydrolase. The cytochrome P-450 fraction gave typical type I and type II difference spectra upon addition of the appropriate substrate, but a peculiarity of this partially purified cytochrome P-450 was that, in contrast to the hepatic system, it required the lipid fraction for complete reduction, even with dithionite. Meanwhile, progress was being made in purification of NADPH-cytochrome c (P-450) reductase (hereafter referred to as the reductase). BUEGE and AUST (1975) isolated the reductase enzymes from rat liver and lung after bromelain digestion and purified them to immunochemical homogeneity. Complete immunologic identity of the two proteins was demonstrated. Similar findings with the lung and liver reductases were reported by PROUGH and BURKE (1975).

Later work by Philpot's group (WOLF et al. 1978) using slightly modified methodology resolved rabbit lung cytochrome P-450 into two forms. Cytochrome P-450$_I$ was purified to 9.6 nmol per milligram protein (77-fold) with a recovery of about 42% while cytochrome P-450$_{II}$ was purified to 6.1 nmol per milligram protein (49-fold) with a recovery of 11%. NADPH-cytochrome P-450 reductase was purified about 100-fold at a recovery of 20%. The two cytochromes were distinguishable by the location of their CO difference peaks, cytochrome P-450$_I$ having an A_{max} at 452 nm and cytochrome P-450$_{II}$ at 450 nm. The addition of sonicated phosphatidylcholine increased the rate and extent of the reduction of cytochrome P-450$_I$ without affecting cytochrome P-450$_{II}$ (WOLF et al. 1978). Cytochrome P-450$_I$ gave typical substrate difference spectra when exposed to type I or type II substrates while cytochrome P-450$_{II}$ gave somewhat anomalous type I spectra. Cytochrome P-450$_I$ was further resolvable on polyacrylamide gels into two proteins (57,000 and 51,000 daltons) while cytochrome P-450$_{II}$ migrated as a single band at 53,000 daltons. Reconstitution required all three components (cytochrome P-450, the reductase, and phosphatidylcholine); only fractions containing cytochrome P-450$_I$ catalyzed the deethylation of 7-ethoxycoumarin and demethylation of benzphetamine. Cytochrome P-450$_{II}$ was inactive with these substrates, but was about 20% more active than cytochrome P-450$_I$ in catalyzing the metabolism of benzo[a]pyrene. It is noteworthy that the two cytochromes produced markedly different metabolite profiles when incubated with reductase, benzo[a]pyrene, and NADPH. It was suggested that the two isozymes of the cytochrome are present in pulmonary microsomes in about equal amounts. GUENGERICH (1977) reported similar studies on the purification of cytochrome P-450 and its reductase (NADPH-cytochrome P-450 reductase) from rabbit lung.

The NADPH-cytochrome P-450 reductases prepared from lung and liver microsomes appeared identical by their apparent subunit molecular weights, isoelectric focusing patterns, activities toward cytochrome c, and abilities to support benzphetamine demethylation with lung and liver cytochrome P-450.

Rabbit lung cytochrome P-450 was resolved into two bands chromatographically: cytochrome P-450 A was purified 55-fold and obtained in 22% yield while cytochrome P-450 B was purified 11-fold and obtained in 6% yield. Both bands were devoid of hemoglobin, methemoglobin, and cytochrome P-420 as well as cytochrome b_5 and NADPH-cytochrme P-450 reductase. Cytochrome P-450 A was homogeneous as determined by SDS–polyacrylamide gel electrophoresis and by isoelectric focusing and was found to have a molecular weight of about 49,000. Electrophoresis of fraction B gave three major bands. The results of reconstitution experiments are reported in Table 6; NADPH, phospholipid (dilauroylphosphatidylcholine), and reductase from either lung or liver were required.

Table 6. Metabolic activity of two cytochrome P-450 fractions purified from rabbit lung toward several substrates

Substrate	Turnover (min^{-1})	
	Fraction A (purified 55-fold)	Fraction B (purified 11-fold)
Benzphetamine	37	2
Cyclohexane	28	2
7-Ethoxycoumarin	1.2	<0.1
Benzo[a]pyrene	0.10	0.03
4-Ipomeanol	3.3	0.04

Taken in part from GUENGERICH (1977)

More careful analysis of the metabolic interaction of pulmonary cytochrome P-450 with benzo[a]pyrene (WOLF et al. 1979) revealed that both forms of rabbit pulmonary cytochrome P-450 catalyzed the total metabolism of benzo[a]pyrene in reconstituted systems at similar rates. Phospholipids were required to obtain maximum activity with cytochrome P-450$_I$, but not with cytochrome P-450$_{II}$. The metabolic profiles of benzo[a]pyrene produced by cytochrome p-450$_I$ and P-450$_{II}$ as determined by high pressure liquid chromatography (HPLC) were markedly different. Moreover, there was differential inhibition of the two cytochromes by the in vitro addition of α-naphthoflavone, (viz., selective for cytochrome P-450$_{II}$) without altering the metabolic profile. It was of further interest that, in the presence of added calf thymus DNA, cytochrome P-450$_I$ and P-450$_{II}$ produced different degrees of covalent binding of benzo[a]pyrene metabolites to the nucleic acid. No significant covalent binding of benzo[a]pyrene metabolites was observed in the presence of cytochrome P-450$_I$. Metabolites that chromatographed with the 3-hydroxyl and quinone standards of benzo[a]pyrene accounted for 95% of the total metabolic activity of cytochrome P-450$_I$. With cytochrome P-450$_{II}$, hydroxylation at positions 9 and 10 accounted for 40%–50% of the total activity. Products that chromatographed with the 3-hydroxy standard were 30%–40% of the total. Formation of the 4,5- or 8,9-dihydrodiol metabolites accounted for less than 5% of the total produced by either cytochrome.

SERABJIT-SINGH et al. (1979) showed that cytochrome P-450$_I$ and P-450$_{II}$ of rabbit lung are immunochemically as well as catalytically distinct. Cytochrome P-450$_I$ was also immunochemically distinct from the cytochrome P-450 induced in rabbit liver by pretreatment with phenobarbital (P-450$_{PB}$), but NADPH-cytochrome P-450 reductase purified from lungs and livers of rabbits were identical as judged by physical, catalytic, and immunochemical criteria. In reconstituted systems consisting of NADPH and reductase (from either liver or lung), pulmonary cytochrome P-450$_I$ was completely responsible for the dealkylation of benzphetamine, aminopyrine, ethylmorphine, and 7-ethoxycoumarin. Cytochrome P-450$_{II}$ had some (slower) activity in the hydroxylation of coumarin, benzo[a]pyrene, p-xylene, and N-hydroxyamphetamine (SERABJIT-SINGH et al. 1979). Demethylase activity of benzphetamine, aminopyrine, etc., catalyzed by cytochrome P-450$_I$ was reduced 40%–50% in the absence of lipid.

Work from Philpot's laboratory (SLAUGHTER et al. 1981) compared the properties of rabbit pulmonary cytochrome P-450$_I$ and P-450$_{II}$ with that of hepatic cytochrome P-450 induced by phenobarbital P-450$_{PB}$). It was reported that:

1. The electrophoretic mobilities of cytochrome P-450$_I$ and P-450$_{PB}$ were the same, but both were different from cytochrome P-450$_{II}$.
2. The molecular weights of cytochrome P-450$_I$ and P-450$_{PB}$ were the same (52,000) whereas that of cytochrome P-450$_{II}$ was 58,000.
3. The amino acid compositions of cytochrome P-450$_I$ and P-450$_{II}$ were different and digestion of the hemoproteins with chymotrypsin or papain yielded peptide patterns in which cytochrome P-450$_I$ and P-450$_{PB}$ were identical and were both different from cytochrome P-450$_{II}$.

It was concluded that the properties of cytochrome P-450$_I$ and P-450$_{II}$ were different in all cases whereas those of cytochrome P-450$_I$ and P-450$_{PB}$ were the same; thus, the protein moieties of cytochrome P-450$_I$ and P-450$_{II}$ are distinct and unrelated and that of cytochrome P-450$_I$ and P-450$_{PB}$ are the same.

Recent studies by UENG and ALVARES (1981) have revealed an interesting species difference in the response of the pulmonary monooxygenase system to Aroclor 1254, a widely used polychlorinated biphenyl mixture. Administration of Aroclor 1254 to rats revealed it to be a powerful inducer of cytochrome P-450 and aryl hydrocarbon hydroxylase (AHH) activity in lung microsomes. However, its administration to rabbits was accompanied by a 40% decrease in pulmonary microsomal cytochrome P-450, a 30% loss in AHH activity, and a 70% reduction in ethylmorphine demethylase. Purification of microsomal cytochrome P-450 by the method of WOLF et al. (1979) from lungs of control and Aroclor 1254-treated rabbits showed a marked decrease in cytochrome P-450$_I$ (70%) with no significant alteration in cytochrome P-450$_{II}$ content. It was also reported that purified cytochrome P-450$_{II}$ was much more stable upon exposure to air at room temperature for 60 min than was cytochrome P-450$_I$.

D. Mixed-Function Oxidase Activity in Specific Pulmonary Cell Types

Early histochemical studies with rat lung yielded discrepant results regarding the distribution of monooxygenase activity. WATTENBERG and LEONG (1962) reported benzo[a]pyrene hydroxylase activity (AHH) localized in the alveolar walls while the bronchi and bronchioles were devoid of activity. On the other hand, GRASSO et al. (1971), found low levels of aniline hydroxylase activity in alveolar epithelial cells, but significant activity in bronchial epithelium.

I. Pulmonary Alveolar Macrophage

PAM is a cell type that can be obtained in a high degree of purity (> 95%).REID and his colleagues (1972) showed that microsomes from rabbit PAM were totally

Table 7. Monooxygenase activities in microsomes from rabbit lung and pulmonary alveolar macrophages (data expressed as nmol product formed per milligram protein per minute)

Activity	Macrophage	Lung
Biphenyl-4-hydroxylase[a]	0.14	4.54
Benzphetamine demethylase[a]	0.29	7.66
Benzo[a]pyrene hydroxylase (AHH)[a]	0.02	2.44
NADPH-cytochrome c reductase[a]	43	127
Cytochrome P-450[a]	0.01	0.27
Cytochrome P-450[b]	0.05	0.32
4-Nitroanisole demethylase[b]	17.1	26.6

[a] Data taken from BEND et al. (1973)
[b] Data taken from FISHER et al. (1977)

incapable of oxidatively metabolizing 7,12-dimethyl-1,2-benzanthacene or bromobenzene under conditions in which lung and liver microsomes from the same animals catalyzed these reactions at brisk rates. BEND et al. (1973) essentially confirmed these results, showing that monooxygenase activity in microsomes from rabbit PAM was < 1% that of whole lung (Table 7). Using a different technique for obtaining PAM, FISHER et al. (1977) found slightly higher levels of cytochrome P-450 than had BEND et al. (1973). In addition, using 4-nitroanisole as a substrate for the monooxygenase system, FISHER et al. (1977) found that microsomes from PAM had about 60% the activity of lung microsomes (Table 7). It does not seem likely, however, that PAM contribute significantly to total pulmonary monooxygenase activity.

II. Dispersed Single Cells Isolated from Whole Lung

Dispersed single cells from rabbit lung were fractionated by centrifugal elutriation, a technique which utilizes differences in cell size (DEVEREUX et al. 1979), which was then followed by density gradient centrifugation. Five heterogeneous fractions were collected and monooxygenase activity was distributed nonuniformly across the various fractions.

III. Type I Pneumocytes

Very limited progress has been made toward preparing high purity type I cells populations from dispersed lung cells. PICCIANO and ROSENBAUM (1978) isolated populations of type I cells that reached 70% purity, but no further progress has been made in this area.

IV. Type II Pneumocytes

Considerable progress has been made in the isolation of highly purified (> 90%) populations of type II cells from enzymatically dispersed rat and rabbit lungs (KIKKAWA et al. 1975; SEVANIAN et al. 1981). TEEL and DOUGLAS (1980) reported on the AHH activity in alveolar type II cells clonally derived from adult rat lung. Although it is difficult to compare the reported activities with those obtained with whole lung homogenates, easily measurable levels of AHH activity were found in these type II cells; moreover, prior exposure (for 24 h) of the cells to 3-methylcholanthrene increased AHH activity 2-fold while exposure to benzo[a]pyrene increased activity 37-fold. Finally, after exposure of the cells to benzo[a]pyrene ^{3}H, about 80% of the retained radioactivity was bound to the nucleus, and the remaining 20% was cytoplasmic.

   DEVEREUX and FOUTS have prepared relatively pure populations of type II and Clara cells for the study of xenobiotic metabolism (DEVEREUX et al. 1979; DEVEREUX and FOUTS 1980 a, b). In a preliminary report (DEVEREUX et al. 1981 a), these workers obtained, from rabbit lung, type II cells estimated to be 80% pure and Clara cells of about 70% purity. The specific activity of 7-ethoxycoumarin-O-deethylase in Clara cells was almost six times that of type II cells (170 compared with 30 pmol per milligram protein). Similarly, AHH and epoxide hydrolase activities were 3–5 times higher in Clara cells: the coumarin hydroxylase activity in Clara cells was 42 compared with 1 pmol per milligram protein per minute in type II cells. Interestingly, the activities of glutathione-S-epoxide transferase were about the same in the two cell populations.

V. Nonciliated Bronchiolar (Clara) Cells

GILLETTE et al. (1974a, b) provided evidence that xenobiotics were being converted in vivo by the cytochrome P-450-dependent monooxygenase system to highly reactive intermediates which covalently bound to vital tissue macromolecules at or very near their site of formation. REID et al. (1973) administered bromobenzene ^{14}C to mice and rats by intraperitoneal injection: 36–48 h later they found:
1. Selective necrosis of the bronchiolar epithelium; no histologic changes were observed in alveolar epithelium or septa.
2. Autoradiograms showed radioactivity heavily concentrated and selectively accumulated in the necrotic bronchiolar epithelium.
3. Incubation of mouse lung microsomes with NADPH and bromobenzene in vitro converted the xenobiotic to an active metabolite which bound covalently to the protein of microsomes.

In the first of a series of studies, BOYD et al. (1975) characterized 4-ipomeanol, a pneumotoxic component of moldy sweet potatoes which, when consumed by cattle, produced severe lung damage. When fed to cattle or administered to experimental animals, severe pulmonary edema and congestion resulted (Fig. 1). Moreover, the material or metabolites selectively accumulated in lung where it bound covalently (BOYD et al. 1975). Some 24 h after administration to rats, radioactivity derived from 4-ipomeanol was covalently bound in lung with a lung : blood ratio of about 60 : 1. As had been shown with bromobenzene earlier, incubation of 4-ipomeanol ^{14}C with lung microsomes and NADPH resulted in covalent binding of radioactivity to microsomes (BOYD 1976).

Using autoradiographic techniques, BOYD (1977) provided evidence that the Clara cell was the primary site of cytochrome P-450-dependent monooxygenase

4-IPOMEANOL

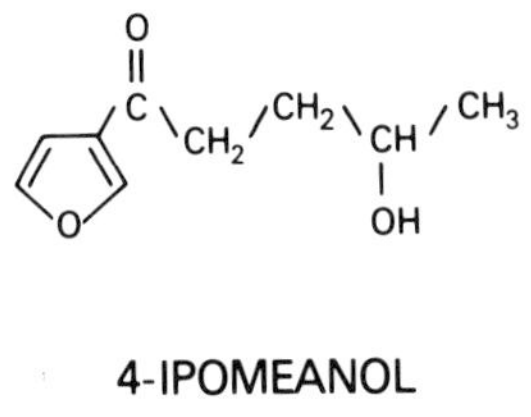

Fig. 1. Structure of 4-ipomeanol

activity in lung. Autoradiograms prepared from animals killed at various times after injection of 4-ipomeanol showed the covalently bound metabolite to be heavily concentrated in the lining cells of the airways. Tissues removed from animals 16 h after dosing showed a striking and specific necrosis of the Clara cells whereas the adjacent ciliated bronchiolar cells and other major pulmonary parenchymal cells were unaffected. Subsequent work (BOYD et al. 1978 b) showed that 3-methylfuran, an analog of 4-ipomeanol, was metabolized in vivo in mice to a potent alkylating agent which also produced selective Clara cell necrosis.

More recent work (BOYD et al. 1980 b) has shown that carbon tetrachloride (CCl_4) which is toxic only after bioactivation by the cytochrome P-450 monooxygenase system binds covalently to lung microsomes from rats and mice and produces striking decreases in lung microsomal cytochrome P-450 and benzphetamine demethylase activity. Electron micrographs from lungs of both species revealed selective necrosis of Clara cells with no discernible effect on adjacent ciliated bronchiolar cells.

Additional evidence that the cytochrome P-450-dependent monooxygenase system of lung is highly localized in Clara cells was provided by SERABJIT-SINGH et al. (1980). Cytochrome P-450$_I$ (the form which catalyzes the dealkylation of benzphetamine and ethoxycoumarin) was purified to homogeneity from rabbit lung and antibodies were raised to it in goats. Employing immunofluorescence techniques, incubation of rabbit lung with the fluorescent antibody revealed that binding occurred almost exclusively to Clara cells. No fluorescent staining was noted in the ciliated bronchiolar epithelium or in the alveolar epithelium. Interestingly, the staining was most intense in the luminal pole of the Clara cell, the location of highest density of smooth endoplasmic reticulum (PLOPPER et al. 1980). Subsequent work employing Ouchterlony double immunodiffusion has shown both isozymes (cytochrome P-450$_I$ and P-450$_{II}$) to be present in microsomes from purified Clara cells and type II cells (DEVEREUX et al. 1981 b). However, when sections of rabbit lung were subjected to immunofluorescence study with antibodies to both isozymes, most of the fluorescence was localized in Clara cells; little if any fluorescence was found in type II cells.

Similar immunofluorescence studies on the localization of NADPH-cytochrome c (P-450) reductase have indicated that this enzyme is also concentrated in the bronchi and bronchioles, but appears to have a much broader distribution than merely in Clara cells (DEES et al. 1980). Fluorescence was intense and diffusely spread throughout bronchiolar cells.

Thus, data available at present obained with a variety of different techniques point strongly to the nonciliated bronchiolar epithelial cell (Clara cell) as the pulmonary cell type in which the cytochrome P-450-dependent monooxygenase system is most highly concentrated. In addition to the compelling evidence for this notion, a phylogenetic peculiarity has provided support. The airways of avian species contain no Clara cells; accordingly, lung microsomes prepared from chickens or Japanese quail were completely unable to catalyze the NADPH-dependent covalent binding of either 4-ipomeanol or benzo[a]pyrene although these reactions occurred in liver or kidney microsomes from these species (BUCKPITT and BOYD 1978, 1982). Correspondingly, the administration of 4-ipomeanol to quail resulted in hepatic necrosis (and covalent binding), but not pulmonary lesions.

E. Induction of the Pulmonary Mixed-Function Oxidase System

I. Phenobarbital

Pretreatment of a variety of animal species with phenobarbital evokes a two- to fourfold induction of cytochrome P-450, NADPH cytochrome c reductase, and drug metabolism in hepatic microsomes (CONNEY 1967). By contrast, as first shown by UEHLEKE (1968), phenobarbital pretreatment is without effect on the pulmonary mixed-function oxidase system. The responsiveness of the hepatic monooxygenase system to induction by phenobarbital and the refractoriness of the pulmonary monooxygenase system in the same animals suggests the possibility of different biochemical regulatory mechanisms in the two organs (Table 8).

Table 8. Pulmonary cytochrome P-450-dependent monooxygenase activities shown *not* to be affected by treatment of animals with phenobarbital

Enzyme activity	Reference
Cytochrome P-450	UEHLEKE (1968), OPPELT et al. (1970), MATSUBARA et al. (1974), LITTERST et al. (1977), KUENZIG et al. (1977), BOYD et al. (1978)
NADPH-cytochrome c reductase	LITTERST et al. (1977), KUENZIG et al. (1977), DEES et al. (1980)
Cytochrome b_5	MATSUBARA et al. (1974)
N-Methylaniline-N-demethylase	UEHLEKE (1968)
N-Methylaniline-4-hydroxylase	UEHLEKE (1968)
Aminopyrine demethylase	OPPELT et al. (1970)
Aniline hydroxylase	OPPELT et al. (1970)
4-Methyltoluene hydroxylase	CARLONE and FOUTS (1974)
Biphenyl-4-hydroxylase	LITTERST et al. (1977)
Bromobenzene hydroxylation	REID et al. (1973)
4-Ipomeanol (covalent binding)	BOYD and BURKA (1978), BOYD et al. (1980)
Benzo[a]pyrene hydroxylase (AHH)	MATSUBARA et al. (1974), WIEBEL et al. (1971), KUENZIG et al. (1977)
Ethoxycoumarin deethylase	KUENZIG et al. (1977)

II. 3-Methylcholanthrene and Other Polycyclic Aromatic Hydrocarbons: Tobacco Smoke, Cannabis

Polycyclic aromatic hydrocarbons, including 3-methylcholanthrene (3-MC), benzo[a]pyrene, dimethylbenzanthracene, and a host of other compounds are potent inducers of the hepatic monooxygenase system (CONNEY 1964; SNYDER and REMMER 1979). GILMAN and CONNEY (1963) demonstrated that 3-MC pretreatment caused a sevenfold stimulation in the demethylation of 3-methyl-4-monomethylaminoazobenzene (3-methyl-MAB) by rat lung microsomes. Pretreatment of animals with 3-MC has also been shown to enhance the oxidative metabolism of other xenobiotic substrates by lung microsomal enzymes; REID et al. (1972) re-

Table 9. Induction of pulmonary benzo[a]pyrene hydroxylase (AHH) activity by 3-methyl-cholanthrene (3-MC)

Species	Control	3-MC	3-MC/control	Reference
Rat	1.0	15.0	15.0	MATSUBARA et al. (1974)
Rat	4.0	18.0	4.5	GELBOIN and BLACKBURN (1964)
Rat	0.72	13.1	18.2	WARREN and BELLWARD (1978)
Rat lung cloned type II cells	0.21	0.59	2.8	TEEL and DOUGLAS (1980)
Rat	2.3	96.0	41.4	HUNDLEY and FREUDEN-THAL (1977)
Rhesus monkey	10.3	72.7	7.1	
Mouse				
C57BL/6J	9.3	190.6	20.5	SEIFRIED et al. (1977)
DBA/2J	4.8	95.8	20.0	
A/HeJ	4.6	259.2	56.3	
Swiss Mouse	15.7	130.7	8.3	WIEBEL et al. (1973)
C3H/He Mouse	0.19	4.32	22.7	WATANABE et al. (1978)
Hamster	0.06	0.20	3.3	BURKE and PROUGH (1976)
Hamster	3.6	77.8	21.6	OKAMOTO et al. (1972)
Rabbit	10.9	35.0	3.2	HULSHOFF et al. (1978)

ported a twofold increase in the hydroxylation of dimethylbenzanthracene. NAKAZAWA and COSTA (1971) found that 3-MC caused a 2.5-fold stimulation in the overall metabolism of Δ^9-tetrahydrocannabinol (Δ^9-THC) by rat lung microsomes. 7-Ethoxyresorufin deethylase activity was enhanced by 3-MC treatment to the extent of nearly 15-fold in rat lung, but only 2-fold in hamster lung (BURKE et al. 1977).

The induction of pulmonary cytochrome P-450 (or cytochrome P-448; form 4) by 3-MC has been reported by numerous authors (MATSUBARA et al. 1974; LITTERST et al. 1977; BOYD et al. 1978; BURKE and PROUGH 1976). The magnitude of the inductive effect has ranged from about 30% to 300%–400%. Cytochrome b_5 has been reported to be induced about fourfold by 3-MC in rat lung (MATSUBARA et al. 1974) whereas NADPH-cytochrome c reductase activity was apparently unaffected (CAPDEVILA et al. 1975).

Pulmonary benzo[a]pyrene hydroxylase (AHH) activity is readily induced by 3-MC, 9,10-dimethyl 1,2-benzanthracene, benzo[a]pyrene, and other hydrocarbons and the magnitude of induction is species and even strain dependent (mice) (Table 9).

GIELEN and associates (1972) discovered that the AHH in the livers of certain strains of mice was unresponsive to the inductive effects of 3-MC and that this resistance has a genetic basis. It is interesting in this regard that a mouse strain (DBA/2J), whose hepatic AHH is unresponsive to 3-MC, responds to the inducer with fivefold increases in AHH activiy in lung and other extrahepatic organs such as kidney, skin, and gut (WIEBEL et al. 1973; SEIFRIED et al. 1977). Moreover, in several strains of mice both responsive and unresponsive to 3-MC (SEIFRIED et al.

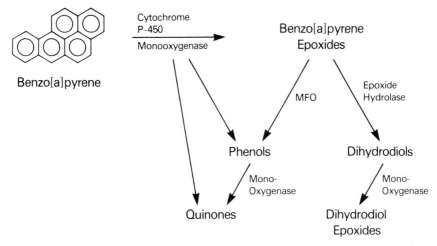

Fig. 2. General scheme for the microsomal metabolism of benzo[*a*]pyrene to a variety of metabolites. (Modified from GELBOIN et al. 1976)

1977), the specific activity of pulmonary epoxide hydrolase was much greater (~ 50-fold) than the monooxygenase activity. Consequently, in studies of the metabolism of benzo[*a*]pyrene in vitro, lung microsomes produced relatively large amounts of dihydrodiols as opposed to phenols and quinones, whereas with liver, phenols and quinones accounted for the bulk of the products and dihydrodiols were comparatively minor metabolites. Since the dihydrodiols are potentially more carcinogenic than the phenols and quinones (see Sect. G.I), this may account for the predominance of pulmonary neplasms after administration of polycyclic aromatic hydrocarbons (Fig. 2). Pulmonary alveolar macrophages isolated from human subjects by bronchial lavage and exposed to 3-MC during cell culture respond within 12–24 h with severalfold increase in AHH (CANTRELL et al. 1973b).

WELCH et al. (1971) examined the effects of cigarette smoke on pulmonary AHH activity. Continuous exposure of rats to a mixture of cigarette smoke and air for as little as 2 h produced a significant increase ($\sim 35\%$) in pulmonary AHH activity which reached about three times control levels after 4 h of exposure. Exposure of pregnant rats to the cigarette smoke–air mixture for 5 h daily for 3 days produced a 12-fold increase in pulmonary AHH activity, a 4-fold increase in placenta, and a doubling of activity in liver (WELCH et al. 1971). Subsequent studies (WELCH et al. 1972) demonstrated that exposure of rats to cigarette smoke for 4 h evoked a maximum induction of AHH activity of about 28-fold in 24 h. The induced activity remained at high levels for an additional 4 days following exposure (induction 24-fold at 5 days) and then fell precipitously to essentially control levels between days 5 and 6. OKAMOTO et al. (1972) instilled benzo[*a*]pyrene, denicotinized tobacco smoke condensate, or marijuana smoke condensate intratracheally into Syrian golden hamsters and studied pulmonary AHH activity. Peak enzyme activities occurred 24 h after instillation and approximately 14-fold increases by benzo[a]pyrene and about 4-fold increases after either of the smoke condensates; activities returned to control levels in 8–12 days. VAN CANTFORT and GIELEN (1975) reported that cigarette smoke induces AHH activity in the lungs of rats and mice whose hepatic AHH is unresponsive to cigarette smoke. Similar results were obtained in mice by ABRAMSON and HUTTON (1975). When C57 Bl/6J mice were exposed to cigarette smoke daily for 8 min (HOLT and KEAST 1973), pulmonary AHH activity was maximally induced ($\sim$4.5-fold) on day 1. After 5 weeks of daily exposure and of discontinuation of exposure, pulmonary AHH activity fell to about 2.5 times control levels and remained significantly elevated at that level for the full 40 weeks of the experiment.

It is worthy of note that the pulmonary AHH activity of virtually all species thus far examined is induced by exposure to cigarette smoke. However, BILIMORIA et al. (1977) reported that exposure of guinea pigs to cigarette smoke failed to enhance pulmonary AHH activity, but, indeed, depressed it. Exposure of rats under identical circumstances evoked a dramatic increase in pulmonary AHH activity. Guinea pigs and rats were then injected with benzo[a]pyrene, 3-MC, or Aroclor 1254 (a polychlorinated biphenyl). In guinea pigs, benzo[a]pyrene administration caused a slight increase in pulmonary AHH, 3-MC had no effect, and Aroclor 1254 produced marked inhibition. Identical doses of these agents administered to rats evoked a three- to eightfold enhancement in pulmonary AHH. Thus, it would appear that there may be something peculiar about the AHH present in guinea pig lung and particularly its responsiveness to enzyme inducers.

CANTRELL et al. (1973 b) studied AHH activity in PAM obtained from human subjects by bronchopulmonary lavage. The number of macrophages obtained under identical circumstances from smokers was about four times that of nonsmokers. In addition, the AHH activity of PAM obtained from smokers (normalized per 10^6 cells) was 11 times that of nonsmokers. In another population of patients studied by these workers (McLEMORE et al. 1977), the difference between nonsmokers and smokers in the AHH activity of alveolar macrophages was about fivefold.

Oral administration to rats of a "crude cannabis resin" caused induction of AHH activity in both lung (threefold) and liver (fivefold) (WITSCHI and ST-FRANCOIS 1972). Exposure of rats to a mixture of cannabis smoke and air significantly enhanced pulmonary AHH activity, but was without effect on the hepatic enzyme (MARCOTTE and WITSCHI 1972). Exposure of animals to a cannabis "placebo" – from which the "cannabinoids" had been removed by solvent extraction – gave results similar to those obtained with untreated cannabis.

III. Flavones

WATTENBERG et al. (1968 a) reported that AHH activity of rat lung and liver was stimulated by a variety of flavones, both naturally occurring and synthetic. Included among the former group were tangeretin, nobilitin, chalcone, and several of its derivatives. In general, AHH activities were stimulated both in liver and lung.

IV. Benzothiazoles

WATTENBERG et al. (1968 b) evaluated the AHH-inducing properties of about 30 substituted benzothiazoles in rats. Most of the compounds tested were effective if not highly active enzyme inducers (one- to eightfold increase over controls) and were unselective in that they stimulated activity in both liver and lung.

V. Phenothiazines

Treatment of rats with phenothiazine and a number of derivatives including chlorpromazine, chlorpromazine sulfoxide, and 10-acetylphenothiazine has been shown to stimulate pulmonary AHH activity five- to eightfold (WATTENBERG et al. 1967). In addition, aminopyrine demethylase was reported to be markedly stimulated in rat lung by pretreatment with phenothiazine (SUNDERMAN and LEIBMAN 1970). Finally, OPPERT et al. (1970) reported that pretreatment of rabbits with chlorpromazine increased pulmonary cytochrome P-450 levels (90%), aminopyrine demethylase (75%), and aniline hydroxylase (65%) activities.

Note Added in Proof: Recent work (JONES et al. 1983) with purified type II cells and Clara cells obtained from rats pretreated with β-naphthoflavone, revealed marked induction in both cell populations of ethoxycoumarin-O-deethylase and AHH activities. Similarly POLAND et al. (1984) showed that the administration of 2,3,7,8-tetrachlorodibenzo-1,4-dioxin (TCDD) enhanced several microsomal monooxygenase parameters in mouse lung.

F. The Role of the Lung in Whole Body Drug Clearance

In the rabbit, the specific activities in liver and lung of benzphetamine demethylase, ethylmorphine demethylase, biphenyl 4-hydroxylase, and NADPH-cytochrome c reductase are nearly the same. However, in most other common laboratory species, this is not the case and specific activities in lung are only 10% –50% those of liver. New Zealand rabbits weighing 2–3 kg have a liver mass of about 70 g and a lung mass of about 10 g. Moreover, rabbit liver yields approximately 2–3 times as much microsomal protein (per gram organ) as does lung. These values permit the simple calculation presented in Table 10. Based on these calculations one might conclude that the overall monooxygenase contribution of the lung is roughly 5% that of liver and therefore, probably trivial. However, these calculations and conclusions are predicated on a number of assumptions, some of which are noted.

1. That the proportion of the total amount of endoplasmic reticulum in the intact organ recovered as the microsomal fraction is nearly the same in lung and liver.
2. That the availability of NADPH and oxygen in the two organs in situ are sufficient to meet the requirements of the monooxygenases.
3. That the kinetic behavior of the monooxygenase systems in vitro are some direct function of their behavior in vivo and that these relationships are similar in lung and liver.

Table 10. Total monooxygenase activity in rabbit lung and liver

	Specific activity	Organ mass (g)	Microsomal protein (mg/g)	Total activity per organ
Liver	1	70	27	1890
Lung	1	10	9	90

4. That the relative organ perfusion, i.e., the rate of delivery of drug substrate to the enzyme, is similar.
5. That the concentration of drug substrate at the enzyme sites, i.e., the uptake or binding of drug by the two organs, do not differ appreciably.

At least two of these assumptions (4 and 5) are demonstrably invalid and the remaining three are not readily evaluated. First, it has been abundantly demonstrated that while the lungs receive 100% of the cardiac output, the hepatic blood flow is much less, in the vicinity of 25% (HILLIKER and ROTH 1980). Moreover, when the difference in the mass of the two organs is taken into account, lung perfusion (ml per gram organ) markedly exceeds that of liver. Thus, perfusion of the two organs in vivo is grossly different. Further, xenobiotics administered intravenously must pass through the pulmonary vascular bed before reaching the general circulation and the liver and would therefore be subject to prior pulmonary uptake or metabolism. This could be very important in the event of a prominent pulmonary "first-pass effect" which has been demonstrated for many endogenous substances (BAKHLE and VANE 1974).

Second, there is abundant evidence that xenobiotics are not uniformly distributed throughout the body. BROWN (1974) and PHILPOT et al. (1977) have shown that many lipophilic basic amines ($pK_a > 8.5$) are highly concentrated in lung. Indeed tissue:plasma ratios ranging from 5:1 to 100:1 or more have been reported for such compounds as imipramine, chlorphentermine, phenothiazines, methadone, chlorcyclizine, and a host of other agents.

Perhaps the first experimental effort to quantify the relative importance of lung and liver in overall drug metabolism was published by UEHLEKE (1968). The findings suggest that the lung has approximately 40% the drug metabolic capacity of liver. ROTH and WIERSMA (1980) have emphasized the importance of organ perfusion as a major determinant of metabolic clearances. Isolated rat liver and lung were perfused at physiologic blood flow rates (lung, 44.8 ml/min; liver, 11.2 ml/min; a lung liver ratio of 4:1) with ^{14}C-labeled 5-hydroxytryptamine (5-HT). The authors found that, despite the paucity of degradative enzyme, the lung probably contributes more to the total body clearance of 5-HT than does the liver. HILLIKER and ROTH (1980) studied the clearance of mescaline (3,4,5-trimethoxyphenethylamine) in rabbits. When expressed on a whole organ basis, the liver had more than seven times the metabolic capacity toward mescaline of the lung, primarily owing to the greater mass of the liver. However, perfusion of the two organs at physiologic rates (lung:liver $\sim 4:1$) revealed that the rabbit lung was capable of clearing mescaline at a rate 72% that of liver. Thus, despite gross differences in degradative enzyme activity of the two organs, and total mass, the lung may contribute substantially to the total body clearance of mescaline.

G. The Role of Pulmonary Xenobiotic Metabolism in Chemically Induced Lung Damage

This section will not attempt to review all aspects of chemically induced lung damage or toxicity, but will concentrate on those instances in which metabolism of the foreign compound results in the formation of a more toxic chemical species which is responsible for the pneumotoxicity.

I. Polycyclic Aromatic Hydrocarbons

This section mainly discusses 3-methylcholanthrene (3-MC), 7,12-dimethylbenz-[*a*]anthracene, dibenz[*a,h*]anthracene, and, in particular, benzo[*a*]pyrene as representative of the polycyclic aromatic hydrocarbons (PAH) from the standpoint of their toxic action (carcinogenesis) on the lung (Fig. 3).

It is widely held (BOYLAND 1980) that the carcinogenic action of PAH is mediated through the formation of highly reactive metabolic products (ultimate carcinogens) which bind covalently to DNA. Benzo[*a*]pyrene was first shown by CONNEY et al. (1957) to be a substrate for the hepatic mixed-function oxidase system yielding hydroxylated phenolic products. This enzyme system, termed benzo[*a*]pyrene hydroxylase, later AHH, was highly inducible by pretreatment of animals with other PAH such as 3-methylcholanthrene (CONNEY et al. 1957). With the advent of HPLC it has been shown that incubation of benzo[*a*]pyrene with liver or lung microsomes and NADPH results in the formation of an array of oxidized products (Table 11); SELKIRK et al. (1974a) including dihydrodiols,

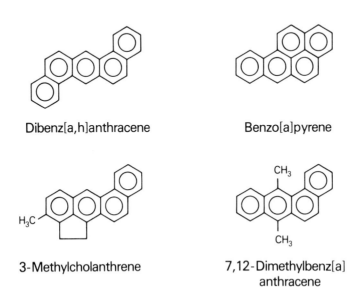

Dibenz[a,h]anthracene   Benzo[a]pyrene

3-Methylcholanthrene   7,12-Dimethylbenz[a]
                                         anthracene

Fig. 3. Structures of some polycyclic aromatic hydrocarbons that are converted by microsomal enzymes to carcinogenic products

Table 11. Some metabolites of benzo[*a*]pyrene produced by hepatic and pulmonary enzymes as determined by high pressure liquid chromatography

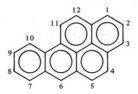

Benzo[*a*]pyrene

Benzo[*a*]pyrene-9,10-dihydrodiol
Benzo[*a*]pyrene-4,5-dihydrodiol
Benzo[*a*]pyrene-7,8-dihydrodiol
Benzo[*a*]pyrene-1,6-quinone
Benzo[*a*]pyrene-3,6-quinone
Benzo[*a*]pyrene-6,12-quinone
Benzo[*a*]pyrene-4,5-epoxide
3-Hydroxybenzo[*a*]pyrene
9-Hydroxybenzo[*a*]pyrene

Abstracted from SELKIRK et al. (1974b).

quinones, epoxides or arene oxides, and phenols (YANG et al. 1975). Presumed intermediates in the formation of these products are the 2,3-epoxide, 4,5-epoxide, 9,10-epoxide, 7,8-epoxide, and 6-hydroxybenzo[*a*]pyrene (GELBOIN et al. 1976). It is now known that the phenols may be formed by spontaneous chemical rearrangement of the appropriate (2,3- or 9,10-) epoxide while the quinones may be formed by oxidation via a 6-hydroxyl intermediate. There is little doubt that the dihydrodiols arise from the hydration of epoxides, as illustrated in Fig. 4.

The first reaction is catalyzed by the microsomal cytochrome P-450-dependent mixed-function oxidase and the second by microsomal epoxide hydrolase. These activation reactions occur both in lung and liver; specific activities in rat lung are as high or higher than in liver (GROVER et al. 1974) while the reverse was true in rhesus monkey (HUNDLEY and FREUDENTHAL 1977b).

The arene oxide or epoxide metabolites of PAH were shown to be more carcinogenic than the parent hydrocarbon or any of its derivatives (HUBERMAN et al. 1972), thus implicating epoxides as reactive carcinogenic species. This finding was supported by the work of SELKIRK et al. (1974b) who found that inhibition of AHH, i.e., mixed-function oxidase activity, reduced the covalent binding of benzo[*a*]pyrene to DNA whereas selective inhibition of epoxide hydrolase increased the binding of benzo[*a*]pyrene-derived radioactivity to DNA and blocked dihydrodiol formation. Similarly, inhibition of epoxide hydrolase enhanced the microsomal catalyzed covalent binding of 3-MC ^{3}H to DNA (BÜRKI et al. 1974).

A significant breakthrough occurred when SIMS et al. (1974) discovered that the metabolic activation of benzo[*a*]pyrene to the ultimate carcinogen apparently takes place in three steps. Thus, mixed-function oxidation of the hydrocarbon initially yields the 7,8-epoxide which, under the influence of epoxide hydrolase, pro-

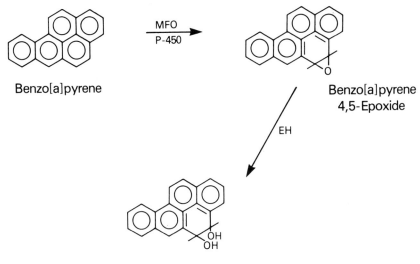

Benzo[a]pyrene

Benzo[a]pyrene
4,5-Epoxide

Benzo[a]pyrene 4,5-Dihydrodiol

Fig. 4. Microsomal conversion of benzo[a]pyrene to a dihydrodiol via an intermediate epoxide. MFO represents the mixed-function oxidase system; EH represents epoxide hydrolase

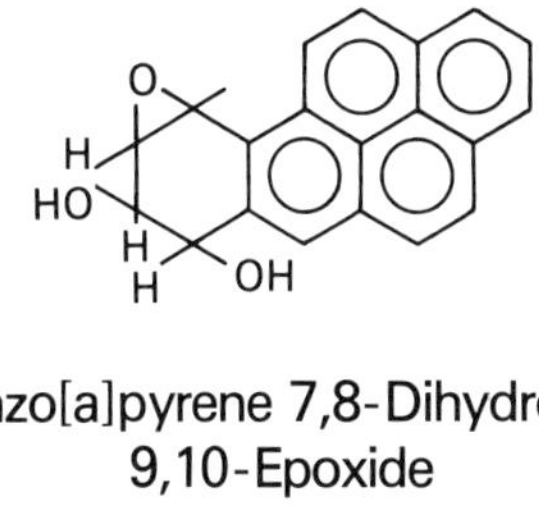

Benzo[a]pyrene 7,8-Dihydrodiol
9,10-Epoxide

Fig. 5. The general structure of the ultimate carcinogenic metabolite of benzo[a]pyrene. With proper stereochemical designation, the compound is *trans*-(+)-7β,8α-dihydroxy-9α,10α-epoxy-7,8,9,10-tetrahydrobenzo[a]pyrene

duces benzo[a]pyrene-7,8-dihydrodiol which is then subject to a second attack by the mixed-function oxidase with the formation of the 7,8-dihydrodiol-9,10-epoxide. Accordingly, ^{3}H-labeled benzo[a]pyrene-7,8-dihydrodiol was incubated with rat liver microsomes, NADPH, and DNA. The DNA was isolated and hydrolyzed and the major radioactive peak cochromatographed with a synthetic sample of benzo[a]pyrene-7,8-dihydrodiol-9,10 epoxide that had been reacted with DNA and thereafter treated similarly (Fig. 5). DAUDEL et al. (1975) reported that when benzo[a]pyrene was painted on the skin of mice and the dermal DNA isolated and purified 24 h later, the fluorescence characteristics were identical to those of a sample of highly purified salmon sperm DNA that had been reacted in vitro with benzo[a]pyrene-7,8-dihydrodiol-9,10-epoxide, the "diol epoxide".

The (+) and (−) enantiomers of benzo[a]pyrene-7,8-epoxide are hydrated stereospecifically at C-8 by microsomal epoxide hydrolase to (−) and (+) *trans*-benzo[a]pyrene-7,8-dihydrodiol (LEVIN et al. 1980). Further epoxidation at C-9 results in the formation of four stereoisomers in which the 7-hydroxyl group is either *cis* (diol epoxides 1) or *trans* (diol epoxides 2) to the 9,10-epoxide. The isomers are thus denoted:

$$(+)\text{-benzo}[a]\text{pyrene-}7\beta,8\alpha\text{-diol-}9\alpha,10\alpha\text{-epoxide 2}$$
$$(-)\text{-benzo}[a]\text{pyrene-}7\beta,8\alpha\text{-diol-}9\beta,10\beta\text{-epoxide 1}$$
$$(-)\text{-benzo}[a]\text{pyrene-}7\alpha,8\beta\text{-diol-}9\beta,10\beta\text{-epoxide 2}$$
$$(+)\text{-benzo}[a]\text{pyrene-}7\alpha,8\beta\text{-diol-}9\alpha,10\alpha\text{-epoxide 1}$$

Tumorigenicity studies with in newborn mice (BUENING et al. 1978) revealed that (+)-7β,8α-dihydroxy-9α,10α-epoxy-7,8,9,10-tetrahydrobenzo[a]pyrene ((+)-benzo[a]pyrene-7β,8α,diol-9α,10α-epoxide 2) had exceptionally high tumorigenic activity whereas benzo[a]pyrene and the other three optically pure isomers of the benzo[a]pyrene-7,8-diol-9,10-epoxides had little or no activity. The striking difference in tumorigenicity between benzo[a]pyrene and its various diol epoxide metabolites is presented in Table 12. The (+)-epoxide 2 apparently possessed all the tumorigenic activity while the other isomers and benzo[a]pyrene at this dose level (14 nmol) were essentially inactive. Similar conclusions were reached with this isomer in studies of skin tumor induction (SLAGA et al. 1979).

Recent work has revealed that mixed-function oxidase activity, heretofore considered to reside exclusively in the endoplasmic reticulum, is also present in the nuclear membrane (KASPER 1971). The question of activation of PAH by purified nuclei from liver and lung has been reviewed by BRESNICK (1979). Nuclei from both organs contain mixed-function oxidase activity toward benzo[a]pyrene (AHH), epoxide hydrolase activity, and are capable of catalyzing the formation of the diol epoxides which bind covalently to nuclear DNA. These activities are usually higher in liver nuclei than in lung, are inducible by pretreatment of animals with 3-MC, and in all ways behave in a fashion similar to that of micro-

Table 12. Pulmonary tumors in mice treated intraperitoneally[a] with diol epoxide metabolites of benzo[a]pyrene

Treatment	Pulmonary tumors	
	(% Mice with tumors)	(Average tumors per mouse)
Control	11	0.12
Benzo[a]pyrene (BP)	14	0.15
(−)-BP-7β,8α-diol-9β,10β-epoxide 1	22	0.25
(+)-BP-7α,8β-diol-9α,10α-epoxide 1	15	0.34
(−)-BP-7α,8β-diol-9β,10β-epoxide 2	12	0.13
(+)-BP-7β,8α-diol-9α,10α-epoxide 2	100	7.67

[a] Each animal received a total dose of 14 nmol test compound in three divided doses; data derived in part from BUENING et al. (1978)

somes. However, considering the physical proximity of this PAH-activating system to the genetic material, its importance can hardly be overestimated.

II. Furans

1. 4-Ipomeanol

The ingestion by cattle of mold-damaged sweet potatoes is associated with severe and often fatal respiratory toxicity. BOYD and his associates isolated, characterized, and synthesized 4-ipomeanol as the lung-toxic factor in moldy sweet potatoes (see Fig. 1). Administration of 4-ipomeanol to common laboratory species (mouse, rat, guinea pig, rabbit) results in toxicity; in all species tested, the lung is the primary target organ. Work with 4-ipomeanol ^{14}C showed that, following its intraperitoneal administration to rats, the toxin was selectively and covalently bound in lung (Table 13; BOYD et al. 1975). Autoradiographic studies in rats, mice, and guinea pigs revealed that 4-ipomeanol ^{14}C was bound covalently almost exclusively in the nonciliated bronchiolar or Clara cell (BOYD 1977). Pretreatment of animals with piperonyl butoxide, an inhibitor of cytochrome P-450-dependent monooxygenase activity prior to 4-ipomeanol resulted in a marked decrease in covalently bound radioactivity in the bronchiolar cells and a total absence of bronchiolar necrosis.

In vitro studies on the metabolic activation of 4-ipomeanol, estimated by covalent binding to tissue constituents, indicated that it was highest in microsomal fractions of both lung and liver and practically nonexistent in nuclei, mitochondria, and cytosol. Microsomal activation was NADPH and oxygen dependent, and was inhibited by anaerobiosis (nitrogen), CO, cytochrome c, and by boiling the microsomes. It was also inhibited by piperonyl butoxide and SKF 525-A, and by pretreatment of animals with $CoCl_2$ – which reduces cytochrome P-450 levels – in vivo. Covalent binding to microsomes was markedly enhanced in liver, but not in lung, by pretreating rats with either phenobarbital or 3-MC. The characteristics of the microsomal system are those of a cytochrome P-450-dependent monooxygenase system. A marked difference between lung and liver microsomes was discovered in the kinetics of covalent binding of 4-ipomeanol. K_m in lung was $0.29 \times 10^{-4} M$, that in liver $4.20 \times 10^{-4} M$, suggesting much higher affinity of the

Table 13. Tissue distribution of radioactivity covalently bound to protein in rats 24 h after intraperitoneal administration of ipomeanol ^{14}C (10 mg/kg)

Organ	Amount bound (nmol per milligram tissue protein)
Lung	2.00
Liver	0.38
Kidney	0.17
Ileum	0.09
Heart	0.04
Blood	0.04
Muscle	0.03

Taken in part from BOYD and BURKA (1978)

lung enzyme for the substrate and providing a possible explanation for the organ specificity of 4-ipomeanol (BOYD and BURKA 1978; BOYD et al. 1978 b). The covalent binding of 4-ipomeanol to lung and liver microsomes was blocked by addition of glutathione, indicating that the activated species is highly electrophilic. Similarly (BOYD and BURKA 1978), pretreatment of rats with diethylmaleate, which depletes tissue glutathione, increased the covalent binding of ipomeanol ^{14}C in liver and lung and markedly increased the toxicity (reduced LD_{50}).

Additional work from Boyd's group (DUTCHER and BOYD 1979) in several different animal species revealed that the organ specificities of covalent binding of 4-ipomeanol correlated very closely with the patterns of organ-specific tissue damage. In all species examined, the lung was a major target for both the covalent binding of 4-ipomeanol and pathologic changes. Studies of both the in vitro and in vivo metabolism of 4-ipomeanol indicated that the covalent binding and the subsequent target organ and cell damage result from the cytochrome P-450-monooxygenase-mediated formation of one or more highly reactive electrophilic 4-ipomeanol metabolites in situ in the target organs. The chemical nature of the reactive metabolites is unknown at present (BOYD 1980 a, b).

2. 3-Methylfuran

This compound is, like 4-ipomeanol, converted by cytochrome P-450-dependent monooxygenase of mouse lung to a highly reactive metabolite which alkylates microsomal protein and produces acute pulmonary bronchiolar necrosis (BOYD et al. 1978 b). 3-Methylfuran produces pulmonary damage after administration by intraperitoneal or inhalation routes. The bronchiolar necrosis can be prevented by pretreatment of mice with piperonyl butoxide.

Note Added in Proof: Recent work (RAVINDRANATH et al. 1984) showed that in the presence of NADPH and microsomes from rat lung or liver, 3-methylfuran undergoes ring opening with the formation of 2-methyl-2-butene-1,4-dial. The latter compound binds covalently to microsomes and presumably mediates the toxicity of 3-methylfuran.

3. Nitrofurantoin

The biochemical mechanisms by which nitrofurantoin produces lung damage may be quite different from those of the furans discussed above. Indeed, nitrofurantoin appears to damage the lung by a mechanism resembling that of paraquat or mitomycin C which will be discussed in Sects. G.V. and G.VI.8. Nitrofurantoin is used clinically to treat urinary tract infections. Its use is accompanied by pulmonary "hypersensitivity reactions" (SOVIJARVI et al. 1977) which range from cough and dyspnea to pulmonary infiltrates, effusion, and fibrosis.

When administered to rats in very large doses (300–500 mg/kg; usual clinical dose 200–400 mg/day), nitrofurantoin produced severe respiratory distress which was fatal in 12–36 h. Animals became tachypneic and cyanotic and at autopsy the lungs were grossly distended, edematous, and hemorrhagic. Histologically, there was widespread interstitial and alveolar edema, vascular congestion and hemorrhagic consolidation (BOYD et al. 1979 a). Interestingly, the lethality of nitrofurantoin could be manipulated widely by factors known to be involved in lipid peroxidation. For example, the lethality was greatly enhanced in rats maintained on a vitamin E-deficient diet which was rich in polyunsaturated fat; the LD_{50} in the latter group was 35 mg/kg compared with 400 mg/kg in controls. Moreover, if vitamin E-deficient rats were repleted with vitamin E, the lethality of nitrofurantoin returned to that of controls. Similarly, a change in the dietary lipid to a more saturated form (corn oil to lard) dramatically reduced the lethality (BOYD et al. 1979a). Finally, the lethality and pulmonary damage produced by nitrofurantoin were significantly enhanced in rats maintained in 100% oxygen after drug administration. It should be noted that in the presence of NADPH, microsomes catalyze a one-electron reduction of the nitro group of nitrofurantoin to yield a nitro free radical (MASON and HOLTZMAN 1975) which spontaneously reacts with oxygen to regenerate the parent nitro compound and simultaneously reduces oxygen to the superoxide radical anion (O_2^-).

SASAME and BOYD (1979) showed that aerobic incubation of nitrofurantoin with NADPH and rat lung microsomes resulted in a 25-fold increase in the formation of superoxide, a 12-fold stimulation in H_2O_2 production, and a 50-fold stimulation in NADPH oxidation. Incubation of microsomes, NADPH, and nitrofurantoin under anaerobic conditions (N_2) blocked superoxide and H_2O_2 formation, but further stimulated NAPDH oxidation as compared with air.

In addition to stimulating the formation of large amounts of reactive oxygen, nitrofurantoin has also been found to bind covalently to microsomes from rat liver and lung in vitro. The covalent binding of nitrofurantoin and 4-ipomeanol was NADPH dependent, but similarities between the binding of the two compounds ended there (BOYD et al. 1979c). For example, binding of 4-ipomeanol was maximal under air and was abolished by N_2 or CO, either alone or in combination. By contrast, the covalent binding of nitrofurantoin to liver and lung microsomes was minimal under an atmosphere of air, but was highest under N_2 or CO, either alone or in combination. The binding of nitrofurantoin was stimulated by flavine adenine dinucleotide; antibody to NADPH-cytochrome c reductase impaired both nitroreduction and covalent binding. Covalent binding of nitrofurantoin by the cytosolic fractions of rat liver and lung was dependent upon NADH or xanthine oxidase/hypoxanthine. Finally, reduced glutathione decreased the covalent binding of nitrofurantoin in microsomes and cytosol of rat liver and lung, but had no effect on nitroreduction. Taken in sum, these data have been interpreted by BOYD (1980a) as indicating that although highly reactive metabolites of nitrofurantoin can be produced by lung cell fractions in vitro and possibly in vivo, the covalent binding of the drug does not appear to be correlated with its acute toxicity in animals. This contrasts nitrofurantoin with other furans such as 4-ipomeanol and 3-methylfuran. Covalent binding of nitrofurantoin can only be demonstrated under anaerobic conditions in vitro; in contrast, under more physiologic conditions (aerobiosis), negligible covalent binding is observed, but large amounts of superoxide are formed in the presence of lung microsomes, NADPH, and nitrofurantoin. Thus, it seems that the pneumotoxicity of this agent is mediated through superoxide and its secondary metabolites H_2O_2 and hydroxyl radical ($\cdot OH$), a family of extremely reactive and toxic substances. This subject will be developed in further detail in relation to paraquat (see Sect. G.V.)

III. Carbon Tetrachloride

Carbon tetrachloride (CCl_4) is a well-known hepatotoxin which produces well-characterized morphological changes such as centrilobular necrosis and lipid infiltration as well as functional changes such as impaired dye (bromsulphalein) clearance, destruction of cytochrome P-450, and marked impairment of the hepatic monooxygenase system and microsomal glucose-6-phosphatase (RECKNAGEL and GLENDE 1973). VALDIVIA and SONNAD (1966) reported that CCl_4 administration to guinea pigs produced alterations in pulmonary alveolar type II cells, consisting of increased cytoplasmic lipid droplets and dilatation of the endoplasmic reticulum. Later work (GOULD and SMUCKLER 1971) confirmed that the primary pathologic effects of CCl_4 on rat lung were at the alveolar level.

Administration of CCl_4 to rats either orally or by inhalation produced profound effects on the pulmonary monooxygenase system; the effects were more pronounced following oral administration. Between 12 and 24 h after CCl_4 administration, pulmonary cytochrome P-450 was decreased by 90% and N,N-dimethylaniline demethylase activity by about 75% (CHEN et al. 1977). These changes were accompanied by alterations in the fine structure of alveolar type II cells. Pulmonary enzyme alterations returned to control levels within about 7 days. Similar reductions in pulmonary cytochrome P-450 levels and biphenyl-4-hydroxylase activity by CCl_4 were reported by LITTERST et al. (1977).

Recent work from Boyd's laboratory (BOYD et al. 1980 b) confirmed earlier findings that CCl_4 administration to rats or mice markedly depresses the pulmonary monooxygenase system. However, in contrast to earlier work, both light and electron microscopic examination of the lungs of CCl_4-poisoned mice and rats, revealed that the morphological changes were limited to the bronchiolar nonciliated epithelial (Clara) cells. Adjacent ciliated bronchiolar cells did not exhibit significant morphological changes. It was remarkable that highly vacuolated obviously necrotic Clara cells were contiguous with ciliated bronchiolar cells whose fine structural appearance was entirely normal. It should be pointed out that the weight of current evidence holds that CCl_4 is not toxic per se, but requires metabolic activation via the cytochrome P-450 monooxygenase system to the trichloromethyl free radical ($\cdot CCl_3$) (RECKNAGEL and GLENDE 1973). Evidence presented in Sect. D.V strongly suggests that pulmonary monooxygenase activity is highly concentrated in Clara cells. Therefore, the argument is made that CCl_4 is metabolically activated, covalently binds, and produces necrosis in the Clara cells, in a manner essentially analogous to 4-ipomeanol.

IV. Butylated Hydroxytoluene

Butylated hydroxytoluene (BHT) (3,5-di-*tert*-butyl-4-hydroxytoluene) is a widely used antioxidant food additive employed at relatively low concentrations ($\sim 0.1\%$). MARINO and MITCHELL (1972) showed that its administration to mice in large doses (~ 500 mg/kg) produced selective pulmonary damage such as general disorganization of the cellular components concomitant with inflammation, edema, and vascular congestion. All other organs examined histologically were considered unaffected. Subsequent work (WITSCHI and SAHEB 1974) showed that BHT administered to mice significantly increased lung mass ($\sim 40\%$)

and DNA synthesis (thymidine ^{14}C incorporation). Fine structural studies (HIRAI et al. 1977) revealed that the initial pathologic effect of BHT in mouse lung was damage to type I alveolar cells, consisting of loss of cytoplasmic organelles and breaks in the plasma membrane, resulting in nearly total necrosis of type I cells by day 3. This was followed by transformation and division of type II cells, and reepithelialization of the alveolus. Marked proliferation of interstitial cells and reduction in the size of alveolar spaces occurred on days 4 and 5. The activity of alveolar macrophages in removing debris was maximum on day 4.

NAKAGAWA et al. (1979) incubated BHT ^{14}C with rat liver microsomes and NADPH and found covalent binding of radiolabeled material to microsomal macromolecules. The binding appeared to be catalyzed by a cytochrome P-450-dependent system as it was oxygen and NADPH dependent and inhibited by CO, SKF 525-A, and by glutathione. Rat lung microsomes had about 40% the activity of liver microsomes while activity in kidney, spleen, and brain was negligible. This system, therefore, shared many characteristics of the microsomal systems which mediate the covalent binding of bromobenzene, acetaminophen, and 4-ipomeanol. The macromolecular targets of BHT covalent binding in rat liver microsomes were primarily RNA and to a lesser extent protein and DNA (NAKAGAWA et al. 1980).

MALKINSON (1979) confirmed earlier results that administration of BHT to mice caused lung damage, but other antioxidants (ethoxyquin, α-tocopherol, pyrogallol, propyl gallate, or butylated hydroxyanisole), substituted phenols (4,5-butylphenol, 2,4-di-t-butylphenol, 2,4,6-trimethylphenol), or BHT metabolites (BHT alcohol, BHT acid, or BHT quinone) did not. Lung damage resulting from BHT was not observed in mice less than 3 weeks of age or in mice exposed to cedar terpenes either in the form of cedarwood shavings or an injection of volatile constituents of cedarwood, cedrene, or cedrol. Cedarwood shavings and its volatile components are known to be inducers of the cytochrome P-450 system (FERGUSON 1966). KEHRER and WITSCHI (1980) reported that BHT-induced pulmonary cellular proliferation in mice was blocked or diminished in a dose-dependent manner by SKF 525-A, piperonyl butoxide, or $CoCl_2$.

Following the administration of BHT ^{14}C, radioactivity was covalently bound to lung, kidney, and liver of mice which exhibited lung damage and rats which did not. The greatest amount of radioactivity was bound by lung tissue of mice; these findings led the authors to postulate that a reactive metabolite of BHT rather than the parent compound produces lung damage in mice. The species difference may be accounted for on the grounds that at the same dose of BHT (400 mg/kg), mouse lung covalently bound more than four times as much radioactivity (per milligram protein) as rat lung. This finding is in accord with the observations of LITTERST et al. (1975a) that monooxygenase activities in mouse lung are much higher than in rat lung. It thus appears that BHT-induced lung damage is mediated by a highly reactive electrophilic metabolite whose formation is catalyzed by the cytochrome P-450-dependent monooxygenase system.

V. Paraquat

Administration of toxic doses of paraquat to rats, mice, guinea pigs, monkeys, dogs, and humans causes death in three stages, each having a different cause. Animals dying within 1–4 h succumb from acute pulmonary insufficiency resulting from massive pulmonary edema and alveolar hemorrhage. In the next phase, animals die in 3–6 days of acute renal failure resulting from widespread necrosis of the proximal renal tubules. Finally, depending upon the dose and species (up to 14–20 days or longer in humans), animals die of chronic respiratory failure resulting from massive pulmonary fibrosis. The pathology of paraquat pneumotoxicity has been described in great detail both at the light and electron microscopic levels (SMITH and HEATH 1976).

The acute pulmonary effects of paraquat – also referred to as the destructive phase – consist initially of massive congestion and pulmonary edema. The lungs are distended and range from bright red to plum in color (ROBERTSON et al. 1971). Histologically, one observes vascular congestion, edema, and hemorrhage associated with a fibrinous alveolar exudate. Alveoli and terminal bronchioles are collapsed in some areas, distended in others. Accompanying all this of course, there is an acute inflammatory reaction with increased numbers of polymorphonuclear leukocytes, lymphocytes, and macrophages (VIJEYARATNAM and CORRIN 1971). The principle event is a widespread necrosis of both type I and type II alveolar epithelial cells which slough into the alveolar space, leaving only the basement membrane covering the denuded capillary endothelium (SMITH et al. 1974; SMITH and HEATH 1974).

The proliferative phase of the paraquat lesion begins with the influx of large numbers of primitive mononuclear cells which have been termed "profibroblasts" (SMITH et al. 1974) which rapidly mature into fibroblasts with well-developed rough endoplasmic reticulum. There is gradual thickening of the alveolar septa as more profibroblasts appear, mature, and proliferate. It is not clear whether paraquat produces interstitial fibrosis or intraalveolar fibrosis so the term "obliterative fibrosis" was coined (SMITH and HEATH 1976). Fibroblastic influx and proliferation progressively thicken the septal walls while the fibroblasts are synthesizing and secreting large amounts of collagen into the extracellular space. The increased septal cellularity, together with massive increases in pulmonary collagen, eventually obliterate the alveolar spaces and the lung becomes a solid glandular-like organ incapable of either inflation or gas exchange. When the thorax is opened, the paraquat lung fails to collapse, exhibits a solid, rubbery consistency, and sinks in water.

The sequence of events described has been produced in a variety of animal species following oral or parenteral administration of paraquat. Interestingly, exposure of rats to paraquat aerosols produces severe congestion, alveolar edema, and pulmonary hemorrhage – in fact more generalized damage to the alveolar epithelium than systemic administration – but it was not possible to produce pulmonary fibrosis by inhalation of paraquat (CONNING et al. 1969). This has led SMITH and HEATH (1976) to the provocative conclusion: "It seems, therefore, that the destructive phase of paraquat poisoning with its fluid exudate is not necessary for the initiation of the proliferative phase which follows independent of it. The cause of the proliferative phase remains an enigma."

Another curiosity concerning paraquat is that all species that have been examined to date, including humans, develop the appalling pulmonary lesions described above; *except* the rabbit. BUTLER and KLEINERMAN (1971) reported that the intraperitoneal administration of paraquat to rabbits in various doses and dosage schedules failed to produce any of the pulmonary effects, particularly pulmonary fibrosis, observed in other species. The intrinsic resistance of rabbits to the toxic pulmonary effects of paraquat have been confirmed (CLARK et al. 1966; ILETT et al. 1974), but not explained.

It is possible that the difference between rats and rabbits in their pulmonary response to paraquat may be related to differences in rates of clearance of paraquat ^{14}C from the lung. ILETT et al. (1974) demonstrated that the initial rates of uptake of paraquat ^{14}C by rat and rabbit lung were quite similar, but the retention by rat lung, a sensitive species, was prolonged whereas the herbicide was cleared very rapidly from rabbit lung. Paraquat is not covalently bound in lung (ILETT et al. 1974; SMITH et al. 1979), although it is avidly taken up by lung both in vivo and in vitro by an active transport process, and this uptake by lung slices can be blocked by a variety of amines.

FISHER et al. (1973) demonstrated a marked enhancement of paraquat toxicity in an oxygen-enriched atmosphere. KEHRER et al. (1979) confirmed that hyperoxia enhances the toxicity of paraquat. On the other hand, hypoxia (10% oxygen compared with the 20% oxygen in room air) offered significant protection against paraquat toxicity (RHODES et al. 1976).

It is obvious that the foregoing studies, and others (AUTOR 1974; BLOCK 1979), implicate oxygen in the pulmonary toxicity of paraquat. GAGE (1968) showed that paraquat markedly stimulated NADPH oxidation by liver microsomes and that this reaction was likely mediated by a flavoprotein. He also demonstrated that, under anaerobic conditions, NADPH reduced paraquat to its free radical and that, aerobically, the oxidation of NADPH involves a cyclic reduction and reoxidation of paraquat. Subsequently, BUS et al. (1974) showed that incubation of mouse lung microsomes with paraquat and NADPH under anaerobic conditions resulted in a one-electron reduction of paraquat to a free radical. This microsomal reaction was shown to be mediated by NADPH cytochrome c reductase as it was markedly inhibited by an antibody to the enzyme. Paraquat markedly stimulated the oxidation of NADPH by lung microsomes. More importantly, addition of paraquat to a system consisting of NADPH cytochrome c reductase, NADPH, and microsomal lipid stimulated lipid peroxidation threefold; the stimulation of peroxidation was blocked by superoxide dismutase. This suggested that paraquat stimulated lipid peroxidation by increasing the formation of superoxide radical anion (O_2^-) or other forms of reactive oxygen. Lipid peroxidation and its damage to biologic membranes is known to be markedly stimulated by O_2^- (PAINE 1978). Therefore, if the reaction sequence depicted in Fig. 6 is valid, one would expect:

1. Stimulation of NADPH oxidation resulting from the futile redox cycling of paraquat, eventually reducing the ratio NADPH:NADP in lung. This has in fact been demonstrated in vitro (GAGE 1968; ILETT et al. 1974) and in vivo (WITSCHI et al. 1977).
2. Massive stimulation of O_2^- formation and resultant lipid peroxidation (FRIDOVICH 1978; SMITH and HEATH 1976; TRUSH et al. 1981).
   Thus, both criteria are met and Fig. 6 appears to be valid.

It has been observed that exposure of rats to 85% oxygen for 7 days causes a 50% increase in rat lung superoxide dismutase activity (CRAPO and TIERNEY

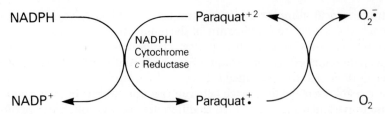

Fig. 6. Paraquat redox cycle (an analogous cycle occurs with aromatic nitro compounds and the nitro radical anion). NADPH-cytochrome c reductase catalyzes an enzymatic one-electron transfer from NADPH to paraquat with the formation of the paraquat radical; under aerobic conditions, the paraquat radical readily reduces (transfers the electron to) oxygen with the formation of superoxide radical. Since paraquat functions catalytically, the rate-limiting component is NADPH and enormous quantities of superoxide and other forms of reactive oxygen can be produced by this reaction sequence

1974). Bus et al. (1976) found that the LT_{50} of paraquat administered to control rats (45 mg/kg intraperitoneally) was 26 h whereas the comparable value in rats previously exposed to 85% oxygen for 7 days was 50 h.

The pulmonary toxicity of paraquat, therefore, is thought to be an oxidative stress resulting from the generation of O_2^- which in turn stimulates lipid peroxidation, resulting in damage to biologic membranes. Accordingly, paraquat toxicity is enhanced by manipulations of factors which impair the body's ability to cope with oxidative stress such as tocopherol (vitamin E) or selenium deficiency, diethyl maleate treatment (which depletes tissue glutathione) or, of course, hyperoxia itself (Bus et al. 1976). Similarly, paraquat toxicity is reduced by hypoxia, supplementation with vitamin E, or superoxide dismutase. Impaired uptake of paraquat in lung by drugs also reduces toxicity.

Although many correlations have been demonstrated, a direct causal relationship between lung injury and drug-induced generation of reactive oxygen (O_2^-, H_2O_2, OH^-, $^1O_2$) has been lacking. Johnson et al. (1981) indicated that the instillation of enzymes that generate reactive oxygen metabolites caused acute and chronic lung injury. For example, intratracheal instillation of xanthine and xanthine oxidase produced acute lung injury which could be blocked by superoxide dismutase, indicating that O_2^- is capable of evoking lung damage. Similarly, glucose and glucose oxidase produced lung injury (changes in vascular permeability to ^{125}I-labeled rat albumin) and this was blocked by catalase, implicating H_2O_2. Interestingly, the combination of glucose, glucose oxidase, and lactoperoxidase produced intense acute lung injury accompanied by hemorrhage and large amounts of intraalveolar fibrin. Animals allowed to survive 14 days after this combination exhibited massive pulmonary hypercellularity, obliteration of alveolar spaces, and extensive interstitial fibrosis. The authors speculated that the offending chemical species might be $^1O_2$ or HOCl.

VI. Miscellaneous Compounds

1. Bromobenzene

The administration of bromobenzene to animals produces a dose-dependent (above a certain critical dose threshold), massive centrilobular hepatic necrosis (GILLETTE 1974 a, b; GILLETTE et al. 1974 c). Other targets for bromobenzene are lung and kidney. REID et al. (1973) reported that necrosis of bronchiolar and bronchial epithelial cells was produced in mice by the injection of bromobenzene or certain other simple halobenzenes. The bronchiolar damage was rather selective and was not accompanied by lesions elsewhere in the lung. Autoradiograms demonstrated a preferential accumulation of radioactive material in the necrotic cells of the bronchi and bronchioles, but it was not possible to discern whether there was selective uptake within specific cell types present in the bronchiolar wall. Incubation of bromobenzene ^{14}C in vitro with NADPH and microsomes from several tissues revealed that significant radioactivity was covalently bound to microsomes from liver, lung, and kidney, organs in which bromobenzene evoked necrosis in vivo, whereas insignificant binding occurred in heart, spleen, and testis, organs not damaged by bromobenzene in vivo.

2. Naphthalene

MAHVI et al. (1977) reported that the effect of naphthalene on mouse lung was to damage the nonciliated bronchiolar (Clara) cells selectively. Employing a dose of 2 mmol/kg (~ 255 mg/kg) administered intraperitoneally and light, as well as scanning and transmission electron microscopy, the earliest effect was observed at 12 h and consisted of extensive enlargement and necrosis of bronchiolar epithelium with exfoliation of Clara cells from large areas of the bronchioles. At 24 h, the bronchioles of most animals were clogged with debris and the few Clara cells seen were strikingly abnornaml in appearance.

This finding, together with the work of BOYD (1980a) and SERABJIT-SINGH et al. (1980), indicating that the pulmonary monooxygenase was highly concentrated in Clara cells, prompted TONG et al. (1981) to investigate the effects of naphthalene on microsomal drug metabolism in mouse lung and liver. Employing a single dose of 250 mg/kg, similar to that used by MAHVI et al. (1977) to produce extensive Clara cell damage in mice, TONG et al. (1981) reported that at 24 h, which coincided with maximum morphological changes, pulmonary cytochrome P-450 was reduced to 45% of control levels. Pulmonary cytochrome b_5, NADPH-cytochrome c reductase, benzphetamine demethylase, 7-ethoxyresorufin deethylase, and aryl hydrocarbon hydroxylase activities were all reduced significantly, but less dramatically. Interestingly, none of these parameters was significantly influenced in the livers of the same animals.

HESSE and MEZGER (1979) found that incubation of rat liver microsomes with NADPH and either naphthalene ^{14}C or l-naphthol ^{14}C resulted in covalent binding of radioactive material to microsomal protein. About twice as much binding occurred with l-naphthol as substrate as with naphthalene, suggesting that covalent binding was more closely related to secondary oxidation of naphthol than to primary monooxygenation of naphthalene. Covalent binding of naphthalene ^{14}C

in vitro by liver microsomes was inhibited by SKF 525-A, anaerobiosis, carbon monoxide, and by the addition of uridine diphosphate glucuronic acid, presumably by conjugation of phenolic products. Addition of glutathione in vitro decreased the binding of naphthalene ^{14}C and of l-naphthol ^{14}C (60%–70%), but did not inhibit the total metabolism of either substrate. Binding was not affected by inhibition of epoxide hydrolase or by superoxide dismutase.

The work of WARREN et al. (1982) has extended this work to mouse lung. Above a distinct dose threshold, naphthalene administration, in a dose-dependent fashion, evoked selective pulmonary bronchial necrosis with no concomitant morphological damage to liver or kidney. In addition, they reported that naphthalene is metabolized to intermediates which bind covalently to tissue macromolecules and induce substantial glutathione depletion in lung, liver, and kidney. Pretreatment of mice with piperonyl butoxide decreased the pulmonary damage, covalent binding, and glutathione depletion produced by naphthalene, whereas pretreatment with diethylmaleate markedly increased the pulmonary damage, enhanced glutathione depletion, and increased covalent binding of naphthalene metabolites in lung and other tissues. Curiously, pretreatment with SKF 525-A had no effect on the lung damage, glutathione depletion, or the covalent binding of naphthalene metabolites in lung. Finally, in contrast to 4-ipomeanol, it is of interest that the tissue specificity for covalent binding in vivo did not parallel tissue damage produced by naphthalene ^{14}C administration. Thus, liver and kidney covalently bound approximately twice as much radioactivity as lung, but did not exhibit pathologic changes while lung was severely damaged. These studies clearly suggested that covalent binding, glutathione depletion, and the pulmonary toxicity of naphthalene are integrated events and that metabolism of naphthalene to highly reactive electrophilic metabolites by cytochrome P-450 monooxygenase enzymes is requisite for toxicity.

3. 3-Methylindole

3-Methylindole (3-MI) is a bacterial metabolite of tryptophan formed in the intestine and is also a component of tobacco smoke. Work published in the early 1970s (CARLSON et al. 1972) showed that administration of 3-MI to cattle and goats produced severe pulmonary edema. Later work showed that either oral or intravenous administration of 3-MI to goats caused a massive protein-rich pulmonary edema, but in addition a vacuolization and necrosis of type I alveolar epithelium and bronchiolar epithelium (HUANG et al. 1977). Some 24–48 h after dosing, the alveoli were denuded of type I cells, type II cells were undamaged, but in the process of transformation into type I cells to repopulate the alveolar surface. Many bronchioles were completey denuded of both ciliated and nonciliated cells. More recent work with smaller doses of 3-MI administered intravenously to goats revealed (BRADLEY and CARLSON 1980) a more selective cytotoxicity which was restricted to alveolar type I and nonciliated bronchiolar (Clara) epithelial cells. The distribution of ^{14}C-labeled 3-MI was studied (BRAY and CARLSON 1980) in rabbits and concentrations were higher in lung at all times from 15 min to 72 h than all other tissues (liver, kidney, heart, fat, plasma, or bile). Subcellular distribution studies showed that in lung, most of the radioactivity was associated with the microsomal fraction, whereas in both liver and kidney, $> 70\%$ of the activity was found in the cytosol. Moreover, about 80% of the radioactivity present in lung microsomes was covalently bound, whereas that found in other lung cell fractions was not. Similar findings were reported by HANAFY and BOGAN (1980) in calves injected with ^{3}H-labeled 3-MI.

4. p-Xylene

Rats administered p-xylene (4-methyltoluene) by intraperitoneal injection, gavage, or by inhalation underwent a 65% loss in pulmonary monooxygenase within 24 h. No corresponding impairment of hepatic monooxygenase activity was observed (PATEL et al. 1978). Pulmonary enzyme activities returned to near control levels 8 days after p-xylene treatment. Maximum inhibition occurred 1–2 days after administration; p-xylene hydroxylase, NADPH-cytochrome c reductase, benzphetamine demethylase, and cytochrome P-450 were reduced to 25%–50% of control levels. Incubation of rabbit lung microsomes with 4-methylbenzaldehyde and NADPH resulted in destruction of about 65%–70% of the cytochrome P-450. NADPH was required for this reaction in lung: no corresponding reaction occurred with liver microsomes. Regardless of concentration or dose, no more than about 70% of the pulmonary P-450 was sensitive to destruction by p-xylene (producing 4-methylbenzaldehyde). The authors proposed a metabolic activation of p-xylene in vivo as depicted in Fig. 7.

It is important to note that the authors were unable to detect either alcohol or aldehyde dehydrogenase activities in rat lung (Fig. 7, reactions 2 and 3) and that reaction 4 occurs only in lung. Thus, in order to elicit lung damage, the al-

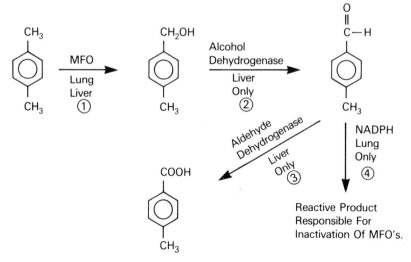

Fig. 7. A scheme for the metabolic activation of p-xylene. As indicated, reaction 1 occurs in both lung and liver, reactions 2 and 3 in liver only, and reaction 4 only in lung. Reaction 4 is assumed to be responsible for the selective destruction in lung of cytochrome P-450 and other monooxygenase components. (Derived from PATEL et al. 1978)

cohol must be transported to the liver where it is oxidized to the aldehyde which in turn diffuses back into the blood and is carried to the lung. The aldehyde is readily detoxified in liver by oxidation to the acid; this reaction, catalyzed by aldehyde dehydrogenase, is apparently deficient in lung where the aldehyde accumulates and is converted in reaction 4 to an unknown toxic product.

5. α-Naphthylthiourea

α-Naphthylthiourea (ANTU) found its first biologic application as a rodenticide as it is highly toxic to rats and mice and much less toxic to cats and rabbits (RICHTER 1945). In susceptible species, ANTU produces lethal toxicity by virtue of massive fibrin-rich pulmonary edema (RICHTER 1952; CUNNINGHAM and HURLEY 1972). Although ANTU is the prototype of this group, thiourea itself and several of its N-substituted derivatives are also lung toxins (Fig. 8). That the toxicity of ANTU and its congeners is related to the integrity of the thiocarbonyl group is demonstrated by the fact that replacement of the sulfur atom by oxygen (α-naphthylurea) abolished the pneumotoxicity (BOYD and NEAL 1976).

In addition to the prominent species differences in thiourea lung toxicity, significant age differences have been observed (DIEKE and RICHTER 1945). Relative to mature animals, young rats are highly resistant to the effects of thioureas. In addition (RICHTER 1946), treatment of adult animals with small nontoxic doses of ANTU resulted in the development of remarkable resistance to the effects of subsequent toxic doses of the agent.

More recent work has clearly implicated covalent binding of ANTU and other thioureas in the pneumotoxicity of these agents. Following the administration to rats of ANTU radiolabeled with either ^{35}S or ^{14}C (in the thiocarbonyl group), significant amounts of radioactivity were covalently bound in lung and liver. Replacement of the sulfur by oxygen abolished the covalent binding and the toxicity (BOYD and NEAL 1976). Similar covalent binding of radioactivity in lungs following administration of thiourea ^{14}C was reported by HOLLINGER et al. (1974), implying a correlation between selective pulmonary toxicity and covalent binding.

Incubation of ^{14}C- or ^{35}S-labeled ANTU with microsomes from rat lung or liver in the presence of NADPH resulted in significant covalent binding of either ^{14}C or ^{35}S (BOYD and NEAL 1976). Somewhat more ^{35}S was bound than ^{14}C, suggesting a crucial role of the sulfur in the covalent binding of ANTU in lung. In

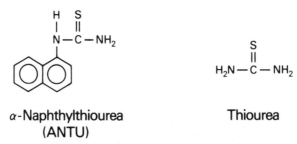

$$\underset{\text{(ANTU)}}{\text{α-Naphthylthiourea}} \qquad\qquad \text{Thiourea}$$

Fig. 8. Structures of α-naphthylthiourea and of thiourea

accord with this finding, LEE et al. (1980) reported that ANTU was metabolized by rat lung and liver microsomes to α-naphthylurea and atomic sulfur and that a portion of the atomic sulfur covalently binds with macromolecules in the microsomes. Approximately half the sulfur bound to lung and liver microsomes was proposed to have reacted with cysteine moieties of the microsomal proteins with the formation of hydrodisulfides. These workers proposed that the pulmonary toxicity of ANTU results from the covalent binding of a monooxygenase-catalyzed metabolite, probably atomic sulfur, to pulmonary macromolecules.

BOYD and NEAL (1976) demonstrated that pretreatment of animals with diethylmaleate reduced pulmonary glutathione to about 20% of control levels and administration of ANTU to these animals resulted in a marked enhancement in the pulmonary toxicity and covalent binding. HOLLINGER et al. (1976), using lung slices and thiourea ^{14}C in vitro, similarly found that covalent binding was modulated by glutathione; covalent binding was reduced by addition of glutathione to the incubation mixture and was markedly increased in slices taken from animals pretreated with diethylmaleate.

Polycyclic hydrocarbons such as benzo[a]pyrene or 3-MC have been abundantly demonstrated to undergo activation in vivo to reactive products (dihydrodiol epoxides) which interact covalently with DNA, thus causing genetic damage which results in carcinogenesis or mutagenesis. It should be pointed out that most of the other compounds discussed in this section (4-ipomeanol, carbon tetrachloride, bromobenzene, naphthalene, ANTU, etc.) have not been shown to interact with nucleic acids (either DNA or RNA), but rather, following their bioactivation, interact with cellular proteins or lipids. Therefore, the precise biochemical events which occur between covalent binding of these xenobiotics and the ultimate event, cellular necrosis, are largely unknown. We write in vague terms about the reactive intermediate interacting with some "vital macromolecule", but is must be admitted that at present we do not understand the cascade of biochemical events which starts with covalent binding of an activated xenobiotic with cellular components and culminates with death of the cell.

6. Pyrrolizidine Alkaloids

Pyrrolizidine alkaloids are a large group of chemically related compounds found in a variety of plant species distributed widely in the world (SCHOENTAL 1968). The basic structure of these alkaloids is shown in Fig. 9. While many of these alkaloids are essentially nontoxic, a number have been identified that are toxic to the lung and liver. Among these are:

Monocrotaline	Fulvine	Indicine
Retrorsine	Jacobine	Lasciocarpine
Heliotrine		

The work of Mattocks and others (MATTOCKS and WHITE 1971; MATTOCKS 1972; JAGO et al. 1970; HSU et al. 1973) has established that the pyrrolizidine alkaloids must undergo metabolic activation in vivo to produce toxicity. MATTOCKS (1972) showed that the parent pyrrolizidine alkaloids are biologically

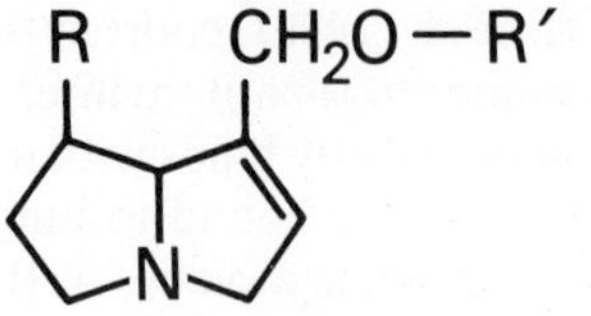

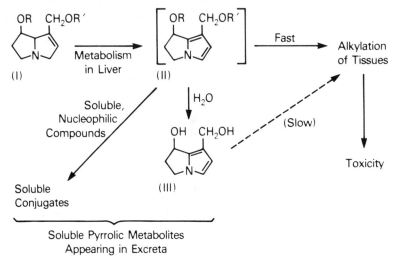

Fig. 9. General structure of the pyrrolizidine alkaloids

Fig. 10. Activation of pyrrolizidine alkaloids. (BOYD 1980 a)

rather inert, but the alkaloids that are toxic undergo dehydrogenation in vivo and in vitro to highly reactive pyrroles. This reaction appeared to be catalyzed by a cytochrome P-450-dependent system in hepatic microsomes. The pyrroles are highly electrophilic molecules which avidly react with macromolecular tissue constituents (Fig. 10) and result from further dehydrogenation of the unsaturated ring.

In an elegantly thorough study, MATTOCKS and WHITE (1971) investigated the conversion of pyrrolizidine alkaloids to pyrrolic (dehydro) products. Using retrorsine and monocrotaline as substrates, the activation reaction was catalyzed by rat liver microsomes, required NADPH and oxygen, was inhibited by CO and by SKF 525-A, and was induced by pretreatment with phenobarbital or DDT. In examining a series of pyrrolizidine alkaloids, their toxicity or lack of toxicity correlated with their ability to form pyrroles (Fig. 10). Of some significance was the observation that the conversion of retrorsine or monocrotaline to pyrroles could *not* be demonstrated with rat lung microsomes. Since monocrotaline is known to produce lung lesions after systemic administration (BUTLER et al. 1970), this finding clearly suggests that activated pyrrole metabolites formed in the liver diffuse back into the blood and are carried to the lungs where they bind covalently and evoke tissue damage (BOYD 1980 c). Finally, the critical role of the hepatic cytochrome P-450-dependent monooxygenase system in modulating the activation of pyrrolizidine alkaloids and thereby modifying their toxicity was clearly demonstrated by ALLEN et al. (1972). If hepatic microsomal enzymes of rats were induced with phenobarbital prior to the administration of monocrotaline, the animals gained less weight, developed more severe lung lesions at an earlier time, and died more rapidly than animals receiving only monocrotaline. By contrast, in rats pretreated with the microsomal inhibitor chloramphenicol, there was an absence of mortality, the growth ratio was unaffected, and the pulmonary lesions were much less severe than in controls receiving monocrotaline alone.

7. Bleomycins

The bleomycins are a family of chemically related glycopeptides produced by *Streptomyces verticillus* which are highly active against a number of malignant tumors in humans (BLUM et al. 1973). The dose-limiting toxicity of bleomycin is pulmonary fibrosis, reported to occur in 5%–20% of treated patients (WILLSON 1978). The initial morphological lesion has been reported to be disruption of the pulmonary capillary endothelium (ADAMSON and BOWDEN 1974) and perivascular edema. This is followed by alveolar epithelial cell necrosis and then a proliferative phase characterized by increased cellularity and thickening of the alveolar septa, the appearance of fibrin in alveolar spaces, and a stimulation in the synthesis and deposition of collagen (JONES and REEVE 1978). Areas of fibrosis are usually patchy in their distribution, but may concentrate in the subpleural area (SIKIC et al. 1978). These changes are accompanied by dyspnea and by compromises in more objective tests of pulmonary function (COLLIS 1980).

The cytotoxic activity of bleomycin results from DNA cleavage. This effect can be duplicated in vitro in reaction mixtures containing Fe^{2+}, bleomycin, and oxygen (SAUSVILLE et al. 1976). In vitro, bleomycin forms a complex with Fe^{2+} and oxygen and this ternary complex, either directly or through the formation of

Table 14. Cytotoxic agents reported to produce lung injury

Bleomycin
Nitrosoureas
BCNU
CCNU
Chlorozotocin
Methyl-CCNU
Neocarcinostatin
Mitomycin C
Cyclophosphamide
Chlorambucil
Melphalan
Busulfan
Procarbazine
6-Mercaptopurine
Thioguanosine
Azathioprine
Uracil mustard

Assembled from: WILLSON (1978), COLLIS (1980), WEISS and MUGGIA (1980)

a new species, degrades DNA. The bleomycin–Fe^{2+}–oxygen complex attacks DNA by cleaving glycosidic bonds with the release of free bases and by attacking the polymeric backbone causing cleavage of the C-3–C-4 bond of deoxyribose (BURGER et al. 1981).

The dual requirement for Fe^{2+} and oxygen for bleomycin activity in vitro, suggests the possibility that reactive oxygen (O_2^-, OH· etc.) might be involved in its antitumor activity, its toxicity, or both. Indeed, recent work in our laboratory (TRUSH et al. 1982a, b) has strongly implicated reactive oxygen in the biologic effects of bleomycin. Thus, it is possible that, like paraquat and nitrofurantoin, bleomycin may express its pulmonary toxicity through some as yet unknown mechanism utilizing reactive oxygen.

8. Oncolytic Agents

A number of agents used in the chemotherapy of neoplastic disease have been reported to cause lung injury. It is not known whether these agents act directly or after metabolic activation. The nature, incidence, severity, and reversibility of the lung injury varies with the agent (WILLSON 1978; COLLIS 1980; WEISS and MUGGIA 1980). These agents are listed in Table 14.

9. O,O,S-Trimethyl Phosphorothioate

An impurity in the insecticide malathion, when administered to rats produces Clara cell necrosis, depletion of lung glutathione, covalent binding, and impairment of pulmonary monooxygenase activities (IMAMURA et al. 1983; IMAMURA and HASEGAWA, 1984).

10. 1,1-Dichloroethylene

Similarly 1,1-dichloroethylene administered to mice, produces selective Clara cell necrosis, impairment of pulmonary monooxygenase activities, and covalent binding. No histologic or monooxygenase alterations were observed in kidney or liver (KRIJGSHELD et al. 1984).

References

Abramson RK, Hutton JJ (1975) Effects of cigarette smoking on aryl hydrocarbon hydroxylase activity in lungs and tissues of inbred mice. Cancer Res 35:23–29

Adamson IYR, Bowden DH (1974) The pathogenesis of bleomycin-induced pulmonary fibrosis in mice. Am J Pathol 77:185–189

Allen JR, Chesney CF, Frazee WJ (1972) Modifications of pyrrolizidine alkaloid intoxication resulting from altered hepatic microsomal enzymes. Toxicol Appl Pharmacol 23:470⁴79

Arinc E, Philpot RM (1976) Preparation and properties of partially purified pulmonary cytochrome P-450 from rabbits. J Biol Chem 251:3213–3220

Autor AP (1974) Reduction of paraquat toxicity by superoxide dismutase. Life Sci 14:1309–1319

Bakhle YS, Vane JR (1974) Pharmacokinetic function of the pulmonary circulation. Physiol Rev 54:1007–1045

Bend JR, Hook GE, Easterling RE, Gram TE, Fouts JR (1972) A comparative study of the hepatic and pulmonary mixed-function oxidase systems in the rabbit. J Pharmacol Exp Ther 183:206–217

Bend JR, Hook GE, Gram TE (1973) Characterization of lung microsomes as related to drug metabolism. Drug Metab Dispos 1:358–367

Bilimoria MH, Johnson J, Hogg JC, Witschi HP (1977) Pulmonary aryl hydrocarbon hydroxylase: tobacco smoke-exposed guinea pigs. Toxicol Appl Pharmacol 41:433–440

Block ER (1979) Potentiation of acute paraquat toxicity by vitamin E deficiency. Lung 156:195–203

Blum RH, Carter SK, Agre K (1983) A clinical review of bleomycin – a new antineoplastic agent. Cancer 31:903–912

Boyd MR (1976) Role of metabolic activation in the pathogenesis of chemically-induced pulmonary disease: mechanism of action of the lung-toxic furan, 4-ipomeanol. Environ Health Perspect 16:127–128

Boyd MR (1977) Evidence for the Clara cell as a site of cytochrome P-450-dependent mixed-function oxidase activity in lung. Nature 269:713–715

Boyd MR (1980a) Biochemical mechanisms of chemical-induced lung injury: role of metabolic activation. CRC Crit Rev Toxicol 7:103–176

Boyd MR (1980b) Biochemical mechanisms in pulmonary toxicity of furan derivatives. Rev Biochem Toxicol 2:71–101

Boyd MR (1980c) Effects of inducers and inhibitors on drug-metabolizing enzymes and on drug toxicity in extrahepatic tissues. Ciba Found 76:43–66

Boyd MR, Burka LT (1978) In vivo studies on the relationship between target organ alkylation and the pulmonary toxicity of a chemically reactive metabolite of 4-ipomeanol. J Pharmacol Exp Ther 207:687–697

Boyd MR, Neal RA (1976) Studies on the mechanisms of toxicity and the development of tolerance to the pulmonary toxin, α-naphthylthiourea (ANTU). Drug Metab Dispos 4:314–322

Boyd MR, Burka LT, Wilson BJ (1975) Distribution, excretion, and binding of radioactivity in the rat after intraperitoneal administration of the lung-toxic furan ^{14}C-4-ipomeanol. Toxicol Appl Pharmacol 32:147–157

Boyd MR, Burka LT, Wilson BJ, Sasame HA (1978a) in vitro studies on the metabolic activation of the pulmonary toxin, 4-ipomeanol, by rat lung and liver microsomes. J Pharmacol Exp Ther 207:677–686

Boyd MR, Statham CN, Franklin RB, Mitchell JR (1978b) Pulmonary bronchiolar alkylation and necrosis by 3-methylfuran, a naturally occurring potential atmospheric contaminant. Nature 272:270–271

Boyd MR, Catignani GL, Sasame HA, Mitchell JR, Stiko AW (1979a) Acute pulmonary injury in rats by nitrofurantoin and modification by vitamin E, dietary fat, and oxygen. Am Rev Resp Dis 120:93–99

Boyd MR, Dutcher JS, Buckpitt AR, Jones RB, Statham CN (1979b) Role of metabolic activation in extrahepatic target organ alkylation in the cytotoxicity by 4-ipomeanol, a furan derivative from moldy sweet potatoes: possible implications for carcinogenesis. In: Miller EC, Miller JA, Hirono I, Sugamura T, Takayama S (eds) Naturally occurring carcinogens – mutagens and modulators of carcinogenesis. University Park Press, Baltimore, pp 35–56

Boyd MR, Stiko AW, Sasame HA (1979c) Metabolic activation of nitrofurantoin – possible implications for carcinogenesis. Biochem Pharmacol 28:601–606

Boyd MR, Sasame HA, Franklin RB (1980a) Comparison of ratios of covalent binding to total metabolism of the pulmonary toxin, 4-ipomeanol, in vitro in pulmonary and hepatic microsomes, and the effects of pretreatments with phenobarbital or 3-methylcholanthrene. Biochem Biophys Res Comm 93:1167–1172

Boyd MR, Statham CN, Longo NS (1980b) The pulmonary Clara cell as a target for toxic chemicals requiring metabolic activation: studies with carbon tetrachloride. J Pharmacol Expt Ther 212:109–114

Boyland E (1980) The history and future of chemical carcinogenesis. Br Med Bull 36:5–10

Bradley BJ, Carlson JR (1980) Ultrastructural pulmonary changes induced by intravenously administered 3-methylindole in goats. Am J Pathol 99:551–560

Bray TM, Carlson JR (1980) Tissue and subcellular distribution and excretion of 3-[^{14}C]methylindole in rabbits after intratracheal infusion. Can J Physiol Pharmacol 58:1399–1405

Bresnick E (1979) Nuclear activation of polycyclic hydrocarbons. Drug Metab Rev 10:209–223

Breyer U (1971) Metabolism of the phenothiazine drug perazine by liver and lung microsomes from various species. Biochem Pharmacol 20:3341–3351

Brodie BB, Reid WD, Cho AK, Sipes G, Krishna G, Gillette JR (1971) Possible mechanism of liver necrosis caused by aromatic organic compounds. Proc Natl Acad Sci USA 68:160–164

Brown EAB (1974) The localization, metabolism, and effects of drugs and toxicants in lung. Drug Metab Rev 3:33–87

Buckpitt A, Boyd M (1978) Xenobiotic metabolism in birds, species lacking pulmonary Clara cells. The Pharmacologist 20:181

Buckpitt AR, Boyd MR (1982) Metabolic Activation of 4-Ipomeanol by Avian Tissue Microsomes. Toxicol Appl Pharmacol 65:53–62

Buege JA, Aust SD (1975) Comparative studies of rat liver and lung NADPH cytochrome c reductase. Biochim Biophys Acta 385:371–379

Buening MK, Wislocki PG, Levin W, Yagi H, Thakker DR, Akagi H, Koreeda M, Jerina DM, Conney AH (1978) Tumorigenicity of the optical enantiomers of the diastereomeric benzo[a]pyrene 7,8-diol-9,10-epoxides in newborn mice: exceptional activity of (+)-7β,8α-dihydroxy-9α,10α-epoxy-7,8,9,10-tetrahydrobenzo[a]pyrene. Proc Natl Acad Sci USA 75:5358–5361

Burger RM, Peisach J, Horwitz SB (1981) Mechanism of bleomycin action: in vitro studies: Life Sci 28:715–727

Burke MD, Prough RA (1976) Some characteristics of hamster liver and lung microsomal aryl hydrocarbon (biphenyl and benzo(a)pyrene) hydroxylation reactions. Biochem Pharmacol 25:2187–2195

Burke MD, Prough RA, Mayer RT (1977) Characteristics of a microsomal cytochrome P-448-mediated reaction: ethoxyresorufin O-deethylation. Drug Metab Dispos 5:1–8

Bürki K, Stroming TH, Bresnick E (1974) Effects of an epoxide hydrase inhibitor on in vitro binding of polycyclic hydrocarbons to DNA and on skin carcinogenesis. J Natl Cancer Inst 52:785–788

Bus JS, Aust SD, Gibson JE (1974) Superoxide and single oxygen-catalyzed lipid peroxidation as a possible mechanism for paraquat (methyl viologen) toxicity. Biochem Biophys Res Commun 58:749–755

Bus JS, Aust SD, Gibson JE (1976) Paraquat toxicity: proposed mechanism of action involving lipid peroxidation. Environ Health Perspect 16:139–146

Butler C, Kleinerman J (1971) Paraquat in the rabbit. Br J Ind Med 28:67–71

Butler WH, Mattocks AR, Barnes JM (1970) Lesions in the liver and lungs of rats given pyrrole derivatives of pyrrolizidine alkaloids. J Pathol 100:169–175

Cantrell ET, Busbee D, Warr G, Martin R (1973a) Induction of aryl hydrocarbon hydroxylase in human leucocytes and pulmonary alveolar macrophages: a comparison. Life Sci 13:1649–1654

Cantrell ET, Warr GA, Busbee DL, Martin RR (1973b) Induction of aryl hydrocarbon hydroxylase in human pulmonary alveolar macrophages by cigarette smoking. J Clin Invest 52:1881–1884

Capdevila J, Jakobsson SW, Jernstrom B, Helia O, Orrenius S (1975) Characterization of a rat lung microsomal fraction obtained by Sepharose 2B ultrafiltration. Cancer Res 35:2820–2829

Carlone MF, Fouts JR (1974) In vitro metabolism of p-xylene by rabbit lung and liver. Xenobiotica 4:705–715

Carlson JR, Yokoyama MT, Dickinson EO (1972) Induction of pulmonary edema and emphysema in cattle and goats with 3-methylindole. Science 176:298–299

Chen W-J, Chi EY, Smuckler EA (1977) Carbon-tetrachloride-induced changes in mixed function oxidases and microsomal cytochromes in the rat lung. Lab Invest 36:388–394

Clark DG, McElligot TF, Hurst EW (1966) The toxicity of paraquat. Br J Ind Med 23:126–132

Collis CH (1980) Lung damage from cytotoxic drugs. Cancer Chemother Pharmacol 4:17–27

Conney AH (1967) Pharmacological implications of microsomal enzyme induction. Pharmacol Rev 19:317–366

Conney AH, Miller EC, Miller JA (1957) Substrate-induced synthesis and other properties of benzpyrene hydroxylase in rat liver. J Biol Chem 228:753–766

Conning DM, Fletcher K, Swann AAB (1969) Paraquat and related bypyridyls. Br Med Bull 25:245–249

Crapo JD, Tierney DF (1974) Superoxide dismutase and pulmonary oxygen toxicity. Am J Physiol 226:1401–1405

Cunningham AL, Hurley JV (1972) Alphanaphthylthiourea-induced pulmonary edema in the rat: a topographical and electronmicroscope study. J Pathol 106:25–34

Daudel P, Duquesne M, Vigny P, Grover PL, Sims P (1975) Fluorescence spectral evidence that benzo[a]pyrene-DNA products in mouse skin arise from diol-epoxides. FEBS Lett 57:250–253

Dees JH, Coe LD, Yasukochi Y, Masters BS (1980) Immunofluorescence of NADPH-cytochrome c (P-450) reductase in rat and minipig tissues injected with phenobarbital. Science 208:1473–1475

Devereux TR, Fouts JR (1974) N-oxidation and demethylation of N,N-dimethylaniline by rabbit liver and lung microsomes: effects of age and metals. Chem Biol Interact 8:91–105

Devereux TR, Fouts JR (1980a) A procedure for isolation of rabbit pulmonary epithelial cells for study of foreign compound metabolism. In: Coon MJ, Conney AH, Estabrook RW, Gelboin HV, Gillette JR, O'Brien PJ (eds) Microsomes, drug oxidations, and chemical carcinogenesis. Academic, New York, pp 825–828

Devereux TR, Fouts JR (1980b) Isolation and identification of Clara cells from rabbit lung. In Vitro 16:958–968

Devereux TR, Hook GE, Fouts JR (1979) Foreign compound metabolism by isolated cells from rabbit lung. Drug Metab Dispos 7:70–75

Devereux T, Smith B, Bend J, Fouts J (1981a) Xenobiotic metabolism in Clara and type II cells isolated from rabbit lung. The Pharmacologist 23:172

Devereux TR, Serabjit-Singh CJ, Slaugher SR, Wolf CR, Philpot RM, Fouts JR (1981b) Identification of cytochrome P-450 isozymes in nonciliated bronchiolar epithelial (Clara) and alveolar type II cells isolated from rabbit lung. Exp Lung Res 2:221–230

Dieke SH, Richter CP (1945) Acute toxicity of thiourea to rats in relation to age, diet, strain, and species variation. J Pharmacol Exp Ther 83:195–201

Dutcher JS, Boyd MR (1979) Species and strain differences in target organ alkylation and toxicity by 4-ipomeanol: predictive value of covalent binding in studies of target organ toxicities by reactive metabolites. Biochem Pharmacol 28:3367–3372

Ferguson HC (1966) Effect of red cedar chip bedding on hexobarbital and pentobarbital sleep time. J Pharm Sci 55:1142–1143

Fisher AB, Huber GH, Furia L (1977) Cytochrome P-450 content and mixed function oxidation by microsomes from rabbit alveolar macrophages. J Lab Clin Med 90:101–108

Fisher HK, Clements JA, Wright RB (1973) Enhancement of oxygen toxicity by the herbicide paraquat. Am Rev Resp Dis 107:246–252

Fouts JR, Devereux TR (1972) Developmental aspects of hepatic and extrahepatic drug-metabolizing enzyme systems: microsomal enzymes and components in rabbit liver and lung during the first month of life. J Pharmacol Expt Ther 183:458–468

Fouts JR, Devereux TR (1973) Use of 10 sec sonication of homogenates to increase microsomal yield in liver and lung from young adult Dutch belt rabbits. Biochem Pharmacol 22:1393–1396

Fridovich I (1978) The biology of oxygen radicals. Sciene 201:875–880

Gage JC (1968) The action of paraquat and diquat on the respiration of liver cell fractions. Biochem J 109:757–761

Gelboin HV, Blackburn NR (1964) The stimulatory effect of 3-methylcholanthrene on benzpyrene hydroxylase activity in several rat tissues: inhibition by actinomycin D and puromycin. Cancer Res 24:356–360

Gelboin HV, Selkirk JK, Yang SK, Wiebel FJ, Namoto, N (1976) Benzo[a]pyrene metabolism by mixed-function oxygenases, hydratases, and glutathione S-transferases: analysis by high pressure liquid chromatography. In: Arias IM, Jakoby WB (eds) Glutathione: metabolism and function. Raven, New York, pp 339–356

Gielen JR, Goujon FM, Nebert DW (1972) Genetic regulation of aryl hydrocarbon hydroxylase induction. II. Simple Mendelian expression in mouse tissues in vivo. J Biol Chem 247:1125–1137

Gillette JR (1974a) A perspective on the role of chemically reactive metabolites of foreign compounds in toxicity. I. Correlation of changes in covalent binding of reactive metabolites with changes in the incidence and severity of toxicity. Biochem Pharmacol 23:2785–2794

Gillette JR (1974b) A perspective on the role of chemically reactive metabolites of foreign compounds in toxicity. II. Alterations in the kinetics of covalent binding. Biochem Pharmacol 23:2927–2938

Gillette JR, Mitchell JR, Brodie BB (1974) Biochemical mechanisms of drug toxicity. Annu Rev Pharmacol 14:271–288

Gilman AG, Conney AH (1963) The induction of aminoazo dye N-demethylase in nonhepatic tissues by 3-methylcholanthrene. Biochem Pharmacol 12:591–593

Gould KG, Clements JA, Jones AL, Felts JM (1972) Dispersal of rabbit lung into individual viable cells: a new model for the study of lung metabolism. Science 178:1209–1210

Gould VE, Smuckler EA (1971) Alveolar injury in acute carbon tetrachloride intoxication. Arch Intern Med 128:109–117

Gram TE (1973) Comparative aspects of mixed function oxidation by lung and liver of rabbits. Drug Metab Rev 2:1–32

Gram TE (1980) The metabolism of xenobiotics by mammalian lung in extrahepatic metabolism of drugs and other foreign compounds. In: Gram TE (ed) Extrahepatic metabolism of drugs and other foreign compounds. SP Medical and Scientific Books, Jamaica, pp 175–209

Grasso P, Williams M, Hodgson R, Gangolli SD (1971) The histochemical distribution of aniline hydroxylase in rat tissues. Histochem J 3:117–126

Grover PL (1974) K-region epoxides of polycyclic hydrocarbons: formation and further metabolism by rat lung preparations. Biochem Pharmacol 23:333–343

Grover PL, Hewer A, Sims P (1973) K-region epoxides of polycyclic hydrocarbons: formation and further metabolism of benz[a]anthracene 5,6-oxide by human lung preparations. FEBS Lett 34:63–68

Grover PL, Hewer A, Sims P (1974) Metabolism of polycyclic hydrocarbons by rat lung preparations. Biochem Pharmacol 23:323–332

Guengerich FP (1977) Preparation and properties of highly purified cytochrome P-450 and NADPH cytochrome P-450 reductase from pulmonary microsomes of untreated rabbits. Mol Pharmacol 13:911–923

Guyton AC (1976) Pulmonary ventilation. In: Textbook of medical physiology, 5th edn. Saunders, Philadelphia, p 523

Hanafy MSM, Bogan JA (1980) The covalent binding of 3-methylindole metabolites to bovine tissue. Life Sci 27:1225–1231

Harper C, Drew RT, Fouts JR (1973) Species differences in benzene hydroxylation to phenol by pulmonary and hepatic microsomes. Drug Metab Dispos 3:381–388

Hesse S, Mezger M (1979) Involvement of phenolic metabolites in the irreversible protein-binding of aromatic hydrocarbons: reactive metabolites of ^{14}C-naphthalene and ^{14}C-l-naphthol formed by rat liver microsomes. Mol Pharmacol 16:667–675

Hilliker KS, Roth RA (1980) Prediction of mescaline clearance by rabbit lung and liver from enzyme kinetic data. Biochem Pharmacol 29:253–255

Hirai K-I, Witschi HP, Coté MG (1977) Electron microscopy of butylated hydroxytoluene-induced lung damage in mice. Exp Mol Pathol 27:295–308

Hollinger MA, Giri SN, Alley M, Budd E, Hwang F (1974) Tissue distribution and binding of radioactivity from ^{14}C-thiourea in the rat. Drug Metab Dispos 2:251–261

Hollinger MA, Giri SN, Hwang F (1976) Binding of radioactivity from ^{14}C-thiourea to rat lung protein. Drug Metab Dispos 4:119–123

Holt PG, Keast D (1973) Induction of aryl hydrocarbon hydroxylase in the lungs of mice in response to cigarette smoke. Experientia 29:1004

Hook GE, Bend JR, Hoel D, Fouts JR, Gram TE (1972) Preparation of lung microsomes and a comparison of the distribution of enzymes between subcellular fractions of rabbit lung and liver. J Pharmacol Exp Ther 182:474–490

Hsu IC, Allen JR, Chesney CF (1973) Identification and toxicological effects of dehydroretronecine, a metabolite of monocrotaline. Proc Soc Exp Biol Med 144:834–842

Huang TW, Carlson JR, Bray TM, Bradley BJ (1977) 3-methylindole-induced pulmonary injury in goats. Am J Pathol 87:647–666

Huberman E, Kuroki T, Marquart H, Selkirk JK, Heidelberger C, Grover PL, Sims P (1972) Transformation of hamster embryo cells by epoxides and other derivatives of polycyclic hydrocarbons. Cancer Res 32:1391–1396

Hulshoff A, Lubauvy WC, Kostenbauder HB (1978) The effect of some cigarette smoke constituents and other compounds on the metabolism of benzo[a]pyrene in rabbit lung 9,000 g supernatant. Xenobiotica 8:711–718

Hundley SG, Freudenthal RI (1977a) A comparison of benzo[a]pyrene metabolism by liver and lung microsomal enzymes from 3-methylcholanthrene-treated rhesus monkeys and rats. Cancer Res 37:3120–3125

Hundley SG, Freudenthal RI (1977b) High-pressure liquid chromatography analysis of benzo[a]pyrene meabolism by microsomal enzymes from rhesus liver and lung. Cancer Res 37:244–249

Ichihara K, Kusunose E, Kusunose M (1969) Microsomal hydroxylation of decane. Biochim Biophys Acta 176:713–719

Ichikawa Y, Yamano T, Fujishima H (1969) Relationships between the interconversion of cytochrome P-450 and P-420 and its activities in hydroxylations and demethylations by P-450 oxidase systems. Biochim Biophys Acta 171:32–46

Ilett KF, Stipp B, Menard RM, Reid WD, Gillette JR (1974) Studies on the mechanism of the lung toxicity of paraquat: comparison of tissue distribution and some biochemical parameters in rats and rabbits. Toxicol Appl Pharmacol 28:216–226

Imamura T, Hasegawa L (1984) Role of metabolic activation, covalent binding and glutathione depletion in pulmonary toxicity produced by an impurity of malathion. Toxicol Appl Pharmacol 72:476–483

Imamura T, Gandy J, Fukuto TR (1983) Selective inhibition of rat pulmonary monooxygenase by O,O,S-trimethyl phosphorothioate treatment. Biochem Pharmacol 32:3191–3195

Jago MV, Edgar JA, Smith LW, Culvenor CC (1970) Metabolic conversion of heliotridine-based pyrrolizidine alkaloids to dehydroheliotridine. Mol Pharmacol 6:402–407

Johannesen K, DePierre JW, Bergstrand A, Dallner G, Ernster L (1977) Preparation and characterization of total, rough, and smooth microsomes from the lungs of control and methylcholanthrene-treated rats. Biochim Biophys Acta 496:115–135

Johnson KJ, Fantone JC, Kaplan J, Ward PA (1981) In vivo damage of rat lungs by oxygen metabolites. J Clin Invest 67:983–993

Jones AW, Reeve NL (1978) Ultrastructural study of bleomycin-induced pulmonary changes in mice. J Pathol 124:227–233

Jones KW, Holland JF, Foureman GL, Bend JR, Fouts JR (1983) Xenobiotic metabolism in Clara cells and alveolar type II cells isolated from lungs of rats treated with β-naphthoflavone. J Pharmacol Exp Ther 225:316–319

Kapitulnik J, Wislocki PG, Levin W, Yagi H, Jerina DM, Conney AH (1978) Tumorigenicity studies with diol-epoxides of benzo[a]pyrene which indicate that ($\pm$) trans-7β,8α-dihydroxy-9α-10α-epoxy-7,8,9,10-tetrahydrobenzo[a]pyrene is an ultimate carcinogen in newborn mice. Cancer Res 38:354–358

Kasper CB (1971) Biochemical distinctions between the nuclear and microsomal membranes from rat hepatocytes. J Biol Chem 246:577–581

Kehrer JP, Haschek WM, Witschi HP (1979) The influence of hyperoxia on the acute toxicity of paraquat and diquat. Drug Chem Toxicol 2:397–408

Kehrer JP, Witschi HP (1980) Effects of drug metabolism inhibitors on butylated hydroxytoluene-induced pulmonary toxicity in mice. Toxicol Appl Pharmacol 53:333–342

Kikkawa Y, Yoneda K, Smith F, Packard B, Suzuki K (1975) The type II epithelial cells of the lung. II. Chemical composition and phospholipid biosynthesis. Lab Invest 32:295–302

Krijgsheld KR, Lowe MC, Mimnaugh EG, Trush MA, Ginsburg E, Gram TE (1984) Selective damage to nonciliated bronchiolar epithelial cells in relation to impairment of pulmonary monooxygenase activities by 1,1-dichloroethylene in mice. Toxicol Appl Pharmacol 74:201–213

Kuenzig W, Tkaczevski V, Kamm JJ, Conney AH, Burns JJ (1977) The effect of ascorbic acid deficiency on extrahepatic microsomal metabolism of drugs and carcinogens in the guinea pig. J Pharmacol Exp Ther 201:527–533

Kuhn C (1976) The cells of the lung and their organelles. In: Crystal RG (ed) The biochemical basis of pulmonary function. Dekker, New York, pp 3–48

Kuhn C (1978) Ultrastructure and cellular function in the distal lung. In: The lung. IAP Monograph, No. 19. Williams and Wilkins, Baltimore, pp 1–20

Lee PW, Arnau T, Neal RA (1980) Metabolism of α-naphthylthiourea by rat liver and lung microsomes. Toxicol Appl Pharmacol 53:164–173

Levin W, Buening MK, Wood AW, Chang RL, Kedzierski B, Thakker DR, Boyd DR, Gadaginamath GS, Armstrong RN, Yagi H, Karle JM, Slaga TJ, Jerina DM, Conney AH (1980) An enantiomeric interaction in the metabolism and tumorigenicity of (+) and (−) benzo[a]pyrene 7,8-oxide. J Biol Chem 255:9067–9074

Litterst CL, Mimnaugh EG, Reagan RL, Gram TE (1975a) Comparison of in vitro drug metabolism by lung, liver and kidney of several common laboratory species. Drug Metab Dispos 3:259–265

Litterst CL, Mimnaugh EG, Reagan RL, Gram TE (1975b) Drug metabolism by microsomes from extrahepatic organs of rat and rabbit prepared by calcium aggregation. Life Sci 17:813–818

Litterst CL, Mimnaugh EG, Gram TE (1977) Comparative alterations in extrahepatic drug metabolism by factors known to affect hepatic activity. Biochem Pharmacol 26:749–755

Lu AYH, Coon MJ (1968) Role of hemoprotein P-450 in fatty acid ω-hydroxylation in a soluble enzyme system from liver microsomes. J Biol Chem 243:1331–1332

Mahvi D, Bank H, Harley R (1977) Morphology of a naphthalene-induced bronchiolar lesion. Am J Pathol 86:559–572

Malkinson AM (1979) Prevention of butylated hydroxytoluene-induced lung damage in mice by cedar terpene administration. Toxicol Appl Pharmacol 49:551–560

Marcotte J, Witschi HP (1972) Induction of pulmonary aryl hydrocarbon hydroxylase by marijuana. Res Commun Chem Pathol Pharmacol 4:561–568

Marino A, Mitchell JT (1972) Lung damage in mice following intraperitoneal injection of butylated hydroxytoluene. Proc Soc Exp Biol Med 140:122–125

Mason HS (1965) Oxidases. Annu Rev Biochem 34:595–634

Mason RP, Holtzman JL (1975) The role of catalytic superoxide formation in the oxygen inhibition of nitroreductase. Biochem Biophys Res Commun 67:1267–1274

Matsubara T, Tochino Y (1971) Electron transport systems of lung microsomes and their physiological functions. I. Intracellular distribution of oxidative enzymes in lung cells. J Biochem (Tokyo) 70:981–991

Matsubara T, Prough RA, Burke MD, Estabrook RW (1974) The preparation of microsomal fractions of rodent respiratory tract and their characterization. Cancer Res 34:2196–2203

Mattocks AR (1972) Toxicity and metabolism of Senecio alkaloids. In: Harborne JB (ed) Phytochemical ecology. Academic, New York

Mattocks AR, White INH (1971) The conversion of pyrrolizidine alkaloids to N-oxides and to dihydropyrrolizidine derivatives by rat liver microsomes in vitro. Chem Biol Interact 3:383–391

McLemore TL, Martin RR, Bushee DL, Richie RC, Springer RR, Toppell KL, Cantrell ET (1977) Aryl hydrocarbon hydroxylase activity in pulmonary macrophages and lymphocytes from lung cancer and noncancer patients. Cancer Res 37:1175–1181

McManus ME, Boobis AR, Pacifici GM, Frempang RY, Brodie MJ, Kahn GC, Whyte C, Davies DS (1980) Xenobiotic metabolism in the human lung. Life Sci 26:481–487

Miranda CL, Mukhtar H, Bend JR, Chhabra RS (1979) Effects of vitamin A deficiency on hepatic and extrahepatic mixed function oxidase and epoxide metabolizing enzymes in guinea pig and rabbit. Biochem Pharmacol 28:2713–2716

Morgan TE (1971) Pulmonary surfactant. N Engl J Med 284:1185–1193

Nakagawa Y, Hiraga K, Suga T (1979) Biological fate of butylated hydroxytoluene (BHT): binding in vitro of BHT to liver microsomes. Chem Pharm Bull (Tokyo) 27:480–485

Nakazawa K, Costa E (1971) Metabolism of Δ^9-tetrahydrocannabinol by lung and liver homogenates of rats treated with methylcholanthrene. Nature 234:48–49

Okamoto T, Chan P-C, So BT (1972) Effect of tobacco, marijuana, and benzo[a]pyrene on aryl hydrocarbon hydroxylase in hamster lung. Life Sci 11:733–741

Oppelt WW, Zange M, Ross WE, Remmer H (1970) Comparison of microsomal drug hydroxylation in lung and liver of various species. Res Commun Chem Pathol Pharmacol 1:43–56

Paine AJ (1978) Excited states of oxygen in biology: their possible involvement in cytochrome P-450 linked oxidations as well as the induction of the P-450 system by many diverse compounds. Biochem Pharmacol 27:1805–1813

Patel JM, Harper C, Drew RT (1978) The biotransformation of p-xylene to a toxic aldehyde. Drug Metab Dispos 6:368–374

Philpot RM, Anderson MW, Eling TE (1977) Uptake, accumulation, and metabolism of chemicals by the lung. In: Bakhle YS, Vane JR (eds) Metabolic functions of the lung. Marcel Dekker, New York, pp 123–171

Picciano P, Rosenbaum RM (1978) The type I alveolar lining cells of the mammalian lung. I. Isolation and enrichment from dissociated adult rabbit lung. Am J Pathol 90:99–122

Plopper CG, Mariassy AT, Hill LH (1980) Ultrastructure of the nonciliated bronchiolar epithelial (Clara) cell of mammalian lung. I. A comparison of rabbit, guinea pig, rat, hamster, and mouse. Exp Lung Res 1:139–154

Poland AP, Glover E, Robinson JR, Nebert DW (1974) Genetic expression of aryl hydrocarbon hydroxylase activity. J Biol Chem 249:5599–5606

Prough RA, Burke MD (1975) The role of NADPH cytochrome c reductase in microsomal hydroxylation reactions. Arch Biochem Biophys 170:160–168

Ravindranath V, Burka LT, Boyd MR (1984) Reactive metabolites from the bioactivation of toxic methylfurans. Science 224:884–886

Recknagel RO, Glende EA (1973) Carbon tetrachloride hepatotoxicity: an example of lethal cleavage. CRC Crit Rev Toxicol 2:263–297

Reid WD, Glick JM, Krishna G (1972) Metabolism of foreign compounds by alveolar macrophages of rabbits. Biochem Biophys Res Commun 49:626–634

Reid WD, Ilett KF, Glick JM, Krishna G (1973) Metabolism and binding of aromatic hydrocarbons in the lung: relationship to experimental bronchiolar necrosis. Am Rev Respir Dis 107:539–551

Reiss OK (1966) Studies of lung metabolism. I. Isolation and properties of subcellular fractions from rabbit lung. J Cell Biol 30:45–57

Rhodes ML, Zavala DC, Brown D (1976) Hypoxic protection in paraquat poisoning. Lab Invest 35:496–500

Richter CP (1945) The development and use of alphanaphthylthiourea (ANTU) as a rat poison. JAMA 129:927–930

Richter CP (1946) Biological factors involved in poisoning rats with alphanaphthylthiourea. Proc Soc Exp Biol Med 63:364–370

Richter CP (1952) The physiology and cytology of pulmonary edema and pleural effusion produced in rats by alphanaphthylthiourea (ANTU). J Thorac Cardiosvase Surg 23:66–72

Robertson B, Enhörning G, Ivemark B, Malmquist J, Modee J (1971) Experimental respiratory distress induced by paraquat. J Pathol 103:239–244

Roth RA, Wiersma DA (1980) Role of the lung in total body clearance of circulating drugs. Clin Pharmacokinet 4:355–367

Sasame HA, Boyd MR (1979) Superoxide and hydrogen peroxide production and NADPH oxidation stimulated by nitrofurantoin in lung microsomes: possible implications for toxicity. Life Sci 24:1091–1096

Sausville EA, Peisach J, Horwitz SB (1976) A role for ferrous ion and oxygen in the degradation of DNA by bleomycin. Biochem Biophys Res Commun 73:814–822

Schoental R (1968) Toxicology and carcinogenic action of pyrrolizidine alkaloids. Cancer Res 28:2237–2246

Seifried HE, Birkett DJ, Levin W, Lu AYH, Conney AH, Jerina DM (1977) Metabolism of benzo[a]pyrene: effect of 3-methylcholanthrene pretreatment on metabolism by microsomes from lungs of genetically "responsive" and "nonresponsive" mice. Arch Biochem Biophys 178:256–263

Selkirk JK, Croy RG, Gelboin HV (1974a) Benzo[a]pyrene metabolites: efficient and rapid separation by high-pressure liquid chromatography. Science 184:169–171

Selkirk JK, Croy RG, Roller PP, Gelboin HV (1974b) High pressure liquid chromatographic analysis of benzo[a]pyrene metabolism and covalent binding and the mechanism of action of 7,8-benzoflavone and 1,2-epoxy-3,3,3-trichloropropane. Cancer Res 34:3474–3480

Serabjit-Singh CJ, Wolf CR, Philpot RM (1979) The rabbit pulmonary monooxygenase system: immunochemical and biochemical characterization of enzyme components. J Biol Chem 254:9901–9907

Serabjit-Singh CJ, Wolf CR, Philpot RM, Plopper CG (1980) Cytochrome P-450: localization in rabbit lung. Science 207:1469–1470

Sevanian A, Kaplan SA, Barrett CT (1981) Phospholipid synthesis in fetal lung organotypic cultures and isolated type II pneumocytes. Biochim Biophys Acta 664:498–512

Sikic BI, Mimnaugh EG, Litterst CL, Gram TE (1977) The effects of ascorbic acid depletion and repletion on pulmonary, renal, and hepatic drug metabolism in the guinea pig. Arch Biochem Biophys 179:663–671

Sikic BI, Young DM, Mimnaugh EG, Gram TE (1978) Quantification of bleomycin pulmonary toxicity in mice by changes in lung hydroxyproline content and morphometric histopathology. Cancer Res 38:787–792

Sims P, Grover PL, Swaisland A, Pal K, Hewer A (1974) Metabolic activation of benzo[a]pyrene proceeds by a diol-epoxide. Nature 252:326–328

Sipal Z, Ablenius T, Bergstrand A, Rodriguez L, Jakobsson SW (1979) Oxidative biotransformation of benzo[a]pyrene by human lung microsomal fractions prepared from surgical specimens. Xenobiotica 9:633–645

Slaga TJ, Bracken WJ, Gleason G, Levin W, Yagi H, Jerina DM, Conney AH (1979) Marked differences in the skin tumor-initiating activities of the optical enantiomers of the diastereomeric benzo[a]pyrene 7,8-diol-9,10-epoxides. Cancer Res 39:67–71

Slaughter SR, Wolf CR, Marciniszyn JP, Philpot RM (1981) The rabbit pulmonary monooxygenase system: partial structural characterization of the cytochrome P-450 components and comparison to the hepatic cytochrome P-450. J Biol Chem 256:2499–2503

Smith BR, Maguire JH, Ball LM, Bend JR (1978) Pulmonary metabolism of epoxides. Fed Proc 37:2480–2484

Smith LL, Rose MS, Wyatt I (1979) The pathology and biochemistry of paraquat. Ciba Found Symp 65:321–336

Smith P, Heath D (1974) The ultrastructure and time sequence of the early stages of paraquat lung in rats. J Pathol 114:177–184

Smith P, Heath D (1976) Paraquat. CRC Crit Rev Toxicol 4:411–445

Smith P, Heath D, Kay JK (1974) The pathogenesis and structure of paraquat induced pulmonary fibrosis in rats. J Pathol 114:57–67

Snyder R, Remmer H (1979) Classes of hepatic microsomal mixed function oxidase inducers. Pharmacol Ther 7:203–244

Sorokin SP (1970) The cells of the lungs. In: Nettesheim P, Hanna MG, Deatherage JW (eds) Morphology of experimental respiratory carcinogenesis. U.S. Atomic Energy Commission, pp 3–43

Sovijarvi ARA, Lemola M, Stenius B, Adanpaan-Heikkila J (1977) Nitrofurantoin induced acute, subacute, and chronic pulmonary reactions. Scand J Respir Dis 58:41–50

Sunderman FW, Leibman KC (1970) Nickel carbonyl inhibition of induction of aminopyrine demethylase activity in liver and lung. Cancer Res 30:1645–1650

Teel RW, Douglas WHJ (1980) Aryl hydrocarbon hydroxylase activity in type II alveolar lung cells. Experientia 36:107

Tierney DF (1974) Lung metabolism and biochemistry. Annu Rev Physiol 36:209–231

Tong SS, Hirokata Y, Trush MA, Mimnaugh EG, Ginsburg E, Lowe MC, Gram TE (1981) Clara cell damage and inhibition of pulmonary mixed-function oxidase activity by naphthalene. Biochem Biophys Res Commun 100:944–950

Trush MA, Mimnaugh EG, Ginsburg E, Gram TE (1981) In vitro stimulation by paraquat of reactive oxygen-mediated lipid peroxidation in rat lung microsomes. Toxicol Appl Pharmacol 60:279–286

Trush MA, Mimnaugh EG, Ginsburg E, Gram TE (1982a) Studies on the interaction of bleomycin A_2 with rat lung microsomes. I. Characterization of factors which influence bleomycin-mediated DNA chain breakage. J Pharmacol Exp Ther 221:152–158

Trush MA, Mimnaugh EG, Ginsburg E, Gram TE (1982b) Studies on the interaction of bleomycin A_2 with rat lung microsomes. II. Involvement of adventitious iron and reactive oxygen in bleomycin-mediated DNA chain breakage. J Pharmacol Exp Ther 221:159–165

Uehleke H (1968) Extrahepatic microsomal drug metabolism. In: Sensitization to drugs. Excerpta Medical International Congress Series No. 181, pp 94–100

Ueng T-H, Alvares AP (1981) Selective loss of pulmonary cytochrome P-450$_1$ in rabbits pretreated with polychlorinated biphenyls. J Biol Chem 256:7536–7542

Valdivia E, Sonnad J (1966) Fatty change of the granular pneumocyte in CCl_4 intoxication. Arch Pathol 81:514–519

Van Cantfort J, Gielen J (1975) Organ specificity of aryl hydrocarbon hydroxylase induction by cigarette smoke in rats and mice. Biochem Pharmacol 24:1253–1256

Vijeyaratnam GS, Corrin B (1971) Experimental paraquat poisoning: a histological and electron-optical study of the changes in the lung. J Pathol 103:123–129

Warren DL, Brown DL, Buckpitt AR (1982) Evidence for cytochrome P-450 mediated metabolism in the bronchiolar damage by naphthalene. Chem Biol Interact 40:287–303

Warren PM, Bellward GD (1978) Induction of aryl hydrocarbon hydroxylase by 3-methylcholanthrene in liver, lung, and kidney of gonadectomized and sham-operated Wistar rats. Biochem Pharmacol 27:2537–2541

Watanabe M, Konno K, Sato H (1978) Properties of aryl hydrocarbon (benzo[a]pyrene) hydroxylase in lung microsomes of mice. Gann 69:1–8

Wattenberg LW, Leong JL (1962) Histochemical demonstration of reduced pyridine nucleotide dependent polycyclic hydrocarbon metabolizing systems. J Histochem Cytochem 10:412–420

Wattenberg LW, Leong JL, Galbraith AR (1967) Induction of increased benzpyrene hydroxylase activity in pulmonary tissue in vitro. Proc Soc Exp Biol Med 127:467–469

Wattenberg LW, Page MA, Leong JL (1968a) Induction of increased benzpyrene hydroxylase activity by flavones and related compounds. Cancer Res 28:934–937

Wattenberg LW, Page MA, Leong JL (1968 b) Induction of increased benzpyrene hydroxylase activity by 2-phenylbenzothiazoles and related compounds. Cancer Res 28:2539–2544

Welch RM, Loh A, Conney AH (1971) Cigarette smoke: stimulatory effect on metabolism of 3,4-benzpyrene by enzymes in rat lung. Life Sci 10:215–221

Welch RM, Cavallito J, Loh A (1972) Effect of exposure to cigarette smoke on the metabolism of benzo[a]pyrene and acetophenetidin by lung and intestine of rats. Toxicol Appl Pharmacol 23:749–758

Weiss RM, Muggia FM (1980) Cytotoxic drug-induced pulmonary disease: update 1980. Am J Med 68:259–266

Wiebel FJ, Lentz JC, Diamond L, Gelboin HV (1971) Aryl hydrocarbon (benzo[a]pyrene) hydroxylase in microsomes from rat tissues: differential inhibition and stimulation by benzoflavones and organic solvents. Arch Biochem Biophys 144:78–86

Wiebel FJ, Leutz JC, Gelboin HV (1973) Aryl hydrocarbon (benzo[a]pyrene) hydroxylase: inducible in extrahepatic tissues of mouse strains not inducible in liver. Arch Biochem Biophys 154:292–294

Willson JKV (1978) Pulmonary toxicity of antineoplastic drugs. Cancer Treat Rep 62:2003–2008

Witschi HP (1976) Proliferation of type II alveolar cells: a review of common responses in toxic lung injury. Toxicology 5:267–277

Witschi HP, Saheb W (1974) Stimulation of DNA synthesis in mouse lung following intraperitoneal injection of butylated hydroxytoluene. Proc Soc Exp Biol Med 147:690–693

Witschi HP, St-Francois B (1972) Enhanced activity of benzpyrene hydroxylase in rat liver and lung after acute cannabis administration. Toxicol Appl Pharmacol 23:165–168

Witschi HP, Kacew S, Hirai K-I, Côté MG (1977) In vivo oxidation of reduced nicotinamide-adenine dinucleotide phosphate by paraquat and diquat in rat lung. Chem Biol Interact 19:143–160

Wolf CR, Szutowski MM, Ball LM, Philpot RM (1978) The rabbit pulmonary monooxygenase system: characteristics and activities of two forms of pulmonary cytochrome P-450. Chem Biol Interact 21:29–43

Wolf CR, Smith BR, Ball LM, Serabjit-Singh C, Bend JR, Philpot RM (1979) The rabbit pulmonary monooxygenase system: catalytic differences between two purified forms of cytochrome P-450 in the metabolism of benzo[a]pyrene. J Biol Chem 254:3658–3663

Yang SK, Selkirk JK, Plotkin EV, Gelboin HV (1975) Kinetic analysis of the metabolism of benzo[a]pyrene to phenols, dihydrodiols, and quinones by high pressure chromatography compared to analysis by aryl hydrocarbon hydroxylase assay, and the effect of enzyme induction. Cancer Res 35:3642–3650

CHAPTER 15

The Surfactant System of the Lung

S. A. ROONEY

A. Introduction

Pulmonary surfactant is the surface tension lowering material which lines the lung alveoli and prevents their collapse on expiration. Its existence was first postulated on theoretical grounds by VON NEERGARD (1929), but it was not actually demonstrated until some 30 years later when PATTLE (1955) found that remarkably stable bubbles were expressed from a lung cut under water and CLEMENTS (1957) showed that lung extracts lowered surface tension at an air–water interface.

The best studied disease entity involving a defect in surfactant is the respiratory distress syndrome of the newborn (hyaline membrane disease). AVERY and MEAD (1959) reported that the lungs of infants who died from hyaline membrane disease were deficient in surfactant. It is now recognized that the respiratory distress syndrome of the newborn is a developmental disorder due to lung immaturity which consequent insufficient surfactant. A number of hormones and other agents have been shown to accelerate fetal lung maturation and stimulate surfactant production in animals (ROONEY 1983); glucocorticoids (ANONYMOUS 1981), thyroxine (MASHIACH et al. 1978), and aminophylline (HADJIGEORGIOU et al. 1979) have been reported to prevent the respiratory distress syndrome in human infants. Endotracheal administration of artificial surfactant has been used to prevent or treat the respiratory distress syndrome in premature infants (FUJIWARA et al. 1980; MORLEY et al. 1981). The history of the discovery of surfactant and its relationship to the respiratory distress syndrome of the newborn has been elegantly reviewed by COMROE (1977 a, b, c).

The objective of this chapter is to review available information on alterations in the surfactant system due to airway-borne toxicants and how such changes may be detected. As background to this, knowledge of surfactant composition, synthesis, secretion, and removal is first summarized. There are numerous reviews on surfactant and these should be consulted for more detailed information on physicochemical aspects (GOERKE 1974; NOTTER and MORROW 1975), biosynthetic aspects (BATENBURG und VAN GOLDE 1979; OHNO et al. 1978; VAN GOLDE 1976), and developmental aspects (FARRELL and HAMOSH 1978; GROSS 1979; HALLMAN and GLUCK 1977; PERELMAN et al. 1981; ROONEY 1983; SMITH and BOGUES 1980).

B. Surfactant Composition

Surfactant for in vitro study can be obtained by endobrachial lavage with saline followed by differential centrifugation (KING and CLEMENTS 1972 a). HARWOOD et al. (1975) studied such materials from rat, rabbit, ox, and sheep lung. All were highly surface active and consisted of lipid (79%–90% by weight) and protein (8%–18%) with only a trace of carbohydrate. The composition of dog lung surfactant was similar (KING and CLEMENTS 1972 b).

Lipids from rabbit lung lavage consist of 80%–90% phospholipids, 10% glycolipids, and 5% neutral lipids (ROONEY et al. 1974). The composition of the phospholipids from lung lavage and lavaged lung tissue are shown in Table 1. The phospholipid composition of surfactant is distinctive and quite different from that of lung tissue. Phosphatidylcholine, more than half of which is disaturated, accounts for over 80% of the total. Phosphatidylethanolamine and sphingomyelin, prominent phospholipids in lung tissue, are relatively minor components of surfactant. Phosphatidylglycerol is the second most abundant phospholipid in surfactant and accounts for up to 11% of the total phospholipid (HALLMAN and GLUCK 1975; MASON et al. 1977 a; PFLEGER et al. 1972; ROONEY et al. 1974; SANDERS and LONGMORE 1975). Palmitic acid is the major fatty acid in surfactant phosphatidylcholine from several species (HARWOOD et al. 1975; KING and CLEMENTS 1972 b; ROONEY et al. 1975 b). Dipalmitoylphosphatidylcholine is, therefore, the major disaturated species of surfactant phosphatidylcholine. Although dipalmitoylphosphatidylcholine and phosphatidylglycerol are characteristic components of surfactant, they are not exclusive markers for it by any means since they also occur in other, nonsurfactant lung fractions. In addition, both disaturated phosphatidylcholine (MASON 1973) and phosphatidylglycerol (WHITE 1973) occur in other mammalian tissues although usually not as abundantly as in surfactant.

Both dipalmitoylphosphatidylcholine (ROONEY et al. 1974) and phosphatidylglycerol (HENDERSON and PFLEGER 1972; ROONEY et al. 1974) are highly surface active. The precise nature of surfactant in vivo, however, is unknown. It is

Table 1. Phospholipid composition of lung lavage and lavaged lung tissue from adult rabbits[a]

Phospholipid	Composition (%total phospholipid phosphorus)	
	Lavage	Lavaged tissue
Phosphatidylcholine	86.2	46.1
Disaturated phosphatidylcholine	46.5	13.2
Phosphatidylethanolamine	3.0	20.1
Sphingomyelin	1.2	18.6
Phosphatidylserine	0.3	8.3
Phosphatidylinositol	2.0	3.2
Phosphatidylglycerol	6.2	2.1
Other	1.2	1.0

[a] These data are adapted from ROONEY et al. (1974, 1977 b)

unlikely to be pure dipalmitoylphosphatidylcholine because of its poor spreading properties (NOTTER et al. 1980). HILDEBRAN et al. (1979) reported that monolayers consisting of at least 90% dipalmitoylphosphatidylcholine with up to 10% cholesterol or monoenoic phosphatidylcholine could function as surfactant. MORLEY et al. (1981) reported that a mixture of 70% dipalmitoylphosphatidylcholine and 30% phosphatidylglycerol was an effective artificial surfactant. A role for protein in lowering surface tension has also been suggested (KING and MACBETH 1979) although others (METCALFE et al. 1980) have reported that it is unnecessary. The exact composition and structure of surfactant which is functional in vivo need to be determined. This is particularly important in the development of an artificial surfactant for use in the treatment of diseases in which surfactant is altered or deficient.

C. Biosynthesis of Surfactant Phospholipids

I. Cellular Site of Surfactant Synthesis

Pulmonary surfactant is produced in the type II alveolar epithelial cell. Early autoradiographic studies (ASKIN and KUHN 1971; BUCKINGHAM et al. 1966) showed that radiolabeled acetate and palmitate were preferentially incorporated into phosphatidylcholine in type II cells. Procedures for isolation and culture of purified type II cells have been described (KIKKAWA and YONEDA 1974; MASON et al. 1977c) and cell lines with morphological characteristics of type II cells have been developed (see Chap. 7). Isolated type II cells are enriched with respect to phosphatidylcholine and phosphatidylglycerol (MASON et al. 1977a), synthesize surfactant phospholipids from nonlipid precursors (BATENBURG et al. 1978; ENGLE et al. 1980; MASON 1978; MASON and DOBBS 1980; SMITH and KIKKAWA 1978, 1979), and secrete disaturated phosphatidylcholine (BROWN and LONGMORE 1981 a; DOBBS and MASON 1978, 1979).

II. Role of Lamellar Bodies in Surfactant Production

Morphologically, type II cells are characterized by the presence of lamellar inclusion bodies. Autoradiographic studies implicated these subcellular organelles in surfactant production (ADAMSON and BOWDEN 1973). Isolated lamellar bodies are rich in phospholipid, the composition of which is very similar to that of surfactant (DiAUGUSTINE 1974; ENGLE et al. 1976; GIL and REISS 1973; PAGE-ROBERTS 1972; ROONEY et al. 1975b). Lamellar bodies have been reported (MEBAN 1972; SPITZER et al. 1975) to contain phosphatidic acid phosphatase, an enzyme involved in the synthesis of phospholipids (see Sect. C. III). However, the lung contains a number of phosphatidic acid phosphatases (CASOLA and POSSMAYER 1981) and the enzyme reported in lamellar bodies was not shown to be involved in glycerolipid synthesis. In addition, lamellar bodies have been reported to lack a number of enzymes of phosphatidylcholine and disaturated phosphatidylcholine biosynthesis (BARANSKA and VAN GOLDE 1977; GARCIA et al. 1976; ROONEY et al. 1975b). Therefore, surfactant phosphatidylcholine does not appear to be synthesized in lamellar bodies. As in the case of mammalian phosphatidylcholine generally, it is synthesized in the endoplasmic reticulum and stored in lamellar inclusions prior to secretion. It has not been established how the phospholipids are transported to the lamellar bodies although recently proteins with the ability to transfer phosphatidylcholine and phosphatidylglycerol between subcellular organelles and between these organelles and liposomes have been identified in lung tissue (ENGLE et al. 1978; LUMB et al. 1980; SPALDING and HOOK 1979; VAN GOLDE et al. 1980; WHITLOW et al. 1980) and isolated type II cells (POST et al. 1980a). Lamellar body contents, containing phospholipids, possibly other components of surfactant, and probably unrelated compounds, are secreted by the process of exocytosis onto the alveolar surface. Electron micrographs of lamellar bodies in the process of secreting their contents have been published (RYAN et al. 1975). After release, lamellar body membranes form tubular myelin (WILLIAMS 1977) which may be a storage form of alveolar surfactant. Tubular myelin appears to exist in a subphase on the surface of which the physiologically active surfactant monolayer is formed (GOERKE 1974).

III. Synthesis of Phosphatidylcholine

1. De Novo Synthesis of Unsaturated Phosphatidylcholine

The synthesis of phosphatidylcholine is illustrated in Fig. 1. Dihydroxyacetone phosphate, an intermediate in the glycolytic pathway, is converted to 1-acylglycerol-3-phosphate, either by initial reduction to glycerol-3-phosphate followed by acylation, or by initial acylation to acyldihydroxyacetone phosphate followed by reduction. MASON (1978) reported that the latter mechanism accounted for synthesis of about 60% of the phosphatidylcholine and phosphatidylglycerol in rat type II cells. Glucose and glycogen are incorporated into phospholipids via dihydroxyacetone phosphate. Glycerol can be incorporated as glycerol-3-phosphate following phosphorylation by glycerol kinase, an enzyme which is present in type II cells (WYKLE and KRAEMER 1977). Fatty acids, synthesized de novo by the lung or from the blood, may be incorporated into phospholipids at a number of acylation steps. Fatty acids may also be metabolized to acetate and thus incorporated into the glycerol backbone of the phospholipids.

Acylation of 1-acylglycerol-3-phosphate yields phosphatidic acid. At this point in the pathway, synthesis of phosphatidylcholine and phosphatidylglycerol diverge. For synthesis of phosphatidylcholine, phosphatidic acid is dephosphorylated to diacylglycerol which reacts with cytidine 5'-diphosphocholine (CDPcholine) to form phosphatidylcholine. Of the three enzymes in the choline incorporation pathway, choline kinase, cholinephosphate cytidylyltransferase, and cholinephosphotransferase, there is accumulating evidence that cholinephosphate cytidylyltransferase may catalyze the rate-limiting step. There is a developmental increase in the activity of this enzyme in the neonatal lung about the time of increased phosphatidylcholine synthesis (BREHIER and ROONEY 1981; MANISCALCO et al. 1978; OLDENBORG and VAN GOLDE 1977; ROONEY et al. 1976b, 1977a; WEINHOLD et al. 1981). Hormones which stimulate phosphatidylcholine synthesis in the fetal lung also increase cholinephosphate cytidylyltransferase activity (BREHIER and ROONEY 1981; GROSS et al. 1980; KHOSLA et al. 1980; POSSMAYER et al. 1981;

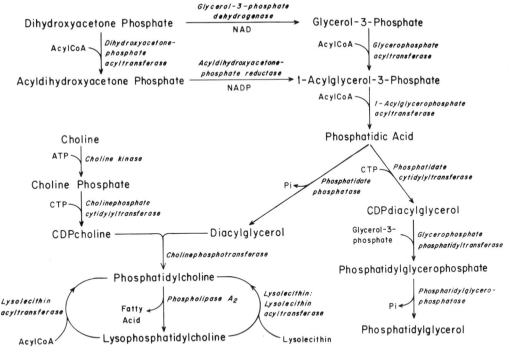

Fig. 1. Pathways of phosphatidylcholine and phosphatidylglycerol biosynthesis. (ROONEY 1979)

ROONEY et al. 1979 a, 1980). Insulin, which antagonizes the dexamethasone-induced stimulation of phosphatidylcholine synthesis in the fetal lung, reduces the stimulatory effect of the hormone on this enzyme (ROONEY et al. 1980). In addition to cholinephosphate cytidylyltransferase, the activities of other enzymes of phosphatidylcholine synthesis in the fetal lung have been reported to increase both developmentally and after hormone treatment (BREHIER and ROONEY 1981; FARRELL and HAMOSH 1978; ROONEY 1979, 1983; VAN GOLDE 1976). Such increases have not been consistently observed, however. The possibility that enzymes other than cholinephosphate cytidylyltransferase play rate-regulatory roles in phosphatidylcholine synthesis cannot be excluded.

2. Disaturated Phosphatidylcholine Biosynthesis

De novo synthesized phosphatidylcholine in the lung, as in other organs, contains predominantly saturated fatty acids on the C-1 position and unsaturated fatty acids on the C-2 position. The lung does not synthesize disaturated phosphatidylcholine de novo (SARZALA and VAN GOLDE 1976; VEREYKEN et al. 1972), but rather by remodeling of unsaturated phosphatidylcholine. This can occur by at least two mechanisms as shown in Fig. 1. Both involve removal of the unsaturated fatty acid on the C-2 position by phospholipase A_2, an enzyme which does occur in the lung (LONGMORE et al. 1979). The resulting lysophosphatidylcholine is then either reacylated with an additional acylCoA in a reaction catalyzed by lysolecithin acyltransferase or, alternatively, two molecules of lysophosphatidylcholine react to form one molecule each of phosphatidylcholine and glycerophosphocholine in a reaction catalyzed by lysolecithin:lysolecithin acyltransferase. Although both of these mechanisms operate in the lung, recent evidence indicates that the first is the more important quantitatively, both in whole lung (VAN HEUSDEN et al. 1980, 1981) and type II cells (BATENBURG et al. 1979; MASON and DOBBS 1980; VOELKER and SNYDER 1979).

3. Other Pathways of Phosphatidylcholine Biosynthesis

Phosphatidylcholine can be synthesized from phosphatidylethanolamine by triple N-methylation and this pathway is of quantitative importance in some organs. Following the reported identification of phosphatidyldimethylethanolamine in lung lavage from dogs (MORGAN et al. 1965a) and rabbits (GLUCK et al. 1967b), there was considerable speculation that the methylation pathway was particularly important in the synthesis of disaturated phosphatidylcholine in the lung (GLUCK and KULOVICH 1973; MORGAN 1969). However, it appears that phosphatidylglycerol was misidentified as phosphatidyldimethylethanolamine (PFLEGER et al. 1972; ROONEY et al. 1974). Subsequent studies showed that the methylation pathway is of little, if any, quantitative importance in the lung (EPSTEIN and FARRELL 1975; ROONEY and MOTOYAMA 1976). AARSMAN and VAN DEN BOSCH (1980) reported de novo synthesis of lysophosphatidylcholine in rat lung microsomes. The reaction involving CDPcholine and monoacylglycerol was analagous to that catalyzed by cholinephosphotransferase (Fig. 1). The contribution of this reaction to overall synthesis of phosphatidylcholine remains to be established.

IV. Synthesis of Phosphatidylglycerol

As shown in Fig. 1, phosphatidylglycerol is also synthesized from phosphatidic acid. Phosphatidylglycerol is usually an intermediate in the synthesis of cardiolipin and does not accumulate to any appreciable extent in most mammalian systems. Liver phosphatidylglycerol synthesis takes place in mitochondria (KIYASU et al. 1963). In lung, however, HALLMAN and GLUCK (1975) reported that surfactant phosphatidylglycerol synthesis takes place in microsomes while cardiolipin synthesis takes place in the mitochondria. Different developmental profiles for the activities of mitochondrial and microsomal glycerophosphate phosphatidyltransferase were also reported, although specific activities were much higher in mitochondria (HALLMAN and GLUCK 1980). In contrast, MAVIS and VANG (1981), using an improved assay, reported that essentially all lung phosphatidylglycerol synthesis takes place in mitochondria. HALLMAN and EPSTEIN (1980) reported that the rate of lung phosphatidylglycerol synthesis is regulated by inositol. Glycerophosphate phosphatidyltransferase activity has been reported to be increased by glucocorticoids in fetal rabbit lung (POSSMAYER et al. 1979; ROONEY et al. 1975a).

D. Control of Surfactant Secretion

As outlined in Sect. C.II, surfactant is believed to be secreted from type II cells by exocytosis. There is evidence that secretion of surfactant is an active process, requiring calcium. Surfactant phospholipid secretion in both isolated type II cells (DOBBS and MASON 1978) and lung slices (MARINO and ROONEY 1980) was inhibited by over 80% at 4 °C. Secretion of surfactant-associated protein from type II cells was inhibited in the cold (KING and MARTIN 1981). Pilocarpine-induced stimulation of the protein secretion was also inhibited by iodoacetate (MASSARO 1975). A role for calcium in surfactant secretion is suggested by the finding that the calcium ionophore A23187 (PRESSMAN 1973) stimulated secretion in type II cells (MASON et al. 1977 b; SHAPIRO et al. 1978) and lung slices from newborn rabbits (MARINO and ROONEY 1980). The stimulation was blocked by ethylenediaminetetraacetate (EDTA) (SHAPIRO et al. 1978).

Intact microtubules and microfilaments are required for surfactant secretion. The microtubule disruptors colchicine and vinblastine (WILSON et al. 1974) have been reported to inhibit secretion of disaturated phosphatidylcholine in hamster lung slices (DELAHUNTY and JOHNSTON 1976) and to inhibit the 12-O-tetradecanoyl-13-phorbol acetate- (DOBBS and MASON 1978) and isoproterenol- (BROWN and LONGMORE 1981 b) stimulated secretion of disaturated phosphatidylcholine in type II cells isolated from rat lung. Colchicine also inhibited surfactant phosphatidylcholine secretion in newborn rabbit lung slices (MARINO and ROONEY 1980) as well as the pilocarpine-induced stimulation of protein into the surfactant fraction of rabbit lung lavage (MASSARO 1975). Cytochalasin-B, a disruptor of microfilaments (DAVIES and ALLISON 1978), inhibited surfactant secretion in newborn rabbit lung slices (MARINO and ROONEY 1980).

Both cholinergic and β-adrenergic mechanisms have been implicated in the control of surfactant secretion. Pilocarpine stimulated surfactant secretion in intact animals and this effect was blocked by atropine (CORBET et al. 1976; GOLDENBERG et al. 1969; MASSARO 1975; OLSEN 1972; ROONEY 1978). The ventilation-induced increase in alveolar phospholipid was blocked by atropine in adult (OYARZUN and CLEMENTS 1977) and newborn (LAWSON et al. 1979) rabbits. The increase in surfactant secretion produced by administration of pilocarpine (CORBET et al. 1977) or oxotremorine (ABDELLATIF and HOLLINGSWORTH 1980) was, however, blocked by propranolol. ABDELLATIF and HOLLINGSWORTH (1980) also reported that the effect of oxotremorine was blocked by adrenalectomy. Although pilocarpine has been reported to stimulate surfactant secretion in isolated lung or lung tissue in some studies (BROWN and LONGMORE 1981 a; HILDEBRAN et al. 1981; PYSHER et al. 1977), cholinergic agents had no such effect in other studies on the isolated perfused lung (ABDELLATIF and HOLLINGSWORTH 1980; MASSARO et al. 1981; NICHOLAS and BARR 1981). ABDELLATIF and HOLLINGSWORTH (1980) and DOBBS and MASON (1979) concluded that cholinomimetic agents stimulate catecholamine release by the adrenal medulla and these, in turn, act directly on the lung to stimulate surfactant secretion. This conclusion is consistent with the findings that cholinomimetic agents had no effect on disaturated phosphatidylcholine secretion in isolated type II cells (BROWN and LONGMORE 1981 a; DOBBS and MASON 1979) and that incubation of newborn rabbit lung slices with pilocarpine or atropine had no effect on phosphatidylcholine secretion (MARINO and ROONEY 1981).

β-Adrenergic agents have been reported to stimulate surfactant secretion in intact animals (ABDELLATIF and HOLLINGSWORTH 1980; CORBET et al. 1977; EN-HORNING et al. 1977; LAWSON et al. 1978; OLSEN 1972; OYARZUN and CLEMENTS 1978; WYSZOGRODSKI et al. 1974), isolated perfused lungs (BROWN and LONG-MORE 1981 a; MASSARO et al. 1981; NICHOLAS and BARR 1981), lung slices from newborn animals (MARINO and ROONEY 1981), and isolated type II cells (BROWN and LONGMORE 1981 a; DOBBS and MASON 1979). β-Mimetic drugs have been reported to lower the incidence of the respiratory distress syndrome in newborn infants (BERGMAN and HEDNER 1978; BOOG et al. 1975; KERO et al. 1973). β-Adrenergic receptors have been demonstrated in type II cells (SHAPIRO and FINKELSTEIN 1981; SOMMERS-SMITH and GIANNOPOULOS 1981) and receptor concentration in fetal lung has been reported to increase toward the end of gestation at the time of increased surfactant production (CHENG et al. 1980; GIANNOPOULOS 1980; WHITSETT et al. 1981).

As in other systems, stimulation of surfactant secretion by β-adrenergic agents appears to be mediated by stimulation of adenylate cyclase and generation of cAMP. BROWN and LONGMORE (1981 a) reported that isoproterenol increased cAMP levels and stimulated disaturated phosphatidylcholine secretion in isolated type II cells. DOBBS and MASON (1979) found that incubation of type II cells with cAMP resulted in increased secretion of disaturated phosphatidylcholine. HALL-MAN (1977) reported that cAMP increased surfactant secretion in neonatal rats. Phosphodiesterase inhibitors increase intracellular cAMP levels by inhibiting its breakdown and one such agent, aminophylline, has been reported to stimulate phosphatidylcholine synthesis in the fetal lung (GROSS et al. 1980; SEVANIAN et al. 1979), although it may also stimulate secretion (BARRETT et al. 1978; CORBET et al. 1978; KAROTKIN et al. 1976). Isoxsuprine has been shown to stimulate phosphatidylcholine synthesis in fetal rabbit lung (KANJANAPONE et al. 1980) and to increase the amount of surfactant in fetal monkey lung lavage at a gestational age when the effect is more likely to be on synthesis than on secretion (ROONEY et al. 1981).

Prostaglandins have also been implicated in surfactant secretion. Labor has been reported to increase the amount of surfactant in newborn rabbit lung lavage (ROONEY et al. 1977 a) and to stimulate surfactant secretion in newborn rabbit lung slices (MARINO and ROONEY 1981). The effect of labor can be mimicked by incubating the slices with prostaglandin E_2 (MARINO and ROONEY 1980) and can be blocked by incubating the slices with indomethacin (MARINO and ROONEY 1981). OYARZUN and CLEMENTS (1978) reported that inhibitors of prostaglandin synthesis prevented the ventilation-induced increase in alveolar phospholipid in adult rabbits. ANDERSON et al. (1978) reported that prostaglandin $F_{2\alpha}$ increased phosphatidylcholine secretion in type II cells.

E. Turnover and Removal of Surfactant

The half-life of surfactant in the alveolar space has been estimated by several investigators. JOBE (1977) injected adult rabbits with palmitic acid ^{14}C and choline

^{3}H and calculated half-lives of 16 and 30 h for lung lavage phosphatidylcholine labeled with ^{14}C and ^{3}H, respectively. The half-life of phosphatidylglycerol was similarly estimated to be 15 h when labeled with palmitic acid or glycerol (HALL-MAN et al. 1981; JOBE et al. 1978). Removal of surfactant has not been as extensively studied as its production. Nevertheless, at least four mechanisms for surfactant removal have been proposed. These include removal by mucociliary transport up the respiratory escalator, phagocytosis by alveolar macrophages, direct catabolism in the alveoli, and reabsorption.

GEIGER et al. (1975) exposed rats to aerosolized dipalmitoylphosphatidylcholine ^{3}H and found that the radioactivity appeared very rapidly in the alveoli. It was also rapidly cleared. Only 12% remained in the alveoli after 12 h. Using autoradiographic techniques, these workers showed radioactivity in alveolar epithelial type I and type II cells as well as alveolar macrophages. Radioactivity was subsequently found in blood and other organs. Tracheal ligation after aerosol deposition did not alter these findings. OYARZUN et al. (1980) carried out similar experiments with dipalmitoylphosphatidylcholine ^{14}C instilled into rabbits in the form of liposomes and reported rapid removal from the alveoli followed by slower removal from lung tissue. Very little labeled phosphatidylcholine was found in the trachea. Although it is possible that surfactant administered as an aerosol or in liposomes may be cleared differently from surfactant generated in vivo, nevertheless these studies have shown that dipalmitoylphosphatidylcholine is rapidly cleared from the alveoli and that removal by mucociliary transport via the trachea is not a major mechanism. FISHER et al. (1979) studied the removal of newly synthesized surfactant in rats. The animals were injected with palmitate ^{3}H and the amount of radioactivity in dipalmitoylphosphatidylcholine in lung and tracheal lavages was measured over 24 h. Although substantial radioactivity appeared in lung lavage, negligible amounts appeared in tracheal lavage. Removal of surfactant via the respiratory escalator does not, therefore, appear to be a major mechanism.

There is considerable evidence that surfactant is removed by alveolar macrophages (HOCKING and GOLDE 1979; NAIMARK 1973). There is a large increase in the number of alveolar macrophages in the newborn rabbit at the time of increased surfactant appearance in the alveoli (ZELIGS et al. 1977). Biochemical (NERURKAR et al. 1977) and morphological (ZELIGS et al. 1977) studies showed that surfactant was taken up by the macrophages. NICHOLS (1976) also reported that alveolar macrophages phagocytosized tubular myelin in adult rabbits. RAO et al. (1981) reported that phospholipases in alveolar macrophages were capable of degrading dipalmitoylphosphatidylcholine. These studies show that phagocytosis of surfactant by alveolar macrophages can occur. However, the quantitative importance of this mechanism of surfactant removal is not clear. GEIGER et al. (1975) reported that type I and type II alveolar epithelial cells removed more dipalmitoylphosphatidylcholine from alveoli than did alveolar macrophages. DESAI et al. (1978) also concluded that cells other than alveolar macrophages may be important in surfactant removal.

Enzymes which hydrolyze phospholipids have been reported in lung lavage. It is therefore possible that surfactant is degraded directly in the alveoli. Lamellar bodies are known to contain a variety of hydrolyases which are probably secreted together with surfactant into the alveolar space (HOOK 1978). Lamellar bodies have been reported to contain phospholipases A_1 and A_2 (HEATH and JACOBSON 1976) as well as phosphatidate phosphatase (MEBAN 1972; SPITZER et al. 1975). Phospholipase A has been reported in lung lavage from patients with alveolar proteinosis (SAHU and LYNN 1977) while phosphatidate phosphatase has been reported to be associated with surfactant in dog (BENSON 1980) and pig (DELA-HUNTY et al. 1979) lung and in amniotic fluid from humans (BLEASDALE et al. 1978; JIMENEZ et al. 1974) and sheep (ROSENFELD et al. 1980). It remains to be established, however, whether these enzymes are involved in surfactant degradation. OYARZUN et al. (1980) reported that when ^{14}C-labeled L- and ^{3}H-labeled D-dipalmitoylphosphatidylcholine liposomes were deposited in rabbit lung alveoli, both isomers were equally well cleared. Such lack of stereospecificity would suggest that enzymatic hydrolysis is not involved in surfactant removal. Furthermore, the ^{14}C:^{3}H ratio in lung tissue saturated phosphatidylcholine was the same as in the original dipalmitoylphosphatidylcholine. These findings would suggest that intact dipalmitoylphosphatidylcholine is absorbed into the lung tissue. The data of GEIGER et al. (1975) are also consistent with this conclusion. HALLMAN et al. (1981) reported that there is a bidirectional flux of surfactant phospholipids between lamellar bodies and alveolar lavage. The mechanism of this reabsorption needs to be investigated.

F. Methods of Measuring Surfactant

I. General Comments

Since it functions at the alveolar surface, the most convenient method of obtaining surfactant for quantitative purposes is by lavaging the lungs with saline via the trachea (ROONEY et al. 1974). Several lavages are required to remove as much material as possible (GLUCK et al. 1967a; MASSARO 1975; ROONEY et al. 1974). Complete removal of surfactant from the alveoli, however, may not be achievable. In addition, lavaging the lungs does not remove intracellular surfactant.

Although lung lavage is a convenient source of surfactant in many studies, surfactant may also be measured in other lung fractions. For assessment of fetal lung maturity in humans, surfactant is measured in amniotic fluid (KULOVICH et al. 1979) and in tracheal or gastric aspirates (MOTOYAMA et al. 1976). Surfactant has been measured in lung minces (CLEMENTS 1957), in material secreted by lung slices (MARINO and ROONEY 1980), in lung explants (PYSHER et al. 1977), and in type II cells in culture (BROWN and LONGMORE 1981a; DOBBS and MASON 1979). Surfactant components have also been measured in lung tissue and subcellular fractions. PACIGA et al. (1980) purified a surfactant fraction from minced lung.

The most direct method of measuring surfactant is to determine surface activity and this can be done in a number of ways as described in Sect. F.II.1. Demonstration of surface activity is the only assurance that the material under study is actually surfactant. Surface avtivity measurements are, however, often tedious and quantitation is sometimes difficult (GOERKE 1974). Chemical methods are less difficult to perform and offer the advantage of easy quantitation. Radiochemical methods are particularly sensitive. When using chemical and radiochemical methods it is important that the material being measured is actually surfactant or at least surfactant related. Ideally, surface activity should be demonstrated. At the very least the material should resemble surfactant in terms of chemical composition or morphological appearance. MARINO and ROONEY (1980), for instance, showed that the material secreted by lung slices from newborn animals was surfactant related because its phospholipid composition was similar to that of lung lavage (Table 1). They then measured the rate of surfactant secretion by measuring the amount of radioactive phosphatidylcholine released. Measurement of radioactive phosphatidylcholine or even disaturated phosphatidylcholine alone would not necessarily be a measure of surfactant since these lipids could be secreted together with lung tissue, rather than surfactant, phospholipids (MARINO and ROONEY 1980).

Measurement of phospholipid synthesis and activities of enzymes of phospholipid synthesis may not reflect surfactant synthesis since the lipids are not exclusive to surfactant. Such measurements can, however, provide useful data on surfactant synthesis if they are correlated with changes in surfactant content determined in a more direct manner.

II. Physical Methods

1. Measurement of Surface Activity

a) The Surface Balance

CLEMENTS (1957) initially demonstrated surface activity of lung extracts on a modified Wilhelmy balance. This method, which is probably the most widely used for measurement of the surface activity of pulmonary surfactant, has been described in detail by GOERKE (1974). The test material is applied to the surface of an aqueous solution in a polytetrafluoroethylene (Teflon) through. The surface area is expanded and compressed and the minimum surface tension is recorded by means of a force transducer. To approximate physiologic conditions, surface activity is measured at 37 °C in a water-saturated atmosphere (GOERKE 1974). Under these conditions, lung surfactant should reduce the minimum surface tension to at least 10 dyn/cm although lower values have also been reported (KOTAS et al. 1977). (The surface tension of a clean water–air interface is 72 dyn/cm.) Dipalmitoylphosphatidylcholine lowers surface tension to approximately zero (HENDERSON and PFLEGER 1972; HILDEBRAN et al. 1979; ROONEY et al. 1974) and phosphatidylglycerol to 0–5 dyn/cm (HENDERSON and PFLEGER 1972; ROONEY et al. 1974). Less surface-active phospholipid lower surface tension to approximately 20–30 dyn/cm (GLUCK et al. 1967a). The amount of material required to reach a particular surface tension can be determined and thus the amount of surfactant in a given preparation quantitated. By suitable calibration, surfactant can be expressed as dipalmitoylphosphatidylcholine equivalents (ABDELLATIF and HOLLINGSWORTH 1980).

b) Surface Activity Measurement In Situ

SCHURCH et al. (1976) measured surface tension in excised rat lungs in situ. Fluorocarbon and silicone droplets have characteristic shapes at certain surface tensions. Droplets were applied to the alveolar surface with a micropipette and viewed with a microscope. With this technique, alveolar surface tension at functional residual capacity was less than 9 dyn/cm.

c) Bubble Stability Measurements

PATTLE (1955) was the first to demonstrate the existence of pulmonary surfactant when he showed that bubbles squeezed from a lung cut under water were unexpectedly stable. Surface tension at the air–water interface can be determined by measuring bubble size as a function of time (PATTLE 1965). The bubble stability ratio – the ratio of bubble diameter at 20 min to that at zero time (PATTLE and BURGESS 1961) – has been used as a measurement of surfactant (MOTOYAMA et al. 1971; WU et al. 1973). ENHORNING (1977) described a pulsating bubble technique which allowed measurement of surface tension at the bubble surface very rapidly and with small amounts of material. Using this technique, METCALFE et al. (1980) reported that canine pulmonary surfactant and lipid extracts thereof lowered surface tension to zero at minimum bubble radius. CLEMENTS et al. (1972) devised a method of measuring the surfactant content of amniotic fluid based on its ability to form stable bubbles in the presence of ethanol. This method compares well with chemical methods of assessing fetal lung maturity (ROSENTHAL et al. 1974). A similar method was developed by PATTLE et al. (1979).

2. Lung Mechanics

Pressure–volume relationships in whole lung have been used to measure surfactant (BACHOFEN et al. 1970; GOERKE 1974). Lung mechanics measurements have been widely used to determine changes in surfactant in the developing neonatal lung (CORBET et al. 1976, 1977, 1978; DELEMOS et al. 1970; KOTAS and AVERY 1971; TAEUSCH et al. 1974).

III. Biochemical Methods

1. Phospholipid Content and Composition

Pulmonary surfactant has a characteristic phospholipid composition which is distinctly different from that of lung tissue (Table 1). Materials rich in surfactant should have a similar phospholipid composition. This has been reported for lung lavage from adult (HALLMAN and GLUCK 1975; ROONEY et al. 1974, 1977b) and newborn (MARINO and ROONEY 1980) rabbits, lamellar bodies (ENGLE et al. 1976; HALLMAN and GLUCK 1974; ROONEY et al. 1975b), the material secreted by lung slices from newborn animals (MARINO and ROONEY 1980), and isolated type II cells (MASON et al. 1977a).

If the material under study has the characteristic surfactant phospholipid composition, the amount of surfactant can be quantitated by measuring total phospholipid, phosphatidylcholine, or disaturated phosphatidylcholine. This is usually done by phosphorus assay (ROONEY et al. 1974, 1976b, 1977b). The data are best expressed per unit tissue or cell protein, DNA, or dry weight.

Changes in phospholipid composition have also been used to detect changes in surfactant content. This is particularly so in the case of amniotic fluid or lung fluids where the volume of liquid is unknown and where lung mass cannot be determined. During development of the fetal lung, there is an increase in the amount of lung lavage phosphatidylcholine expressed as a percentage of total phospholipid and a concomitant decrease in the amount of sphingomyelin (ROONEY et al. 1976 b). There is, therefore, a marked increase in the phosphatidylcholine (lecithin):sphingomyelin (L:S) ratio. The L:S ratio in human amniotic fluid can be used to predict the degree of fetal lung maturity (KULOVICH et al. 1979). Measurement of the percentages of disaturated phosphatidylcholine, phosphatidylglycerol, and phosphatidylinositol leads to greater accuracy in predicting the degree of fetal lung maturity, especially in complicated pregnancies (KULOVICH et al. 1979; KULOVICH and GLUCK 1979). The phospholipid composition of tracheal and gastric liquids may also be used to assess the degree of fetal lung maturity (MOTOYAMA et al. 1976). Changes in the phospholipid composition of lung fluids from adult humans might likewise be used to assess the status of the surfactant system. Expression of phospholipid content per unit protein in lavage fluid may also be useful.

The fatty acid composition of phosphatidylcholine in surfactant-rich material may also be used. SHELLY et al. (1979) evaluated the surfactant content of newborn infants by fatty acid analysis of phosphatidylcholine from the surfactant fraction of tracheal and pharyngeal aspirates. Amniotic fluid fatty acid analysis has also been used in the prediction of fetal lung maturity (WARREN et al. 1974).

2. Phospholipid Synthesis

a) Rate of Precursor Incorporation

Rates of incorporation of a variety of radiolabeled precursors into surfactant components have been measured in intact animals, isolated perfused lungs, minces and slices of whole lung, lung explants in culture, and isolated type II cells. Rates of incorporation of choline, palmitate, acetate, glycerol, glucose, phosphate, and lysophosphatidylcholine into total and disaturated phosphatidylcholine have been measured. However, there are two major problems with studies of this type in terms of measuring the rate of surfactant synthesis. First, unless the rate of incorporation into phosphatidylcholine in a surfactant-like fraction is measured, it cannot be stated that surfactant synthesis is being measured. Second, unless the pool size of all precursors and intermediates is known, the true rate of synthesis is not being measured. The measurement is merely that of rate of incorporation of radioisotope into product. In most studies neither of these provisos are met. Nevertheless, measurement of precursor rate of incorporation can provide useful information on surfactant synthesis when substantiated by measurement of surfactant content. In fetal rabbit lung slices, for instance, the developmental increase in the rate of choline incorporation into phosphatidylcholine (ROONEY et al. 1979 a) correlated well with the increased amount of surfactant in lung lavage (ROONEY et al. 1976 b). In the fetal monkey, the rate of choline incorporation into phosphatidylcholine in lung slices increases concomitantly which increased surfactant as determined in lung extracts on a surface balance and from pressure–volume relationships (KOTAS et al. 1977).

b) Enzyme Activities

When surfactant production has been shown to be altered by the methods described, it is of interest to determine if activities of enzymes of phospholipid synthesis are also changed. Activities of enzymes which catalyze rate-limiting steps would be expected to be altered when rates of synthesis are altered. Most of the enzymes of phospholipid synthesis have been assayed in lung and optimal conditions have been developed (Hallman and Gluck 1975, 1980; Khosla et al. 1980; Oldenborg and van Golde 1976, 1977; Possmayer et al. 1979, 1981; Rooney et al. 1976b, 1979a). Enzyme activities have usually been measured in whole lung homogenates or subcellular fractions. Thus, activities of enzymes involved in surfactant and membrane phospholipid synthesis are not distinguished. Nevertheless, changes in surfactant production in fetal lung have been correlated with changes in the activities of enzymes of lung phospholipid biosynthesis, although there are extensive discrepancies between different studies (Brehier and Rooney 1981; Rooney 1979, 1983; van Golde 1976). Some enzymes of phospholipid synthesis have been assayed in isolated type II cells (Batenburg et al. 1979), but altered surfactant synthesis has not yet been correlated with alterations in enzyme activities in such cells.

3. Surfactant Secretion

Secretion of surfactant has been measured in a number of models, including the intact lung in vivo, the isolated perfused lung in vitro, lung slices and explants, and isolated type II cells. The physiologic control of surfactant secretion is probably best studied in the intact animal in vivo. However, measurements of surfactant in lung lavage or tracheal fluid (Mescher et al. 1975) cannot readily distinguish between effects on synthesis and effects on secretion. Similarly, in whole animals, it is impossible to distinguish between a direct effect on the lung and those mediated via other organs. The isolated type II cell would appear to be the ideal model in which to study surfactant secretion. However, there are potential disadvantages with isolated cells too. Cells can loose receptors during the trypsin treatment used in their isolation (Dobbs and Mason 1979). To overcome this, Dobbs et al. (1980) isolated type II cells with elastase rather than trypsin. In addition, receptors may also be regenerated in culture. The cell cytoskeleton in culture may differ from that in vivo and this may alter its response to secretagogues. Intercellular contact is different in culture. Certain effects on surfactant production may be mediated via other lung cells and thus cannot be demonstrated in pure type II cells. Smith (1978), for instance, reported that a factor from lung fibroblasts – fibroblast pneumocyte factor – is required for type II cell responsiveness to cortisol. The isolated perfused lung, lung slices, and lung explants overcome a number of the disadvantages of whole animals and isolated type II cells although they have other disadvantages. Use of a combination of models of varying degrees of complexity offers advantages over reliance on any single model although for specific questions particular models may offer advantages.

In many studies, secretion of surfactant components, usually disaturated phosphatidylcholine, has been measured (Brown and Longmore 1981a; Delahunty and Johnston 1976, 1979; Dobbs and Mason 1979). Secretion of surfactant phospholipids has been measured by lavaging intact lungs (ABDELLATIF and HOLLINGSWORTH 1980; GILFILLAN et al. 1980; ROONEY et al. 1977a). If lung lavage is to be used to detect changes in surfactant secretion, unaltered synthesis should be demonstrated independently. Secretion of surfactant can be conveniently measured in lung slices from newborn animals (MARINO and ROONEY 1980, 1981). KELLER and LADDA (1979), on the other hand, reported that surfactant secretion did not occur in slices of adult rat lung. In that study however, it is likely that secreted surfactant was lost on centrifugation at 16,000 g. Secretion of disaturated phosphatidylcholine did occur in lung slices from adult hamsters (DELAHUNTY and JOHNSTON 1976).

IV. Other Methods

Although the role of protein in surfactant is unclear, surfactant-associated proteins have been measured by immunochemical means. KING et al. (1974) developed a radioimmunoassay for measurement of surfactant apoprotein. Antibodies against surfactant protein were also described by other workers (KATYAL and SINGH 1979; SUEISHI et al. 1977). WILLIAMS and BENSON (1981) recently reported an immunocytochemical method for localization of surfactant proteins.

G. The Fetal Lung as an Example of Altered Surfactant Production

Many of the methods of surfactant measurement described in Sect. F have been used in studying the effects of hormones on surfactant production in the fetal lung. These studies are described briefly here since they provide a convenient example of approaches which might be used in studying alterations in surfactant in other systems. A more detailed discussion of hormone-accelerated fetal lung development can be found in other reviews (FARRELL and HAMOSH 1978; GROSS 1979; ROONEY 1983; SMITH and BOGUES 1980).

LIGGINS (1969) first reported that administration of glucocorticoid to fetal lambs resulted in partial lung aeration on premature delivery and suggested that this might be due to accelerated appearance of surfactant. This was soon shown to be the case by DELEMOS et al. (1970) in the fetal lamb and by KOTAS and AVERY (1971) in the fetal rabbit. Increased surfactant was demonstrated by the pressure–volume technique as well as by surface balance measurements on lung extracts. In addition to the pressure–volume and surface balance methods, MOTOYAMA et al. (1971) showed imreased surfactant in lung lavage from cortisol-treated fetal rabbits by use of the bubble stability ratio. Thyroxine was shown to have a similar effect by the same technique (WU et al. 1973). CORBET et al. (1976, 1977, 1978), using the pressure–volume method, reported that glucocorticoids, aminophylline, cholinergic agents, and β-adrenergic agents increased surfactant production in the fetal rabbit.

Glucocorticoids (ROONEY et al. 1976a, 1979a), estrogen (KHOSLA and ROONEY 1979), and thyrotropin-releasing hormone (ROONEY et al. 1979b) increased the amount of surfactant in fetal rabbit lung lavage as shown by increased amounts of total phospholipid and phosphatidylcholine per unit lung dry weight, an increase in phosphatidylcholine as percentage of total phospholipid, a decrease in the percentage of sphingomyelin, and an increase in the L : S ratio.

Glucocorticoids increased the rate of choline incorporation into phosphatidylcholine in lung slices from the fetal rabbit (BREHIER et al. 1977; FARRELL and ZACHMAN 1973; POSSMAYER et al. 1979; ROONEY et al. 1979 a), rat (FARRELL et al. 1977), and mouse (BREHIER and ROONEY 1981). Estrogen had a similar effect in the fetal rabbit (KHOSLA et al. 1980; POSSMAYER et al. 1981). Estrogen (GROSS et al. 1979) as well as dexamethasone and thyroxine (GROSS et al. 1980) increased the rate of choline incorporation into total and disaturated phosphatidylcholine in fetal rat lung explants. Glucocorticoids and thyroxine increased the rate of choline incorporation into phosphatidylcholine in mixed fetal rabbit lung cells in monolayer culture (SMITH and TORDAY 1974). Glucocorticoids increased the rate of precursor incorporation into phosphatidylcholine and phosphatidylglycerol in purified cultures of fetal (SANDERS et al. 1981) and adult (POST et al. 1980 b) rat type II cells.

Glucocorticoids increased the activity of fetal lung cholinephosphate cytidylyltransferase in the rabbit in vivo (ROONEY et al. 1976 a, 1979 a) and in vitro (MENDELSON et al. 1980; KHOSLA et al. 1983), in the rat in vitro (GROSS et al. 1980), and in the mouse in vivo (BREHIER and ROONEY 1981). Estrogen had a similar effect in the fetal rabbit in vivo (KHOSLA et al. 1980; POSSMAYER et al. 1981) and in vitro (KHOSLA et al. 1983). In some studies, however, the stimulatory effect of glucocorticoids on cholinephosphate cytidylyltransferase was not observed (FARRELL 1973; OLDENBORG and VAN GOLDE 1977; TSAO et al. 1979). Other enzymes of phospholipid synthesis were also reported to be stimulated by glucocorticoids in some studies and not in others (ROONEY 1979, 1983; VAN GOLDE 1976). Clearly, the detailed mechanism by which hormones stimulate surfactant production yet remains to be elucidated. Further studies in pure type II cell cultures will hopefully accomplish this.

In addition to stimulating surfactant production in the fetus, hormones such as glucocorticoids, estrogen, and thyroxine also accelerate fetal lung maturation as determined by morphological criteria (KHOSLA et al. 1981; MOTOYAMA et al. 1971; WU et al. 1973) and by decreased lung glycogen content (GROSS et al. 1979, 1980; KHOSLA et al. 1981, 1983; ROONEY et al. 1979 a). Although these parameters may be related to surfactant production in the fetus, they are probably of little use in determining changes in surfactant in adults.

H. Altered Surfactant Due to Toxicants in the Airways

The effects of a variety of toxic agents on the surfactant system have been examined (Table 2). Although only agents delivered to the lungs via the airways are included in Table 2, agents delivered to the lungs via the vasculature also influence surfactant (DASTON 1981; MALMQUIST 1980; MANKTELOW 1981; RYAN et al. 1981). Alcohol consumption may result in altered surfactant (HEINEMANN 1977) and radiation has been reported to produce a similar effect (BELLET-BARTHAS et al. 1980; GROSS 1978; RUBIN et al. 1980). In addition, various pathologic conditions such as, for instance, adult respiratory distress syndrome (PETTY et al.

Table 2. Toxic agents which have been reported to alter surfactant

Toxic agent	Species	Parameter measured	Effect	Reference
Cigarette smoke	Human	Lung lavage, surface balance measurements	Decreased surfactant	Cook and Webb (1966)
	Human	Lung lavage, surfactant phospholipid content	Decreased	Finley and Ladman (1972)
	Human	Lung lavage, phospholipid content and composition	Decreased phospholipid: albumin ratio	Low et al. (1978)
	Human	Lung lavage, phosphatidylcholine content	No change	Pre et al. (1980)
	Rat	Lung lavage, surface balance measurements	Decreased surface tension, increased surface compressibility	Miller and Bondurant (1962)
	Rat	Lung lavage, surfactant by weight	Decreased	Le Mesurier et al. (1980)
	Rat	Lung tissue, glucose incorporation into lipid	Increased	Hamosh et al. (1979)
	Dog	Lung extracts, surface balance measurements; lung lavage, palmitate incorporation into lipids	No change	Giammona et al. (1971)
Smoke (wood and kerosine)	Dog	Lung tissue mince, surface balance measurements	Decreased surfactant	Nieman et al. (1980)
HCl	Rat	Lung lavage, surface balance measurements, phospholipid content	Decreased surfactant and phosphatidylcholine	Krishnan and Rao (1981)
	Rat	Lung lavage and tissue, palmitate incorporation into phospholipids	Decreased	Krishnan et al. (1979)
	Goat	Pressure–volume curves	Decreased surfactant	Stothert et al. (1981)
H_2SO_4	Rat	Lung homogenates, surface balance measurements, bubble stability ratio, phospholipid content	Little change	Krishnan et al. (1974)
Gasoline, trichloroethylene, carbon tetrachloride	Rat	Lung lavage, surfactant by weight	Decreased	Le Mesurier et al. (1980)

Table 2 (continued)

Toxic agent	Species	Parameter measured	Effect	Reference
Welding fume particles	Rat	Lung lavage, surfactant by weight	Increased	White et al. (1981)
Quartz	Rat and hamster	Lung lavage, surface tension measurements, pressure–volume curves	Decreased surfactant	Gabor et al. (1971)
	Rat	Lung lavage, surface tension measurements, phospholipid content	Increased surfactant	Gabor et al. (1978)
Asbestos	Rat	Lung lavage, surfactant by weight	Increased	Tetley et al. (1977)
	Rat	Lung tissue, cholinephosphotransferase activity	Increased	Tetley et al. (1977)
	Rabbit	Lung lavage, phosphatidylcholine fatty acid composition	Increased unsaturated fatty acids	Oblin et al. (1978)
Anesthetics	Human	Lung extracts, surface balance measurements	No effect	Miller and Thomas (1967)
	Human	Tracheal aspirates, phosphatidylcholine fatty acid composition	No effect	Namba et al. (1981)
	Mouse	Bubble stability after in vitro exposure	No effect when clinical concentrations were used	Pattle et al. (1972)
	Rabbit	Lung extracts, surface balance measurements, pressure–volume curves	Enflurane – no effect: methoxyflurane – decreased surfactant	Landauer et al. (1975, 1976)
	Dog	Pressure–volume curves	Decreased surfactant	Woo et al. (1971)
NO$_2$	Rat	Lung lavage, surface balance and phospholipid measurements	Increased surfactant	Williams et al. (1971)
	Rat	Lung lavage, surface balance measurements, pressure–volume curves	Decreased surfactant	Arner and Rhoades (1973)
	Rat	Lung tissue, phospholipid content and composition, rate of palmitate incorporation into phospholipids	Increased disaturated phosphatidylcholine and phosphatidylglycerol, increased palmitate incorporation	Blank et al. (1978)

	Animal	Method	Result	Reference
	Rat	Lung tissue, phospholipid fatty acid composition	Minor changes	Kobayashi et al. (1980)
	Rat	Activities of enzymes of phospholipid synthesis	Increased	Wright and Mavis (1981)
	Hamster	Isolated type II cells, rate of precursor incorporation into phosphatidylcholine	Increased	Pfleger and Rebar (1979)
CO_2	Guinea pig	Lung minces, surface balance measurements	Decreased surfactant	Schaefer et al. (1964)
O_3	Rat	Lung lavage, phosphatidylcholine fatty acid composition	Decreased palmitic and increased arachidonic acids	Shimasaki et al. (1976)
	Rabbit	Lung lavage and tissue, rate of fatty acid incorporation into phosphatidylcholine	Increased in lavage, decreased in tissue	Kyei-Aboagye et al. (1973)
O_2	Rat	Lung transudate, phosphatidylcholine content, pressure–volume curves	Decreased surfactant	Beckman and Weiss (1969)
	Rat	Lung lavage, rate of phosphate incorporation into phospholipids	Decreased	Valimaki et al. (1975)
	Cat, rabbit	Lung minces, surface balance measurements	Decreased surfactant	Giammona et al. (1965)
	Rabbit	Lung slices, precursor rate of incorporation into phosphatidylcholine	Decreased	Gilder and McSherry (1976)
	Rabbit	Activities of cholinephosphotransferase and lysolecithin acyltransferase	Both decreased	Gilder and McSherry (1976)
	Dog	Lung lavage, surface balance measurements, phospholipid content and composition	Increased surface tension, increased phospholipid, decreased palmitic acid content of phosphatidylcholine, phospholipid composition unchanged	Morgan et al. (1965 b)

1977, 1979), infection (SHIMIZU and MAHOUR 1976; STINSON et al. 1976; VON
WICHERT and WILKE 1976), hemorrhagic pancreatitis (MACIVER et al. 1977), and
shock (BALIBREA et al. 1979; HENRY 1968; VON WICHERT and KOHL 1977) can result in altered surfactant. PATTLE and BURGESS (1961), however, measured the
bubble stability ratio of lung extracts in a variety of pathologic conditions, including inhalation and intratracheal administration of a number of toxicants, and
concluded that, although there were some abnormalities, the degree of surfactant
deficiency in the newborn respiratory distress syndrome was never observed.

In most studies included in Table 2, altered surfactant was demonstrated by
measurement of the parameters discussed in Sect. F. There are also many studies
in which only changes in whole lung phospholipids were demonstrated. Since
such changes are not necessarily reflective of altered surfactant, these studies are
not included. Altered lung phospholipids in toxic and diseased states has been reviewed by AKINO and OHNO (1981).

There is a considerable degree of inconsistency in the data in Table 2. Several
toxic agents increased the amount of surfactant while others decreased it. The
same agent in different studies had opposite effects. Many such differences are
probably due to the level of toxicant used, frequency and duration of exposure,
and possibly the method of surfactant measurement.

The mechanism by which alterations in surfactant occur are generally not
understood. Some agents may have a direct effect on surfactant in the alveoli.
MILLER and BONDURANT (1962) reported that the surface tension of lung extracts
was increased when measured in the presence of cigarette smoke. High concentrations of anesthetics have been reported to decrease the surface activity of lung
extracts in vitro (PATTLE et al. 1972). Dipalmitoylphosphatidylcholine is adsorbed
by kaolin dust (WALLACE et al. 1975). The relevence of such in vitro studies to
in vivo exposure is not clear, however. Although exposure to cigarette smoke has
been reported to decrease surfactant in many studies, exposure to clinical concentrations of anesthetics generally had little effect on surfactant while exposure to
dusts tended to increase the amount of surfactant. Increased phagocytosis by alveolar macrophages in response to the presence of toxic materials may lead to increased surfactant removal. PLOWMAN and FLEMANS (1980), for instance, reported increased amounts of surfactant in macrophages from smokers.

Although the effects of toxic agents on surfactant could be due to direct effects
on surfactant synthesis, secretion, or removal, it is also possible that many such
effects are secondary to cellular damage. Decreased surfactant on exposure to
CO_2 (SCHAEFER et al. 1964) may very well be secondary to acidemia. Damage to
type I epithelial cells by toxic concentration of NO_2, O_2, and O_3 leads to proliferation of type II cells (ADAMSON et al. 1970; EVANS et al. 1975; HOOK and DIAU-
GUSTINE 1976; WITSCHI 1976). Such proliferation could lead to increased surfactant and, indeed, increased amounts of surfactant have been observed on exposure to NO_2 and O_3 in some studies. Hyperoxia, however, led to decreased surfactant (Table 2) as well as decreased synthesis of lung phosphatidylcholine (GIL-
DER and MCSHERRY 1976).

Clearly, the mechanisms of altered surfactant on exposure to toxic agents need
to be elucidated. Changes in the amount of surfactant, whether determined by
surface activity or phospholipid measurements, may not be apparent until consid-

erable cellular damage has occurred. However, subtle changes in rates of synthesis or secretion of surfactant may be detectable earlier and may serve as early indicators of lung damage. Exposure of isolated type II cells to toxic agents in vitro may be useful in elucidating mechanisms of surfactant alteration. However, exposure of a cell in vitro is clearly not the same as in vivo exposure and caution should be exercised in the application of in vitro findings to the in vivo situation.

Acknowledgment. Work in the author's laboratory was supported by grant HD-10192 from the National Institute of Child Health and Human Development, United States Public Health Service.

References

Aarsman AJ, H Bosch van den (1980) Does de novo synthesis of lysophosphatidylcholine occur in rat lung microsomes? Biochim Biophys Acta 620:410–417

Abdellatif MM, Hollingsworth M (1980) Effect of oxotremorine and epinephrine on lung surfactant secretion in neonatal rabbits. Pediatr Res 14:916–920

Adamson IWR, Bowden DH (1973) The intracellular site of surfactant synthesis. Autoradiographic studies on murine and avian lung explants. Exp Mol Pathol 18:112–124

Adamson IWR, Bowden DH, Wyatt JP (1970) Oxygen poisoning in mice. Ultrastructural and surfactant studies during exposure and recovery. Arch Pathol 90:463–472

Akino T, Ohno K (1981) Phospholipids of the lung in normal, toxic and diseased states. Crit Rev Toxicol 9:201–274

Anderson GG, Cidlowski JA, Absher PM, Hewitt AR, Douglas WHJ (1978) The effect of dexamethasone and prostaglandin, $F_{2\alpha}$ on production and release of surfactant in type II alveolar cells. Prostaglandins 16:923–929

Anonymous (1981) Effect of antenatal dexamethasone administration on the prevention of respiratory distress syndrome. Am J Obstet Gynecol 141:276–286

Arner EC, Rhoades RA (1973) Long-term nitrogen dioxide exposure. Effects on lung lipids and mechanical properties. Arch Environ Health 26:156–160

Askin FB, Kuhn C (1971) The cellular origin of pulmonary surfactant. Lab Invest 25:260–268

Avery ME, Mead J (1959) Surface properties in relation to atelectasis and hyaline membrane disease. Am J Dis Child 97:517–523

Bachofen H, Hildebrandt J, Bachofen M (1970) Pressure-volume curves of air- and liquid-filled excised lungs – surface tension in situ. J Appl Physiol 29:422–431

Balibrea JL, Garcia-Barreno B, Garcia-Barreno P, Municio AM (1979) Pulmonary lung and surfactant lipid biosynthesis in dogs under septic and hypovolemic shock syndromes. Int J Biochem 10:91–96

Baranska J, Golde LMG van (1977) Role of lamellar bodies in the biosynthesis of phosphatidylcholine in mouse lung. Biochim Biophys Acta 488:285–293

Barrett CT, Sevanian A, Phelps DL, Gilden C, Kaplan SA (1978) Effects of cortisol and aminophylline upon survival, pulmonary mechanics, and secreted phosphatidylcholine of prematurely delivered rabbits. Pediatr Res 12:38–42

Batenburg JJ, Golde LMG van (1979) Formation of pulmonary surfactant in whole lung and in isolated type II alveolar cells. Rev Perinat Med 3:73–114

Batenburg JJ, Longmore WJ, Golde LMG van (1978) The synthesis of phosphatidylcholine by adult rat lung alveolar type II epithelial cells in primary culture. Biochim Biophys Acta 529:160–170

Batenburg JJ, Longmore WJ, Klazinga W, Golde LMG van (1979) Lysolecithin acyltransferase and lysolecithin: lysolecithin acyltransferase in adult rat lung alveolar type II epithelial cells. Biochim Biophys Acta 573:136–144

Beckman DL, Weiss HS (1969) Hyperoxia compared to surfactant washout on pulmonary compliance in rats. J Appl Physiol 26:700–709

Bellet-Barthas M, Barthelemy L, Bellet M (1980) Effects of [60]CO radiation on the rabbit lung surfactant system. Int J Radiat Oncol Biol Phys 6:1169–1177

Benson BJ (1980) Properties of an acid phosphatase in pulmonary surfactant. Proc Natl Acad Sci USA 77:808–811

Bergman B, Hedner T (1978) Antepartum administration of terbutaline and the incidence of hyaline membrane disease in preterm infants. Acta Obstet Gynecol Scand 57:217–221

Blank ML, Dalbey W, Nettesheim P, Price J, Creasia D, Snyder F (1978) Sequential changes in phospholipid composition and synthesis in lungs exposed to nitrogen dioxide. Am Rev Respir Dis 117:273–280

Bleasdale JE, Davis CS, Agranoff BW (1978) Measurement of phosphatidate phosphohydrolase in human amniotic fluid. Biochim Biophys Acta 528:331–343

Boog G, Ben-Brahim M, Gandar R (1975) Beta-mimetic drugs and possible prevention of respiratory distress syndrome. Br J Obstet Gynaecol 82:285–288

Brehier A, Rooney SA (1981) Phosphatidylcholine synthesis and glycogen depletion in fetal mouse lung: Developmental changes and the effects of dexamethasone. Exp Lung Res 2:273–287

Brehier A, Benson BJ, Williams MC, Mason RJ, Ballard PL (1977) Corticosteroid induction of phosphatidic acid phosphatase in fetal rabbit lung. Biochem Biophys Res Commun 77:883–890

Brown LAS, Longmore WJ (1981a) Adrenergic and cholinergic regulation of lung surfactant secretion in the isolated perfused rat lung and in the alveolar type II cell in culture. J Biol Chem 256:66–72

Brown LS, Longmore WJ (1981b) Effects of antimicrotubular and antimicrofilament agents in alveolar type II cells. Fed Proc 40:407

Buckingham S, Heinemann HO, Sommers SC, McNary WF (1966) Phospholipid synthesis in the large pulmonary alveolar cell. Its relation to lung surfactants. Am J Pathol 48:1027–1038

Casola PG, Possmayer F (1981) Separation and characterization of the membrane-bound and aqueously dispersed phosphatidate phosphatidic acid phosphohydrolase activities in rat lung. Biochim Biophys Acta 664:298–315

Cheng JB, Goldfien A, Ballard PL, Roberts JM (1980) Glucocorticoids increase pulmonary β-adrenergic receptors in the fetal rabbit. Endocrinology 107:1646–1648

Clements JA (1957) Surface tension of lung extracts. Proc Soc Exp Biol Med 95:170–172

Clements JA, Platzker ACG, Tierney DF, Hobel CJ, Creasy RK, Margolis AJ, Thibeault DW, Tooley WH, Oh W (1972) Assessment of the risk of the respiratory distress syndrome by a rapid test for surfactant in amniotic fluid. N Engl J Med 286:1077–1081

Comroe JH Jr (1977a) Premature science and immature lungs. Part I. Some premature discoveries. Am Rev Respir Dis 116:127–135

Comroe JH Jr (1977b) Premature science and immature lungs. Part II. Chemical warfare and the newly born. Am Rev Respir Dis 116:311–323

Comroe JH Jr (1977c) Premature science and immature lungs. Part III. The attack on immature lungs. Am Rev Respir Dis 116:497–518

Cook WA, Webb WR (1966) Surfactant in chronic smokers. Ann Thorac Surg 2:327–333

Corbet AJS, Flax P, Rudolph AJ (1976) Reduced surface tension in lungs of fetal rabbits injected with pilocarpine. J Appl Physiol 41:7–14

Corbet AJS, Flax P, Rudolph AJ (1977) Role of autonomic nervous system controlling surface tension in fetal rabbit lungs. J Appl Physiol 43:1039–1045

Corbet AJ, Flax P, Alston C, Rudolph AJ (1978) Effect of aminophylline and dexamethasone on secretion of pulmonary surfactant in fetal rabbits. Pediatr Res 12:797–799

Daston GP (1981) Toxicity of minimal amounts of cadmium to the developing rat lung and pulmonary surfactant. Toxicol Lett 9:125–130

Davies P, Allison AC (1978) Effects of cytochalasin B on endocytosis and exocytosis. In: Tannenbaum SW (ed) Cytochalasins – biochemical and cell biological aspects. Elsevier/North-Holland, New York, pp 143–160

Delahunty TJ, Johnston JM (1976) The effect of colchicine and vinblastine on the release of pulmonary surface active material. J Lipid Res 17:112–116

Delahunty TJ, Johnston JM (1979) Neurohumoral control of pulmonary surfactant secretion. Lung 157:45–51

Delahunty TJ, Spitzer HL, Jimenez JM, Johnston JM (1979) Phosphatidate phosphohydrolase activity in porcine pulmonary surfactant. Am Rev Respir Dis 119:75–80

deLemos RA, Shermeta DW, Knelson JH, Kotas R, Avery ME (1970) Acceleration of appearance of pulmonary surfactant in the fetal lamb by administration of corticosteroids. Am Rev Respir Dis 102:459–461

Desai R, Tetley TD, Curtis GC, Powell GM, Richards RJ (1978) Studies on the fate of pulmonary surfactant on the lung. Biochem J 176:455–462

DiAugustine RP (1974) Lung concentric laminar organelle. Hydrolase activity and compositional analysis. J Biol Chem 249:584–593

Dobbs LG, Mason RJ (1978) Stimulation of secretion of disaturated phosphatidylcholine from isolated alveolar type II cells by 12-O-tetradecanoyl-13-phorbol acetate. Am Rev Respir Dis 118:705–713

Dobbs LG, Mason RJ (1979) Pulmonary alveolar type II cells isolated from rats. Release of phosphatidylcholine in response to β-adrenergic stimulation. J Clin Invest 63:378–387

Dobbs LG, Geppert EF, Williams MC, Greenleaf RD, Mason RJ (1980) Metabolic properties and ultrastructure of alveolar type II cells isolated with elastase. Biochim Biophys Acta 618:510–523

Engle MJ, Sanders RL, Longmore WJ (1976) Phospholipid composition and acyltransferase activity of lamellar bodies isolated from rat lung. Arch Biochem Biophys 173:586–595

Engle MJ, Golde LMG van, Wirtz KWA (1978) Transfer of phospholipids between subcellular fractions of the lung. FEBS Lett 86:277–281

Engle MJ, Sanders RL, Douglas WHJ (1980) Type II alveolar cells in organotypic culture. A model system for the study of surfactant synthesis. Biochim Biophys Acta 617:225–236

Enhorning G (1977) Pulsating bubble technique for evaluating pulmonary surfactant. J Appl Physiol 43:198–203

Enhorning G, Chamberlain D, Contreras C, Burgoyne R, Robertson B (1977) Isoxsuprine-induced release of pulmonary surfactant in the rabbit fetus. Am J Obstet Gynecol 129:197–202

Epstein MF, Farrell PM (1975) The choline incorporation pathway: primary mechanism for de novo lecithin synthesis in fetal primate lung. Pediatr Res 9:658–665

Evans MJ, Cabral LJ, Stevens RJ, Freeman G (1975) Transformation of alveolar type 2 cells to type 1 cells following exposure to NO_2. Exp Mol Pathol 22:142–150

Farrell PM (1973) Regulation of pulmonary lecithin synthesis. In: Villee CA, Villee DB, Zuckerman J (eds) Respiratory distress syndrome. Academic, New York, pp 311–341

Farrell PM, Hamosh M (1978) The biochemistry of fetal lung development. Clin Perinatol 5:197–229

Farrell PM, Zachman RD (1973) Induction of choline phosphotransferase and lecithin synthesis in the fetal lung by corticosteroids. Science 179:297–298

Farrell PM, Blackburn WR, Adams AJ (1977) Lung phosphatidylcholine synthesis and cholinephosphotransferase activity in anencephalic rat fetuses with corticosteroid deficiency. Pediatr Res 11:770–773

Finley TN, Ladman AJ (1972) Low yield of pulmonary surfactant in cigarette smokers. N Engl J Med 286:223–227

Fisher RK, Hyman MH, Ashcraft SJ (1979) Alveolar surfactant phospholipids are not cleared via trachea. Fed Proc 38:1373

Fujiwara T, Chida S, Whatabe Y, Maeta H, Morita T, Abe T (1980) Artificial surfactant therapy in hyaline membrane disease. Lancet I:55–59

Gabor S, Frits T, Bohm B, Anca Z, Coldea V, Zugravu E (1971) Les forces de surface alveolaire et la composition du surfactif pulmonaire dans la silicose experimentale. Int Arch Arbeitsmed 28:312–320

Gabor S, Zugravu E, Kovats A, Bohm B, Andrasoni D (1978) Effects of kuartz on lung surfactant. Environ Res 16:443–448

Garcia A, Sener SF, Mavis RD (1976) Lung lamellar bodies lack certain key enzymes of phospholipid metabolism. Lipids 11:109–112

Geiger K, Gallagher ML, Hedley-Whyte J (1975) Cellular distribution and clearance of aerosolized dipalmitoyl lecithin. J Appl Physiol 39:759–766

Giammona ST, Kerner D, Bondurant S (1965) Effect of oxygen breathing and atmospheric pressure on pulmonary surfactant. J Appl Physiol 20:855–858

Giammona ST, Tocci P, Webb WR (1971) Effects of cigarette smoke on incorporation of radioisotopically labelled palmitic acid into pulmonary surfactant and on surface activity of canine lung extracts. Am Rev Respir Dis 104:358–367

Giannopoulos G (1980) Identification and ontogeny of β-adrenergic receptors in fetal rabbit lung. Biochem Biophys Res Commun 95:388–394

Gil J, Reiss OK (1973) Isolation and characterization of lamellar bodies and tubular myelin from rat lung homogenates. J Cell Biol 58:152–171

Gilder H, McSherry CK (1976) Phosphatidylcholine synthesis and pulmonary oxygen toxicity. Biochim Biophys Acta 441:48–56

Gilfillan AM, Harkes A, Hollingsworth M (1980) Secretion of lung surfactant following delivery after uterine section. J Develop Physiol 2:101–110

Gluck L, Kulovich MV (1973) Fetal lung development. Current concepts. Pediatr Clin North Am 20:367–379

Gluck L, Motoyama EK, Smiths HL, Kulovich MV (1967a) The biochemical development of surface activity in mammalian lung. I. The surface-active phospholipids; the separation and distribution of surface-active lecithin in the lung of the developing rabbit fetus. Pediatr Res 1:237–246

Gluck L, Sribney M, Kulovich MV (1967b) The biochemical development of surface activity in mammalian lung. II. The biosynthesis of phospholipids in the lung of the developing rabbit fetus and newborn. Pediatr Res 1:247–265

Goerke J (1974) Lung surfactant. Biochim Biophys Acta 344:241–261

Goldenberg VE, Buckingham S, Sommers SC (1969) Pilocarpine stimulation of granular pneumocyte secretion. Lab Invest 20:147–158

Gross I (1979) The hormonal regulation of fetal lung maturation. Clin Perinatol 6:377–395

Gross I, Wilson CM, Ingleson LD, Brehier A, Rooney SA (1979) The influence of hormones on the biochemical development of fetal rat lung in organ culture. I. Estrogen. Biochim Biophys Acta 575:375–383

Gross I, Wilson CM, Ingleson LD, Brehier A, Rooney SA (1980) Fetal lung in organ culture. III. Comparison of dexamethasone, thyroxine, and methylxanthines. J Appl Physiol 48:872–877

Gross NJ (1978) Early physiologic and biochemical effects of thoracic X-irradiation on the pulmonary surfactant system. J Lab Clin Med 91:537–544

Hadjigeorgiou E, Kitsiou S, Psaroudakis A, Segos C, Nicolopoulos D, Kaskarelis D (1979) Antepartum aminophylline treatment for prevention of the respiratory distress syndrome in premature infants. Am J Obstet Gynecol 135:257–260

Hallman M (1977) Induction of surfactant phosphatidylglycerol in the lung of fetal and newborn rabbit by dibutyryl adenosine 3':5'-monophosphate. Biochem Biophys Res Commun 77:1094–1102

Hallman M, Epstein BL (1980) Role of myo-inositol in the synthesis of phosphatidylglycerol and phosphatidylinositol in the lung. Biochem Biophys Res Commun 92:1151–1159

Hallman M, Gluck L (1975) Phosphatidylglycerol in lung surfactant. II. Subcellular distribution and mechanism of biosynthesis in vitro. Biochim Biophys Acta 409:172–191

Hallman M, Gluck L (1977) Development of the fetal lung. J Perinat Med 5:3–31

Hallman M, Gluck L (1980) Formation of acidic phospholipids in rabbit lung during perinatal development. Pediatr Res 14:1250–1259

Hallman M, Epstein BL, Gluck L (1981) Analysis of labeling and clearance of lung surfactant phospholipids in rabbit. Evidence of bidirectional surfactant flux between lamellar bodies and alveolar lavage. J Clin Invest 68:742–751

Hamosh M, Shechter Y, Hamosh P (1979) Effect of tobacco smoke on the metabolism of rat lung. Arch Environ Health 34:17–23

Harwood JL, Desai R, Hext P, Tetley T, Richards R (1975) Characterization of pulmonary surfactant from ox, rabbit, rat and sheep. Biochem J 151:707–714

Heath MF, Jacobson W (1976) Phospholipases A_1 and A_2 in lamellar inclusion bodies of alveolar epithelium of rabbit lung. Biochim Biophys Acta 441:443–452

Heinemann HO (1977) Alcohol and the lung. A brief review. Am J Med 63:81–85

Henderson RF, Pfleger RC (1972) Surface tension studies of phosphatidyl glycerol isolated from the lungs of beagle dogs. Lipids 7:492–494

Henry JN (1968) The effect of shock on pulmonary alveolar surfactant. Its role in refractory respiratory insufficiency of the critically ill or severely injured patient. J Trauma 8:756–773

Hildebran JN, Goerke J, Clements JA (1979) Pulmonary surface film stability and composition. J Appl Physiol 47:604–611

Hildebran JN, Goerke J, Clements JA (1981) Surfactant release in excised rat lung is stimulated by air inflation. J Appl Physiol 51:905–910

Hocking WG, Golde DW (1979) The pulmonary-alveolar macrophage. N Engl J Med 310:580–587 and 639–645

Hook GER (1978) Extracellular hydrolases of the lung. Biochemistry 17:520–528

Hook GER, DiAugustine RP (1976) Secretory cells of the peripheral pulmonary epithelium as targets for toxic agents. Environ Health Perspect 16:147–156

Jimenez JM, Schultz FM, MacDonald PC, Johnston JM (1974) Fetal lung maturation. II. Phosphatidic acid phosphohydrolase in human amniotic fluid. Gynecol Invest 5:245–251

Jobe A (1977) The labeling and biological half-life of phosphatidylcholine in subcellular fractions of rabbit lung. Biochim Biophys Acta 489:440–453

Jobe A, Kirkpatrick E, Gluck L (1978) Labeling of phospholipids in the surfactant and subcellular fractions of rabbit lung. J Biol Chem 253:3810–3816

Kanjanapone V, Hartig-Beecken I, Epstein MF (1980) Effect of isoxsuprine on fetal lung surfactant in rabbits. Pediatr Res 14:278–281

Karotkin EH, Kido M, Cashore WJ, Redding RA, Douglas WJ, Stern L, Oh W (1976) Acceleration of fetal lung maturation by aminophylline in pregnant rabbits. Pediatr Res 10:722–724

Katyal SL, Singh G (1979) An immunologic study of the apoproteins of rat lung surfactant. Lab Invest 40:562–567

Keller GH, Ladda RL (1979) Quantitation of phosphatidylcholine secretion in lung slices and primary cultures of rat lung cells. Proc Natl Acad Sci USA 76:4102–4106

Kero P, Hirvonen T, Valimaki L (1973) Prenatal and postnatal isoxsuprine and respiratory distress syndrome. Lancet 2:198

Khosla SS, Rooney SA (1979) Stimulation of fetal lung surfactant production by administration of 17β-estradiol to the maternal rabbit. Am J Obstet Gynecol 133:213–216

Khosla SS, Gobran LI, Rooney SA (1980) Stimulation of phosphatidylcholine synthesis by 17β-estradiol in fetal rabbit lung. Biochim Biophys Acta 617:282–290

Khosla SS, Smith GJW, Parks PA, Rooney SA (1981) Effects of estrogen on fetal rabbit lung maturation: morphological and biochemical studies. Pediatr Res 15:1274–1281

Khosla SS, Brehier A, Eisenfeld AJ, Ingleson LD, Parks PA, Rooney SA (1983) Influence of sex hormones on lung maturation in the fetal rabbit. Biochim Biophys Acta 750:112–126

Kikkawa Y, Yoneda K (1974) The type II epithelial cell of the lung. I. Method of isolation. Lab Invest 30:76–84

King RJ, Clements JA (1972 a) Surface-active materials from dog lung. I. Method of isolation. Am J Physiol 223:707–714

King RJ, Clements JA (1972 b) Surface-active materials from dog lung. II. Composition and physiological correlations. Am J Physiol 223:715–726

King RJ, MacBeth MC (1979) Physicochemical properties of dipalmitoyl phosphatidylcholine after interaction with an apolipoprotein of pulmonary surfactant. Biochim Biophys Acta 557:86–101

King RJ, Martin HM (1981) Effects of inhibiting protein synthesis on the secretion of surfactant by type II cells in primary culture. Biochim Biophys Acta 663:289–301

King RJ, Gikas E, Ruch J, Clements JA (1974) The radioimmunoassay of pulmonary surface active material in sheep lung. Am Rev Respir Dis 110:273–281

Kiyasu JY, Pieringer RA, Paulus H, Kennedy EP (1963) The biosynthesis of phosphatidyl-glycerol. J Biol Chem 238:2293–2298

Kobayashi T, Noguchi T, Kikuno M, Kubota K (1980) Effect of acute nitrogen dioxide exposure on the composition of fatty acids in lung and liver phospholipids. Toxicol Lett 6:149–155

Kotas RV, Avery ME (1971) Accelerated appearance of pulmonary surfactant in the fetal rabbit. J Appl Physiol 30:358–361

Kotas RV, Farrell PM, Ulane RE, Chez RA (1977) Fetal rhesus monkey lung development: lobar differences and discordances between stability and distensibility. J Appl Physiol 43:92–98

Krishnan B, Rao AS (1981) Surface activity and phospholipid content of saline extracts from control and hydrogen chloride exposed lungs. Indian J Exp Biol 19:637–639

Krishnan B, Nambinarayanan TK, Sivasankaran VP (1974) Effect of sulphuric acid fumes on lung surfactant. Indian J Exp Biol 12:524–527

Krishnan B, Rao AS, Balasubramanian A, Ramakrishnan S (1979) Palmitate 1-^{14}C incorporation in rat lung surfactant and phospholipid content in chronic hydrogen chloride exposure. Indian J Exp Biol 17:689–690

Kulovich MV, Gluck L (1979) The lung profile. II. Complicated pregnancy. Am J Obstet Gynecol 135:64–70

Kulovich MV, Hallman M, Gluck L (1979) The lung profile. I. Normal pregnancy. Am J Obstet Gynecol 135:57–63

Kyei-Aboagye K, Hazucha M, Wyszogrodski I, Rubinstein D, Avery ME (1973) The effect of ozone exposure in vivo on the appearance of lung tissue lipids in the endobronchial lavage of rabbits. Biochem Biophys Res Commun 54:907–913

Landauer B, Tolle W, Kolb E (1975) Beeinflussung der Oberflächenspannung der Lunge durch das Inhalationsanaestheticum Enfluran (Ethrane®) Anaesthesist 24:432–436

Landauer B, Tolle W, Zanker K, Blumel G (1976) Beeinflussung der Oberflächenspannung der Lunge durch das Inhalationsanaestheticum Methoxyfluran (Penthrane®). Anaesthesist 25:431–439

Lawson EE, Brown AR, Torday JS, Madansky DL, Taeusch HW Jr (1978) The effect of epinephrine on tracheal fluid flow and surfactant efflux in fetal sheep. Am Rev Respir Dis 118:1023–1026

Lawson EE, Birdwell RL, Huang PS, Taeusch HW Jr (1979) Augmentation of pulmonary surfactant secretion by lung expansion at birth. Pediatr Res 13:611–614

Le Mesurier SM, Lykke AWJ, Stewart BW (1980) Reduced yield of pulmonary surfactant: patterns of response following administration of chemicals to rats by inhalation. Toxicol Lett 5:89–93

Liggins GC (1969) Premature delivery of foetal lambs infused with glucocorticoids. J Endocrinol 45:515–523

Longmore WJ, Oldenborg V, Golde LMG van (1979) Phospholipase A$_2$ in rat lung microsomes: substrate specificity towards endogenous phosphatidylcholines. Biochim Biophys Acta 572:452–460

Low RB, Davis GS, Giancola MS (1978) Biochemical analyses of bronchoalveolar lavage fluids of healthy human volunteer smokers and nonsmokers. Am Rev Respir Dis 118:863–875

Lumb RH, Cottle DA, White LC, Hoyle SN, Pool GL, Brumley GW (1980) Lung phosphatidylcholine transfer in six vertebrate species. Correlations with surfactant parameters. Biochim Biophys Acta 620:172–175

Maciver AG, Metcalfe IL, Possmayer F, Harding PGR, Passi RB (1977) Alteration of surfactant chemistry in experimental hemorrhagic pancreatitis. J Surg Res 23:311–314

Malmquist E (1980) The influence of paraquat on the in vivo incorporation of lecithin precursors in lung tissue and "alveolar" lecithin. Scand J Clin Lab Invest 40:233–237

Maniscalco WM, Wilson CM, Gross I, Gobran L, Rooney SA, Warshaw JB (1978) Development of glycogen and phospholipid metabolism in fetal and newborn rat lung. Biochim Biophys Acta 530:333–346

Manktelow BW (1981) The loss of pulmonary surfactant in paraquat poisoning: a model for the study of the respiratory distress syndrome. Br J Exp Pathol 48:366–369

Marino PA, Rooney SA (1980) Surfactant secretion in a newborn rabbit lung slice model. Biochim Biophys Acta 620:509–519

Marino PA, Rooney SA (1981) The effect of labor on surfactant secretion in newborn rabbit lung slices. Biochim Biophys Acta 664:389–396

Mashiach S, Barkai G, Sack J, Stern E, Goldman B, Brish M, Serr DM (1978) Enhancement of fetal lung maturity by intra-amniotic administration of thyroid hormone. Am J Obstet Gynecol 130:289–293

Mason RJ (1973) Disaturated lecithin concentration of rabbit tissues. Am Rev Respir Dis 107:678–679

Mason RJ (1978) Importance of the acyldihydroxyacetone phosphate pathway in the synthesis of phosphatidylglycerol and phosphatidylcholine in alveolar type II cells. J Biol Chem 253:3367–3370

Mason RJ, Dobbs LG (1980) Synthesis of phosphatidylcholine and phosphatidylglycerol by alveolar type II cells in primary culture. J Biol Chem 255:5101–5107

Mason RJ, Dobbs LG, Greenleaf RD, Williams LC (1977a) Alveolar type II cells. Fed Proc 36:2697–2702

Mason RJ, Williams MC, Dobbs LG (1977b) Secretion of disaturated phosphatidylcholine by primary cultures of type II alveolar cells. In: Sanders CL, Schneider RP, Dagle GE, Ragan HA (eds) Pulmonary macrophage and epithelial cells. National Technical Information Service, Springfield, Viriginia, pp 280–297

Mason RJ, Williams MC, Greenleaf RD, Clements JA (1977c) Isolation and properties of type II alveolar cells from rat lung. Am Rev Respir Dis 115:1015–1026

Massaro D (1975) In vivo protein secretion by lung. Evidence for active secretion and interspecies differences. J Clin Invest 56:263–271

Massaro D, Clerch L, Massaro GD (1981) Studies on the regulation of surfactant secretion. Fed Proc 40:408

Mavis RD, Vang MJ (1981) Optimal assay and subcellular location of phosphatidylglycerol synthesis in lung. Biochim Biophys Acta 664:409–415

Meban C (1972) Localization of phosphatidic acid phosphatase activity in granular pneumonocytes. J Cell Biol 53:249–252

Mendelson CR, Norwood S, Snyder JM, Johnston JM (1980) CTP:cholinephosphate cytidylyltransferase (CYTase) activity in developing fetal rabbit lung: effect of cortisol. Pediatr Res 14:458

Mescher EJ, Platzker ACG, Ballard PL, Kitterman JA, Clements JA, Tooley WH (1975) Ontogeny of tracheal fluid, pulmonary surfactant, and plasma corticoids in the fetal lamb. J Appl Physiol 39:1017–1021

Metcalfe IL, Enhorning G, Possmayer F (1980) Pulmonary surfactant-associated proteins: their role in the expression of surface activity. J Appl Physiol 49:34–41

Miller D, Bondurant S (1962) Effects of cigarette smoke on the surface characteristics of lung extracts. Am Rev Respir Dis 85:692–696

Miller RN, Thomas PA (1967) Pulmonary surfactant: determinations from lung extracts of patients receiving diethyl ether or halothane. Anesthesiology 28:1089–1095

Morgan TE (1969) Isolation and characterization of lipid N-methyltransferase from dog lung. Biochim Biophys Acta 178:21–34

Morgan TE, Finley TN, Fialkow H (1965a) Comparison of the composition and surface activity of "alveolar" and whole lung lipids in the dog. Biochim Biophys Acta 106:403–413

Morgan TE, Finley TN, Huber GL, Fialkow H (1965b) Alterations in pulmonary surface active lipids during exposure to increased oxygen tension. J Clin Invest 44:1737–1744

Morley CJ, Miller N, Bangham AD, Davis JA (1981) Dry artificial lung surfactant and its effect on very premature babies. Lancet 1:64–68

Motoyama EK, Orzalesi MM, Kikkawa Y, Kaibara M, Wu B, Zigas CJ, Cook CD (1971) Effect of cortisol on the maturation of fetal rabbit lungs. Pediatrics 48:547–555

Motoyama EK, Namba Y, Rooney SA (1976) Phosphatidylcholine content and fatty acid composition of tracheal and gastric liquids from premature and full-term newborn infants. Clin Chim Acta 70:449–454

Naimark A (1973) Cellular dynamics and lipid metabolism in the lung. Fed Proc 32:1967–1971

Namba Y, Motoyama EK, Rooney SA (1981) Effect of anesthetics on pulmonary surfactant – fatty acid composition of tracheal liquid (in Japanese). J Clin Anesth 5:907–911

Nerurkar LS, Zeligs BJ, Bellanti JA (1977) Maturation of the rabbit alveolar macrophage during animal development. II. Biochemical and enzymatic studies. Pediatr Res 11:1202–1207

Nicholas TE, Barr HA (1981) Control of release of surfactant phospholipids in the isolated perfused rat lung. J Appl Physiol 51:90–98

Nichols BA (1976) Normal rabbit alveolar macrophages. I. The phagocytosis of tubular myelin. J Exp Med 144:906–919

Nieman GF, Clark WR, Wax SD, Webb WR (1980) The effect of smoke inhalation on pulmonary surfactant. Ann Surg 191:171–181

Notter RH, Morrow PE (1975) Pulmonary surfactant: a surface chemistry viewpoint. Ann Biomed Eng 3:119–159

Notter RH, Tabak SA, Mavis RD (1980) Surface properties of binary mixtures of some pulmonary surfactant components. J Lipid Res 21:10–22

Oblin A, Warnet JM, Jaurand MC, Bignon J, Claude JR (1978) Biological effects of chrysolite after SO_2 sorption. III. Effects on the biochemical components of alveolar washing. Br J Exp Pathol 59:32–36

Ohno K, Akino T, Fujiwara T (1978) Phospholipid metabolism in perinatal lung. Rev Perinat Med 2:227–318

Oldenborg V, Golde LMG van (1976) Activity of cholinephosphotransferase, lysolecithin: lysolecithin acyltransferase and lysolecithin acyltransferase in the developing mouse lung. Biochim Biophys Acta 441:433–442

Oldenborg V, Golde LMG van (1977) The enzymes of phosphatidylcholine biosynthesis in the fetal mouse lung. Effects of dexamethasone. Biochim Biophys Acta 49:454–465

Olsen DB (1972) Neurohumoral-hormonal secretory stimulation of pulmonary surfactant in the rat. Physiologist 15:230

Oyarzun MJ, Clements JA (1977) Ventilatory and cholinergic control of pulmonary surfactant in the rabbit. J Appl Physiol 43:39–45

Oyarzun MJ, Clements JA (1978) Control of lung surfactant by ventilation, adrenergic mediators, and prostaglandins in the rabbit. Am Rev Respir Dis 117:879–891

Oyarzun MJ, Clements JA, Baritussio A (1980) Ventilation enhances pulmonary alveolar clearance of radioactive dipalmitoyl phosphatidylcholine in liposomes. Am Rev Respir Dis 121:709–721

Paciga JE, Shelley SA, Balis JU (1980) Secretory IgA is a component of rabbit lung surfactant. Biochim Biophys Acta 631:487–494

Page-Roberts BA (1972) Preparation and partial characterization of a lamellar body fraction from rat lung. Biochim Biophys Acta 260:334–338

Pattle RE (1955) Properties, function and origin of the alveolar lining layer. Nature 175:1125–1126

Pattle RE (1965) Surface lining of lung alveoli. Physiol Rev 45:48–79

Pattle RE, Burgess F (1961) The lung lining film in some pathological conditions. J Pathol Bacteriol 82:315–331

Pattle RE, Schock C, Battensby J (1972) Some effects of anesthetics on lung surfactant. Br J Anaesth 44:1119–1127

Pattle RE, Kratzing CC, Parkinson CE, Graves L, Robertson RD, Robards GJ, Currie JO, Parsons JH, Sutherland PD (1979) Maturity of fetal lungs tested by production of stable microbubbles in amniotic fluid. Br J Obstet Gynaecol 86:615–622

Perelman RH, Engle MJ, Farrell PM (1981) Perspectives on fetal lung development. Lung 159:53–80

Petty TL, Reiss OK, Paul GW, Silvers GW, Elkins ND (1977) Characteristics of pulmonary surfactant in adult respiratory distress syndrome associated with trauma and shock. Am Rev Respir Dis 115:531–536

Petty TL, Silvers GW, Paul GW, Stanford RE (1979) Abnormalities in lung elastic properties and surfactant function in adult respiratory distress syndrome. Chest 75:571–574

Pfleger RC, Rebar AH (1979) Indices of lung cell damage in Syrian hamsters' pulmonary alveolar type II cells and macrophages following inhalation of NO_2. Fed Proc 38:1436

Pfleger RC, Henderson RF, Waide J (1972) Phosphatidyl glycerol – a major component of pulmonary surfactant. Chem Phys Lipids 9:51–58

Plowman PN, Flemans RJ (1980) Human pulmonary macrophages: the relationship of smoking to the presence of sea blue granules and surfactant turnover. J Clin Pathol 33:738–743

Possmayer F, Casola P, Chan F, Hill S, Metcalfe IL, Stewart-DeHaan PJ, Wong T, Las Heras J, Gammal EB, Harding PGR (1979) Glucocorticoid induction of pulmonary maturation in the rabbit fetus. The effect of maternal injection of betamethasone on the activity of enzymes in fetal lung. Biochim Biophys Acta 574:197–211

Possmayer F, Casola PG, Chan F, MacDonald P, Ormseth MA, Wong T, Harding PGR, Tokmakjian S (1981) Hormonal induction of pulmonary maturation in the rabbit fetus. Effects of maternal treatment with estradiol-17β on the endogenous levels of cholinephosphate, CDP-choline and phosphatidylcholine. Biochim Biophys Acta 664:10–21

Post M, Batenburg JJ, Schuurmans EAMG, Golde LMG van (1980a) Phospholipid-transfer activity in type II cells isolated from adult rat lung. Biochim Biophys Acta 620:317–321

Post M, Batenburg JJ, Golde LMG van (1980b) Effects of cortisol and thyroxine on phosphatidylcholine and phosphatidylglycerol synthesis by adult rat lung alveolar type II cells in primary culture. Biochim Biophys Acta 618:308–317

Pre J, Bladier B, Battesti JP (1980) An improved method for the determination of lecithin content of human bronchoalveolar lavages. Values for smokers and nonsmokers. IRCS Med Sci 8:225

Pressman BC (1973) Properties of ionophores with broad range cation selectivity. Fed Proc 32:1698–1703

Pysher TJ, Konrad KD, Reed GB (1977) Effects of hydrocortisone and pilocarpine on fetal rat lung explants. Lab Invest 37:588–594

Rao RH, Waite M, Myrvik QN (1981) Deacylation of dipalmitoyllecithin by phospholipases A in alveolar macrophages. Exp Lung Res 2:9–15

Rooney SA (1978) Pilocarpine stimulates pulmonary surfactant secretion in the newborn rabbit. Am Rev Respir Dis 117, no 4, part 2:386

Rooney SA (1979) Biosynthesis of lung surfactant during fetal and early postnatal development. Trends Biochem Sci 4:189–191

Rooney SA (1983) Biochemical development of the lung. In: Warshaw JB (ed) The biological basis of reproductive and development medicine. Elsevier Biomedical, New York, pp 239–287

Rooney SA, Motoyama EK (1976) Studies on the biosynthesis of pulmonary surfactant. The role of the methylation pathway of phosphatidylcholine biosynthesis in primate and non-primate lung. Clin Chim Acta 69:525–531

Rooney SA, Canavan PM, Motoyama EK (1974) The identification of phosphatidylglycerol in the rat, rabbit, monkey and human lung. Biochim Biophys Acta 360:56–67

Rooney SA, Gross I, Gassenheimer LN, Motoyama EK (1975a) Stimulation of glycerol phosphate phosphatidyltransferase activity in fetal rabbit lung by cortisol administration. Biochim Biophys Acta 398:433–441

Rooney SA, Page-Roberts BA, Motoyama EK (1975b) Role of lamellar inclusions in surfactant production: studies on phospholipid composition and biosynthesis in rat and rabbit lung subcellular fractions. J Lipid Res 16:418–425

Rooney SA, Gobran L, Gross I, Wai-Lee TS, Nardone LL, Motoyama EK (1976a) Studies on pulmonary surfactant. Effects of cortisol administration to fetal rabbits on lung phospholipid content, composition and biosynthesis. Biochim Biophys Acta 450:121–130

Rooney SA, Wai-Lee TS, Gobran L, Motoyama EK (1976b) Phospholipid content, composition and biosynthesis during fetal lung development in the rabbit. Biochim Biophys Acta 431:447–458

Rooney SA, Gobran LI, Wai-Lee TS (1977a) Stimulation of surfactant production by oxytocin-induced labor in the rabbit. J Clin Invest 60:754–759

Rooney SA, Nardone LL, Shapiro DL, Motoyama EK, Gobran L, Zaehringer N (1977b) The phospholipids of rabbit type II alveolar epithelial cells: comparison with lung lavage, lung tissue, alveolar macrophages and a human alveolar tumor cell line. Lipids 12:438–442

Rooney SA, Gobran LI, Marino PA, Maniscalco WM, Gross I (1979a) Effects of betamethasone on phospholipid content, composition and biosynthesis in the fetal rabbit lung. Biochim Biophys Acta 572:64–76

Rooney SA, Marino PA, Gobran LI, Gross I, Warshaw JB (1979b) Thyrotropin-releasing hormone increased the amount of surfactant in lung lavage from fetal rabbits. Pediatr Res 13:623–625

Rooney SA, Ingleson LD, Wilson CM, Gross I (1980) Insulin antagonism of dexamethasone-induced stimulation of cholinephosphate cytidylyltransferase in fetal rat lung in organ culture. Lung 158:151–155

Rooney SA, Gross I, Marino PA, Schwartz R, Sehgal PK, Susa JB, Warshaw JB, Widness JA, Zeller WP (1981) Effect of insulin and isoxsuprine on lung surfactant production in the fetal rhesus monkey. Pediatr Res 15:729

Rosenfeld CR, Andujo O, Johnston JM, Jimenez JM (1980) Phosphatidic acid phosphohydrolase and phospholipids in the tracheal and amniotic fluids during normal ovine pregnancy. Pediatr Res 14:891–893

Rosenthal AF, Vargas MG, Schiff SV (1974) Comparison of four indexes to fetal pulmonary maturity. Clin Chem 20:486–491

Rubin P, Shapiro DL, Finklestein JM, Penney DP (1980) The early release of surfactant following lung irradiation of alveolar type II cells. Int J Radiat Oncol Biol Phys 6:75–77

Ryan SF, Liau DF, Bell ALL, Hashim SA, Barrett CR (1981) Correlation of lung compliance and quantities of surfactant phospholipids after acute alveolar injury from N-nitroso-N-methylurethane in the dog. Am Rev Respir Dis 123:200–204

Ryan US, Ryan JW, Smith DS (1975) Alveolar type II cells: studies on the mode of release of lamellar bodies. Tissue Cell 7:587–599

Sahu S, Lynn WS (1977) Phospholipase A in pulmonary secretions of patients with alveolar proteinosis. Biochim Biophys Acta 487:354–360

Sanders RL, Longmore WJ (1975) Phosphatidylglycerol in rat lung. II. Comparison of occurrence, composition and metabolism in surfactant and residual lung fractions. Biochemistry 14:835–840

Sanders RL, Engle MJ, Douglas WHJ (1981) Effect of dexamethasone upon surfactant phosphatidylcholine and phosphatidylglycerol synthesis in organotypic cultures of type II cells. Biochim Biophys Acta 664:380–388

Sarzala MG, Golde LMG van (1976) Selective utilization of endogenous unsaturated phosphatidylcholines and diacylglycerols by cholinephosphotransferase of mouse lung microsomes. Biochim Biophys Acta 441:423–432

Schaefer KE, Avery ME, Bensch K (1964) Time course of changes in surface tension and morphology of alveolar epithelial cells in CO_2-induced hyaline membrane disease. J Clin Invest 43:2080–2093

Schurch S, Goerke J, Clements JA (1976) Direct determination of surface tension in the lung. Proc Natl Acad Sci USA 73:4698–4702

Sevanian A, Gilden C, Kaplan SA, Barrett CT (1979) Enhancement of fetal lung surfactant production by aminophylline. Pediatr Res 13:1336–1340

Shapiro DL, Finkelstein JN (1981) The beta-adrenergic receptor in the type II pneumocyte. Pediatr Res 15:730

Shapiro DL, Nardone LL, Rooney SA, Motoyama EK, Munoz JL (1978) Phospholipid biosynthesis and secretion by a cell line (A549) which resembles type II alveolar epithelial cells. Biochim Biophys Acta 530:197–207

Shelley SA, Kovacevic M, Paciga JE, Balis JU (1979) Sequential changes of surfactant phosphatidylcholine in hyaline membrane, disease of the newborn. N Engl J Med 300:112–116

Shimasaki H, Takatori T, Anderson WR, Horton HL, Privett OS (1976) Alteration of lung lipids in ozone exposed rats. Biochem Biophys Res Commun 68:1256–1262

Shimizu CSN, Mahour GH (1976) Effect of endotoxin on rabbit alveolar phospholipids. J Surg Res 20:25–32

Smith BT (1978) Fibroblast-pneumonocyte factor: intracellular mediator of glucocorticoid effect on fetal lung. In: Stern L (ed) Neonatal intensive care. Mason, Boston, pp 25–32

Smith BT, Bogues WG (1980) Effects of drugs and hormones on lung maturation in experimental animal and man. Pharmacol Therap 9:51–74

Smith BT, Torday JS (1974) Factors affecting lecithin synthesis by fetal lung cells in culture. Pediatr Res 8:848–851

Smith FB, Kikkawa Y (1978) The type II epithelial cells of the lung. III. Lecithin synthesis: a comparison with pulmonary macrophages. Lab Invest 38:45–51

Smith FB, Kikkawa Y (1979) The type II epithelial cells of the lung. V. Synthesis of phosphatidyl glycerol in isolated type II cells and pulmonary alveolar macrophages. Lab Invest 40:172–177

Sommers-Smith SK, Giannopoulos G (1981) Beta-adrenergic receptor binding in isolated fetal, neonatal and adult alveolar type II cells. Fed Proc 40:407

Spalding JW, Hook GER (1979) Phospholipid exchange between subcellular organelles of rabbit lung. Lipids 14:606–613

Spitzer HL, Rice JM, MacDonald PC, Johnston JM (1975) Phospholipid biosynthesis in lung lamellar bodies. Biochem Biophys Res Commun 66:17–23

Stinson SF, Ryan DP, Hertweck MS, Hardy JD, Hwang-Kow SY, Loosli CH (1976) Epithelial and surfactant changes in influenzal pulmonary lesions. Arch Pathol Lab Med 100:147–153

Stothert J, Winn R, Nadir B, Hildebrandt J (1981) Mechanical properties of goat lung following single intratracheal instillation of pH 1 HCl. Fed Proc 40:386

Sueishi K, Tanaka K, Oda T (1977) Immunoultrastructural study of surfactant system. Distribution of specific protein of surface active material in rabbit lung. Lab Invest 37:136–142

Taeusch HW Jr, Wyszogrodski I, Wang NS, Avery ME (1974) Pulmonary pressure-volume relationships in premature fetal and newborn rabbits. J Appl Physiol 37:809–813

Tetley TD, Richards RJ, Harwood JL (1977) Changes in pulmonary surfactant and phosphatidylcholine metabolism in rats exposed to chrysotile asbestos dust. Biochem J 166:323–329

Tsao FHC, Gutcher GR, Zachman RD (1979) Effect of hydrocortisone on the metabolism of phosphatidylcholine in maternal and fetal rabbit lungs and livers. Pediatr Res 13:997–1001

Valimaki M, Pelliniemi TT, Niinikoski J (1975) Oxygen-induced changes in pulmonary phospholipids in the rat. J Appl Physiol 39:780–787

van Golde LMG (1976) Metabolism of phospholipids in the lung. Am Rev Respir Dis 114:977–1000

van Golde LMG, Oldenborg V, Post M, Batenburg JJ, Poorthuis BJHM, Wirtz KWA (1980) Phospholipid transfer proteins in rat lung. Identification of a protein specific for phosphatidylglycerol. J Biol Chem 255:6011–6013

van Heusden GPH, Vianen GM, Bosch H van den (1980) Differentiation between acyl coenzyme A: lysophosphatidylcholine acyltransferase and lysophosphatidylcholine: lysophosphatidylcholine transacylase in the synthesis of dipalmitoylphosphatidylcholine in rat lung. J Biol Chem 255:9312–9318

van Heusden GPH, Noteborn HPJM, Bosch H van den (1981) Selective utilization of palmitoyl lysophosphatidylcholine in the synthesis of disaturated phosphatidylcholine in rat lung. A combined in vitro and in vivo approach. Biochim Biophys Acta 664:49–60

Vereyken JM, Montfoort A, Golde LMG van (1972) Some studies on the biosynthesis of the molecular species of phosphatidylcholine from rat lung and phosphatidylcholine and phosphatidylethanolamine from rat liver. Biochim Biophys Acta 260:72–81

Voelker DR, Snyder F (1979) Subcellular site and mechanism of synthesis of disaturated phosphatidylcholine in alveolar type II cell adenomas. J Biol Chem 254:8628–8633

von Neergaard K (1929) Neue Auffassungen über einen Grundbegriff der Atemmechanik. Die Retraktionskraft der Lunge, abhängig von der Oberflächenspannung in den Alveolen. Z Gesamte Exp Med 66:373–394

von Wichert P, Kohl FV (1977) Decreased dipalmitoyllecithin content found in lung specimens from patients with so-called shock-lung. Intensiv Care Med 3:27–30

von Wichert P, Wilke A (1976) Alveolar stability and phospholipid content in normal pig lungs and in pig lungs with Mycoplasma pneumonia. Scand J Respir Dis 57:25–30

Wallace WE Jr, Headley MC, Weber KC (1975) Dipalmitoyl lecithin surfactant adsorption by kaolin dust in vitro. J Colloid Interface Sci 51:535–537

Warren C, Holton JB, Allen JT (1974) Assessment of fetal lung maturity by estimation of amniotic fluid palmitic acid. Br Med J 1:94–96

Weinhold PA, Feldman DA, Quade MM, Miller JC, Brooks RL (1981) Evidence for a regulatory role of CTP:cholinephosphate cytidylyltransferase in the synthesis of phosphatidylcholine in fetal lung following premature birth. Biochim Biophys Acta 665:134–144

White DA (1973) The phospholipid composition of mammalian tissues. In: Ansell GB, Hawthorne JN, Dawson RMC (eds) Form and function of phospholipids. Elsevier, Amsterdam, pp 441–482

White LR, Hunt J, Tetley TD, Richards RJ (1981) Biochemical and cellular effects of welding fume particles in the rat lung. Ann Occup Hyg 24:93–101

Whitlow CD, Pool GL, Brumley GW, Lum RH (1980) Protein-catalyzed transfer of phosphatidylglycerol by sheep lung soluble fraction. FEBS Lett 113:221–224

Whitsett JA, Manton MA, Darovec-Beckerman C, Adams KG, Moore JJ (1981) β-Adrenergic receptors in the developing rabbit lung. Am J Physiol 240:E351–E357

Williams MC (1977) Conversion of lamellar body membranes into tubular myelin in alveoli of fetal rat lungs. J Cell Biol 72:260–277

Williams MC, Benson BJ (1981) Immunocytochemical localization and identification of the major surfactant protein in adult rat lung. J Histochem Cytochem 29:291–305

Williams RA, Rhoades RA, Adams WS (1971) The response of lung tissue and surfactant to nitrogen dioxide exposure. Arch Intern Med 128:101–108

Wilson L, Bamburg JR, Mizel SB, Grisham LM, Creswell KM (1974) Interaction of drugs with microtubule proteins. Fed Proc 33:158–166

Witschi H (1976) Proliferation of type II alveolar cells: a review of common responses in toxic lung injury. Toxicology 5:267–277

Woo SW, Berlin D, Hedley-Whyte J (1969) Surfactant function and anesthetic agents. J Appl Physiol 26:571–577

Wright ES, Mavis RD (1981) Changes in pulmonary phospholipid biosynthetic enzymes after nitrogen dioxide exposure. Toxicol Appl Pharmacol 58:262–268

Wu B, Kikkawa Y, Orzalesi MM, Motoyama EK, Kaibara M, Zigas CJ, Cook CD (1973) The effect of thyroxine on the maturation of fetal rabbit lungs. Biol Neonate 22:161–168

Wykle RL, Kraemer WF (1977) Glycerol kinase activiy in adenoma alveolar type II cells. FEBS Lett 78:83–85

Wyszogrodski I, Taeusch HW Jr, Avery ME (1974) Isoxsuprine-induced alterations of pulmonary pressure-volume relationships in premature rabbits. Am J Obstet Gynecol 119:1107–1111

Zeligs BJ, Nerurkar LS, Bellanti JA (1977) Maturation of the rabbit alveolar macrophage during animal development. I. Perinatal influx into alveoli and ultrastructural differentiation. Pediatr Res 11:197–208

CHAPTER 16

Effects of Pneumotoxins
on Lung Connective Tissue

J. A. LAST and K. M. REISER

A. Introduction

In this chapter, the toxicologic effects of inhaled materials on lung collagen and elastin are reviewed. Since the term "inhaled" is ambiguous in a practical sense, we have interpreted the term to include intratracheal instillation. In addition to assembling a bibliography of toxic effects of inhaled and/or instilled agents on lung connective tissue in experimental animal models, we have also included selected case reports of effects of lung toxins on humans. References to systemic toxins causing pulmonary fibrosis and/or emphysema are also collated.

To make this chapter useful as a reference, we have assembled the literature in the form of tables. A few fibrotic agents (bleomycin, paraquat, radiation, and silica) are listed in indidivual tables; the remainder are divided into gaseous and nongaseous agents and listed alphabetically. Agents inducing emphysema are listed in separate tables. The tables list the species of animals, the duration of exposure, and the types of assays used (B = biochemistry, H = histology, P = physiology). The chapter itself provides a critical evaluation of the methods most commonly used to evaluate changes in lung connective tissue, as it would clearly be impossible to critique each reference individually. In addition, several theories on the mechanism of pneumotoxin-induced lung injury are discussed, and key review articles are cited.

B. Pneumotoxins and Lung Collagen

Collagen is a group of complex, heterogeneous macromolecules widely distributed throughout the body. It is highly insoluble, the better to subserve its primary role as the major structural protein of both soft and ossified tissues and organs. Several characteristic features of collagen are the result of extensive posttranslational modifications of this protein, including hydroxylation of certain proline and lysine residues and the formation of inter- and intramolecular crosslinks. A number of recent reviews have summarized current information on collagen structure and biosynthesis (EYRE 1980; NIMNI 1980; PROCKOP et al. 1979).

Collagen is the predominant protein in the mammalian lung, comprising approximately 10%–20% of the dry weight of the lung. However, analysis of lung collagen has been difficult, even in normal lungs, for several reasons. First, lung collagen is extremely insoluble, even as compared with the solubility of collagen in many other tissues. With the use of solubilizing agents such as pepsin, less than 20% of total lung collagen can usually be extracted from normal mature lungs as intact chains; less than 1% of total lung collagen can be extracted with acetic acid or neutral salt solutions (Hance and Crystal 1976). Second, lung contains all five of the molecular species (at least ten different chains) of collagen identified thus far, several of which are still poorly characterized. Finally, the lung contains at least 40 cell types; it is still not known how many are involved in collagen synthesis (Kuhn 1976). Despite these difficulties, a great many studies have been done on the effects of toxic substances on lung collagen, using histologic, morphological, biochemical, and physiologic assays. Before one can attempt to develop a cohesive picture of lung response to injury, one must have an appreciation of the limitations and pitfalls inherent in the various assays used to detect and quantitate toxin-induced aberrations of collagen structure, synthesis, and/or content.

I. Histologic Studies

Many early studies on pulmonary toxins evaluated changes in collagen by histologic techniques. Studies using nonspecific stains such as hematoxylin–eosin provide no direct evidence about changes in collagen. However, changes are sometimes inferred from such phenomena as thickening of alveolar septa or "consolidation". More recent studies have used so-called specific stains, such as Masson's trichrome, van Gieson's, or silver impregnation. Even with these stains, there is no consensus on what types of collagen are being stained. Several studies attempting to correlate collagen staining characteristics with specific antibody immunofluorescence have been done; such studies have provided evidence that type I collagen stains with van Gieson's and Masson's trichrome, whereas type III collagen is better visualized with silver impregnation stains. There is also evidence that newly synthesized collagen may have different staining characteristics from mature collagen; it is possible that newly synthesized type I collagen may stain with silver impregnation (Bateman et al. 1981; Gay et al. 1976; Meigel et al. 1977; Remberger et al. 1975). In addition, nothing is known about the staining characteristics of the other parenchymal lung collagen types, types IV and V. Since toxin-induced lung injury may include such events as increases in newly synthesized collagen and changes in lung collagen types (Reiser and Last 1981; Reiser et al. 1982), the lack of precision and uncertainty inherent in conventional histologic staining techniques remains a serious drawback when histologic techniques alone are used to assess complex changes in lung collagen. In addition, problems of random sampling inherent in routine histologic evaluation of lung tissue place constraints on the value of the data obtained by such methods.

II. Morphometric Studies

Quantitative morphometric studies generally involve selecting specific areas of the lung to study in detail; inference about changes in connective tissue are made from observations of changes in such parameters as alveolar wall thickness, fibroblast accumulation, and vessel wall changes (Bachofen and Weibel 1974; Cassan et al. 1974). Although such techniques provide quantitative data, in contrast to routine histologic techniques, only a small part of the whole lung is usually studied. Inferring changes in the composition of the remainder of the lung from a detailed study of small selected sections is certainly a potential source of error. In addition, there are two other important problems in interpretation of morphometric studies of lung connective tissue. First, the morphological definition of collagen or of elastin is imprecise: it is not synonymous with biochemically defined collagen or elastin. This difficulty is further compounded when acutely damaged lungs are examined (HANCE and CRYSTAL 1976; HORWITZ et al. 1976). Second, there is a serious denominator problem in data normalization to either area (e. g., cells per field) or relative percentage (e. g., cells per thousand cells), in that the edema and the cellular inflammation that accompany acute lung damage may affect such a normalization denominator (GREENBERG et al. 1978 a, b).

III. Electron Microscopy

Collagen fibrils have certain distinguishing features, including characteristic cross-striations with a regular periodicity of 67 nm for the major bands, when examined by electron microscopy. Individual fibrils (40–200 nm) or fibrils aggregated as fibers are observed. Fibrillar material that does not contain banding has also been observed in the lung; it is unknown if this material is collagenous and, if collagenous, which collagen type it may be composed of (HANCE and CRYSTAL 1976). Electron microscopy cannot be used to distinguish between different collagen types. Again, only small portions of the lung may be studied, and the procedures are extremely labor intensive.

IV. Immunofluorescent Studies

Various collagen types have been purified and specific antibodies to these collagen types for immunofluorescence studies have been produced. All five of the known collagen types have been observed in normal lung, and changes in the distribution of these collagens have been reported in certain disease states (MADRI and FURTHMAYR 1980). The accuracy of such assays is dependent in part on the care with which the collagen antigens were purified (NOWACK et al. 1976). Although this approach can provide information about the location of collagen types in the lung, it is at best a semiquantitative technique. In addition, it is not known whether antibodies prepared against soluble collagen stain both soluble and insoluble collagens with fidelity.

V. Physiologic Studies

Physiologic studies related to lung connective tissue generally involve the measurement of quasistatic or dynamic lung compliance. Use of saline-filled rather than air-filled lungs for such determinations is preferred, so as to eliminate potential confounding effects of changes in compliance secondary to changes in surface-active properties of the small airways and/or of the alveoli. Probably as much as 90% of the change in compliance of an air-filled lung is related to expansion against surface forces rather than to stretching of the connective tissue matrix, whereas essentially all of the change in compliance of a saline-filled lung is thought to reflect the distension of structural proteins (HORWITZ et al. 1976).

It is thought that compliance changes ascertained between functional residual capacity (FRC) and about 75% or more of the total lung capacity (TLC) are related to distension of elastic fibers (elastin), whereas compliance changes at higher lung volumes are related to the stretching of collagen fibers (HOGG et al. 1969; JOHANSON et al. 1972; KOO et al. 1974; MEAD 1961; RADFORD 1964; TURINO and LOURENCO 1972). While there are theoretical considerations and experimental data (mainly based on pressure–volume curves obtained with lungs digested with crude collagenolytic or elastolytic enzymes) that support this assumption, it is by no means proven that elastin and collagen have specific roles in determining changes in lung compliance at defined distending pressures. Nothing is known about the effects of collagen or elastin interactions with other matrix proteins on lung compliance, nor do we understand what role, if any, is played by intermolecular cross-links of collagen in determining the compliance of a lung. Since aging of an animal is associated with increases both in collagen cross-linking and lung "stiffness", this is an important area for further study.

VI. Biochemical Studies

A great many biochemical assays dealing with various aspects of collagen metabolism have been used to study effects of lung toxins. Hydroxyproline is a fairly specific marker for collagen; the amount present in lung elastin and the C1q component of complement in the normal lung is negligible by comparison. Thus, lung collagen content can be measured by assaying hydroxyproline in lung hydrolysates. The Woessner assay (WOESSNER 1961) is most often used. Even in this fairly straightforward assay there are pitfalls. If hydroxyproline is expressed as a concentration (per gram protein, for example) rather than on a per lung basis, net increases in total lung collagen may be masked by transient changes in the lung protein content secondary to edema and inflammation, which often accompany the acute phase of lung injury (GREENBERG et al. 1978a). Hydroxyproline also provides a useful marker for determinations of collagen synthesis rates. If radiolabeled proline is used as the isotope, the rate of production of hydroxyproline is a good index of the net rate of collagen synthesis. Such synthesis rate determinations can be performed in cell lines isolated from the lung or in short-term lung explant cultures (GREENBERG et al. 1978a; HANCE and CRYSTAL 1976; HESTERBERG et al. 1981). Accumulation of newly synthesized collagen per unit time can also be determined, both in cultures and in lungs from animals administered radiolabeled proline in vivo (HASCHEK et al. 1982). To avoid potential difficulties in these assays, one generally determines specific activity of the isotope by determining proline pool sizes in total lung homogenates (GREENBERG et al. 1978a). Prolyl hydroxylase and lysyl oxidase, two enzymes involved in posttranslational modifications of collagen, have also been used as markers of "lung fibrosis" or injury (HOLLINGER and CHVAPIL 1977; MURAD et al. 1981; ORTHOEFER et al. 1976), but the rationale for their use other than as nonspecific markers of inflammation is open to question.

Changes in lung collagen types can also be determined biochemically. Early studies measured collagen type ratios only in the soluble fraction, using such techniques as differential salt precipitation and chromatographic separation; such studies do not appear to reflect accurately the collagen type ratios in the whole lung (HUANG 1977; MADRI and FURTHMAYR 1979). Complete solubilization of lung collagen followed by peptide mapping appears to be the only way to assay a representative sample of the collagen. Tryptic digestion and two-dimensional electrophoresis have been used for this purpose (KELLY et al. 1981); more commonly, cyanogen bromide digestion, followed by chromatography and/or electrophoresis of the peptides is used (EPSTEIN 1974; REISER and LAST 1980, 1981; SEYER et al. 1976). Types I, III, and V collagen have been quantitated in the lung by such techniques (REISER and LAST 1983).

Changes in reducible collagen cross-links can also be assayed biochemically by reductive labeling with such compounds as NaB^3H_4 or $NaCNB^3H_3$ (ROBINS and BAILEY 1977). Even in mature lung, reducible cross-links are present in sufficient amount for quantitation. Changes in lung collagen cross-links have been reported in certain fibrotic diseases (SEYER et al. 1981).

VII. Specific Fibrotic Agents

As can be seen in Tables 1–4, a few fibrotic agents have been extensively studied in animals. Perhaps the most venerable of these models, silica-induced lung fibrosis, has been studied for at least 40 years (see ZAIDI 1969 and REISER and LAST 1979 for reviews). Asbestos, another pneumoconiosis-inducing agent, has also been reviewed (CRAIGHEAD and MOSSMAN 1982; MILLER 1978). Fibrosis induced in lungs by ionizing radiation is also a field with a long history and has been reviewed by GROSS (1977, 1981). More recently, interest has developed in experimental pulmonary fibrosis induced by bleomycin. As a model, it appears to resemble, both histologically and morphologically, such human entities as idiopathic pulmonary fibrosis more closely than do other animal models (HESTERBERG et al. 1981). Furthermore, bleomycin-induced fibrosis in humans has become an increasing problem in certain patients receiving bleomycin in the course of cancer chemotherapy (COMIS 1978; FINCH et al. 1980; SCHLEIN et al. 1981). Similarly, experimental fibrosis induced by the herbicide paraquat has recently received attention, as the danger to humans exposed to it has become increasingly apparent (SMITH and HEATH 1976). Several recent case reports have documented that fatal pulmonary fibrosis can occur in humans after percutaneous absorption of this agent, as well as after inhalation (LEVIN et al. 1979; NEWHOUSE et al. 1978). Oxygen has been used to induce experimental fibrosis for some time (see Table 5); recent attention has been focused on its role in the evolution of adult respiratory distress syndrome (KATZENSTEIN et al. 1976; PRATT et al. 1979). Pertinent reviews include those by KATZENSTEIN et al. (1976) and CLARK and LAMBERTSEN (1971). Finally, recent reviews of pulmonary fibrosis in general have attempted to integrate data from animal toxicology studies with observations from the clinic (BITTERMAN et al. 1981; KARLINSKY and GOLDSTEIN 1980; RINALDO and ROGERS 1982). Real progress seems to be occurring in the integration of these often disparate approaches.

C. Pneumotoxins and Lung Elastin

Elastin has been less well defined chemically than collagen, in part because, unlike collagen, it is extremely difficult to solubilize in intact form from any of the tissues in which it is found. There is general agreement that elastin is characterized by large amounts of nonpolar amino acids (glycine, alanine, valine, and proline), a small amount of hydroxyproline, and the absence of hydroxylysine. Like collagen, elastin contains cross-links derived from lysine groups. Some of these cross-links, such as lysinonorleucine, are also present in collagen. However, elastin also contains at least two cross-links that are not found in collagen: desmosine and isodesmosine. Recent reviews of elastin structure and synthesis have appeared (RUCKER and TINKER 1977; SANDBERG et al. 1981). As discussed later in this section, the problems in defining precisely what constitutes elastin have made accurate assessment of changes in this connective tissue protein in disease very difficult.

Histologically, elastic fibers have long been characterized by their ability to take up such stains as Verhoeff–hematoxylin, resorcin–fuchsin, and orcein; stainability has been attributed to the presence of unreacted aldehyde groups and/or the presence of the strongly hydrophobic regions of the molecule (LILLIE et al. 1972; McCALLUM 1973). Electron microscopy stains such as uranyl acetate and lead citrate stain the microfibrillar component surrounding the amorphous component of elastic fibers. Unfortunately, it has by no means been determined that such histologically and ultrastructurally defined entities are equivalent to biochemically defined elastin. Thus, even semiquantitative assessment of elastin content by histologic or morphological methods remains impractical. Correlation of biochemical with histologic observations is even more fraught with difficulty for elastin than for collagen.

Biochemical quantitation of elastin levels in lung tissue is made difficult by the lack of consensus on a standard method of assay for this insoluble molecule. Because of the many approaches to quantitating elastin, estimations of elastin content of normal lung have ranged from 1% to 34% of the acellular dry weight (HORWITZ et al. 1976). Probably the most widely used method for quantitating elastin is the Lansing procedure, in which elastin is isolated on the basis of its insolubility in boiling NaOH. Several variations of the method exist in which insoluble nonelastin material is separated from elastin in the final precipitate, including solubilization of elastin with KOH (BRISCOE and LORING 1958) and elastase digestion (FITZPATRICK and HOSPELHORN 1962). Another approach is to measure nitrogen content of the final precipitate and assume elastin is 16.34% nitrogen (PIERCE and HOCOTT 1960). Enzymatic methods for quantitating elastin have also been used, such as digestion of crude tissue preparations with trypsin and collagenase (HOSPELHORN and FITZPATRICK 1961). A more elaborate version of this method has been published, describing sequential treatment of the lung with guanidine, collagenase, guanidine plus a reducing agent, and 6 M urea with sodium dodecylsulfate (RICHMOND 1974). All of these methods suffer from the potential loss of elastin during the harsh extraction procedures and/or the persistence of nonelastin material in the final product. These difficulties are especially pronounced when examining a complex organ such as lung, particularly when the effects of disease processes and pneumotoxins on the biochemical properties of elastin are not fully understood.

More recently, methods for quantitating elastin content have been described in which crude tissue is hydrolyzed in HCl, and desmosine and isodesmosine are quantitated on an amino acid analyzer (STARCHER 1977). Recently, a radioimmunoassay for quantitating desmosine has also been developed (STARCHER and MECHAM 1981). Since desmosine and its isomer appear to be cross-links unique to elastin, this approach avoids the problem of including nonelastin material in the final calculation. However, the assumption has to be made that the elastin being quantitated is fully cross-linked, and that the number of desmosines per chain is constant. We do not really know that this is the case during lung injury and lung repair.

Correlation of physiologic measurements (mainly of dynamic or quasistatic lung compliance) with changes in lung biochemistry and/or histology has also proven to be very difficult. Dogma suggests that changes in lung volume in response to changes in distending pressure at the midrange of pressure–volume curves (25%–75% between FRC and TLV) are mainly related to stretching of elastic fibers (elastin) in the alveolar interstitium. However, the exact roles of lung collagen, elastin, structural glycoproteins, and other substances of the intercellular matrix in determining the expansion and contraction properties of the lung are far from well understood. Much speculation on the postulated role of elastin in determining lung structure and function in health and disease (predominantly emphysema) has come from studies of lung from animals exposed to proteolytic enzymes, especially papain or elastases, either inhaled as aerosols or injected intratracheally (see Sect. D.V for references). In Table 8, we have collated much of the literature on induction of experimental emphysema by administration of proteolytic enzymes to animals. Animal models of emphysema have been reviewed by KARLINSKY and SNIDER (1978).

D. Mechanisms of Pneumotoxin-Induced Damage to Connective Tissue

There are many ways of analyzing lung connective tissue. As can be seen in Tables 1–8, various combinations of these techniques have been used to study pneumotoxins for at least 60 years. The most fundamental question is determining how many ways the lung can respond to injury. To approach this question, we must first deal with the problem of defining injury, a problem greatly exacerbated by the fact that each discipline has tended to develop its own vocabulary to describe the various abnormalities seen in damaged lungs. For example, there is no consensus on the definition of fibrosis. Is it a final, fixed state, defined by the presence of abnormal deposition of collagen detected histologically? Is it a process, defined biochemically as observed aberrations in collagen biosynthesis rates, which may or may not continue long enough to result in deposition of biochemically measurable or histologically observable collagen? Is it a change in mechanical properties of the lung, defined physiologically by alterations in pressure–volume curves? Clearly, it is necessary to determine what is meant by "fibrosis" in a given experimental context. There is less controversy over the use of the term "emphysema", the term usually used for lung injury involving loss of lung structural elements, thought to be secondary to degradation of lung elastin. A generally accepted definition of emphysema (SANDBERG et al. 1981) is: "an anatomic alteration of the lung characterized by an abnormal enlargement of the air spaces distal to the terminal nonrespiratory bronchiole, accompanied by destructive changes of the alveolar walls."

I. Central Role of Free Radicals in Fibrosis

A number of investigators have postulated that many pneumotoxic agents act primarily by generating free radicals in the lung, which initiate the damage. Such a mechanism has been proposed for many toxins, ranging from ozone (and other oxidant gases) to paraquat (BUS et al. 1975; KELLOGG and FRIDOVICH 1975; McCORD and FRIDOVICH 1978; PETRONE et al. 1980; YASAKA et al. 1981; YOST and FRIDOVICH 1976).

Central to such arguments has been the observation of the role (or roles) of superoxide and various peroxides and free radical forms of oxygen as mediators of lung injury. Such toxic oxygen species may arise directly, as from the peroxidation of lipids by ozone, or may arise secondarily, as a by-product of phagocytosis or other metabolic activities of macrophages or neutrophils. These highly reactive compounds are thought to damage cell membranes or other essential cellular components, thereby initiating (and amplifying) a sequence of events leading to death of cells and their replacement by acellular substances such as collagen. Such pathways of fibrotic injury are probably universal in that radiation and other nonchemical damaging agents share common properties of generation of free radicals and other highly reactive short-lived species at their sites of interaction with lung tissue. After tissue is damaged, it may presumably be repaired with restoration of its original structure and cellular distribution. Alternatively, damage may be exacerbated and progress through an amplification phase involving recruitment of and infiltration by inflammatory cells from the circulating blood (PETRONE et al. 1980).

II. Central Role of "Fibrogenic Factors"

Recruitment of neutrophils, other leukocytes, and ultimately of fibroblasts to sites of lung injury is thought to be controlled, at least in part, by release of chemotactic factors by pulmonary alveolar macrophages (NATHAN et al. 1980) and by other inflammatory cells such as lymphocytes (COHEN 1981). Platelets, macrophages, and lymphocytes also elaborate factors capable of stimulating fibroblast proliferation, thereby indirectly stimulating collagen synthesis at sites of injury (ANTONIADES et al. 1979; BITTERMAN et al. 1982; DeLUSTRO et al. 1980; LIEBOVICH and ROSS 1976). Important roles in recruitment and/or proliferation of inflammatory cells have also been ascribed to the complement system, the fibrin system, and to several other circulating factors.

In addition, specific factors have been directly implicated in the direct regulation of collagen synthesis by fibroblasts. This mechanism has been most extensively investigated in silica-induced lung injury. It has been proposed that the first event is the ingestion of silica by macrophages, resulting in the death of the macrophage (ALLISON et al. 1966). The dying macrophages then release a "fibrogenic factor" that specifically stimulates collagen synthesis by fibroblasts (AALTO and KULONEN 1979; BURRELL and ANDERSON 1973; HEPPLESTON and STYLES 1967; NOURSE et al. 1975). Since the silica is released unchanged when the macrophage dies, the process is self-perpetuating once the silica has reached the lungs. The long-term evolution of silicotic damage is obviously complex, as the silica becomes increasingly sequestered in acellular collagenous nodules, leaving much of the parenchyma relatively normal. What directs this apparently adaptive response, in contrast to the diffuse fibrosis seen after asbestos exposure, for example, is unknown. In addition to the obvious marked histologic differences of this nodular disease, silica-induced fibrosis differs from other types of experimental fibroses in several important biochemical and immunologic respects (REISER and LAST 1979; REISER et al. 1983).

III. Central Role of Immunologic Factors

It has been proposed that the key event in some forms of fibrosis is the production of autoantibodies to collagen (BURRELL 1981; VIGLIANI and PERNIS 1963). Such an event could occur secondarily to generalized toxic injury to lung cells, in which collagen not normally accessible to lymphocytes is exposed. The subsequent production of autoantibodies to collagen would then have several effects, one of which might be the stimulation of macrophages to produce a fibroblast "fibrogenic factor". Indeed, such a sequence of events has been demonstrated in tissue culture (LEWIS and BURRELL 1976). Although some investigators still think that such complex immunologic events may underlie pneumotoxin-induced fibrosis, most workers feel that immunologic abnormalities in diseases such as silicosis are probably secondary phenomena.

IV. Synergism in Pneumotoxin-Induced Lung Injury

In some examples of experimental fibrosis, synergism between fibrogenic agents has been observed. One group has published a number of papers describing a model of pulmonary fibrosis in mice induced by intraperitoneal injection of butylated hydroxytoluene (BHT) followed by exposure to 70% oxygen (HASCHEK and WITSCHI 1979; HASCHEK et al. 1983; KEHRER and WITSCHI 1980). They found that BHT alone produced increases in hydroxyproline content and a transient pneumonitis. Some 3 weeks later the lungs were virtually normal with only slight thickening of alveolar septa. However, if the mice were exposed to 70% O_2 for 5 days immediately after receiving the BHT, there was a dramatic increase in hydroxyproline content, and histologically there was disruption in alveolar septa by 3 weeks. Mice given O_2 alone did not show any evidence of lung damage. The authors conclude that the severe fibrosis seen after the combination of BHT and oxygen is the result of a synergistic interaction. They suggest that when lung damage is caused by BHT there is an initial phase of epithelial proliferation. If the mice are exposed to 70% oxygen during this period, the epithelial type II cells are either inhibited from dividing or killed. The authors speculate that damage to the epithelial cells then leads to uninhibited interstitial cell growth; they suggest that this mechanism may also underlie other types of lung injury.

Synergistic interactions between particulates and gases have also been studied. McJilton and Charles (1976) studied the effects of sodium chloride aerosols and sulfur dioxide on guinea pigs. When the mixture was at a high humidity, they found decreases in flow resistance. Normally, SO_2 does not penetrate the deep lung. However, in this study it was proposed that the highly soluble SO_2 dissolved in the droplets, and thus was able to "piggyback" into the lower respiratory tract. This area has been reviewed by Ellison and Waller (1978). The interaction of particulates and oxidant gases has also been studied. Gardner et al. (1977) found that combinations of ozone and ammonium sulfate aerosols were more toxic than either agent alone, based on mortality rates of mice exposed to *Streptococcus pyogenes*. Juhos et al. (1978) also found evidence for synergism between ozone and ammonium sulfate, based on histologic evaluations of rat lungs. Synergism between ozone and ammonium sulfate has also been suggested as responsible for decreased maximal flow rates observed during human exposures at near ambient levels (Hazuka and Bates 1975). Recently, we (Last et al. 1983) studied the effects of ammonium sulfate aerosols in combination with ozone or with nitrogen dioxide on collagen metabolism in rat lungs. Rats were exposed to varying concentrations of the oxidant gases for 1 week; collagen synthesis rates in lung explants were then measured. Ammonium sulfate aerosols alone had no effect on collagen synthesis rates; however, they significantly potentiated the effects of the oxidant gases. The mechanism for this synergy is unclear. Since the mechanisms of injury of individual pneumotoxins are so poorly understood, it is hardly surprising that mechanisms underlying synergistic interactions remain highly speculative.

V. Mechanisms of Injury in Experimental Emphysema

As shown in Tables 7 and 8, experimental emphysema has been produced both by proteases and by a variety of miscellaneous agents. Although the "mechanism" in this sort of injury is thought to be more straightforward than for fibrosis (the elastase either directly instilled or induced destroys the elastin), what governs ensuing events is unclear. Studies on enzyme-induced emphysema indicate that, although there are initial disruptions in elastin content and elastin synthesis, elastin content then returns to normal (Kilburn et al. 1971). Most studies on emphysematous human lungs have also shown a normal elastin concentration (Wright et al. 1960; Johnson and Andrews 1970). However, a recent study in which elastin content was measured by quantitating desmosine reported decreased elastin content in human emphysematous lungs (Chrzanowski et al. 1980).

Based on experiments with both acute and chronic exposure of lungs to pneumotoxins, several investigators (Haschek et al. 1982; Niehwohner 1982) have suggested the possibility that fibrosis and emphysema may not be mutually exclusive responses of the lung to injury, but rather different aspects of what could be a common response. While much more work remains to be done in this area before we truly understand the mechanisms of cause and effect in chronic lung disease, the suggestion of common mechanisms in the etiology of emphysema and fibrosis certainly should stimulate further experiments in these areas.

In summary, then, there is little consensus on the "mechanisms" of pneumotoxin-induced connective tissue injury to the lung; not enough is known about the regulation of synthesis, deposition, and degradation of collagen and elastin, or of the complex interrelationships between the many cell populations of the lung. Tables 1–8 list the pneumotoxic agents alphabetically.

Table 1. Bleomycin-inducing lung fibrosis

Species	Maximum duration (weeks)	Assays used[a]	Reference
Baboon	38	B, H	COLLINS et al. (1981)
Baboon	38	B, P	FINE et al. (1981)
Baboon	52	B, H, P	MCCULLOUGH et al. (1978a)
Baboon	22	Lavage	MCCULLOUGH et al. (1978b)
Guinea pig	6	H	UPRETI et al. (1979)
Hamster	4	B	STARCHER et al. (1978)
Hamster	26	H	SNIDER et al. (1978b)
Hamster	26	P	SNIDER et al. (1978a)
Hamster	13	B, P	GOLDSTEIN et al. (1979)
Hamster	3	B	CLARK et al. (1980b)
Hamster	4	B, H, P	FEDULLO et al. (1980)
Hamster	4	B, H, P	RILEY et al. (1981)
Hamster	4	B, H, P	RILEY et al. (1982)
Hamster	4	B, H	GIRI et al. (1980)
Hamster	2	B	ZUCKERMAN et al. (1980)
Human lung fibroblasts		B	CLARK et al. (1980a)
Mouse	20	H	ADAMSON and BOWDEN (1974)
Mouse	8	H	ADAMSON (1976)
Mouse	8	B, H	SIKIC et al. (1978a)
Mouse	8	B, H	SIKIC et al. (1978b)
Mouse	4	H	JONES and REEVE (1978)
Mouse	8	H	SZAPIEL et al. (1979)
Mouse	6	B	LAZO (1981)
Mouse	3	H	RAISFELD (1980)
Mouse	3	B	HAKKINEN et al. (1982)
Rabbit	8	B, H	LAURENT et al. (1981)
Rat	8	B, H, P	HESTERBERG et al. (1981)
Rat	1	B	REISER and LAST (1981)
Rat	8	B, H	THRALL et al. (1979)
Rat	4	B	PHAN et al. (1980)
Rat	1	B	PHAN and THRALL (1982b)
Rat		B	PHAN and THRALL (1982a)
Rat	4	B, H	THRALL et al. (1981)
Rat	6	B	PHAN et al. (1981)
Rat	6	B, H	TOM and MONTGOMERY (1980)
Rat	46	B	COUNTS et al. (1981)
Rat	4	B	STERLING et al. (1982)
Rat	4	B, H, P	KELLEY et al. (1980)
Rat	4	H, P	EVANS et al. (1982)

[a] B = biochemistry; H = histology; P = physiology

Table 2. Paraquat-induced lung fibrosis

Species	Dose (mg/kg)	Duration (days)	Assays used[a]	Reference
Chick embryo			H	Lutz-Ostertag and Henou (1975)
Dog			H	Kelly et al. (1976)
Guinea pig	20–25, p.o.	7	H	Murray and Gibson (1972)
Hamster	3–12, s.c.	84	H	Butler (1975)
Human			H	Russel et al. (1981)
Human			H	Higenbottam et al. (1979)
Human		22	H	Dearden et al. (1978)
Human			H	Smith and Heath (1974a)
Monkey	35–126, p.o.	21	H	Murray and Gibson (1972)
Mouse		28	H	Popenoe (1979)
Mouse	750 ppm, p.o.	280	H	Niden and Khurana (1976)
Rabbit	10^{-1}–10^{-12} g, intrabronchial	14	H	Zavala and Rhodes (1978)
Rat	101–252, p.o.	14	H	Murray and Gibson (1972)
Rat	24, i.p.	3	B	Greenberg et al. (1978a)
Rat	24, i.p.	7	B, H	Greenberg et al. (1978b)
Rat	25, i.p.	9	B	Kuttan et al. (1979)
Rat	25, i.p.	8	H	Roujeau et al. (1973)
Rat	25, i.p.	21	B	Hollinger and Chvapil (1977)
Rat	25–35, i.p.	18–25	B	Hollinger et al. (1978)
Rat	5–10, i.p., multiple	28	H	Cegla et al. (1975)
Rat	20, i.p.	7	B	Thompson and Patrick (1978)
Rat	5, i.p., multiple	10	B	Griffin et al. (1979)
Rat	25, i.p.	42	H	Vijeyaratnam and Corrin (1971)
Rat	20–100, i.p.	45	H	Smith et al. (1974)
Rat	30–40, i.p.	4	H	Smith and Heath (1974b)
Rat	24, i.p.	7	B	Reiser and Last (1981)
Rat	10^{-5}–10^{-12} g, intrabronchial	14	H	Wyatt et al. (1981)
Rat, human	32–133 mg, percutaneously	84	H	Levin et al. (1979)
Rat	10–30, i.p.	8	H	Wasan and McElligot (1972)
Rat	3–6, i.v., 150–400, p.o.	13	H	Kimbrough and Gaines (1970)
Rat			B	Hussain and Bhatnagar (1979)
Rat	25	3	H	Thurlbeck and Thurlbeck (1976)

[a] B = biochemistry; H = histology; i.p. = intraperitoneal; i.v. = intravenous; p.o. = peroral; s.c. = subcutaneous

Table 3. Radiation-induced lung fibrosis

Species	Dose (rad $\times 10^{-3}$)	Duration (months)	Assays used [a]	Reference
Baboon	3–4	12	B, H, P	COLLINS et al. (1978 b)
Baboon, rat	50–150 nCi/g	24	B, H	METIVIER et al. (1977)
Baboon	3–4	12	B, P	FINE et al. (1979)
Baboon		28	B, H	METIVIER et al. (1974)
Dog	20–55	6	B	PICKRELL et al. (1975)
Dog	8–86	23	B, H, P	PICKRELL et al. (1978)
Dog	1.2	4.5	P	TYREE et al. (1966)
Dog	4.9–12	11	P	MAUDERLY et al. (1973)
Hamster	2–14	6	B, H, P	PICKRELL et al. (1976 b)
Hamster	90	4.5	H	DIEL and SHORT (1979)
Hamster	90	4	B, H, P	PICKRELL et al. (1976 a)
Hamster	2–6	9	B, H	PICKRELL et al. (1975)
Mouse	2–4	11	B	LAW et al. (1976)
Mouse	0.2	0.5	B, H	HASCHEK et al. (1980)
Mouse, Rat	0.65–1.1 3	6	H	ADAMSON et al. (1970)
Rat			B	DR'OZDZ et al. (1981 a)
Rat			B	DR'OZDZ et al. (1981 b)
Rat	0.75–1.5	5	B, P	DUBRAWSKY et al. (1978)
Rat	0.5–1	1	B	GERBER et al. (1961)
Rat	2.4		H	KUROHARA and CASARETT (1972)
Rat	50–150 nCi/g	24	B	METIVIER et al. (1980)
Rat	0.4–0.8	0.2	B	THYAGARAJAN et al. (1976)
Rat	0.15–0.16	5	B	TSEVELA (1974)
Rat	1–3	8	H	WATANABE (1974)

[a] B = biochemistry; H = histology; P = physiology

Table 4. Silica-induced lung fibrosis

Species	Duration (months)	Assays used [a]	Reference
Guinea pig	6	B, H	DAUBER et al. (1980)
Guinea pig	16	B, H	KAW and ZAIDI (1969)
Hamster	16	H	GROSS et al. (1967)
Mouse	7	H	SAHU et al. (1975)
Rabbit	6	B	DALE (1973)
Rabbit	4	H	POWELL and GOUGH (1959)
Rat	7	B, H	KAW and ZAIDI (1970)
Rat	10	B, H	ZAIDI and KAW (1970)
Rat	6	H	SHANKER et al. (1975)
Rat	5	B, H	SINGH et al. (1977)
Rat	6	B	LINDY et al. (1970)
Rat	4	B, H	HURYCH et al. (1980)
Rat	5	B	HURYCH et al. (1981)
Rat	2	B	MIREJOVSKA et al. (1981)
Rat	12	H	LE BOUFFANT et al. (1977)
Rat	8	B, H	RENNE et al. (1980)
Rat	3	B, H	KYSELA et al. (1973)
Rat	11	H	DAVIS et al. (1981)

Table 4 (continued)

Species	Duration (months)	Assays used[a]	Reference
Rat	6	H	Green et al. (1981)
Rat	0.4	B	Junge-Hulsing et al. (1968)
Rat	13	B	Vasileva and Miagkaia (1970)
Rat	6	B, H	Halme et al. (1970)
Rat	15	H	King et al. (1953)
Rat	14	H	King et al. (1950)
Rat	12–24	B, H	Le Bouffant et al. (1975)
Rat	24	B, H	Martin et al. (1975)
Rat	10	B, P	McDermott et al. (1975)
Rat	19	H	Heppleston et al. (1970)
Rat, hamster, guinea pig	14	H	Gross and de Treville (1968)
Rat		H	Heppleston (1975)
Rat	28	H	Corrin and King (1969)
Rat	4	B, H, P	Kuncova et al. (1972)
Rat	1	B	Chvapil et al. (1979)
Rat	4	B	Chvapil (1967)
Rat	11	B	Rodkina (1974)
Rat	4	B	Babuskina (1975)
Rat	20	B	Belobragina and Medvedev (1975)
Rat			Huang et al. (1981)
Rat	8	B	Swensson (1970)
Rat		H	Arutiunov et al. (1975)
Rat	5	B, H	Levene et al. (1968)
Rat	8	B, H	Daniel-Moussard et al. (1970)
Rat		B	Konno et al. (1975)
Rat, guinea pig, monkey	18	B, H, P	Groth et al. (1981)
Rat	0.5	B, H	Reiser et al. (1982)
Rat	12	B, H, P	Reiser et al. (1983)

[a] B = biochemistry; H = histology; P = physiology

Table 5. Miscellaneous gaseous agents reported to produce lung fibrosis

Agent	Species	Duration (months)	Assays used[a]	Reference
NO$_2$	Human, rodents		H	Guidotti (1978)
NO$_2$	Human		P	Horvath et al. (1978)
NO$_2$	Rat	12	B	Pickrell et al. (1981)
NO$_2$	Rat	24	H	Stephens et al. (1971)
Oxygen	Guinea pig	0.3	B	Richmond and D'Aoust (1976)
Oxygen	Human	1	H	Gould et al. (1972)
Oxygen	Mouse	0.25	H	Adamson and Bowden (1976)
Oxygen	Mouse	0.5	B, H	Witschi et al. (1981)
Oxygen	Rat	0.5	B	Riley et al. (1980)
Oxygen	Rat	1	H	Frank and Roberts (1979)
Oxygen	Rat	1	B, H	Valimaki et al. (1975)

Table 5 (continued)

Agent	Species	Duration (months)	Assays used[a]	Reference
Oxygen	Rat	3	B	CHVAPIL and PENG (1975)
Oxygen	Rat	0.3	H	PARIENTE et al. (1969)
Ozone	Dog	100	B	ORTHOEFER et al. (1976)
Ozone	Dog	18	H	FREEMAN et al. (1973)
Ozone	Guinea pig, rat, hamster	14	H	STOKINGER et al. (1957)
Ozone	Monkey	0.25	B	LAST et al. (1981)
Ozone	Rabbit		B	BUELL et al. (1965)
Ozone	Rat	0.25	B	HUSSAIN et al. (1976)
Ozone	Rat	0.75	B, H	LAST et al. (1979)
Ozone	Rat	8	B	LAST and GREENBERG (1980)
Ozone	Rat	0.25	B	REISER and LAST (1981)
Ozone	Rat	1	P	BARTLETT et al. (1974)
Ozone	Rat	0.25	B	CROSS et al. (1981)
Ozone	Rat	0.25	B	HESTERBERG and LAST (1981)
Ozone	Rat	6	H	FREEMAN et al. (1974)
Ozone	Rat	3	H	BOORMAN et al. (1980)

[a] B = biochemistry; H = histology; P = physiology

Table 6. Miscellaneous non-gaseous agents reported to produce lung fibrosis

Agents	Species	Duration (months)	Assays used[a]	Reference
Alumina	Rat	15	H	KING et al. (1955)
Aluminum powder, intratracheal	Hamster, guinea pig	24	H	GROSS et al. (1973)
Asbestos	Guinea pig	18	H	HOLT (1974)
Asbestos	Guinea pig	18	H	HOLT et al. (1966)
Asbestos	Guinea pig	3	B	JAISWAL (1981)
Asbestos	Rat	12	H, P	CRAPO et al. (1980)
Asbestos	Guinea pig, rat	18	H	BOTHAM and HOLT (1972)
Asbestos	Human		H	MORGENROTH (1974)
Asbestos	Human		H	WOITOWITZ (1972)
Asbestos	Guinea pig	4	B, H	SINGH et al. (1976)
Asbestos	Rat	5	B	RAHMAN et al. (1975)
Asbestos	Rat	15	B, H	DAVIS and REEVES (1971)
Beryllium	Rat		B	IVANOVA (1971)
Busulfan	Human	120	H, P	BURNS et al. (1970)
Busulfan	Human		H	KAY (1970)
Butylated hydroxytoluene (BHT)	Mouse	0.3	H	ADAMSON et al. (1977)
BHT	Mouse		H	BRODY et al. (1981)
BHT	Mouse	12	B, H	HASCHEK et al. (1981)
BHT	Mouse	0.5	B, H	HASCHEK et al. (1980)
BHT	Mouse	0.75	H	HASCHEK and WITSCHI (1979)
BHT	Mouse	0.5	B	KEHRER (1982)

Table 6 (continued)

Agents	Species	Duration (months)	Assays used[a]	Reference
BHT	Mouse	0.5	B	KEHRER and WITSCHI (1981)
BHT	Mouse	0.5	B	KEHRER and WITSCHI (1980)
BHT	Mouse	0.25	H	SMITH and BRODY (1981)
BHT	Mouse	0.5	B, H	WITSCHI et al. (1981)
BHT	Mouse		H	WITSCHI et al. (1980)
Cadmium	Rat	10	H	MILLER et al. (1974)
Cadmium	Human		P	SMITH et al. (1976)
CdCl$_2$	Rat	0.75	H	DERVAN and HAYES (1979)
CdCl$_2$	Rat	10	H	MILLER et al. (1974)
CdCl$_2$	Hamster	1.25	H, P	NIEWOEHNER and HOIDAL (1982)
CdCl$_2$	Rat	0.3	H	PALMER et al. (1976)
Carrageenan	Rat	17	H	BOWERS et al. (1980)
Cemented tungsten carbide	Rat	6	H	KITAMURA (1980)
Cigarette smoke	Mouse	0.7	B	ROSENKRANTZ et al. (1969)
Coal dust	Human		B	LOXLEY (1979)
Coal dust	Human		B	WAGNER et al. (1975)
Cobalt	Pig		H, P	KERFOOT et al. (1975)
Concanavalin A	Rabbit	2	H	WILLOUGHBY et al. (1979)
Cyclophosphamide	Mouse	0.75	B	HAKKINEN et al. (1982)
Cyclophosphamide	Rat	1	H	GOULD and MILLER (1975)
Dehydromono-crotaline	Dog	1	H	RACZNIAK et al. (1979)
Fluoride	Rabbit		B	SUSHEELA and MUKERJEE (1981)
Fluoride	Rat	3	B	DR'OZDZ et al. (1979)
Freund's adjuvant	Guinea pig	0.6	H	VON WICHERT and MORGENROTH (1976)
Hair spray	Human		H	WRIGHT and COCKCROFT (1981)
Hay dust	Guinea pig	6	H	ZAIDI et al. (1971)
Methylcyclopenta-dienyl manganese tricarbonyl	Mouse	0.75	B, H	WITSCHI et al. (1981)
Methysergide	Human	24–36	H	GRAHAM (1967)
Methysergide	Human	72	H	HINDLE et al. (1981)
Methysergide	Human	9–54	H	GRAHAM et al. (1966)
Mineral oil	Rat	1.5	H	ECKERT et al. (1979)
N-nitroso-N-methylurethane	Hamster	20	H	RYAN (1972)
Nitrofurantoin	Human	16	H	HAINER and WHITE (1981)
Nitrofurantoin	Rat		H	BOYD et al. (1979)
Oil shale	Rat	24	B, H	RENNE et al. (1980)
Penicillamine	Rat	2	B, P	HOFFMAN et al. (1972)
Phorbol myristate acetate	Rat	0.20	H	JOHNSON and WARD (1982)
Polyvinylchloride	Human	276	H	ARNAUD et al. (1978)
Titanium phosphate	Rat, hamster	18	H	GROSS et al. (1977)
Trypsin aerosol	Rat	0.1	B	COUNTS and KNIGHTEN (1977)
Volcanic ash	Rat	6	H	GREEN et al. (1981)
Welding dust residue	Rat	9	B	NAUMENKO (1966)

[a] B = biochemistry; H = histology; P = physiology

Table 7. Protease-induced emphysema

Species	Protease used	Duration (weeks)	Assays used [a]	Reference
Dog	Elastase neutrophil, human		H	JANOFF et al. (1977)
Dog	Papain	12	B, H	OSMAN et al. (1980)
Dog	Elastase leukocyte, human		B, H	JANOFF et al. (1979)
Dog	Elastase pancreatic, pig		P	POLZIN et al. (1979)
Dog	Papain aerosol	5	H, P	MARCO et al. (1972)
Hamster	Papain	3	H	SNIDER et al. (1974)
Hamster	Elastase pancreatic, pig	16	B, H	KUHN et al. (1976)
Hamster	Elastase leukocyte, human	8	B, H	SENIOR et al. (1977)
Hamster	Elastase pancreatic, pig	4	B	YU et al. (1978)
Hamster	Elastase pancreatic, pig	4	B	YU and KELLER (1978)
Hamster	Elastase pancreatic, pig	8	B, H	KUHN and STARCHER (1980)
Hamster	Elastase pancreatic, pig		B, H	KUHN et al. (1980)
Hamster	Papain aerosol $+NO_2$	1.5	H, P	NIEWOEHNER and KLEINERMAN (1973)
Hamster	Papain	1	H	MARTORANA (1976)
Hamster	Elastase pancreatic, pig	3	H, P	SNIDER et al. (1977)
Hamster	Papain	9	B, H	KILBURN et al. (1971)
Hamster	Elastase pancreatic, pig	3	H, P	SNIDER and KORTHY (1978)
Hamster	Elastase pancreatic, pig	3	H, P	SCHUYLER et al. (1978)
Hamster	Elastase pancreatic, pig	3	B, H	STONE et al. (1976)
Hamster	Elastase pancreatic, pig	3	B	GOLDSTEIN and STARCHER (1978)
Hamster	Elastase		B	AKIRA and YEH (1978)

Table 7 (continued)

Species	Protease used	Duration (weeks)	Assays used [a]	Reference
Hamster	Papain		B	ZIMMERMAN et al. (1981)
Hamster	Elastase pancreatic, pig	2	B	STONE et al. (1982)
Hamster	Elastase pancreatic, pig	17	B, H	KLEINERMAN et al. (1980)
Rabbit	Proteases, *Pseudomonas*	1	H	GRAY and KREGER (1979)
Rabbit	Papain	4	B	COLLINS et al. (1978 a)
Rabbit	Papain	35	H, P	CALDWELL (1971)
Rat	Papain	26	H	JOHANSON et al. (1973)
Rat	Papain	66	H, P	JOHANSON and PIERCE (1973)
Rat	Papain aerosol	5	P	SAHEBJAMI and VASSALLO (1976)

[a] B = biochemistry; H = histology; P = physiology

Table 8. Miscellaneous agents reported to produce emphysema

Agent	Species	Duration (weeks)	Assays used [a]	Reference
Betamethasone	Monkey fetus		H	BECK et al. (1980)
$CdCl_2$	Hamster	5	H, P	NIEWOHNER and HOIDAL (1982)
$CdCl_2$	Rat, mouse		B	SINGHAL et al. (1976)
$CdCl_2$	Rat		H	SNIDER et al. (1973)
Carbon disulfide	Rat	56	B	WEGROWSKI (1980)
Cigarette smoke	Rat		H	BLUE and JANOFF (1978)
Cigarette smoke	Rat		B	JANOFF et al. (1978)
Kerosene	Rat	2	H, P	SCHARF et al. (1981)
NO_2	Guinea pig	26	B, H	DR'OZDZ et al. (1977)
NO_2	Hamster	4	B	KLEINERMAN and SORENSEN (1982)
NO_2	Hamster	70	H	KLEINERMAN (1977)
NO_2	Hamster	6	B	KLEINERMAN and IP (1979)
NO_2	Mouse	8	H, P	RANGA and KLEINERMAN (1981)
NO_2	Rat	70	H	JUHOS et al. (1980)
NO_2	Rat	100	H	STEPHENS et al. (1971)
NO_2	Rat	52	H	PICKRELL et al. (1981)
NO_2	Review			GUIDOTTI (1978)
Ozone	Guinea pig	14	H	STOKINGER et al. (1957)

[a] B = biochemistry; H = histology; P = physiology

References

Aalto M, Kulonen E (1979) Fractionation of connective-tissue-activating factors from the culture medium of silica-treated macrophages. Acta Pathol Microbiol Scand [C]87:241–250

Adamson IY (1976) Pulmonary toxicity of bleomycin. Environ Health Perspect 16:119–125

Adamson IYR, Bowden DM (1974) The pathogenesis of bleomycin-induced pulmonary fibrosis in mice. Am J Pathol 77:185–198

Adamson YI, Bowden DH (1976) Pulmonary injury and repair. Organ culture studies of murine lung after oxygen. Arch Pathol Lab Med 100:640–643

Adamson IYR, Bowden DH, Wyatt JP (1970) A pathway to pulmonary fibrosis: An ultrastructural study of mouse and rat following radiation to the whole body and hemithorax. Am J Pathol 58:481–498

Adamson IYR, Bowden DH, Cote MG, Witschi H (1977) Lung injury induced by butylated hydroxytoluene. Lab Invest 36:26–32

Akira Y, Yeh YS (1978) Study on the metabolism of insoluble elastin in hamster lungs during experimental (elastase induced) emphysema. Nippon Kyobu Shikkan Gakkai Zasshi 16:151–156

Allison AC, Harington JS, Birbeck M (1966) An examination of the cytotoxic effects of silica on macrophages. J Exp Med 124:141–154

Antoniades HN, Scher CD, Stiles CD (1979) Purification of human platelet derived growth factor. Proc Natl Acad Sci USA 76:1790–1813

Arnaud A, Pommier de Santi PP, Garbe L, Payan H, Charpin J (1978) Polyvinyl chloride pneumoconiosis. Thorax 33(1):19–25

Arutiunov VD, Batsura ID, Kruglikov GG (1975) The structure of fibroblasts and the fibrous structures of connective tissue according to raster electron microscopic findings. Arkh Patol 37:10–15

Babuskina LG (1975) The effect of polyvinylpyridine-N-oxide on lipid metabolism indices in healthy and silicotic rats. Farmakol Toksikol 38:337–341

Bachofen M, Weibel ER (1974) Basic pattern of tissue repair in human lungs following unspecific injury. Chest [Suppl] 65:19S–21S

Bartlett D Jr, Faulkner CS, Cook K (1974) Effect of chronic ozone exposure on lung elasticity of young rats. J Appl Physiol 37:92–96

Bateman E, Turner-Warwick M, Adelmann-Grill BC (1981) Immunohistochemical study of collagen types in human foetal lung and fibrotic lung disease. Thorax 36:645–653

Beck JC, Mitzner W, Johnson JWC, Hutchins GM, Foidart J, London WT, Palmer AE, Scott R (1980) Betamethasone and the rhesus fetus: effect on lung morphometry and connective tissue. Pediatr Res 15:235–240

Belobragina GV, Medvedev LA (1975) Collagen fractions in the lung tissue of white rats with experimental silicosis caused by crystallized and condensate silicon dioxide. Gig Sanit 3:119–120

Bitterman PB, Rennard SI, Crystal RG (1981) Environmental lung disease and the interstitium. Clin Chest Med 2:393–412

Bitterman PB, Rennard SE, Hunninghake GW, Crystal RG (1982) Human alveolar macrophage, growth factor for fibroblasts. J Clin Invest 70:806–822

Blue M, Janoff A (1978) Possible mechanisms of emphysema in cigarette smokers. Am Rev Respir Dis 117:317–325

Boorman GA, Schwartz LW, Dungworth DL (1980) Pulmonary effects of prolonged ozone insult in rats. Lab Invest 43:108–115

Botham SK, Holt PF (1972) The effects of inhaled crocidolites from Transvaal and northwest cape mines on the lungs of rats and guinea-pigs. Br J Exp Pathol 53:612–620

Bower RR, Houstin F, Clinton R, Lewis M, Ballard R (1980) A histological study of the carrageenan-induced granuloma in the rat lung. J Pathol 132(3):243–253

Boyd MR, Catignani GL, Sasame HA, Mitchell JR, Stiko AW (1979) Acute pulmonary injury in rats by nitrofurantoin and modification by vitamin E, dietary fat, and oxygen. Am Rev Respir Dis 120:93–99

Briscoe AM, Loring WE (1958) Elastin content of the human lung. Proc Soc Exp Biol Med 99:162–164

Brody AR, Soler P, Basset F, Haschek WM, Witschi H (1981) Epithelial-mesenchymal associations of cells in human pulmonary fibrosis and in BHT-oxygen-induced fibrosis in mice. Exp Lung Res 2(3):207–220

Buell GC, Tokiwa Y, Mueller PK (1965) Potential crosslinking agents in lung tissue. Formation and isolation after in vivo exposure to ozone. Arch Environ Health 10:213–219

Burns WA, McFarland W, Matthews MJ (1970) Busulfan-induced pulmonary disease. Am Rev Respir Dis 101:408–413

Burrell R (1981) Immunologic aspects of silica. In: Dunnom DD (ed) Health effects of synthetic silica particulates. American Society for Testing and Materials, Philadelphia, pp 82–92

Burrell R, Anderson M (1973) The induction of fibrogenesis by silica-treated alveolar macrophages. Environ Res 6:389–394

Bus JS, Aust SD, Gibson JE (1975) Lipid peroxidation: a possible mechanism for paraquat toxicity. Res Commun Chem Pathol Pharmacol 11:31–38

Butler C (1975) Pulmonary interstitial fibrosis from paraquat in the hamster. Arch Pathol Lab Med 99:503–507

Caldwell EJ (1971) Physiologic and anatomic effects of papain on the rabbit lung. J Appl Physiol 31:458–465

Cassan SM, Divertie MB, Brown AL (1974) Fine structural morphometry on biopsy specimens of human lungs. Chest 65:269–274

Cegla UH, Kroidl RF, Kronberger H, Weber H (1975) Experimental animal model of lung fibrosis in the rat by the injection of paraquat. Pneumonologie 152:65–74

Chrzanowski P, Keller S, Cereta J, Mandl I, Turino GM (1980) Elastin content of normal and emphysematous lung parenchyma. Am J Med 69:351–359

Chvapil M (1967) Conflicting hypotheses on experimental silicotic fibrogenesis: new experimental data. Environ Res 1:89–101

Chvapil M, Peng YM (1975) Oxygen and lung fibrosis. Arch Environ Health 30:528–532

Chvapil M, Eskelson CD, Stiffel V, Owen JA (1979) Early changes in the chemical composition of the rat lung after silica administration. Arch Environ Health 34:402–406

Clark JG, Starcher BC, Uitto J (1980a) Bleomycin-induced synthesis of type I procollagen by human lung and skin fibroblasts in culture. Biochim Biophys Acta 631:359–370

Clark JG, Overton JE, Marino BA, Uitto J, Starcher BC (1980b) Collagen biosynthesis in bleomycin-induced pulmonary fibrosis in hamsters. J Lab Clin Med 96:943–953

Clark JM, Lambertsen CJ (1971) Pulmonary oxygen toxicity: a review. Pharmacol Rev 23:37–114

Cohen S (1981) Regulation of lymphokine-dependent reactions. Fed Proc 40:51–53

Collins JF, Durnin LS, Johanson WG Jr (1978a) Papain-induced lung injury: alterations in connective tissue metabolism without emphysema. Exp Mol Pathol 29:29–36

Collins JF, Johanson WG Jr, McCullough B, Jones MA, Waugh HJ Jr (1978b) Effects of compensatory lung growth in irradiation-induced regional pulmonary fibrosis in the baboon. Am Rev Respir Dis 117:1079–1089

Collins JF, McCullough B, Coalson JJ, Johanson WG Jr (1981) Bleomycin-induced diffuse interstitial pulmonary fibrosis in baboons. II. Further studies on connective tissue changes. Am Rev Respir Dis 123:305–312

Comis RL (1978) Bleomycin pulmonary toxicity. In: Carter SK, Crooke ST, Umezawa H (eds) Bleomycin. Academic, New York, pp 279–291

Corrin B, King E (1969) Experimental endogenous lipid pneumonia and silicosis. J Pathol 97:325–330

Counts DF, Knighten P (1977) Collagen and noncollagen protein synthesis in the lungs of rats exposed to a trypsin aerosol. Conn Tissue Res 5:165–170

Counts DF, Evans JN, Dipetrillo TA, Sterling KM Jr, Kelley J (1981) Collagen lysyl oxidase activity in the lung increases during bleomycin-induced lung fibrosis. J Pharmacol Exp Ther 219:675–678

Craighead JE, Mossman BT (1982) The pathogenesis of asbestos-associated diseases. N Engl J Med 306:1446–1482

Crapo JD, Barry BE, Brody AR, O'Neil JJ (1980) Morphological, morphometric and x-ray microanalytical studies on lung tissue of rats exposed to chrysotile asbestos in inhalation chambers. Biol Eff Miner Fibres 1:273–283

Cross CE, Hesterberg TW, Reiser KM, Last JA (1981) Ozone toxicity as a model of lung fibrosis. Chest 80:52–54

Dale K (1973) A method for inducing unilateral silicosis in rabbits by an injection technique with some observations on lung clearance and quantitative evaluation of experimental silicosis. Scand J Respir Dis 54:157–167

Daniel-Moussard H, Martin JC, Le Bouffant L (1970) Experimental study of the action of nitrous vapours on the dust-containing lung. Poumon Coeur 26:905–912

Dauber JH, Rossman MD, Pietra GG, Jimenez SA, Daniele RP (1980) Experimental silicosis; morphologic and biochemical abnormalities produced by intratracheal instillation of quartz into guinea pig lungs. Am J Pathol 101:595–612

Davis HW, Reeves AL (1971) Collagen biosynthesis in rat lungs during exposure to asbestos. Am Ind Hyg Assoc J 32:599–602

Davis GS, Hemenway DR, Evans JN, Lapenas DJ, Brody AR (1981) Alveolar macrophage stimulation and population changes in silica-exposed rats. Chest [Suppl] 80:8S–10S

Dearden LC, Fairshter RD, McRae DM, Smith WR, Glauser FL, Wilson AF (1978) Pulmonary ultrastructure of the late aspects of human paraquat poisoning. Am J Pathol 93:667–680

DeLustro F, Sherer GK, Le Roy EC (1980) Human monocyte stimulation of fibroblast growth by a soluble mediator(s). J Reticuloendothel Soc 28:579–532

Dervan PA, Hayes JA (1979) Peribronchiolar fibrosis following acute experimental lung damage by cadmium aerosol. J Pathol 128:143–149

Diel JH, Short RK (1979) Collagen localization in lung parenchyma irradiated by inhaled $^{238}PuO_2$ particles. Radiat Res 79:417–423

Dr'ozdz M, Kucharz E, Szyja J (1977) Effect of chronic exposure to nitrogen dioxide on collagen content in lung and skin of guinea pigs. Environ Res 13:369–377

Dr'ozdz M, Kuchar'z E, Bara'nska-Cachowska M, Grucka-Mamczar E, Piewowarczyk B (1979) Collagen metabolism in animals exposed to hydrogen fluoride. Gig Tr Prof Zabol 11:35–58

Dr'ozdz M, Antoniewicz M, Kucharz E (1981 a) Study of the collagen structure in the subacute radiation syndrome with white rats. Z Gesamte Hyg 27:753–755

Dr'ozdz M, Piwowarczyk B, Olozyk K (1981 b) Effect of ionizing radiation on the contents of total collagen and collagen fractions and activity of collagenolytic enzymes in rat tissues. Med Pr 32:317–322

Dubrawsky C, Dubravsky NB, Withers HR (1978) The effect of colchicine on the accumulation of hydroxypyroline and on lung compliance after irradiation. Radiat Res 73:111–120

Eckert H, Jerochin S, Winsel K (1979) Ultrastructural and autoradiographical investigations of early changes in experimental lung fibrosis. Z Erkr Atmungsorgane 152(1):37–41

Ellison JM, Waller RE (1978) A review of sulphur oxides and particulate matter as air pollutants with particular reference to effects on health in the United Kingdom. Environ Res 17:302–325

Epstein EH (1974) [α_1(III)3] human skin collagen. Release by pepsin digestion and preponderance in fetal life. J Biol Chem 249:3225–3231

Evans JN, Kelley J, Low RB, Adler KB (1982) Increased contractility of isolated lung parenchyma in an animal model of pulmonary fibrosis induced by bleomycin. Am Rev Respir Dis 125:89–94

Eyre DR (1980) Collagen: Molecular diversity in the body's protein scaffold. Science 207:1315–1322

Fedullo AJ, Karlinsky JB, Snider GL, Goldstein RH (1980) Lung statics and connective tissues after penicillamine in bleomycin-treated hamsters. J Appl Physiol 49:1083–1090

Finch WR, Rodnan GP, Buckingham RB, Prince RK, Winkelstein A (1980) Bleomycin-induced scleroderma. J Rheumatol 7:651–659

Fine R, McCullough B, Collins JF, Johanson WG Jr (1979) Lung elasticity in regional and diffuse pulmonary fibrosis. J Appl Physiol 47:138–144

Fitzpatrick M, Hospelhorn VD (1962) Studies on human pulmonary connective tissue. I. Amino acid composition of elastin isolated by alkaline digestion. J Lab Clin Med 60:799–810

Frank L, Roberts RJ (1979) Endotoxin protection against oxygen-induced acute and chronic lung injury. J Appl Physiol Respir Environ Exercise Physiol 47:577–581

Freeman G, Stephens RJ, Coffin DL, Stara JF (1973) Changes in dogs' lungs after long-term exposure to ozone. Arch Environ Health 26:209–216

Freeman G, Juhos LT, Furiosi NJ, Mussenden R, Stephens RJ, Evans MJ (1974) Pathology of pulmonary disease from exposure to interdependent ambient gases (NO_2 and O_3). Arch Environ Health 29:203–210

Gardner DE, Miller JF, Illing JW, Kirtz JM (1977) Increased infectivity with exposure to ozone and sulfuric acid. Toxicol Lett 1:59–74

Gay S, Muller PK, Meigel WM (1976) Polymorphie des Kollagens. Neue Aspekte für Struktur und Funktion des Bindegewebes. Hautarzt 27:196–205

Gerber GB, Gerber G, Altman KK, Hempelmann LH (1961) Studies on the metabolism of tissue proteins. II. Influence of x-irradiation and starvation on the metabolism of collagen. Int J Radiol Biol 4:609–614

Giri SN, Schwartz LW, Hollinger MA, Freywald ME, Schiedt MJ, Zuckerman JE (1980) Biochemical and structural alterations of hamster lungs in response to intratracheal administration of bleomycin. Exp Mol Pathol 33:1–14

Goldstein RA, Starcher BC (1978) Urinary excretion of elastin peptides containing desmosine after intratracheal injection of elastase in hamsters. J Clin Invest 61:1286–1290

Goldstein RH, Lucey EC, Franzblau C, Snider GL (1979) Failure of mechanical properties to parallel changes in lung connective tissue composition in bleomycin-induced pulmonary fibrosis in hamsters. Am Rev Respir Dis 120:67–73

Gould VE, Miller J (1975) Sclerosing alveolitis induced by cyclophosphamide. Ultrastructural observations of alveolar injury and repair. Am J Pathol 81(3):513–530

Gould VE, Tsoco R, Wheelis RF, Gould NS, Kapanci Y (1972) Oxygen pneumonitis in man. Lab Invest 26:499–508

Graham JR (1967) Cardiac and pulmonary fibrosis during methysergide therapy for headache. Am J Med Sci 254:1–12

Graham JR, Suby HI, LeCompte PR, Sadowsky NL (1966) Fibrotic disorders associated with methysergide therapy for headache. N Engl J Med 274:359–368

Gray L, Kreger A (1979) Microscopic characterization of rabbit lung damage produced by Pseudomonas aeruginosa proteases. Infect Immun 23:150–159

Green FHY, Vallyathan V, Mentnech MS, Tucker JH, Merchant JA, Kiessling PJ, Antonius JA, Parshley P (1981) Is volcanic ash a pneumoconiosis risk? Nature 293:216–217

Greenberg DB, Lyons SA, Last JA (1978a) Paraquat-induced changes in the rate of collagen biosynthesis by rat lung explants. J Lab Clin Med 92:1033–1042

Greenberg DB, Reiser KM, Last JA (1978b) Correlation of biochemical and morphologic manifestations of acute pulmonary fibrosis in rats administered paraquat. Chest 74:421–425

Griffin M, Smith LL, Wynne J (1979) Changes in transglutaminase activity in an experimental model of pulmonary fibrosis induced by paraquat. Br J Exp Pathol 60:653–661

Gross NJ (1977) Pulmonary effects of radiation therapy. Ann Intern Med 86:81–92

Gross NJ (1981) The pathogenesis of radiation induced lung damage. Lung 159:115–125

Gross P, Treville RTP de (1968) Alveolar proteinosis. Arch Pathol Lab Med 86:255–261

Gross P, Villiers AJ de, Treville RTP de (1967) Experimental silicosis: The "atypical" reaction in the Syrian hamster. Arch Pathol Lab Med 84:87–94

Gross P, Harky RA Jr, Treville RTP de (1973) Pulmonary reaction to metallic aluminum powders. Arch Environ Health 26:227–236

Gross P, Kociba RJ, Sparschu GL, Norris JM (1977) The biologic response to titanium phosphate. A new synthetic mineral fiber. Arch Pathol Lab Med 101:550–554

Groth DH, Moorman WJ, Lynch DW, Stettler LE, Wagner WD, Hornung RW (1981) Chronic effects of inhaled amorphous silica in animals. In: Dunnom DD (ed) Health effects of synthetic silica particulates. ASTM, Philadelphia, pp 118–143 (STP 732)

Guidotti TL (1978) The higher oxides of nitrogen: Inhalation toxicology. Environ Res 15:443–472

Hainer BL, White AA (1981) Nitrofurantoin pulmonary toxicity. J Fam Pract 13:817–823

Hakkinen PJ, Whiteley JW, Witschi HR (1982) Hyperoxia, but not thoracic x-irradiation, potentiates bleomycin- and cyclophosphamide-induced lung damage in mice. Am Rev Respir Dis 126:281–285

Halme J, Uitto J, Kahanpää K, Karhunen P, Lindy S (1970) Protocollagen proline hydroxylase activity in experimental pulmonary fibrosis of rats. J Lab Clin Med 75:535–541

Hance AJ, Crystal RG (1976) Collagen. In: Crystal RD (ed) The biochemical basis of pulmonary function. Marcel Dekker, New York, pp 215–271

Haschek WM, Witschi H (1979) Pulmonary fibrosis: A possible mechanism. Toxicol Appl Pharmacol 51:475–487

Haschek WM, Meyer KR, Ullrich RL, Witschi H (1980) Potentiation of chemically induced lung fibrosis by thorax irradiation. Int J Radiat Oncol Biol Phys 6:449–455

Haschek WM, Klein-Szanto AJP, Last JA, Reiser KM, Witschi H (1982) Long-term morphologic and biochemical features of experimentally-induced lung fibrosis in the mouse. Lab Invest 46:438–449

Haschek WM, Reiser KM, Klein-Szanto AJP, Kehrer JP, Smith LH, Last JA, Witschi HP (1983) Potentiation of butylated hydroxytoluene-induced acute lung damage by oxygen. Cell kinetics and collagen metabolism. Am Rev Respir Dis 127:28–34

Hazuka M, Bates DV (1975) Combined effects of ozone and sulphur dioxide on human pulmonary function. Nature 257:50–51

Heppleston AG (1975) Pulmonary alveolar lipo-proteinosis. Am J Pathol 78:171–174

Heppleston AG, Styles JA (1967) Activity of a macrophage factor in collagen formation by silica. Nature 214:521–522

Heppleston AG, Wright NA, Stewart JA (1970) Experimental alveolar lipo-proteinosis following the inhalation of silica. J Pathol 101:293–307

Hesterberg TW, Last JA (1981) Ozone-induced acute pulmonary fibrosis in rats. Prevention of increased rates of collagen synthesis by methylprednisolone. Am Rev Respir Dis 123:47–52

Hesterberg TW, Gerriets JE, Reiser KM, Jackson AC, Cross CE, Last JE (1981) Bleomycin-induced pulmonary fibrosis: correlation of biochemical, physiological, and histological changes. Toxicol Appl Pharmacol 60:360–367

Higenbottam T, Crome P, Parkinson C, Nunn J (1979) Further clinical observations on the pulmonary effects of paraquat ingestion. Thorax 34:161–165

Hindle W, Posner E, Sweetnam MT, Tan RSH (1981) Pleural effusion and fibrosis during treatment with methysergide. Br Med J 1:605–606

Hoffman L, Blumenfeld OO, Mondshine RB, Park SS (1972) Effect of DL-penicillamine on fibrous proteins of rat lung. J Appl Physiol 33:42–45

Hogg JX, Nepszy SJ, Macklem PT, Thurlbeck WM (1969) Elastic properties of the centrilobular space. J Clin Invest 48:1306–1312

Hollinger MA, Chvapil M (1977) Effect of paraquat on rat lung prolyl hydroxylase. Res Commun Chem Pathol Pharmacol 16:159–162

Hollinger MA, Zuckerman JE, Giri SN (1978) Effect of acute and chronic paraquat on rat lung collagen content. Res Commun Chem Pathol Pharmacol 21:295–306

Holt PF (1974) Small animals in the study of the pathological effects of asbestos. Environ Health Perspect 9:205–211

Holt PF, Mills J, Young DK (1966) Experimental asbestosis in the guinea-pig. J Pathol Bacteriol 92:185–195

Horvath EP, DoPico GA, Barbee RA, Dickie HA (1978) Nitrogen dioxide-induced pulmonary disease. J Occup Med 20:103–110

Horwitz AL, Elson NA, Crystal RG (1976) Proteoglycans and elastic fibers. In: Crystal RG (ed) The biochemical basis of pulmonary function. Marcel Dekker, New York, pp 273–311

Hospelhorn VS, Fitzpatrick MJ (1961) The isolation of elastic tissue from the lung. Biochim Biophys Acta 351:173–177

Huang TG, Zhao XN, Liu YY, Li YR (1981) Characteristics of collagen from lungs of rats with experimental silicosis. Chung Kuo I Hsueh Ko Hsueh Yuan Huseh Pao 3:7–9

Huang TW (1977) Chemical and histochemical studies of human alveolar collagen fibers. Am J Pathol 86:81–98

Hurych J, Holusa R, Effenbergerova E, Mirejovska E (1980) Attempt to influence silicotic fibrosis by means of N-(2-hydroxyethyl) palmitamide (Impulsin). Czech Med 3:218–225

Hurych J, Mirejovska E, Kobrle V, Rencova J (1981) Enzyme changes during experimental silicotic fibrosis. I. PZ peptidase and collagen deposition in the lungs. Environ Res 25:424–433

Hussain MZ, Bhatnagar RS (1979) Involvement of superoxide in the paraquat-induced enhancement of lung collagen synthesis in organ culture. Biochem Biophys Res Commun 89:71–76

Hussain MZ, Mustafa MG, Chow CK, Cross CE (1976) Ozone-induced increase of lung proline hydroxylase activity and hydroxyproline content. Chest 69:273–275

Ivanova AS (1971) Change in the protein-carbohydrate components of lung connective tissue in experimental berylliosis. Gig Tr Prof. Zabol 15(6):32–35

Jaiswal AK (1981) Biochemical studies in infective amosite pneumoconiosis. Toxicology 22(1):59–68

Janoff A, Sloan B, Weinbaum G, Damiano V, Sandhaus RA, Elias J, Kimbel P (1977) Experimental emphysema induced with purified human neutrophil elastase: tissue localization of the instilled protease. Am Rev Respir Dis 115:461–478

Janoff A, Carp H, Lee DK, Drew RT (1978) Cigarette smoke inhalation decreases antitrypsin activity in rat lung. Science 206:1313–1314

Janoff A, White R, Carp H, Harel S, Dearing R, Lee D (1979) Lung injury induced by leukocytic proteases. Am J Pathol 97:111–136

Johanson WG, Pierce AK (1972) Effects of elasase, collagenase, and papain on structure and function of rat lungs in vitro. J Clin Invest 51:288–293

Johanson WG, Pierce AK (1973) Lung structure and function with age in normal rats and rats with experimental emphysema. J Clin Invest 52:2921–2927

Johanson WG Jr, Reynolds RC, Scott TC, Pierce AK (1973) Connective tissue damage in emphysema. An electron microscopic study of papain-induced emphysema in rats. Am Rev Respir Dis 107:589–595

Johnson KJ, Ward PA (1982) Acute and progressive lung injury after contact with phorbol myristate acetate. Am J Pathol 107:29–35

Johnson R, Andrews FA (1970) Lung scleroproteins in age and emphysema. Chest 47:239–244

Jones AW, Reeve NL (1978) Ultrastructural study of bleomycin-induced changes in mice. J Pathol 124:227–233

Juhos LT, Evans MJ, Mussenden-Harvey R, Furiosi NJ, Lapple CE, Freeman G (1978) Limited exposure of rats to H_2SO_4 with and without ozone. J Environ Sci Health C13:33–47

Juhos LT, Green DP, Furiosi NJ, Freeman G (1980) A quantitative study of stenosis in the respiratory bronchiole of the rat in NO_2-induced emphysema. Am Rev Respir Dis 121:541–549

Junge-Hulsing G, Wagner H, Einbrodt HJ (1968) Studies of the effect of polyvinylpyridine-N-oxide (P204) on the metabolism of the connective tissue. Beitr Silikoseforsch 94:41–57

Karlinsky JB, Goldstein RH (1980) Fibrotic lung disease: A perspective. J Lab Clin Med 96:939–942

Karlinsky JB, Snider GL (1978) Animal models of emphysema. Am Rev Respir Dis 117:1109–1133

Katzenstein ALA, Bloor CM, Leibow AA (1976) Diffuse alveolar damage – the role of oxygen, shock, and related factors. Am J Pathol 86:210–221

Kaw JL, Zaidi SH (1969) Effect of ascorbic acid on pulmonary silicosis of guinea pigs. Arch Environ Health 19:74–83

Kaw JL, Zaidi SH (1970) Pathogenesis of pulmonary silicosis in rats fed stock and multideficient diet since weaning. Environ Res 3:199–211

Kay JM (1970) Busulphan lung: electron microscopy. Thorax 25(2):257

Kehrer JP (1982) Collagen production rates following acute lung damage induced by butylated hydroxytoluene. Biochem Pharmacol 31:2053–2058

Kehrer JP, Witschi H (1980) In vivo collagen accumulation in an experimental model of pulmonary fibrosis. Exp Lung Res 1:259–270

Kehrer JP, Witschi H (1981) The effect of indomethacin, prednisolone and cis-4-hydroxy-proline on pulmonary fibrosis produced by butylated hydroxytoluene and oxygen. Toxicology 20(4):281–288

Kelley J, Newman RA, Evans JN (1980) Bleomycin-induced pulmonary fibrosis in the rat. J Lab Clin Med 96:954–964

Kellogg EW, Fridovich I (1975) Superoxide, hydrogen peroxide, and singlet oxygen in lipid peroxidation by a xanthine oxidase system. J Biol Chem 250:8812–8817

Kelly DR, Morgan DG, Darke PGG, Gibbs C, Pearson H, Weaver BMQ (1976) Pathology of acute respiratory distress in the dog associated with paraquat poisoning. J Comp Pathol 88:275–294

Kelly PT, Mark K von der, Conrad GW (1981) Identification of collagen types I, II, III and V by two-dimensional fingerprinting of ^{125}I-labeled peptides. Anal Biochem 112:105–116

Kerfoot EJ, Fredrick WG, Domeier E (1975) Cobalt metal inhalation studies in miniature swine. Am Ind Hyg Assoc J 36(1):17–25

Kilburn KH, Dowell AR, Pratt PC (1971) Morphological and biochemical assessment of papain-induced emphysema. Arch Int Med 127:884–890

Kimbrough RD, Gaines TB (1970) Toxicity of paraquat to rats and its effect on rat lungs. Toxicol Appl Pharmacol 17:679–690

King EJ, Wright BM, Ray SC, Harrison CV (1950) Effect of aluminum on the silicosis producing action of inhaled quartz. Br J Ind Med 7:27–36

King EJ, Mohanty GP, Harrison CV, Nagelschmidt G (1953) The action of different forms of pure silica on the lungs of rats. Br J Ind Med 10:9–17

King EJ, Harrison CV, Mohanty GP, Nagelschmidt G (1955) The effect of various forms of alumina on the lung of rats. J Pathol Bacteriol 49:81–93

Kitamura H (1980) Cemented tungsten carbide pneumoconiosis: Human case and experimental approach. Yokahama Med Bull 31(4–6)103–126

Kleinerman J (1977) Some effects of nitrogen dioxide on the lung. Fed Proc 36:1714–1718

Kleinerman J, Ip MPC (1979) Effects of nitrogen dioxide on elastin and collagen contents of lung. Arch Environ Health 34:228–232

Kleinerman J, Sorensen J (1982) Nitrogen dioxide exposure and alveolar macrophage elastase in hamsters. Am Rev Respir Dis 125:203–207

Kleinerman J, Ranga V, Rynbrandt D, Sorensen J, Powers JC (1980) The effect of the specific elastase inhibitor alanyl alanyl prolyl alanine chloromethylketone, on elastase-induced emphysema. Am Rev Respir Dis 121:381–387

Konno K, Motomiya M, Oizumi K, Isawa T, Ariji F, Sato J, Hayashi I, Okubo K, Takeda S, Yokosawa A, Arai H (1975) The study on pulmonary fibrosis collagen metabolism of the lung. Jpn J Med 14:59

Koo KW, Hayes JA, Kagen HM, Leith DE, Franzblau C, Snider GL (1974) Lung volumes and mechanics following elastase and collagenase in hamsters. Clin Res 22:508A

Kuhn C (1976) The cells of the lung and their organelles. In: Crystal R (ed) The biochemical basis of pulmonary function. Marcel Dekker, New York, pp 3–37

Kuhn C, Starcher BC (1980) The effect of lathyrogens on the evolution of elastase-induced emphysema. Am Rev Respir Dis 122:453–460

Kuhn C, Yu SH, Chraplyvy M, Linder HE, Senior RM (1976) The induction of emphysema with elastase. II. Changes in connective tissue. Lab Invest 34:372 380

Kuhn C, Slodkowska J, Smith T, Starcher B (1980) The tissue response to exogeneous elastase. Bull Eur Physiopathol Respir 16:127–139

Kuncova M, Havrankova J, Kunc L, Holusa R, Palecek F (1972) Silicosis: Evolution of functional, biochemical, and morphological changes in the rat. Arch Environ Health 24:281–287

Kurohara SS, Casarett GW (1972) Effects of single thoracic x-ray exposure in rats. Radiat Res 52:263–290

Kuttan R, Lafranconi M, Sipes IG, Meezan E, Brendel K (1979) Effect of paraquat treatment on prolyl hydroxylase activity and collagen synthesis of rat lung and kidney. Res Commun Chem Pathol Pharmacol 25:257–268

Kysela B, Jirakova D, Holusa R, Skoda V (1973) The influence of the size of quartz dust particles on the reaction of lung tissue. Ann Occup Hyg 16:103–109

Last JA, Greenberg DB (1980) Ozone-induced alterations in collagen metabolism of rat lungs. II. Long-term exposures. Toxicol Appl Pharmacol 55:108–114

Last JA, Greenberg DB, Castleman WL (1979) Ozone-induced alterations in collagen metabolism of rat lungs. Toxicol Appl Pharmacol 51:247–258

Last JA, Hesterberg TW, Reiser KM, Cross CE, Amis TC, Gunn C, Steffey EP, Grandy J, Henrickson R (1981) Ozone-induced alterations in collagen metabolism of monkey lungs: Use of biopsy-obtained lung tissue. Toxicol Appl Pharmacol 60:579–585

Last JA, Gerriets JE, Hyde DM (1983) Synergistic effects on rat lungs of mixtures of oxidant air pollutants (ozone or nitrogen dioxide) and respirable aerosols. Am Rev Respir Dis 128:539–544

Laurent GJ, McAnulty RJ, Corrin B, Cockerill P (1981) Biochemical and histological changes in pulmonary fibrosis induced in rabbits with intratracheal bleomycin. Eur J Clin Invest 11:441–448

Law MP, Hornsey S, Field SB (1976) Collagen content of lungs of mice after x-ray irradiation. Radiat Res 65:60–70

Lazo JS (1981) Angiotensin converting enzyme activity in mice after subacute bleomycin administration. Toxicol Appl Pharmacol 59:395–404

Le Bouffant L, Daniel H, Martin JC (1975) The therapeutic action of aluminium compounds on the development of experimental lesions produced by pure quartz or mixed dust. Inhaled Part 4:389–401

Le Bouffant L, Daniel H, Martin JC, Bruyere S (1977) Variation in the toxicity of various silicas in relation to the duration of presence in the body. CR Acad Sci 285:599–602

Leibovich SJ, Ross R (1976) A macrophage-dependent factor that stimulates the proliferation of fibroblasts in vitro. Am J Pathol 84:501–514

Levene CI, Bye I, Saffriotti U (1968) The effect of β-aminopropionitrile on silicotic pulmonary fibrosis in the rat. Br J Exp Pathol 49:152–159

Levin PJ, Klaff LJ, Rose AG, Ferguson AD (1979) Pulmonary effects of contact exposure to paraquat: A clinical and experimental study. Thorax 34:150–160

Lewis DM, Burrell R (1976) Induction of fibrogenesis by lung antibody-treated macrophages. Br J Ind Med 33:25–28

Lillie RD, Pizzolato P, Donaldson PT (1972) Elastin IV: lysinal aldehyde relations, blocking and extraction tests, staining mechanisms. Acta Histochem (Jena) 44:215–225

Lindy S, Kahanpaa K, Karhunen P, Halme J, Uitto J (1970) Lactate dehydrogenase isoenzymes during the development of experimental fibrosis. J Lab Clin Med 76:756–760

Loxley R (1979) Determination of the amino acid contents of coalworkers' lungs after correction for blood, fat, dust and collagen. Analyst 104(1242):860–864

Lutz-Ostertag Y, Henou C (1975) Paraquat: Embryonic mortality and effects on pulmonary apparatus of chick and quail embryos. CR Acad Sci 281:439–442

Marco V, Meranze DR, Yoshida M, Kimbel P (1972) Papain-induced experimental emphysema in the dog. J Appl Physiol 33:293–299

Madri JA, Furthmayr H (1979) Isolation and localization of AB_2 collagen in the lung. Am J Pathol 94:171–184

Madri JA, Furthmayr H (1980) Collagen polymorphism in the lung: an immunochemical study of pulmonary fibrosis. Hum Pathol 11:353–366

Martin JC, Daniel H, Bouffant L Le(1975) Short- and long-term experimental study of the toxicity of coal-mine dust and of some of its constituents. Inhaled Part 4:361–371

Martorana PA (1976) The hamster as a model for experimental pulmonary emphysema. Lab Anim Sci 26:352–354

Mauderly JL, Pickrell JA, Hobbs CH, Benjamin SA, Hahn FF, Jones RK, Barnes JE (1973) The effects of inhaled ^{90}Y fused clay aerosol on pulmonary function and related parameters of the Beagle dog. Radial Res 56:83–96

McCallum DK (1973) Positive schiff reactivity of aortic elastin without prior HIO_4 oxidation; influence of maturity and a suggested source of the aldehyde. Stain Technol 48:117–122

McCord JM, Fridovich I (1978) The biology and pathology of oxygen radicals. Ann Intern Med 89:122–127

McCullough B, Collins JF, Jethanson WG Jr, Grover FL (1978a) Bleomycin-induced diffuse interstitial pulmonary fibrosis in baboons. J Clin Invest 61:79–88

McCullough B, Schneider S, Greene ND, Johanson WG Jr (1978b) Bleomycin-induced lung injury in baboons: Alteration of cells and immunoglobulins recoverable by bronchoalveolar lavage. Lung 155:337–358

McDermott M, Wagner JC, Tetley T, Harwood J, Richards RJ (1975) The effects of inhaled silica and chrysotile on the elastic properties of rat lungs; physiological, physical, and biochemical studies of lung surfactant. Inhaled Part 4:415–427

McJilton CE, Charles RJ (1976) Influence of relative humidity on functional effects of an inhaled sulphur dioxide aerosol mixture. Am Rev Respir Dis 113:163–169

Mead J (1961) Mechanical properties of lungs. Physiol Rev 41:281–330

Meigel WN, Gay S, Weber L (1977) Dermal architecture and collagen type distribution. Arch Dermathol Res 259:1–10

Metivier H, Nolibe D, Masse R, Lafuma J (1974) Excretion and acute toxicity of $^{239}PuO_2$ in baboons. Health Phys 27:512–514

Metivier H, Masse R, Nolibe D, Lafuma J (1977) Plutonium-239 dioxide aerosol inhalation with emphasis on pulmonary connective tissue modifications. Inhaled Part 4(2):583–595

Metivier H, Junqua S, Masse R, Legendre N, Lafuma J (1980) Pulmonary connective tissue modifications induced in the rat by inhalation of $^{239}PuO_2$ aerosol. In: Sanders CL, Cross FT, Dagle GE, Mahaffey JA (eds) Pulmonary toxicology of respirable particles. U. S. Department of Energy, CONF-791002, Springfield, Va, pp 392–403

Miller K (1978) The effects of asbestos on macrophages. CRC Crit Rev Toxicol 9:319–354

Miller ML, Murthy L, Sorenson JR (1974) Fine structure of connective tissue after ingestion of cadmium. Observations on interstitium of male rat lung. Arch Pathol 98(6):386–392

Mirejovska E, Bass A, Hurych J, Teisinger J (1981) Enzyme changes during experimental silicotic fibrosis. II. Intermediary metabolism enzymes of the lungs. Environ Res 25:434–440

Morgenroth K (1974) Cellular reaction in the human lung caused by inhalation of asbestos dust over long periods. Beitr Pathol 148(2):199–210

Murad S, Sivarajah A, Pinnel SR (1981) Regulation of prolyl and lysyl hydroxylase activities in cultured human skin fibroblasts by ascorbic acid. Biochem Biophys Res Comm 101:868–875

Murray RE, Gibson JE (1972) A comparative study of paraquat intoxication in rats, guinea pigs, and monkeys. Exp Mol Pathol 17:317–325

Nathan CF, Murray HW, Cohn ZA (1980) The macrophage as effector cell. N Engl J Med 303:622–626

Naumenko IM (1966) Effects of electric welding on the content of collagen and ascorbic acid in the pulmonary tissue. Vrach Delo 1:92–94

Newhouse M, McEvoy D, Rosenthal D (1978) Percutaneous paraquat absorption. Arch Dermatol 114:1516–1519

Niden AH, Khurana MML (1976) An animal model for diffuse interstitial pulmonary fibrosis-chronic low dose paraquat ingestion. Fed Proc 35:631 (abstract)

Niewoehner DE, Hoidal JR (1982) Lung fibrosis and emphysema: divergent responses to a common injury. Science 217:359–360

Niewoehner DE, Kleinerman J (1973) Effects of experimental emphysema and bronchiolitis on lung mechanics and morphometry. J Appl Physiol 35:25–31

Nimni ME (1980) The molecular organization of collagen and its role in determining the biophysical properties of the connective tissues. Biorheology 17:51–82

Nourse LD, Nourse PN, Botes H, Schwartz HM (1975) The effects of macrophages isolated from the lungs of guinea pigs dusted with silica on collagen biosynthesis by guinea pig fibroblasts in cell culture. Environ Res 9:115–127

Nowack H, Gay S, Wick G, Becker U, Timpl R (1976) Preparation and use in immunohistology of antibodies for type I and type III collagen and procollagen. J Immunol Methods 12:117–124

Orthoefer JH, Bhatnager RS, Rahman A, Yang YY, Lee SD, Stara JF (1976) Collagen and prolyl hydroxylase levels in lungs of beagles exposed to air pollutants. Environ Res 12:299–305

Osman M, Keller S, Cerreta JM, Leuenberger P, Mandl I, Turnino GM (1980) Effect of papain-induced emphysema on canine pulmonary elastin. Proc Soc Exp Biol Med 164:471–477

Palmer KC, Snider GL, Hayes JA (1976) An association between alveolar cell proliferation and interstitial fibrosis following acute lung injury. Chest 69:307–309

Pariente R, Legrand M, Brouet G (1969) Ultrastructural aspects of the lung in oxygen poisoning at atmospheric pressure in the rat. Presse Med 77:1073–1076

Petrone WF, English DK, Wong K, McCord JM (1980) Free radicals and inflammation: Superoxide-dependent activation of a neutrophil chemotactic factor in plasma. Proc Natl Acad Sci USA 77:1159–1163

Phan SH, Thrall RS (1982a) The role of soluble factors in bleomycin-pulmonary fibrosis. Am J Pathol 106:156–164

Phan SH, Thrall RS (1982b) Inhibition of bleomycin-induced pulmonary fibrosis by cobra venom factor. Am J Pathol 107:25–28

Phan SH, Thrall RS, Ward PA (1980) Bleomycin-induced pulmonary fibrosis in rats: biochemical demonstration of increased rate of collagen synthesis. Am Rev Respir Dis 121:501–506

Phan SH, Thrall RS, Williams C (1981) Bleomycin-induced pulmonary fibrosis. Effects of steroid on lung collagen metabolism. Am Rev Respir Dis 123:428–434

Pickrell JA, Harris DV, Hahn FF, Belaisch JJ, Jones RK (1975a) Biological alterations resulting from chronic lung irradiation. III. Radiat Res 62:133–144

Pickrell JA, Harris DB, Pfleger RC, Benjamin SA, Belasich JJ, Jones RK, McClellan RO (1975b) Biological alterations resulting from chronic lung irradiation. II. Connective tissue alterations following inhalation of cerium-144 fused clay aerosol in beagle dogs. Radiat Res 63:299–309

Pickrell JA, Harris DV, Mauderly JL, Hahn FF (1976a) Altered collagen metabolism in radiation-induced interstitial pulmonary fibrosis. Chest 69:311–316

Pickrell JA, Harris DV, Benjamin SA, Cuddihy RG, Pfleger RC, Mauderly JL (1976b) Pulmonary collagen metabolism after lung injury from inhaled ^{90}Y in fused clay particles. Exp Mol Pathol 25:70–81

Pickrell JA, Schnizlein CT, Hahn FF, Snipes MB, Jones RK (1978) Radiation-induced pulmonary fibrosis: Study of changes in collagen constituents in different lung regions of beagle dogs after inhalation of Beta-emitting radionuclides. Radiat Res 74:363–377

Pickrell JA, Hahn FF, Rebar AH, Damon EG, Beethe RL, Pfleger RC, Hobbs CH (1981) Pulmonary effects of exposure to 20 ppm NO_2. Chest [Suppl] 80:50–52

Pierce JA, Hocott JB (1960) Studies on the collagen and elastin content of the human lung. J Clin Invest 39:8–14

Pierce JA, Hocott JB, Hefley BF (1961a) Elastic properties and the geometry of the lungs. J Clin Invest 40:1515–1524

Pierce JA, Hocott HB, Ebert RV (1961b) The collagen and elastin content of the lung in emphysema. Ann Intern Med 55:210–222

Polzin JK, Napier JS, Taylor JC, Rodarte JR (1979) Effect of elastase and ventilation on elastic recoil of excised dog lungs. Am Rev Respir Dis 119:377–381

Popenoe D (1979) Effects of paraquat aerosol on mice. Arch Pathol Lab Med 103:331–334

Powell DEB, Gough J (1959) The effect on experimental silicosis of hypersensitivity induced by horse serum. Br J Exp Pathol 40:40–43

Pratt PC, Vollmer RT, Shelburne JD, Crapo JD (1979) Pulmonary morphology in a multihospital collaborative extracorporeal membrane oxygenation project. Am J Pathol 95:191–214

Prockop DJ, Kivirikko KI, Tuderman L, Guzman N (1979) The biosynthesis of collagen and its disorders. N Engl J Med 302:13–23, 77–95

Raczniak TJ, Shumaker RC, Allen JR, Will JA, Lalich JJ (1979) Pathophysiology of dehydromonocrotaline-induced pulmonary fibrosis in the beagle. Respiration 37:252–260

Radford EP (1964) Static mechanical properties of mammalian lungs. In: Handbook of physiology, Sect 3: Respiration vol 1. American Physiological Society, Washington, DC, pp 429–449

Rahman Q, Beg MU, Viswanathan PN, Zaidi SH (1975) Biochemical changes caused by asbestos dust in the lungs of rats. Scand J Work Environ Health, 1:50–53

Raisfeld IH (1980) Pulmonary toxicity of bleomycin analogs. Toxicol Appl Pharmacol 56:326–336

Ranga V, Kleinerman J (1981) Lung injury and repair in the blotchy mouse. Effects of nitrogen dioxide inhalation. Am Rev Respir Dis 123:90–97

Reiser KM, Last JA (1979) Silicosis and fibrogenesis: Fact and artifact. Toxicology 13:51–72

Reiser KM, Last JA (1980) Quantitation of specific collagen types from lungs of small mammals. Anal Biochem 104:87–98

Reiser KM, Last JA (1981) Pulmonary fibrosis in experimental acute respiratory disease. Am Rev Respir Dis 123:58–63

Reiser KM, Last JA (1983) Type V collagen: Quantitation in normal lungs and in lungs of rats with bleomycin-induced pulmonary fibrosis. J Biol Chem 258:269–275

Reiser KM, Hesterberg TW, Haschek WM, Last JA (1982) Experimental silicosis. I. Acute effects of intratracheally instilled quartz on collagen metabolism and morphology of rat lungs. Am J Pathol 107:176–185

Reiser KM, Haschek WM, Hesterberg TW, Last JA (1983) Experimental silicosis. II. Long-term effects of intratracheally instilled quartz on collagen metabolism and morphologic characteristics of rat lungs. Am J Pathol 110:30–40

Remberger K, Gay S, Fietzek PP (1975) Immunohistochemical characterization of collagen in liver cirrhosis. Virchows Arch Pathol 367:231–240

Renne RA, Smith LG, McDonald KE, Shields CA, Gandolfi AJ, Lund JE (1980) Morphologic and biochemical effects of intratracheally administered oil shale in rats. J Environ Pathol Toxicol 3:397–406

Richmond V (1974) Lung parenchymal elastin isolated by nondegradative means. Biochim Biophys Acta 351:173–177

Richmond V, D'Aoust BG (1976) Effects of intermittent hyperbaric oxygen on guinea pig lung elastin and collagen. J Appl Physiol 41:295–301

Riley DJ, Berg RA, Edelman NH, Prockop DJ (1980) Prevention of collagen deposition following pulmonary oxygen toxicity in the rat by cis-4-hydroxy-L-proline. J Clin Invest 65:643–651

Riley DJ, Kerr JS, Berg RA, Ianni BD, Pietra GG, Edelman NH, Prockop DJ (1981) Prevention of bleomycin-induced pulmonary fibrosis in the hamster by cis-4-hydroxy-L-proline. Am Rev Respir Dis 123:388–393

Riley DJ, Kerr JS, Berg RA, Ianni BD, Pietra GG, Edelman NH, Prockop DJ (1982) beta-Aminopropionitrile prevents bleomycin-induced pulmonary fibrosis in the hamster. Am Rev Respir Dis 125:67–73

Rinaldo JE, Rogers RM (1982) Adult respiratory distress syndrome. Changing concept of lung injury and repair. N Engl J Med 306:900–909

Robins SP, Bailey AJ (1977) The chemistry of the collagen cross-links. Biochem J 163:339–346

Rodkina BS (1974) Hydroxyproline content in the peptide makeup of the lung tissue of animals with experimental silicosis. Ukr Biokhim Zh 46:393–397

Rosenkrantz H, Esber HJ, Sprague R (1969) Lung hydroxyproline levels in mice exposed to cigarette smoke. Life Sci 8:571–576

Roujeau J, Pfister A, Nogues C, Leclerc JP (1973) Pulmonary fibroses and poisoning. Poumon Coeur 29:643–647

Rucker RB, Tinker D (1977) Structure and metabolism of arterial elastin. Int Rev Exp Pathol 17:1–47

Russell LA, Stone BE, Rooney PA (1981) Paraquat poisoning: Toxicologic and pathologic findings in three fatal cases. Clin Toxicol 18:915–928

Ryan SF (1972) Experimental fibrosing alveolitis. Am Rev Respir Dis 105:776–791

Sahebjami H, Vassallo CL (1976) Exercise stress and enzyme-induced emphysema. J Appl Physiol 41:332–335

Sahu AP, Shanker R, Dogra RK, Zaidi SH (1975) Effect of quartz dust on the lungs of mice. Exp Pathol 10:83–85

Sandberg LB, Soskel NT, Leslie JH (1981) Elastin structure, biosynthesis, and relation to disease states. N Engl J Med 304:566–579

Scharf SM, Heimer D, Goldstein J (1981) Pathologic and physiologic effects of aspiration of hydrocarbons in the rat. Am Rev Respir Dis 124:625–629

Schlein A, Schurig JE, Baca C, Bradner WT, Crooks ST (1981) Pulmonary toxicity studies of bleomycin and talisomycin. Cancer Treat Rep 65:291–297

Schuyler MR, Rynbrandt DJ, Kleinerman J (1978) Physiologic and morphologic observations of the effects of intravenous elastase on the lung. Am Rev Respir Dis 117:97–102

Senior RM, Tegner H, Kuhn C, Ohlsson K, Starcher BC, Pierce JA (1977) The induction of pulmonary emphysema with human leukocyte elastase. Am Rev Respir Dis 116:469–475

Seyer JM, Hutcheson ET, Kang AH (1976) Collagen polymorphism in idiopathic chronic pulmonary fibrosis. J Clin Invest 57:1408–1507

Seyer JM, Kang AH, Rodnan G (1981) Investigation of type I and type III collagens of the lung in progressive systemic sclerosis. Arthritis Rheum 24:625–631

Shanker R, Sahu AP, Dogra RK, Zaidi SH (1975) A study of the age factor in experimental silicosis in rats. Environ Physiol Biochem 5:158–164

Sikic BI, Young DM, Mimnaugh EG, Gram TE (1978 a) Quantification of bleomycin pulmonary toxicity in mice by changes in lung hydroxyproline content and morphometric histopathology. Cancer Res 38:787–792

Sikic BI, Mimnaugh EG, Gram TE (1978 b) Development of quantifiable parameters of bleomycin toxicity in the mouse lung. In: Carter SK, Crooke ST, Umezawa H (eds) Bleomycin: Current status and new developments. Academic, New York, pp 293–297

Singh J, Beg MU, Kaw JL, Viswanathan PN, Zaidi SH (1976) Biochemical changes and pulmonary response of guinea pigs to asbestos dust. Acta Pharmacol Toxicol 39:77–86

Singh J, Kaw JL, Pandey SD, Viswanathan PN, Zaidi SH (1977) Amino acid changes and pulmonary response of rats to silica dust. Environ Res 14:452–462

Singhal RL, Merali Z, Hridina PD (1976) Aspects of the biochemical toxicology of cadmium. Fed Proc 35:75–80

Smith LJ, Brody JS (1981) Influence of methylprednisolone on mouse alveolar type 2 cell response to acute lung injury. Am Rev Respir Dis 123:459–464

Smith P, Heath C (1974a) Paraquat lung: A reappraisal. Thorax 29:643–653

Smith P, Heath D (1974b) The ultrastructure and time sequence of the early stages of paraquat lung in rats. J Pathol 114:177–184

Smith P, Heath D (1976) Paraquat. CRC Crit Rev Toxicol 4:411–445

Smith P, Heath D, Kay JM (1974) The pathogenesis and structure of paraquat-induced pulmonary fibrosis in rats. J Pathol 114:57–67

Smith TJ, Pettu TL, Reading JC, Lakshminarayan S (1976) Pulmonary effects of chronic exposure to airborne cadmium. Am Rev Respir Dis 114:161–169

Snider GL, Korthy AL (1978) Internal surface area and number of respiratory air spaces in elastase-induced emphysema in hamsters. Am Rev Respir Dis 117:685–693

Snider GL, Hayes JA, Korthy AL, Lewis GP (1973) Centrilobular emphysema experimentally induced by cadmium chloride aerosol. Am Rev Respir Dis 108:40–48

Snider GL, Hayes JA, Franzblau C, Kagan HM, Stone PS, Korthy AL (1974) Relationship between elastolytic activity and experimental emphysema-induced properties of papain preparations. Am Rev Respir Dis 110:254–262

Snider GL, Sherter CB, Koo KW, Karlinsky JB, Hayes JA, Franzblau C (1977) Respiratory mechanics in hamsters following treatment with endotracheal elastase or collagenase. J Appl Physiol 42:206–215

Snider GL, Celli BR, Goldstein RH, O'Brien JJ, Lucey EC (1978 a) Chronic interstitial pulmonary fibrosis produced in hamsters by endotracheal bleomycin. Lung volumes, volume-pressure relations, carbon monoxide uptake, and arterial gas studies. Am Rev Respir Dis 117:289–297

Snider GL, Hayes JA, Korthy AL (1978 b). Chronic interstitial pulmonary fibrosis produced in hamsters by endotracheal bleomycin. Am Rev Respir Dis 117:1099–1108

Starcher BC (1977) Determination of the elastin content of tissues by measuring desmosine and isodesmosine. Anal Biochem 79:11–15

Starcher BC, Mecham RP (1981) Desmosine radioimmunoassay as a means of studying elastogenesis in cell culture. Connect Tissue Res 8:255–258

Starcher BC, Kuhn C, Overton JE (1978) Increased elastin and collagen content in the lungs of hamsters receiving an intratracheal injection of bleomycin. Am Rev Respir Dis 117:299–305

Stephens RJ, Freeman G, Evans MJ (1971) Ultrastructural changes in connective tissue in lungs of rats exposed to NO_2. Arch Intern Med 127:873–883

Sterling KM Jr, DiPetrillo T, Cutroneo KR, Prestayko A (1982) Inhibition of collagen accumulation by glucocorticoids in rat lung after intratracheal bleomycin instillation. Cancer Res 42:405–408

Stokinger HE, Wagner WD, Dobrogorski OJ (1957) Ozone toxicity studies. III. Chronic injury to lungs of animals following exposure at a low level. Arch Environ Health 16:514–522

Stone PJ, Pareira W Jr, Biles D, Snider GL, Kagan HM, Franzblau C (1977) Studies on the fate of pancreatic elatase in the hamster lung: ^{14}C-guanidinated elastase. Am Rev Respir Dis 116:49–56

Stone PJ, Calore JD, Snider GL, Franzblau C (1982) Role of alpha-macroglobulin-elastase complexes in the pathogenesis of elastase-induced emphysema in hamsters. J Clin Invest 69:920–931

Susheela AK, Mukerjee D (1981) Fluoride poisoning and the effect on collagen biosynthesis of osseous and nonosseous tissues or rabbit. Toxicol Eur Res 3(2):99–104

Swensson A (1970) Experimental evaluation of the fibrogenic power of mineral dusts. In Ahlmark A, Franburg B (eds) Swedish-Yugoslavian Symposium on Pneumoconiosis. National Institute of Occupational Health, Stockholm, pp 86–97 (WF 654–59)

Szapiel SV, Elson NA, Fulmer JD, Hunninghake GW, Crystal RG (1979) Bleomycin-induced interstitial pulmonary disease in the nude, athymic mouse. Am Rev Respir Dis 120:893–899

Thompson WS, Patrick RS (1978) Collagen prolyl hydroxylase levels in experimental paraquat poisoning. Br J Exp Pathol 59:288–291

Thrall RS, McCormick JR, Jack RM, McReynolds RA, Ward PA (1979) Bleomycin-induced pulmonary fibrosis in the rat: inhibition by indomethacin. Am J Pathol 95:117–130

Thrall RS, Phan SH, McCormick JR, Ward PA (1981) The development of bleomycin-induced pulmonary fibrosis in neutrophil-depleted and complement-depleted rats. Am J Pathol 105:76–81

Thurlbeck WM, Thurlbeck SM (1976) Pulmonary effects of paraquat poisoning. Chest [Suppl] 69:276–280

Thyagarajan P, Vakil UK, Sreenivasan A (1976) Effects of whole-body x-irradiation on some aspects of collagen metabolism in the rat. Radiat Res 66:576–586

Tom W, Montgomery MR (1980) Biochemical and morphological assessments of bleomy-cin pulmonary toxicity in rats. Toxicol Appl Pharmacol 53:64–74

Tsevela IA (1974) Collagen biosynthesis in the lungs of rats with radiation injury. Vop Med Khim 20:640–643

Turino GM, Lourenco RV (1972) The connective tissue basis of pulmonary mechanics. In: Mittman C (ed) Pulmonary emphysema and proteolysis. Academic, New York, pp 509–524

Tyree EB, Glicksman AS, Nickson JJ (1966) Effect of L-triiodothyronine on radiation-in-duced pulmonary fibrosis in dogs. Radiat Res 28:30–36

Upreti RK, Sahu AP, Shukla L, Srivastava SN, Shanker R (1979) Bleomycin induced changes in lungs and lymph nodes of guinea pigs. Indian J Exp Biol 17:922–925

Valimaki M, Juva K, Rantanen J, Ekfors T, Niinikoski J (1975) Collagen metabolism in rat lungs during chronic intermittent exposure to oxygen. Aviat Space Environ Med 46:684–690

Vasileva GN, Miagkaia GL (1970) The composition of insoluble collagen in the lungs of rats under normal conditions and in experimental silicosis. Vopr Med Khim 16:286–289

Vigliani EC, Pernis B (1963) Immunological aspects of silicosis. Adv Tuberc Res 12:230–279

Vijeyaratnam GS, Corrin B (1971) Experimental paraquat poisoning: A histological and electron optical study of the changes in the lung. J Pathol 103:123–129

von Wichert P, Morgenroth K (1976) Comparison between pathological and biochemical investigations on an experimental model of fibrosing alveolitis. Respiration 33:36–46

Wagner JC, Wusteman FS, Edwards JH, Hill RJ (1975) The composition of massive lesions in coal miners. Thorax 30(4):82–88

Wasan SM, McElligot TF (1972) An electron microscopic study of experimentally induced pulmonary fibrosis. Am Rev Respir Dis 105:276–282

Watanabe S, Watanabe K, Ohishi T, Aiba M, Kageyama K (1974) Mast cells in the rat alveolar septa undergoing fibrosis after ionizing radiation. Lab Invest 31:555–567

Wegrowski J (1980) Effects of carbon disulfide on the metabolism of connective tissue of rats. Med Pr 31:13–19

Willoughby WF, Willoughby JB, Cantrell BB, Wheelis R (1979) In vivo response to inhaled proteins: II. Induction of interstitial pneumonitis and enhancement of immune com-plex-mediated alveolitis by inhaled concanavalin A. Lab Invest 40(3):399–414

Witschi H, Haschek WM, Meyer KR, Ullrich RL, Dalbey WE (1980) A pathogenic mech-anism in lung fibrosis. Chest 78(2) [Suppl] 395–399

Witschi HR, Haschek WM, Klein-Szanto AJ, Hakkinen PJ (1981) Potentiation of diffuse lung damage by oxygen: determining variables. Am Rev Respir Dis 123:98–103

Woessner JF (1961) The determination of hydroxyproline in tissue and protein samples containing small proportions of this imino acid. Arch Biochem Biophys 93:440–447

Woitowitz HJ (1972) Importance of asbestos for industrial medicine and ecology. Dtsch Med Wochenschr 97(9):346–410

Wright GW, Kleinerman J, Zorn EM (1960) The elastin and collagen content of normal and emphysematous human lung. Am Rev Respir Dis 81:938–950

Wright JL, Cockcroft DW (1981) Lung disease due to abuse of hairspray. Arch Pathol Lab Med 105(7):363–366

Wyatt I, Doss AW, Zavala DC, Smith LL (1981) Intrabronchial instillation of paraquat in rats: Lung morphology and retention study. Br J Ind Med 38:42–48

Yasaka T, Ohya I, Matsumoto J, Shiramizu T, Sasaguri Y (1981) Acceleration of lipid peroxidation in human paraquat poisoning. Arch Intern Med 141:1169–1171

Yost FJ, Fridovich I (1976) Superoxide and hydrogen peroxide in oxygen damage. Arch Biochem Biophys 175:514–519

Yu SY, Keller NR (1978) Synthesis of lung collagen in hamsters with elastase-induced em-physema. Exp Mol Pathol 29:37–43

Yu SY, Keller NR, Yoshida A (1978) Biosynthesis of insoluble elastin in hamster lungs during elastase-emphysema. Proc Soc Exp Biol Med 157:369–373

Zaidi SH (1969) Experimental pneumoconiosis, 2nd edn. Johns Hopkins, Baltimore

Zaidi SH, Kaw JL (1970) Effect of general dietary deficiency and protein malnutrition on the fibrogenesis caused by silica dust in rats. Br J Ind Med 27:250–259

Zaidi SH, Dogra RKS, Shanker R, Chandra SV (1971) Experimental farmer's lung in guinea-pigs. J Pathol 105(1):41–48

Zavala DC, Rhodes ML (1978) The effect of paraquat on the lungs of rabbits and its implications in smoking contaminated marijuana. Chest 74:418–420

Zimmerman M, Ashe BM, Mulvey D, Frankshun R, Jones H, Martorana P, Share N (1981) Inhibition of elastase by heterocyclic acylating agents: in vitro and in vivo activities. Semin Arthritis Rheum 11:75–76

Zuckerman JE, Hollinger MA, Giri SN (1980) Evaluation of antifibrotic drugs in bleomycin-induced pulmonary fibrosis in hamsters. J Pharmacol Exp Therap 213:425–431

Subject Index

Handbook of Experimental Pharmacology

Continuation of "Handbuch der experimentellen Pharmakologie"

Editorial Board
G. V. R. Born, A. Farah,
H. Herken, A. D. Welch

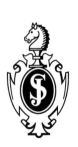

Springer-Verlag
Berlin
Heidelberg
New York
Tokyo

Handbook of Experimental Pharmacology

Continuation of
"Handbuch der
experimentellen
Pharmakologie"

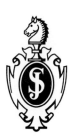

Springer-Verlag
Berlin
Heidelberg
New York
Tokyo